ORAL PATHOLOGY

Clinical Pathologic
Correlations

fourth edition

ORAL PATHOLOGY

Clinical Pathologic Correlations

JOSEPH A. REGEZI, DDS, MS
Professor, Oral Pathology
Department of Stomatology
School of Dentistry;
Professor, Pathology
Department of Pathology
School of Medicine
University of California San Francisco
San Francisco, California

JAMES J. SCIUBBA, DMD, PhD
Professor
Departments of Otolaryngology, Head and Neck Surgery; Pathology; Dermatology
The Johns Hopkins School of Medicine;
Director, Dental Oral Medicine
Department of Otolaryngology, Head and Neck Surgery
The Johns Hopkins Medical Center
Baltimore, Maryland

RICHARD C.K. JORDAN, DDS, MSc, PhD, FRCD(C)
Associate Professor, Oral Pathology
Department of Stomatology
School of Dentistry;
Associate Professor, Pathology
Department of Pathology
School of Medicine
University of California San Francisco
San Francisco, California

with 927 illustrations

SAUNDERS
An Imprint of Elsevier Science

SAUNDERS

An Imprint of Elsevier Science

11830 Westline Industrial Drive
St. Louis, Missouri 63146

Oral Pathology: Clinical Pathologic Correlations   0-7216-9805-0

Notice

Dentistry is an ever-changing field. Standard safety precautions must be followed, but as new research and clinical experience broaden our knowledge, changes in treatment and drug therapy may become necessary or appropriate. Readers are advised to check the most current product information provided by the manufacturer of each drug to be administered to verify the recommended dose, the method and duration of administration, and contraindications. It is the responsibility of the licensed prescriber, relying on experience and knowledge of the patient, to determine dosages and the best treatment for each individual patient. Neither the publisher nor the author assumes any liability for any injury and/or damage to persons or property arising from this publication.

Previous editions copyrighted 1999, 1993, 1989.

Library of Congress Cataloging-in-Publication Data
Regezi, Joseph A.
    Oral pathology : clinical pathologic correlations / Joseph A. Regezi, James J. Sciubba,
Richard C.K. Jordan.—4th ed.
        p. ; cm.
    Includes bibliographical references and index.
    ISBN 0-7216-9805-0 (alk. paper)
    1. Mouth–Diseases. 2. Teeth–Diseases. I. Sciubba, James J. II. Jordan, Richard C.K.
III. Title.
    [DNLM: 1. Tooth Diseases–pathology. 2. Mouth Diseases–pathology. WU 140 R333o 2003]
RC815 .R39 2003
617.5′22–dc21   2002029929

Publishing Director: Linda L. Duncan
Senior Acquisitions Editor: Penny Rudolph
Senior Developmental Editor: Kimberly Alvis
Publishing Services Manager: Pat Joiner
Project Manager: Rachel E. Dowell
Designer: Mark A. Oberkrom

BS/WPC

Printed in the United States of America

Last digit is the print number: 9 8 7 6 5 4 3 2 1

CONTRIBUTORS

ERIC R. CARLSON, DMD, MD
Professor and Chairman
Department of Oral and Maxillofacial Surgery;
Director, Oral and Maxillofacial Surgery Residency
    Program
University of Tennessee Graduate School of Medi-
    cine
Knoxville, Tennessee

JOHN KIM, MD, FRCPC
Assistant Professor
Department of Radiation Oncology
Princess Margaret Hospital, University Health
    Network
University of Toronto
Toronto, Ontario, Canada

GINAT WINTERMEYER MIROWSKI, DMD, MD
Associate Professor of Oral Medicine
Department of Oral Pathology, Medicine, and
    Radiology
Indiana University School of Dentistry;
Associate Professor of Dermatology
Department of Dermatology
Indiana University School of Medicine
Indianapolis, Indiana

TODD W. ROZYCKI, MD
Senior Resident Associate
Department of Dermatology
Mayo Clinic, Mayo Foundation
Rochester, Minnesota

JEFFERY C.B. STEWART, DDS, MS
Associate Professor
Department of Pathology
School of Dentistry
Oregon Health & Science University
Portland, Oregon

RICHARD J. ZARBO, DMD, MD
Professor
Department of Pathology
Case Western Reserve University
Henry Ford Health Sciences Center;
Chairman
Department of Pathology
Henry Ford Hospital and Medical Group;
Senior Vice President for Pathology and Laboratory
    Medicine
Henry Ford Health System
Detroit, Michigan

PREFACE

The textbook carries on the tradition of presenting oral pathology in a clinically useful format in which diseases are classified according to appearance (as opposed to etiology). This practical approach to understanding oral diseases will assist the clinician in the recognition of specific conditions and in the development of differential diagnoses. Microscopic features, an invaluable component to understanding oral diseases, are described throughout the text. Knowledge of microscopy helps the clinician to develop a pathologic foundation that is the basis of clinical appearance; it provides insight to the understanding of disease mechanisms; and it assists the clinician in the interpretation of biopsy reports.

The fourth edition marks major improvements to the text. The addition of a third author (Richard C.K. Jordan) brings new energy and a refreshing perspective that is evident throughout the book. Two new contributors (Eric R. Carlson and John Kim) make significant contributions to the treatment side of oral cancers.

The addition of the molecular basis of cancer and a chapter on molecular methods elevates the text into mainstream thinking, reflecting the revolution occurring in molecular medicine. Understanding this area of disease will help the clinician appreciate the current literature and help in the understanding of developing therapeutic strategies that will be seen in the coming decades.

The most obvious change in the fourth edition is the full-color format. The digitized images will significantly enhance the clinical and microscopic recognition of oral conditions. The addition of all new tables and drawings will give the reader a convenient summary of the key features of many of the diseases discussed.

An accompanying CD-ROM features color clinical images from the overview section plus complementary photomicrographs, 30 "unknown" cases, and a test bank containing 680 multiple-choice questions and an answer key. The case studies on the CD-ROM are available in PowerPoint format and can be reconfigured for presentations or for individual study. It should be useful not only for the reader, but also for the instructor who may wish to develop computer-assisted lectures.

ABOUT THE COVER

The cover image is a stylized version of Figure 3-45 which illustrates the diagnostic features of lichen planus. Discussion of this disease can be found beginning on p. 92 of the text.

HOW TO USE THIS BOOK

The narrative or latter part of this book provides the body of information that is oral and maxillofacial pathology. It is the starting point for comprehensive study of this discipline. The overview, or front section, is a distillation of the clinical aspects found in the main text and is designed to be used as a quick reference or as a rapid review. The CD-ROM provides the reader with a contemporary alternative review opportunity, as well as a format from which presentations can be developed.

Joseph A. Regezi
James J. Sciubba
Richard C.K. Jordan

Acknowledgments

The authors wish to express their love and appreciation to their families, who have had to live with preoccupied and often difficult academic authors. Without their understanding and support, this body of work would not have been produced.

The authors also gratefully acknowledge the contributions made by the talented professional staff at Elsevier Science. In particular to Penny Rudolph, Kimberly Alvis, Rachel Dowell, and Judith Bange, we offer a special thank you. Their exceptional efforts made the production of this book possible.

Joseph A. Regezi
James J. Sciubba
Richard C.K. Jordan

CONTENTS

ORAL PATHOLOGY

Clinical Pathologic Correlations

CLINICAL OVERVIEW

MUCOSAL (SURFACE) LESIONS

Vesiculobullous Diseases

Ulcerative Conditions

White Lesions

Red-Blue Lesions

Pigmented Lesions

Verrucal-Papillary Lesions

SUBMUCOSAL SWELLINGS (BY REGION)

Gingiva

Floor of Mouth

Lips and Buccal Mucosa

Tongue

Palate

Neck

DIFFERENTIAL DIAGNOSIS APPROACH TO JAW LESIONS

Cysts of the Jaws and Neck

Odontogenic Tumors

Benign Nonodontogenic Tumors

Inflammatory Jaw Lesions

Malignancies of the Jaws

Metabolic and Genetic Diseases

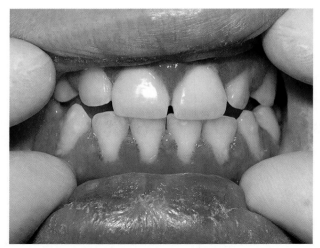

Figure 1   Primary herpes simplex infection.

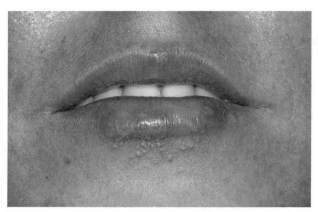

Figure 2   Secondary herpes simplex infection of the lips.

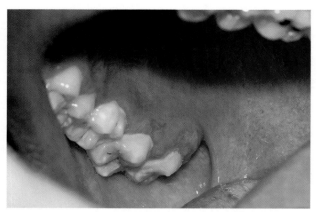

Figure 3   Secondary herpes simplex infection of the palate.

Vesiculobullous Diseases

Disease	Clinical Features	Cause	Significance
Herpes simplex infections			
Primary herpetic gingivostomatitis	Multiple painful oral ulcers preceded by vesicles; may have similar perioral and skin lesions; fever and gingivitis usually present; usually affects children under 5 years of age	Herpes simplex virus type 1 (occasionally type 2)	Self-limited; heals in about 2 weeks; reactivation of latent virus results in secondary infections; circulating antibodies provide only partial immunity
Secondary herpes simplex infection	Multiple small ulcers preceded by vesicles; prodromal symptoms of tingling, burning, or pain; most common on lip, intraorally on palate and attached gingiva; adults and young adults usually affected; very common; called *herpetic whitlow* when occurs around fingernail	Herpes simplex virus—represents reactivation of latent virus and not reinfection; commonly precipitated by stress, sunlight, cold temperature, low resistance, and immunodeficiency	Self-limited; heals in about 2 weeks without scar; lesions infectious during vesicular stage; patient must be cautioned against autoinoculation; herpes type 1 infections have not been convincingly linked to oral cancer; any site affected in AIDS patients
Varicella	Painful pruritic vesicles and ulcers in all stages on trunk and face; few oral lesions; common childhood disease	Varicella-zoster virus	Self-limited; recovery uneventful in several weeks
Herpes zoster	Unilateral multiple ulcers preceded by vesicles distributed along a sensory nerve course; very painful; usually on trunk, head, and neck; rare intraorally; adults	Reactivation of varicella-zoster virus	Self-limited, but may have a prolonged, painful course; seen in debilitation, trauma, neoplasia, and immunodeficiency
Hand-foot-and-mouth disease	Painful ulcers preceded by vesicles on hands, feet, and oral mucosa; usually children; rare	Coxsackie viruses	Self-limited; recovery uneventful in about 2 weeks
Herpangina	Multiple painful ulcers in posterior oral cavity and pharynx; lesions preceded by vesicles; children most commonly affected; seasonal occurrence; rare	Coxsackie viruses	Self-limited; recovery uneventful in less than a week

AIDS, Acquired immunodeficiency syndrome.

Continued

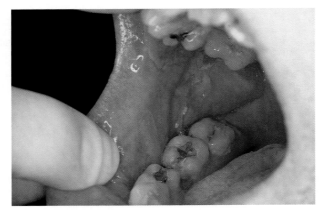

Figure 4 Pemphigus vulgaris.

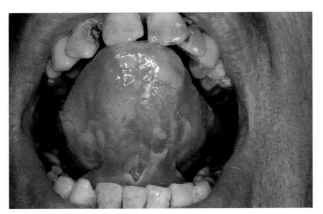

Figure 5 Pemphigus vulgaris.

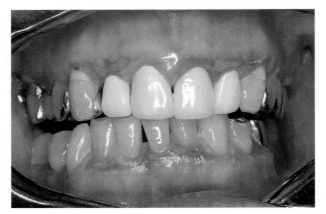

Figure 6 Mucous membrane pemphigoid.

Vesiculobullous Diseases *Continued*

Disease	Clinical Features	Cause	Significance
Measles (rubeola)	Koplik's spots precede maculopapular skin rash; fever, malaise, plus other symptoms of systemic viral infection; children most commonly affected	Measles virus	Self-limited; recovery uneventful in about 2 weeks
Pemphigus vulgaris	Multiple painful ulcers preceded by bullae; middle age; positive Nikolsky's sign; progressive disease; remissions or control with therapy; rare	Autoimmune; antibodies directed against desmosome-associated protein, desmoglein 3	Without treatment, may be fatal; significant morbidity from steroid therapy; oral lesions precede skin lesions in half the cases; prognosis improved if treated early
Mucous membrane pemphigoid	Multiple painful ulcers preceded by vesicles and bullae; lesion may heal with scar; positive Nikolsky's sign; may affect mucous membranes of oral cavity, eyes, and genitals; middle-aged or elderly women; uncommon; clinically may be confused with lichen planus, chronic lupus of gingiva, and hypersensitivity	Autoimmune; antibodies directed against basement membrane antigens, laminin 5, and BP180	Protracted course; may cause significant morbidity if severe; ocular scarring may lead to symblepharon or blindness; death uncommon
Bullous pemphigoid	Skin disease (trunk and extremities) with infrequent oral lesions; ulcers preceded by bullae; no scarring; elderly persons	Basement membrane autoantibodies are detected in tissue and serum	Chronic course; remissions; uncommon
Dermatitis herpetiformis	Skin disease with rare oral involvement; vesicles and pustules; pruritic exacerbations and remissions are typical; young and middle-aged adults	Unknown; IgA deposits in site of lesions; usually associated with gluten enteropathy	Chronic course that may require diet restriction or drug therapy
Epidermolysis bullosa	Multiple ulcers preceded by bullae; positive Nikolsky's sign; recessive; adult inheritance pattern determines age of onset during childhood and severity; may heal with scar; primarily a skin disease, but oral lesions often present; rare	Hereditary, autosomal dominant or recessive; acquired adult form also exists	Severe, debilitating disease that may be fatal in recessive form; simple operative procedures may elicit bullae; acquired form less debilitating

BP, Bullous pemphigoid antigen; *Ig,* immunoglobulin.

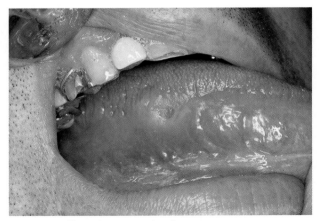

Figure 7   Chronic traumatic ulcer.

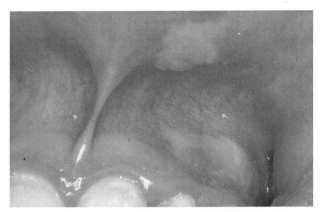

Figure 8   Acute ulcers (cotton roll injury).

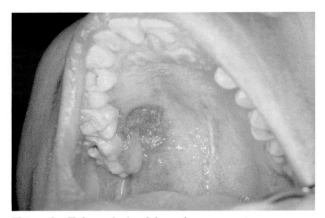

Figure 9   Tuberculosis of the palate.

Ulcerative Conditions

Disease	Clinical Features	Cause	Significance
Reactive lesions	Painful ulcer covered by yellow fibrin membrane; diagnosis usually evident from appearance when combined with history; common; traumatic factitial injuries are diagnostic challenge	Trauma, chemicals, heat, radiation	Self-limited; heals in days to weeks; factitial injuries follow unpredictable course
Syphilis	*Primary* (chancre)—single, indurated, nonpainful ulcer at site of spirochete entry; spontaneously heals in 4 to 6 weeks *Secondary*—maculopapular rash on skin; oral ulcers covered by membrane (mucous patches) orally *Tertiary*—gummas, cardiovascular and central nervous system lesions *Congenital*—dental abnormalities (mulberry molars, notched incisors), deafness, interstitial keratitis (Hutchinson's triad)	Spirochete—*Treponema pallidum*	Primary and secondary forms are highly infectious; mimics other diseases clinically; if untreated, secondary form develops in 2 to 10 weeks; a minority of patients develop tertiary lesions; latency periods, in which there is no clinically apparent disease seen between primary and secondary stages and between secondary and tertiary stages; untreated, 30% progress to tertiary stage
Gonorrhea	Typically, genital lesions, with rare oral manifestations; painful erythema or ulcers, or both	*Neisseria gonorrhoeae*	May be confused with many oral ulcerative diseases
Tuberculosis	Indurated, chronic ulcer that may be painful—on any mucosal surface	*Mycobacterium tuberculosis*	Lesions are infectious; oral lesions almost always secondary to lung lesions; differential diagnosis includes oral cancer and chronic traumatic ulcer
Leprosy	Skin disease, with rare oral nodules/ulcers	*Mycobacterium leprae*	Rare in United States but relatively common in Southeast Asia, India, South America
Actinomycosis	Typically seen in mandible, with draining skin sinus; wood-hard nodule with sulfur granules	*Actinomyces israelii*	Infection follows entry through a surgical site, periodontal disease, or open root canal

Continued

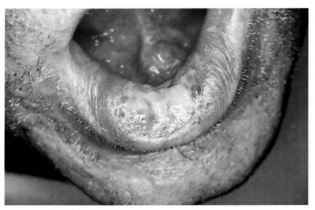

Figure 10   Histoplasmosis of the lip.

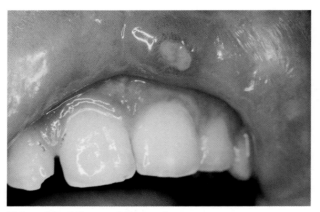

Figure 11   Minor aphthous ulcer.

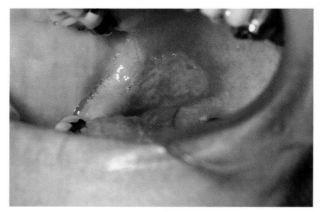

Figure 12   Major aphthous ulcer.

Ulcerative Conditions *Continued*

Disease	Clinical Features	Cause	Significance
Noma	Necrotic, nonhealing ulcer of gingiva or buccal mucosa; rare; affects children	Anaerobes in patient whose systemic health is compromised	Often associated with malnutrition; may result in severe tissue destruction
Deep fungal diseases	Indurated, nonhealing, frequently painful, chronic ulcer, usually following implantation of organism from lung	*Histoplasma capsulatum, Coccidioides immitis,* others	Oral lesions are secondary to systemic lesions; some types are endemic
Subcutaneous fungal diseases	Nonspecific ulcers of skin and, rarely, mucosa	Usually *Sporothrix schenckii*	Sporotrichosis usually follows inoculation via thorny plants
Opportunistic fungal infections	Occurs in compromised host; necrotic; nonhealing ulcer(s)	*Mucormycosis, Rhizopus,* others	Known collectively as *phycomycosis;* may mimic syphilis, midline granuloma, others; frequently fatal
Aphthous ulcers	Recurrent, painful ulcers found on tongue, vestibular mucosa, floor of mouth, and faucial pillars; not found on skin, vermilion, attached gingiva, or hard palate; usually round or oval; ulcers not preceded by vesicles; *minor type*—usually solitary, less than 0.5 cm in diameter; common; *major type*—severe, heals in up to 6 weeks with scar greater than 0.5 cm in diameter; *herpetiform type*—multiple, recurrent crops of ulcers	Unknown; probably an immune defect mediated by T cells; not caused by virus; precipitated by stress, trauma, other factors	Painful nuisance disease; rarely debilitating, except in major type; recurrences are the rule; more severe in patients with AIDS; may be seen in association with Behçet's syndrome, Crohn's disease, or gluten-sensitive enteropathy (celiac sprue)
Behçet's syndrome	Minor aphthae; eye lesions (uveitis, conjunctivitis); genital lesions (ulcers); arthritis occasionally seen	Probably an immune defect; HLA-B51	Biopsy and laboratory studies give nonspecific results; complications may be significant

AIDS, Acquired immunodeficiency syndrome; *HLA,* human leukocyte antigen.

Continued

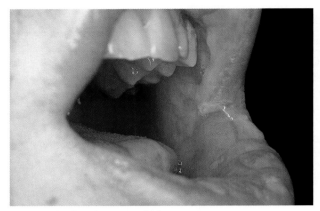

Figure 13   Erythema multiforme.

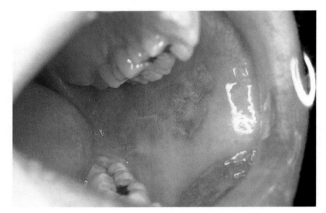

Figure 14   Lupus erythematosus.

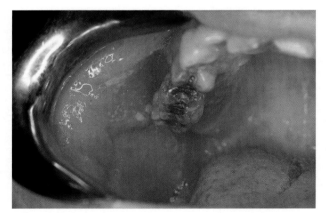

Figure 15   Contact hypersensitivity, buccal and palatal gingiva.

Ulcerative Conditions *Continued*

Disease	Clinical Features	Cause	Significance
Reiter's syndrome	Arthritis, urethritis, conjunctivitis or uveitis; oral ulcers; usually in white men in third decade	Unknown; immune response to bacterial antigen; usually follows STD or *Shigella* dysentery; HLA-B27	Duration of weeks to months; may be recurrent
Erythema multiforme	Sudden onset; painful, widespread, superficial ulcers; crusted ulcers on vermilion of lips; usually self-limited; young adults; may also have target or iris lesions of skin; may be recurrent, especially in spring and fall; some cases become chronic; uncommon	Unknown; may be hypersensitivity; may follow drug ingestion or an infection such as herpes labialis or *Mycoplasma* pneumonia	Cause should be investigated; can be debilitating, especially in severe forms, erythema multiforme major (Stevens-Johnson syndrome) and toxic epidermal necrolysis
Lupus erythematosus	Usually painful erythematous and ulcerative lesions on buccal mucosa, gingiva, and vermilion; radiating white keratotic areas may surround lesions; chronic *discoid type*—generally affects skin and mucous membrane only; acute *systemic type*—skin lesions may be erythematous with scale (classic sign is butterfly rash across bridge of nose); also may have joint, kidney, and heart lesions; middle-aged women; uncommon	Immune defect; patient develops autoantibodies, especially antinuclear antibodies	*Discoid type* may cause discomfort and cosmetic problems; *systemic type* has variable prognosis from mild to severe
Drug reactions	May affect skin or mucosa; erythema, white lesions, vesicles, ulcers may be seen; history of recent drug ingestions is important	Potentially any drug via stimulation of immune system	Reactions, such as anaphylaxis or angioedema, may require emergency care; highly variable clinical picture can make diagnosis difficult
Contact allergy	Lesions due to direct contact with foreign antigen; erythema, vesicles, ulcers may be seen	Potentially any foreign antigen that contacts skin or mucosa; cinnamon frequently cited	Patch testing may be helpful for diagnosis; history is important

STD, Sexually transmitted disease.

Continued

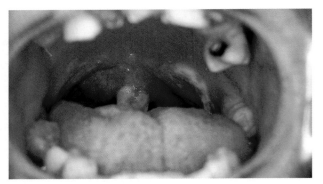

Figure 16   Midline granuloma.

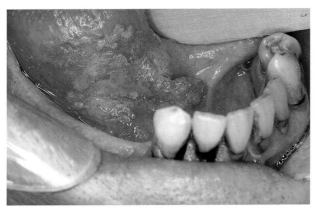

Figure 17   Squamous cell carcinoma, floor of mouth.

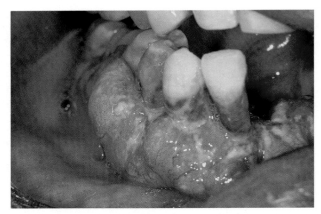

Figure 18   Squamous cell carcinoma, gingiva.

Ulcerative Conditions *Continued*

Disease	Clinical Features	Cause	Significance
Wegener's granulomatosis	Inflammatory lesions (necrotizing vasculitis) of lung, kidney, and upper airway; may affect gingiva when intraoral; rare	Unknown; possibly immune defect, or infection	May become life threatening as a result of tissue destruction in any of the three involved sites
Midline granuloma	Destructive, necrotic, nonhealing lesions of nose, palate, and sinuses; biopsy shows nonspecific inflammation; distinct from Wegener's granulomatosis; rare	Represents NK/T-cell lymphoma	Poor prognosis; death may follow erosion into major blood vessels
Chronic granulomatous disease	Recurrent infections in various organs; oral ulcers; males; rare	Genetic disease (X linked)	Altered neutrophil and macrophage function results in inability to kill bacteria and fungi
Cyclic neutropenia	Oral ulcers with periodicity; infections; adenopathy; periodontal disease	Mutations in neutrophil elastase gene	Rare blood dyscrasia
Squamous cell carcinoma	Indurated, nonpainful ulcer with rolled margins; most commonly found on lateral tongue and floor of mouth; males affected twice as often as females; clinical appearance may also be as a white or red patch or mass	DNA alterations due to carcinogens such as tobacco, UV light, some viruses; alcohol acts as cocarcinogen	Overall 5-year survival rate is 45% to 50%; improved prognosis if found in early stages, poor prognosis if metastasis to regional lymph nodes
Carcinoma of maxillary sinus	Patient may have symptoms of sinusitis or referred pain to teeth; may cause malocclusion or mobile teeth; may appear as ulcerative mass in palate or alveolus	Unknown	Prognosis only fair; metastases are not uncommon

UV, Ultraviolet.

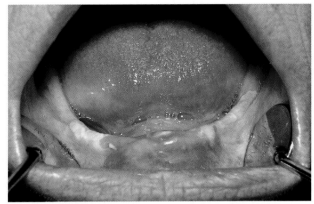

Figure 19   Hyperkeratosis, edentulous ridge.

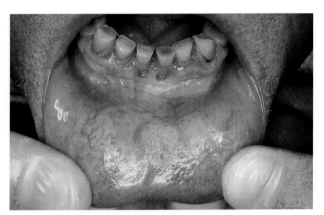

Figure 20   Hyperkeratosis, snuff dipper's pouch.

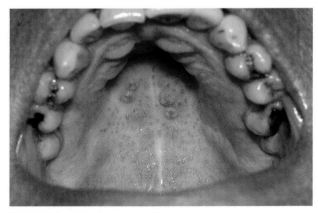

Figure 21   Nicotine stomatitis.

White Lesions

Disease	Clinical Features	Cause	Significance
Leukoedema	Common uniform opacification of buccal mucosa bilaterally	Unknown	Remains indefinitely; no ill effects
White sponge nevus	Asymptomatic, bilateral, dense, shaggy, white or gray, generalized opacification; primarily buccal mucosa affected, but other membranes may be involved; rare	Hereditary, autosomal dominant (keratin 4 and/or 13)	Remains indefinitely; no ill effects
Hereditary benign intraepithelial dyskeratosis	Asymptomatic, diffuse, shaggy white lesions of buccal mucosa, as well as other tissues; eye lesions—white plaques surrounded by inflamed conjunctiva; rare	Hereditary, autosomal dominant, duplication of chromosome 4q35	Remains indefinitely
Follicular keratosis	Keratotic papular lesions of skin and, infrequently, mucosa; lesions are numerous and asymptomatic	Genetic, autosomal dominant, mutation in *ATP2A2* gene	Chronic course with occasional remissions
Focal (frictional) hyperkeratosis	Asymptomatic white patch, commonly on edentulous ridge, buccal mucosa, and tongue; does not rub off; common	Chronic irritation, low-grade trauma	May regress if cause eliminated
White lesions associated with smokeless tobacco	Asymptomatic white folds surrounding area where tobacco is held; usually found in labial and buccal vestibules; common	Chronic irritation from snuff or chewing tobacco	Increased risk for development of verrucous and squamous cell carcinoma after many years
Nicotine stomatitis	Asymptomatic, generalized opacification of palate with red dots representing salivary gland orifices; common	Heat and smoke associated with combustion of tobacco	Rarely develops into palatal cancer

Continued

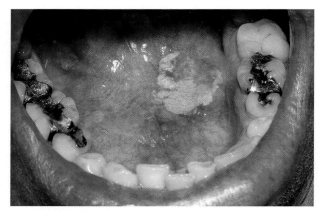

Figure 22   Idiopathic leukoplakia.

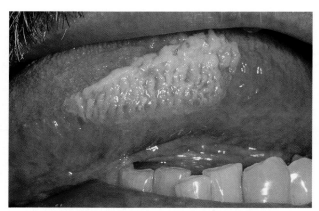

Figure 23   Hairy leukoplakia.

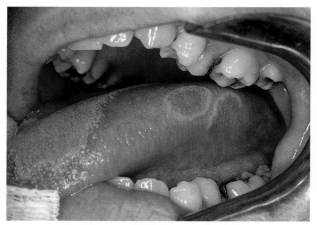

Figure 24   Geographic tongue.

White Lesions Continued

Disease	Clinical Features	Cause	Significance
Solar cheilitis	Lower lip—atrophic epithelium, poor definition of vermilion-skin margin, focal zones of keratosis; common	UV light (especially UVB, 2900–3200 nm)	May result in squamous cell carcinoma
Idiopathic leukoplakia	Asymptomatic white patch; cannot be wiped off; males affected more than females	Unknown; may be related to tobacco and alcohol use	May recur after excision; 5% are malignant, and 5% become malignant; higher risk of carcinoma if dysplasia present
Hairy leukoplakia	Filiform to flat patch on lateral tongue, often bilateral, occasionally on buccal mucosa; asymptomatic	Epstein-Barr virus infection	Seen in 20% of HIV-infected patients; marked increase in AIDS; may occur in non–AIDS-affected immunosuppressed patients and rarely in immunocompetent patients
Hairy tongue	Elongation of filiform papillae; asymptomatic	Unknown; may follow antibiotic, corticosteroid use, tobacco habit	Benign process; may be cosmetically objectionable
Geographic tongue (erythema migrans)	White annular lesions with atrophic red centers; pattern migrates over dorsum of tongue; varies in intensity and may spontaneously disappear; occasionally painful; common	Unknown	Completely benign; spontaneous regression after months to years

UV, Ultraviolet; *UVB*, ultraviolet B; *HIV*, human immunodeficiency virus; *AIDS*, acquired immunodeficiency syndrome.

Continued

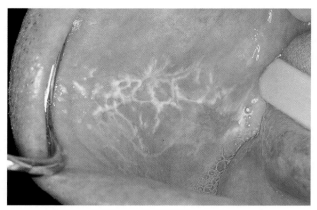

Figure 25   Lichen planus.

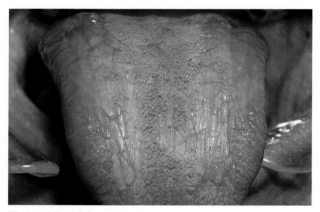

Figure 26   Lichen planus.

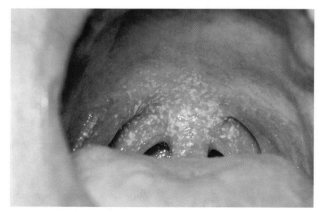

Figure 27   Candidiasis.

White Lesions *Continued*

Disease	Clinical Features	Cause	Significance
Lichen planus	Bilateral white striae (Wickham's); asymptomatic except when erosions are present; seen in middle age; buccal mucosa most commonly affected, with lesions occasionally on tongue, gingiva, and palate; skin lesions occasionally present and are purple pruritic papules; forearm and lower leg most common skin areas	Unknown; may be precipitated by stress; may be hyperimmune condition mediated by T cells	May regress after many years; treatment may only control disease; rare malignant transformation
Dentifrice-associated slough	Asymptomatic, slough of filmy parakeratotic cells	Mucosal reaction to components in toothpaste	None
Candidiasis	Painful elevated plaques (fungus) that can be wiped off, leaving eroded, bleeding surface; associated with poor hygiene, systemic antibiotics, systemic diseases, debilitation, reduced immune response; chronic infections may result in erythematous mucosa without obvious white colonies; common	Opportunistic fungus— *Candida albicans* and rarely other *Candida* species	Usually disappears in 1 to 2 weeks after treatment; some chronic cases require long-term therapy
Mucosal burns	Painful white fibrin exudate covering superficial ulcer with erythematous ring; common	Chemicals (aspirin, phenol), heat, electrical burns	Heals in days to weeks
Submucous fibrosis	Areas of opacification with loss of elasticity; any oral region affected; rare	May be due to hypersensitivity to dietary constituents such as areca (betel nut), capsaicin	Irreversible; predisposes to oral cancer

Continued

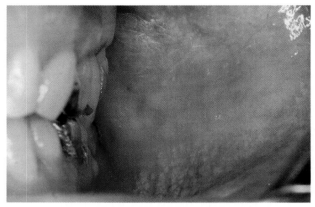

Figure 28   Fordyce's granules (bottom).

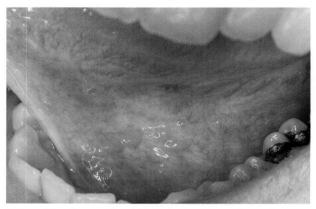

Figure 29   Ectopic lymphoid tissue, floor of mouth.

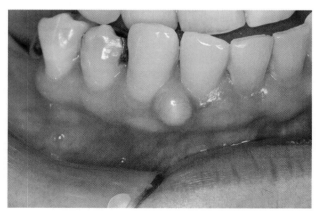

Figure 30   Gingival cyst.

White Lesions *Continued*

Disease	Clinical Features	Cause	Significance
Fordyce's granules	Multiple asymptomatic, yellow, flat or elevated spots seen primarily in buccal mucosa and lips; seen in a majority of patients; many consider them to be a variation of normal	Developmental	Ectopic sebaceous glands of no significance
Ectopic lymphoid tissue	Asymptomatic elevated yellow nodules less than 0.5 cm in diameter; usually found on tonsillar pillars, posterolateral tongue, and floor of mouth; covered by intact epithelium; common	Developmental	No significance; lesions remain indefinitely and are usually diagnostic clinically
Gingival cyst	Small, usually white to yellow nodule; multiple in infants, solitary in adults; common in infants, rare in adults	Proliferation and cystification of dental lamina rests	In infants lesions spontaneously rupture or break; recurrence not expected in adults
Parulis	Yellow-white gingival swelling due to submucosal pus	Periodontitis or tooth abscess	Periodic drainage until primary cause is eliminated
Lipoma	Asymptomatic, slow-growing, well-circumscribed, yellow or yellow-white mass; benign neoplasm of fat; occurs in any area	Unknown	Seems to have limited growth potential intraorally; recurrence not expected after removal

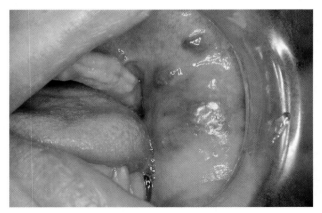

Figure 31   Vascular malformation.

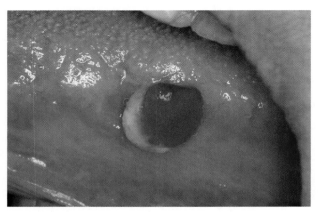

Figure 32   Pyogenic granuloma.

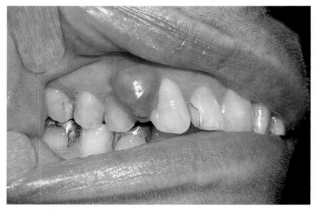

Figure 33   Peripheral giant cell granuloma.

Red-Blue Lesions

Disease	Clinical Features	Cause	Significance
Congenial hemangiomas and vascular malformations	Red or blue lesion that blanches when compressed; extent of lesion usually difficult to determine; skin, lips, tongue, and buccal mucosa most commonly affected; common on skin, uncommon in mucous membrane, rare in bone; part of Sturge-Weber syndrome; telangiectasias (small focal dilations of terminal blood vessels) blanch when compressed; commonly found in sun-damaged skin and seen with hereditary hemorrhagic telangiectasia (HHT)	Some are benign congenital neoplasms, others are due to abnormal vessel morphogenesis (vascular malformation); *HHT—* autosomal dominant; *venous varix—*congenital or induced by UV light	May remain quiescent or gradually enlarge; hemorrhage may be a significant complication; often a cosmetic problem; *HHT—*epistaxis and GI bleeding may be a problem
Pyogenic granuloma	Asymptomatic red mass composed of granulation tissue; most commonly seen in gingiva; may occur during pregnancy; may be secondarily ulcerated; common	Trauma or chronic irritation; size modified by hormonal changes	Remains indefinitely; recurrence if incompletely excised; reduction in size if cause removed or after pregnancy
Peripheral giant cell granuloma	Asymptomatic red mass of gingiva composed of fibroblasts and multinucleated giant cells; found mostly in adults in the former area of deciduous teeth; produces found in up-shaped lucency when edentulous areas; uncommon	Trauma or chronic irritation	Remains indefinitely if untreated; a reactive lesion; clinical appearance similar to that of pyogenic granuloma
Erythroplakia	Asymptomatic red velvety patch found usually in floor of mouth or retromolar area in adults; seen in older adults; red lesions may have foci or white hyperkeratosis (speckled erythroplakia)	Tobacco and alcohol	Most (90%) are in situ or invasive squamous cell carcinoma
Kaposi's sarcoma	May be part of AIDS; usually on skin, but may be oral, especially in palate; red to blue macules or nodules; rare, except in immunodeficiency	Endothelial cell proliferation related to cytokine/growth factor imbalance; HHV8 is part of etiology	Fair prognosis; poor when part of AIDS; incidence on the decline in AIDS patients

UV, Ultraviolet; *GI*, gastrointestinal.

Continued

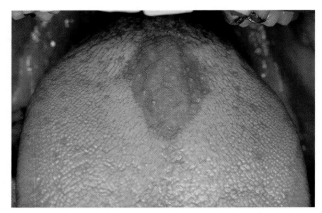

Figure 34   Median rhomboid glossitis (hyperplastic candidiasis).

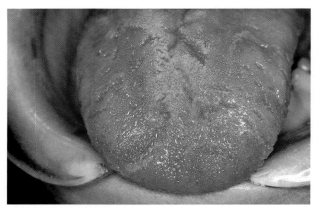

Figure 35   Geographic tongue.

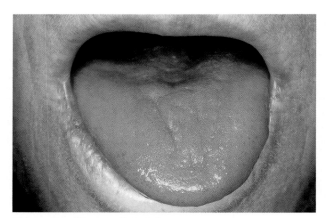

Figure 36   Vitamin B deficiency.

Red-Blue Lesions *Continued*

Disease	Clinical Features	Cause	Significance
Median rhomboid glossitis	Red lobular elevation anterior to circumvallate papillae in midline	Chronic *Candida* infection	Little; treat *Candida albicans* infection
Geographic tongue	White annular lesions with atrophic, red centers; white (keratotic) areas may be poorly developed, leaving red patches on dorsum of tongue; occasionally painful; common	Unknown	Little significance except when painful; not premalignant
Psoriasis	Chronic skin disease with rare oral lesions; red skin lesions covered with silvery scales; oral lesions red to white patches	Unknown	Must have skin lesions to confirm oral disease; exacerbations and remissions are typical
Vitamin B deficiency	Generalized redness of tongue due to atrophy of papillae; may be painful; may have an associated angular cheilitis; rare in United States	B complex deficiency	Remains until therapeutic levels of vitamin B are administered
Anemia (pernicious and iron deficiency)	May result in generalized redness of tongue due to atrophy of papillae; may be painful; patients may have angular cheilitis; females more commonly affected than males; Plummer-Vinson syndrome—anemia (iron deficiency), mucosal atrophy, predisposition for oral cancer	Some forms acquired, some hereditary	Some types may be life threatening; oral manifestations disappear with treatment; complication of oral cancer with Plummer-Vinson syndrome
Burning mouth syndrome	Wide range of oral complaints, usually without any visible tissue changes; especially middle-aged women; uncommon in males	Multifactorial—e.g., *C. albicans*, vitamin B deficiency anemias, xerostomia, idiopathic, psychogenic	May persist despite treatment
Scarlet fever	Pharyngitis, systemic symptoms, strawberry tongue	Group A streptococci	Complications of rheumatic fever and glomerulonephritis

HHV8, Human herpesvirus 8; *AIDS*, acquired immunodeficiency syndrome.

Continued

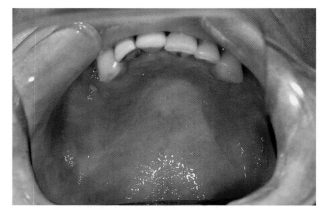

Figure 37   Erythematous candidiasis.

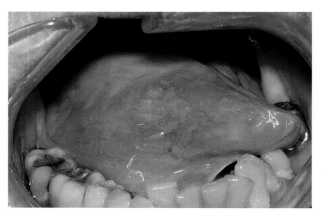

Figure 38   Drug reaction.

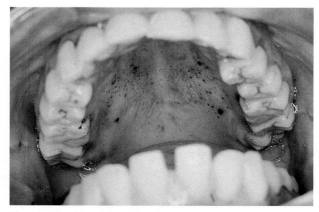

Figure 39   Petechiae, blood dyscrasia.

Red-Blue Lesions *Continued*

Disease	Clinical Features	Cause	Significance
Erythematous candidiasis	Painful, hyperemic palate under denture; angular cheilitis; red, painful mucosa	Chronic *C. albicans* infection; poor oral hygiene, ill-fitting denture are frequent predisposing factors	Discomfort may prevent wearing denture; not allergic or premalignant
Plasma cell gingivitis	Red, painful tongue; angular cheilitis; red gingiva	Possible allergic reactions to dietary antigen such as mint- or cinnamon-flavored chewing gum	Gingival lesions similar to lupus, lichen planus, and pemphigoid lesions
Drug reactions and contact allergies	Red, vesicular, or ulcerative eruption	Hypersensitivity reaction to allergen	Hypersensitivity reactions to drugs or HSV may produce erythema multiforme pattern clinically
Petechiae and ecchymoses			
Traumatic lesions	Hemorrhagic spot (red, blue, purple, black) composed of extravasated blood in soft tissue; does not blanch with compression; may be seen anywhere in skin or mucous membranes after trauma; changes color as blood is degraded and resorbed	Follows trauma such as that caused by tooth extraction, tooth bite, fellatio, chronic cough, vomiting	Resolves in days to weeks; no sequelae
Blood dyscrasias	Hemorrhagic spots (small—petechiae, large—ecchymoses) on mucous membranes due to extravasated blood; may be spontaneous or follow minor trauma; spots do not blanch with compression; color varies with time; uncommon in general practice, but dental personnel may be first to observe	Lack of clotting factor, reduced numbers of platelets for various reasons, or lack of vessel integrity	May be life threatening; must be investigated, diagnosed, and treated

HSV, Herpes simplex virus.

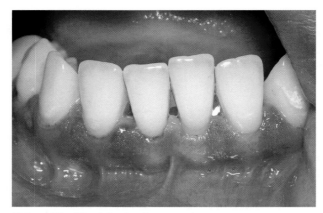

Figure 40   Physiologic pigmentation.

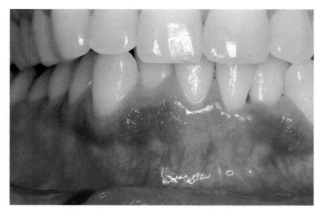

Figure 41   Smoking-associated melanosis.

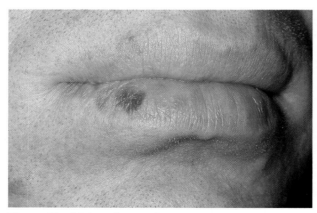

Figure 42   Melanotic macule.

Pigmented Lesions

Disease	Clinical Features	Cause	Significance
Physiologic pigmentation	Symmetric distribution; does not change in intensity; does not alter surface morphology	Normal melanocyte activity	None
Smoking-associated melanosis	Gingival pigmentation; especially women taking birth control pills	Component in smoke stimulates melanocytes	Cosmetic; may herald smoking-associated lesions elsewhere
Oral melanotic macule	Flat oral pigmentation less than 1 cm in diameter; lower lip, gingiva, buccal mucosa, palate usually affected; may represent oral ephelis, perioral lesions associated with Peutz-Jeghers syndrome, Addison's disease, or postinflammatory pigmentation	Unknown; postinflammatory; trauma	Remains indefinitely; no malignant potential
Neuroectodermal tumor of infancy	Pigmented, radiolucent, benign neoplasm in maxilla of newborns; pigment is melanin; rare	Unknown; tumor cells of neural crest origin	Recurrence unlikely

UV, Ultraviolet.

Continued

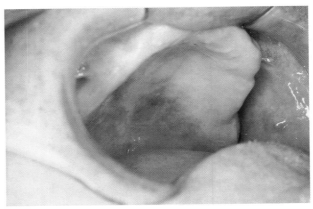

Figure 43   Blue nevus.

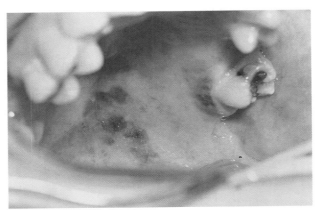

Figure 44   Melanoma.

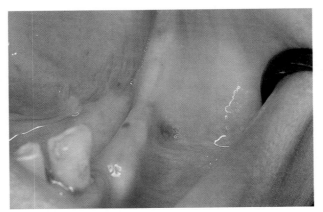

Figure 45   Amalgam tattoo.

Pigmented Lesions *Continued*

Disease	Clinical Features	Cause	Significance
Nevomelanocytic nevus	Elevated pigmentations; often nonpigmented when intraoral; uncommon orally; blue nevi seen in palate	Unknown; due to nests of nevus cells	Remains indefinitely; cannot be separated from melanoma clinically
Melanoma	Malignancy of melanocytes; some have a radial growth phase of years' duration (in situ type) before vertical growth phase, but invasive type has only vertical growth phase; oral melanomas may appear first as insignificant spot, especially on palate and gingiva; adults affected	UV light may be carcinogenic on skin; unknown for oral lesions	Skin—65% 5-year survival; oral—20% 5-year survival; in situ melanomas have better prognosis than invasive melanomas; unpredictable metastatic behavior
Amalgam tattoo	Asymptomatic gray-pigmented macule found in gingiva, tongue, palate, or buccal mucosa adjacent to amalgam restoration; may be seen radiographically if particles are large; no associated inflammation; common	Traumatic implantation of amalgam	Remains indefinitely and changes little; no ill effects
Heavy-metal pigmentation	Dark line along marginal gingiva due to precipitation of metal; rare	Intoxication by metal vapors (lead, bismuth, arsenic, mercury) from occupational exposure	Exposure may affect systemic health; gingiva pigmentation of cosmetic significance
Minocycline pigmentation	Gray pigmentation of palate, skin, scars, bone, and, rarely, of formed teeth	Ingestion of minocycline	Must differentiate from melanoma; drug may cause intrinsic staining of teeth

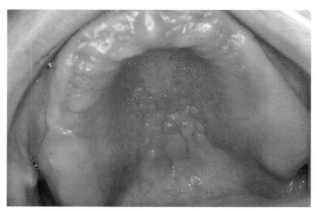

Figure 46   Papillary hyperplasia.

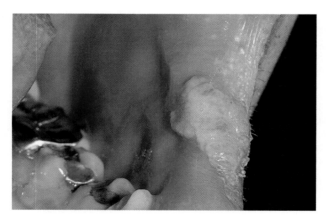

Figure 47   Condyloma latum.

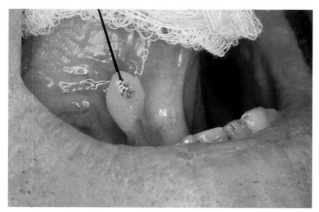

Figure 48   Papilloma.

Verrucal-Papillary Lesions

Disease	Clinical Features	Cause	Significance
Papillary hyperplasia	Painless papillomatous "cobblestone" lesion of hard palate in denture wearers; usually red as a result of inflammation; common	Soft tissue reaction to ill-fitting denture and probable fungal overgrowth	Lesion is not premalignant; may show significant regression if denture taken away from patient; topical antifungals may help
Condyloma latum	Clinically similar to papillary hyperplasia; part of secondary syphilis	*Treponema pallidum*	Prognosis good with treatment
Squamous papilloma	Painless exophytic granular to cauliflower-like lesions; predilection for tongue, floor of mouth, palate, uvula, lips, faucial pillars; generally solitary; soft texture; white or same color as surrounding tissue; young adults and adults; common	Most due to papillomavirus; some unknown	Lesion has no known malignant potential; recurrences rare
Oral verruca vulgaris	Painless papillary lesion usually with white surface projections because of keratin production; may be regarded as a type of papilloma; children and young adults; common on skin, uncommon intraorally	Human papillomavirus	Little significance; may be multiple and a cosmetic problem
Condyloma acuminatum	Painless, pedunculated to sessile, exophytic, papillomatous lesion; adults; same color as or lighter than surrounding tissue; patient's sexual partner has similar lesions; rare in oral cavity	Human papillomavirus	Oral lesions acquired through autoinoculation or sexual contact with infected partner; recurrences common

Continued

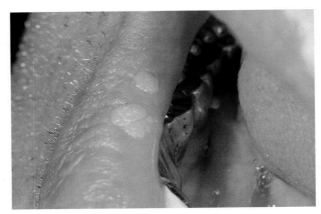

Figure 49   Focal epithelial hyperplasia.

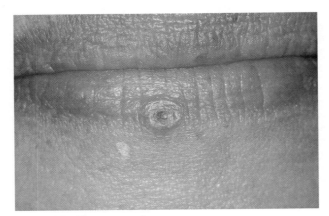

Figure 50   Keratoacanthoma.

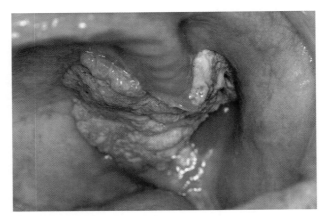

Figure 51   Verrucous carcinoma.

Verrucal-Papillary Lesions *Continued*

Disease	Clinical Features	Cause	Significance
Focal epithelial hyperplasia	Multiple soft nodules on lips, tongue, buccal mucosa; asymptomatic	Papillomavirus (HPV 13 and 32)	Little significance; may be included in differential diagnosis of mucosal nodules
Keratoacanthoma	Well-circumscribed, firm, elevated lesion with central keratin plug; may cause pain; develops rapidly over 4 to 8 weeks and involutes in 6 to 8 weeks; found on sun-exposed skin and lips; rare intraorally; predilection for men	Unknown	Difficult to differentiate clinically and microscopically from squamous cell carcinoma; may heal with scar
Verrucous carcinoma	Broad-based, exophytic, indurated lesions; usually found in buccal mucosa or vestibule; men most frequently affected; uncommon	May be associated with use of tobacco HPV present in some lesions	Slow-growing malignancy; well differentiated, with better prognosis than usual squamous cell carcinoma; growth pattern is more expansile than invasive; metastasis uncommon
Pyostomatitis vegetans	Multiple small pustules in oral mucosa; males more than females	Unknown	May be associated with bowel disease such as ulcerative colitis or Crohn's disease
Verruciform xanthoma	Solitary, pebbly, elevated or depressed lesion occurring anywhere in oral mucous membrane; color ranges from white to red; rare	Unknown	Limited growth potential; does not recur

HPV, Human papillomavirus.

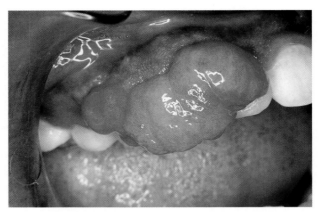

Figure 52   Pyogenic granuloma.

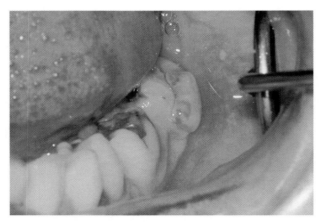

Figure 53   Peripheral (ossifying) fibroma.

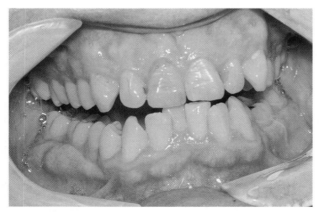

Figure 54   Exostoses.

Gingival Swellings

Disease	Clinical Features	Cause	Significance
Pyogenic granuloma	Asymptomatic red mass found primarily on gingiva but may be found anywhere on skin or mucous membrane where trauma has occurred; common	Reaction to trauma or chronic irritation	May recur if incompletely excised; usually does not cause bone resorption
Peripheral giant cell granuloma	Asymptomatic red mass of gingiva; cannot be clinically separated from pyogenic granuloma; uncommon	Reaction to trauma or chronic irritation	Completely benign behavior; unlike central counterpart; recurrence not anticipated
Peripheral fibroma	Firm mass; color same as surrounding tissue; no symptoms; common; may be pedunculated or sessile	Reaction to trauma or chronic irritation	Represents overexuberant repair process with proliferation of scar; occasional recurrence seen with peripheral ossifying fibroma
Parulis	Red mass (or yellow if pus filled) occurring usually on buccal gingiva of children and young adults; usually without symptoms	Sinus tract from periodontal or periapical abscess	Cyclic drainage occurs until underlying problem is eliminated
Exostosis	Bony hard nodule(s) covered by intact mucosa found attached to buccal aspect of alveolar bone; asymptomatic; common; usually appears in adulthood	Unknown	No significance except in denture construction

Continued

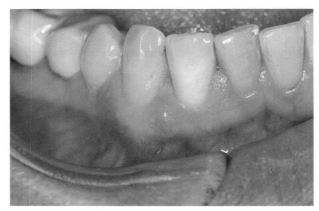

Figure 55   Gingival cyst.

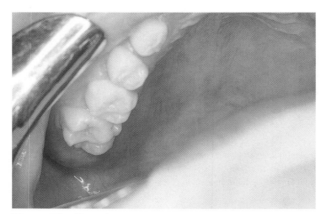

Figure 56   Eruption cyst.

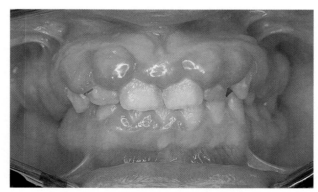

Figure 57   Generalized gingival hyperplasia.

Gingival Swellings *Continued*

Disease	Clinical Features	Cause	Significance
Gingival cyst	Small, elevated, yellow to pink nodule(s); multiple in infants, solitary in adults; common in infants, rare in adults	Proliferation and cystification of dental lamina rests	Known as *Bohn's nodules* or *Epstein's pearls* in infants; lesions are unroofed during mastication; adult lesions do not occur
Eruption cyst	Bluish (fluid- or blood-filled) sac over crown of erupting tooth; uninflamed and asymptomatic; uncommon	Hemorrhage into follicular space between tooth crown and reduced enamel epithelium	None; should not be confused with neoplasm
Congenital epulis of newborn	Firm, pedunculated or sessile mass attached to gingiva in infants; same color as or lighter than surrounding tissue; rare	Unknown	Benign neoplasm of granular cells similar to granular cell tumor of adult; does not recur
Generalized hyperplasia	Firm, increased bulk of free and attached gingiva; usually asymptomatic; pseudopockets; nonspecific type common, others (drug induced, hormone modified, leukemia induced, genetically influenced) uncommon to rare	Local gingival irritants plus systemic drugs (phenytoin [Dilantin], nifedipine, cyclosporine), hormone imbalance, leukemia, or hereditary factors/syndromes	Cosmetic, as well as hygienic, problem; causative factors should be eliminated if possible; improvement can be made by control of local factors

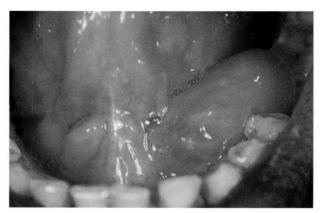

Figure 58   Mucus retention cyst (ranula).

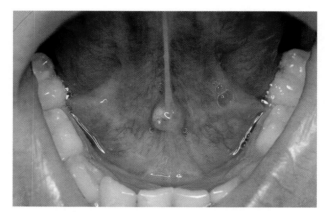

Figure 59   Lymphoepithelial cyst, lingual frenum.

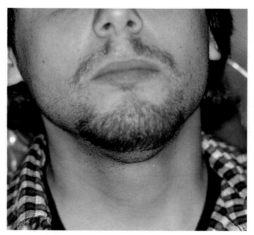

Figure 60   Dermoid cyst, midline of neck.

Floor-of-Mouth Swellings

Disease	Clinical Features	Cause	Significance
Mucus retention cyst (ranula)	Elevated, fluctuant, bluish white mass in lateral floor of mouth; cyclic swelling often; usually painful; uncommon	Sialolith blockage of duct or traumatic severance of duct	Most are due to sialoliths, some are due to severance of duct with extravasation of mucin into soft tissues; recurrence not uncommon
Lymphoepithelial cyst	Asymptomatic nodules covered by intact epithelium less than 1 cm in diameter; any age; characteristically found on faucial pillars, floor of mouth, ventral and posterior-lateral tongue; yellowish pink; uncommon within oral cavity, common in major salivary glands	Developmental defect	Ectopic lymphoid tissue of no significance; recurrence not expected
Dermoid cyst	Asymptomatic mass in floor of mouth (usually midline) covered by intact epithelium of normal color; young adults; feels doughy on palpation; rare	Proliferation of multipotential cells; stimulus unknown	Recurrence not expected; called *teratoma* when tissues from all three germ layers are present, and *dermoid* when secondary skin adnexa is present
Salivary gland tumor	Solitary, firm, asymptomatic mass usually covered by epithelium; malignant tumors may cause pain, paresthesia, or ulceration; young adults and adults; most common intraorally in palate, followed by tongue, upper lip, and buccal mucosa; uncommon	Unknown	Approximately half of minor salivary gland tumors are malignant; malignancies may metastasize to bones and lungs, as well as regional lymph nodes; pleomorphic adenoma is most common benign neoplasm
Mesenchymal neoplasm	Firm, asymptomatic tumescence covered by intact epithelium; may arise from any connective tissue cell	Unknown	Benign tumors not expected to recur; malignancies rare

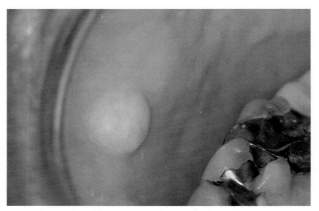

Figure 61   Focal fibrous hyperplasia.

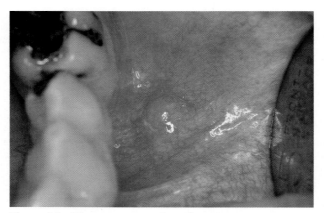

Figure 62   Mucus extravasation phenomenon, mandibular vestibule.

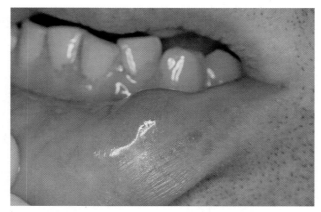

Figure 63   Mucus extravasation phenomenon.

Lip and Buccal Mucosa Swellings

Disease	Clinical Features	Cause	Significance
Focal fibrous hyperplasia (oral fibroma)	Firm, asymptomatic nodule covered by epithelium unless secondarily traumatized; usually found along line of occlusion in buccal mucosa and lower lip; common	Reaction to trauma or chronic irritation	Represents hyperplastic scar; limited growth potential, and no malignant transformation seen
Salivary gland tumor	Solitary, firm, asymptomatic mass usually covered by epithelium; malignant tumors may cause pain, paresthesia, or ulceration; young adults and adults; most common intraorally in palate, followed by tongue, upper lip, and buccal mucosa; uncommon	Unknown	Approximately half of minor salivary gland tumors are malignant; malignancies may metastasize to bones and lungs, as well as regional lymph nodes; pleomorphic adenoma is most common benign neoplasm
Mucus retention cyst	Solitary, usually asymptomatic, mobile, nontender; covered by intact epithelium; color same as surrounding tissue; adults over 50 years of age; common in palate, cheek, floor of mouth; uncommon in upper lip, rare in lower lip	Blockage of salivary gland excretory duct by sialolith	Recurrence not anticipated if associated gland removed; clinically indistinguishable from more significant salivary gland neoplasms
Mucus extravasation phenomenon	Bluish nodule (normal color if deep) usually covered by epithelium; may be slightly painful and have associated acute inflammatory reaction; most frequently seen in lower lip and buccal mucosa, rare in upper lip; adolescents and children; common	Traumatic severance of salivary gland excretory duct	Recurrence expected if contributing salivary gland not removed or if adjacent ducts are severed
Mesenchymal neoplasm	Firm, asymptomatic tumescence covered by intact epithelium; may arise from any connective tissue cell	Unknown	Benign tumors not expected to recur; malignancies rare

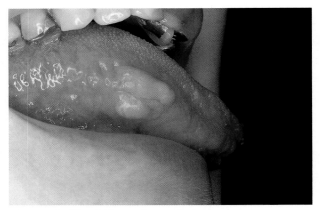

Figure 64   Focal fibrous hyperplasia.

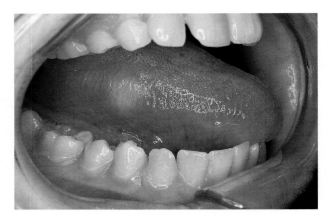

Figure 65   Granular cell tumor, lateral tongue.

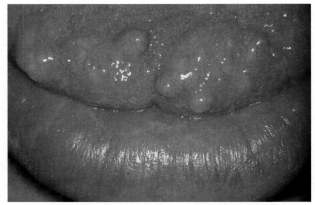

Figure 66   Mucosal neuromas of multiple endocrine neoplasia syndrome type III.

Tongue Swellings

Disease	Clinical Features	Cause	Significance
Focal fibrous hyperplasia	Firm, asymptomatic nodule covered by epithelium unless secondarily traumatized; usually found along line of occlusion in buccal mucosa and lower lip; common	Reaction to trauma or or chronic irritation	Represents hyperplastic scar; limited growth potential, and no malignant transformation seen
Pyogenic granuloma	Asymptomatic red mass found primarily on gingiva but may be found anywhere on skin or mucous membranewhere trauma has occurred; common	Reaction to trauma or chronic irrition	May recur if incompletely excised; usually does not cause bone resorption
Granular cell tumor	Painless elevated tumescence covered by intact epithelium; color same as or lighter than surrounding tissue; strong predilection for dorsum of tongue but may be found anywhere; any age; uncommon	Unknown; cell of origin undetermined; Schwann cell; granularity due to cytoplasmic autophagosomes	Does not recur; of significance in that it must be differentiated from other lesions; no malignant potential
Neurofibroma/palisaded encapsulated neuroma	Soft, single or multiple, asymptomatic nodules covered by epithelium; same as or lighter than surrounding mucosa; most frequently seen on tongue, buccal mucosa, and vestibule but may be seen anywhere; any age; uncommon	Unknown; cell of origin is probably Schwann cell; NF-1 gene mutation if part of neurofibromatosis syndrome	Recurrence not expected; multiple neurofibromas should suggest neurofibromatosis-1 (von Recklinghausen's disease of nerve) which includes neurofibromas and >6 café-au-lait macules); palisaded encapsulated neuromas are not syndrome associated
Mucosal neuroma	Multiple; lips, tongue, buccal mucosa; may be associated with MEN III syndrome	Unknown; MEN III syndrome is autosomal dominant	MEN III syndrome (pheochromocytoma, medullary carcinoma of thyroid, and mucosal neuromas)
Salivary gland tumor	Solitary, firm, asymptomatic mass usually covered by epithelium; malignant tumors may cause pain, paresthesia, or ulceration; young adults and adults; most common intraorally in palate, followed by tongue, upper lip, and buccal mucosa; uncommon	Unknown	Approximately half of minor salivary gland tumors are malignant; malignancies may metastasize to bones and lungs, as well as regional lymph nodes; pleomorphic adenoma is most common benign neoplasm
Lingual thyroid	Nodular mass in base of tongue; may cause dysphagia; young adults; rare	Incomplete descent of thyroid anlage to neck	Lingual thyroid may be patient's only thyroid tissue

MEN III, Multiple endocrine neoplasia syndrome type III.

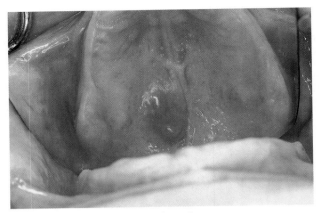

Figure 67   Mucus extravasation phenomenon.

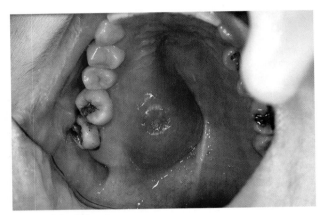

Figure 68   Mixed tumor.

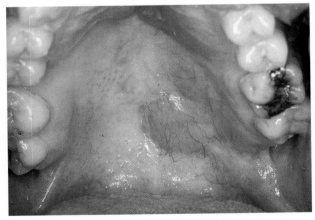

Figure 69   Lymphoma.

Palatal Swellings

Disease	Clinical Features	Cause	Significance
Mucus extravasation phenomenon	Bluish nodule (normal color if deep) usually covered by epithelium; may be slightly painful and have associated acute inflammatory reaction; most frequently seen in lower lip and buccal mucosa, rare in upper lip; adolescents and children; common	Traumatic severance of salivary gland excretory duct	Recurrence expected if contributing salivary salivary gland not removed or if adjacent ducts are severed
Salivary gland tumor	Solitary, firm, asymptomatic mass usually covered by epithelium; malignant tumors may cause pain, paresthesia, or ulceration; young adults and adults; most common intraorally in palate, followed by tongue, upper lip, and buccal mucosa; uncommon	Unknown	Approximately half of minor salivary gland tumors are malignant; malignancies may metastasize to bones and lungs, as well as regional lymph nodes; pleomorphic adenoma is most common benign neoplasm
Palatal abscess from periapical lesion	Painful, pus-filled, fluctuant tumescence of hard palate; color same as or redder than surrounding tissue; associated with nonvital tooth	Extension of periapical abscess through palatal bone	Pus may spread to other areas, seeking path of least resistance
Lymphoma	Asymptomatic, spongy to firm tumescence of hard palate; rare in adults; increased frequency in patients with AIDS	Unknown	May represent primary lymphoma (non-Hodgkin's type); lymphoma workup indicated; high-grade lesions seen in patients with AIDS
Torus	Asymptomatic, bony, hard swelling of hard palate (torus palatinus); bony, exophytic growths along lingual aspect of mandible (torus mandibularis); torpid growth; young adults and adults; affects up to 25% of population	Unknown	No significance; should not be confused with other palatal lesions
Neoplasm of maxilla or maxillary sinus	Palatal swelling with or without ulceration; pain or paresthesia; may cause loosening of teeth or malocclusion; denture may not fit; any age; rare	Unknown	May represent benign or malignant jaw neoplasm or carcinoma of maxillary sinus; poor prognosis for malignant lesions

AIDS, Acquired immunodeficiency syndrome.

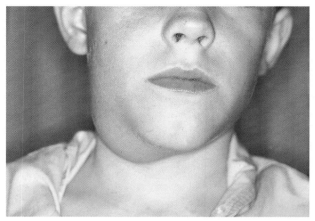

Figure 70   Branchial (cervical lymphoepithelial) cyst.

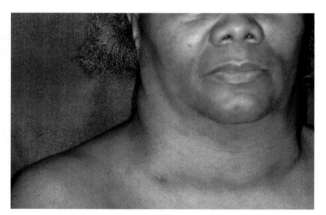

Figure 71   Metastatic carcinoma to multiple neck nodes.

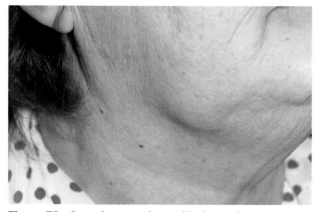

Figure 72   Lymphoma, submandibular node.

Neck Swellings

Disease	Clinical Features	Cause	Significance
Branchial cyst	Asymptomatic uninflamed swelling in lateral neck; soft or fluctuant; children and young adults; rare	Developmental, proliferation of epithelial remnants within lymph nodes	Clinical diagnostic problem
Lymphadenitis—nonspecific, bacterial, fungal	Single or multiple painful nodules (lymph nodes) in neck, especially submandibular and jugulodigastric areas; lesions are usually soft when acute and usually not fixed to surrounding tissue; nonspecific type common	Any oral inflammatory condition, especially dental abscess; oral tuberculosis, syphilis, or deep fungus may affect neck nodes	Neck disease often reflects oral disease
Metastatic carcinoma to lymph nodes	Usually single but may be multiple (rarely bilateral), indurated masses; fixed and nonpainful; most frequently affects submandibular and jugulodigastric nodes; adults	Metastatic oral cancer; may occasionally come from nasopharyngeal lesion	Signifies advanced disease with poorer prognosis
Lymphoma	Single or bilateral swellings in lateral neck; indurated, asymptomatic, and often fixed; patient may have weight loss, night sweats, and fever; young adults and adults; uncommon	Unknown	After diagnostic biopsy, staging procedures are done; prognosis poor to excellent, depending on stage and classification; increased frequency in patients with AIDS
Parotid lesion	When tail of parotid affected, neck mass may occur; *neoplasm*—indurated, asymptomatic, single lump (Warthin's tumor—may be bilateral); *Sjögren's syndrome*—bilateral, diffuse, soft swelling plus sicca complex, affects primarily older women; *infection*—unilateral, diffuse, soft, painful mass	*Neoplasm*—unknown; *Sjögren's syndrome*—autoimmune; *infection*—viral, bacterial, or fungal; *metabolic disease*—diabetes, alcoholism	Requires diagnosis and treatment by experienced clinician

AIDS, Acquired immunodeficiency syndrome.

Continued

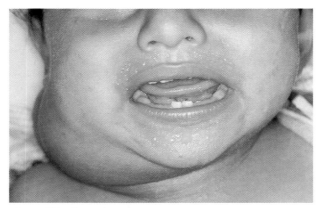

Figure 73   Lymphangioma.

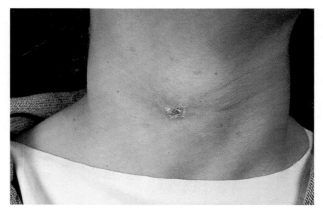

Figure 74   Thyroglossal tract cyst (sinus tract opening).

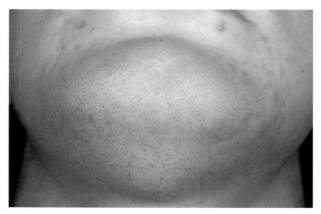

Figure 75   Dermoid cyst.

Neck Swellings *Continued*

Disease	Clinical Features	Cause	Significance
Carotid body tumor	Firm, movable mass in neck at carotid bifurcation; bruit and thrill may be apparent; adults; rare	Neoplastic transformation of carotid body (chemoreceptor) cells	Morbidity from surgery may be profound because of tumor attachment to carotid sheath
Epidermal cyst	Elevated nodule in skin of neck (or face); usually uninflamed and asymptomatic; up to several centimeters in size; covered by epidermis and near skin surface; common	Epithelial rest proliferation	Recurrence not expected; more superficially located than other neck lesions discussed
Lymphangioma	Spongy, diffuse, painless mass in dermis; may become large; lighter than surrounding tissue to red-blue; crepitance; children; rare	Developmental	May be disfiguring or cause respiratory distress
Thyroglossal tract cyst	Midline swelling in neck above level of thyroid gland; often moves when swallowing; may develop sinus tract; most common developmental cyst of neck	Failure of complete descent of thyroid tissue from foramen caecum with subsequent cystification	Recurrence not uncommon because of tortuous course of cystic lesion
Thyroid gland tumor	Midline swelling in area of thyroid gland; firm, asymptomatic; uncommon	Unknown	Prognosis poor to excellent, depending on stage and histologic type of tumor
Dermoid cyst	Swelling in floor of mouth or midline of neck; young adults	Unknown	Recurrence not expected

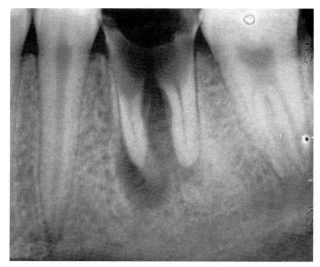

Figure 76   Periapical cyst associated with a carious tooth.

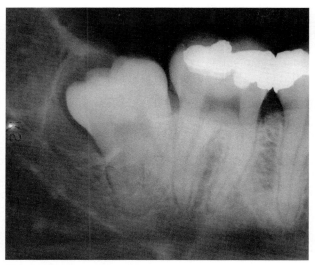

Figure 77   Dentigerous cyst.

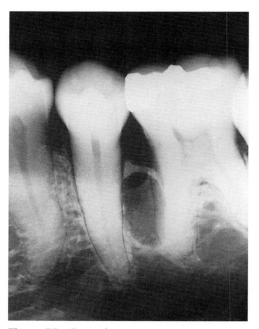

Figure 78   Lateral root cyst.

Cysts of the Jaws and Neck

Disease	Clinical Features	Radiographic Appearance	Other Features
Periapical (radicular) cyst	Any age; peaks in third through sixth decades; common; apex of any nonvital erupted tooth, especially anterior maxilla	Well-defined lucency at apex of nonvital tooth	Cannot be distinguished radiographically from periapical granuloma; develops from inflammatory stimulation of rests of Malassez; incomplete enucleation results in *residual cyst*; chronic process and usually asymptomatic; common
Dentigerous cyst	Young adults; associated most commonly with impacted mandibular third molars and maxillary third molars and cuspids	Well-defined lucency around crown of impacted teeth	Some become very large, with rare possibility of pathologic fracture; complication of neoplastic transformation of cystic epithelium to ameloblastoma and, rarely, to squamous cell or mucoepidermoid carcinoma; common; *eruption cyst*—gingival tumescence developing as a dilation of follicular space over crown of erupting tooth
Lateral periodontal cyst	Adults; lateral periodontal membrane, especially mandibular cuspid and premolar area	Well-defined lucency; usually unilocular but may be multilocular	Usually asymptomatic; associated tooth is vital; origin from rests of dental lamina; some keratocysts are found in a lateral root position; gingival cyst of adult may be soft tissue counterpart
Gingival cyst of newborn	Newborn; gingival soft tissues	Usually not apparent on radiograph	Newborns—common, multiple, no treatment; adult gingival cyst is rare, solitary, and treated by local excision

Continued

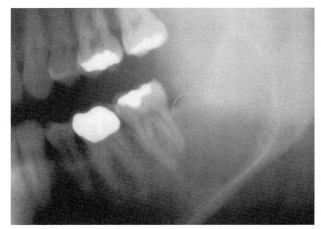

Figure 79   Odontogenic keratocyst.

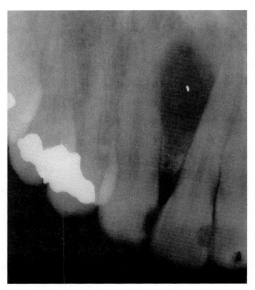

Figure 80   Globulomaxillary lesion.

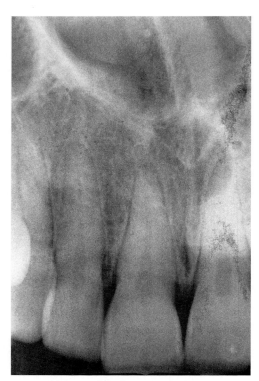

Figure 81   Nasopalatine canal cyst.

Cysts of the Jaws and Neck *Continued*

Disease	Clinical Features	Radiographic Appearance	Other Features
Odontogenic keratocyst	Any age, especially adults; mandibular molar-ramus area favored; may be found in position of dentigerous, lateral root, periapical cyst	Well-defined lucency; unilocular or multilocular	Recurrence rate of 5% to 62%; may have aggressive behavior; may be part of nevoid basal cell carcinoma syndrome (keratocysts, skeletal anomalies, basal cell carcinomas)
Calcifying odontogenic cyst	Any age; maxilla favored; gingiva second most common site	Well-defined lucency; may have opaque foci	Origin and behavior are in dispute; ghost cell keratinization characteristic; may have aggressive behavior; rare
Glandular odontogenic cyst	Any age; mandible favored	Well-defined lucency	Recurrence potential
Globulomaxillary lesion	Any age; between roots of maxillary cuspid and lateral incisor	Well-defined oval or pear-shaped lucency	Teeth are vital; asymptomatic; anatomic designation; represents one of several different odontogenic cysts/tumors
Nasolabial cyst	Adults; soft tissue of upper lip, lateral to midline	No change	Origin likely from remnants of nasolacrimal duct; rare
Nasopalatine canal cyst	Any age; nasopalatine canal or papilla	Well-defined midline maxillary lucency; may be oval or heart shaped	Teeth are vital; may be symptomatic if secondarily infected; may be difficult to differentiate from normal canal; common

Continued

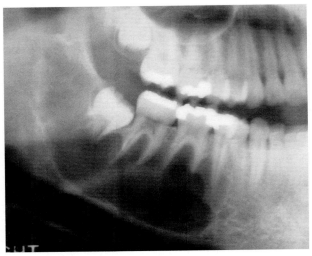

Figure 82   Traumatic bone cyst.

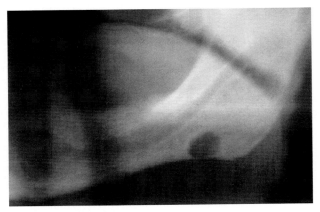

Figure 83   Static bone cyst.

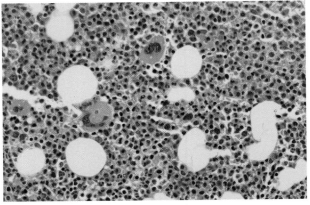

Figure 84   Hematopoietic bone marrow defect.

Cysts of the Jaws and Neck *Continued*

Disease	Clinical Features	Radiographic Appearance	Other Features
Median mandibular lesion	Any age; midline of mandible	Well-defined lucency	Teeth are vital; asymptomatic; represents one of several different odontogenic cysts/tumors
Aneurysmal bone cyst	Second decade favored; either jaw; also long bones and vertebrae	Lucency, may be poorly defined; may have honeycomb or soap bubble appearance	Represents vascular lesion in bone consisting of blood-filled sinusoids; blood wells up when lesion is entered; cause and pathogenesis unknown; rare; follow-up important
Traumatic (simple) bone cyst	Second decade favored; mandible favored	Well-defined lucency often extending between roots of teeth	Represents dead space in bone without epithelial lining; cause and pathogenesis unknown; uncommon in oral region; often part of florid osseous dysplasia
Static (Stafne) bone cyst	Developmental defect that should be apparent from childhood; mandibular molar area below alveolar canal	Well-defined oval lucency; does not change with time	Represents lingual depression of mandible; filled with salivary gland or other soft tissue from floor of mouth; asymptomatic; an incidental finding that requires no biopsy or treatment; uncommon
Focal osteoporotic bone marrow defect	Adults; mandible favored	Lucency; often in edentulous areas	Contains hematopoietic marrow; probably represents unusual healing in bone; must be differentiated from other, more significant lesions; uncommon

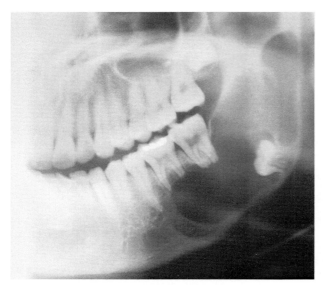

Figure 85 Ameloblastoma.

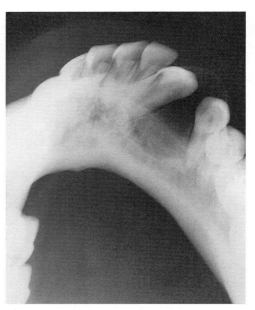

Figure 86 Adenomatoid odontogenic tumor.

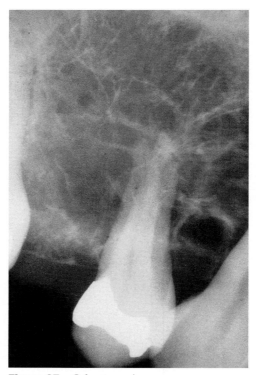

Figure 87 Odontogenic myxoma.

Odontogenic Tumors

Disease	Clinical Features	Radiographic Appearance	Other Features
Ameloblastoma	Fourth and fifth decades; mandibular molar-ramus area favored	Lucent; usually well circumscribed; unilocular or multilocular	May arise in wall of dentigerous cyst; may exhibit aggressive behavior; rarely metastasizes (usually to lung); recurrence rate lower for cyst; ameloblastoma usually asymptomatic; uncommon
Squamous odontogenic tumor	Mean age of 40 years; second through seventh decades; alveolar process; anterior more than posterior	Lucency	Conservative therapy; few recurrences
Calcifying epithelial odontogenic tumor (Pindborg tumor)	Mean age around 40 years; second through tenth decades; mandibular molar-ramus area favored	Lucent with or without opaque foci; usually well circumscribed; unilocular or multilocular	Behavior and prognosis are similar to those for ameloblastoma; rare
Clear cell odontogenic tumor	Seventh decade; mandible, maxilla	Lucency	Rare
Adenomatoid odontogenic tumor	Second decade; anterior jaws	Well-defined lucency; may have opaque foci	Usually associated with crown of impacted tooth; no symptoms
Odontogenic myxoma	Mean age of about 30 years; ages 10 to 50 years; any area of jaws	Lucent lesion; often multilocular or honeycombed; may be poorly defined peripherally	Tumors may exhibit aggressive behavior; no symptoms; uncommon; recurrence not uncommon
Central odontogenic fibroma	Any age; any area of jaws	Lucency; usually multilocular	Two microscopic subtypes exhibit same benign clinical behavior; differentiate from desmoplastic fibroma
Cementifying fibroma	Fourth and fifth decades; posterior mandible	Well-defined lucent lesion; may have opaque foci	Asymptomatic; grows by local expansion; recurrence unlikely; rare

Continued

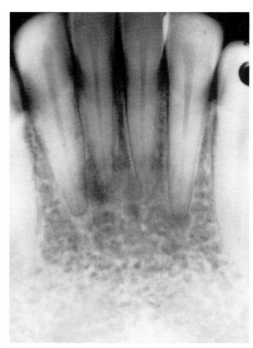

Figure 88   Periapical cementoosseous dysplasia.

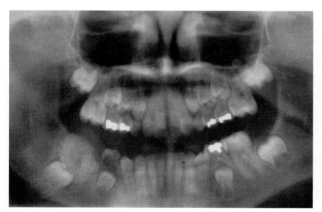

Figure 89   Odontoma.

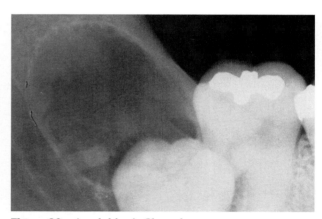

Figure 90   Ameloblastic fibroodontoma.

Odontogenic Tumors *Continued*

Disease	Clinical Features	Radiographic Appearance	Other Features
Cementoblastoma	Second and third decades; root of posterior teeth; mandible more than maxilla	Opaque lesion; attached to and replaces root; opaque spicules radiate from central area	May cause cortical expansion; tooth and lesion removed together; no symptoms; rare
Periapical cementoosseous dysplasia	Fifth decade; mandible, especially apices of anterior teeth; usually more than one tooth affected	Starts as periapical lucencies that eventually become opaque in months to years	May be a reactive process; always associated with vital teeth; requires no treatment; asymptomatic; common; rare variant known as *florid cemento-osseous dysplasia* represents severe form that may affect one to four quadrants and may have complications of chronic osteomyelitis and traumatic bone cysts
Odontoma	Second decade; any location, especially anterior mandible and maxilla	Opaque; *compound type*—tooth shapes apparent; *complex type*—uniform opaque mass	May block eruption of a permanent tooth; *complex type* rarely causes cortical expansion, no recurrence; *compound type* appears as many miniature teeth; *complex type* is conglomeration of enamel and dentin; probably represents hamartoma rather than neoplasm; common
Ameloblastic fibroma and ameloblastic fibroodontoma	First and second decades; mandibular molar-ramus area; often in a dentigerous relationship with tooth	Well-defined lucency; may be multilocular and large; fibroodontoma may have associated opaque mass representing an odontoma	Well encapsulated; recurrence not expected; no symptoms; if odontoma present, lesion is called *ameloblastic fibroodontoma*; rare

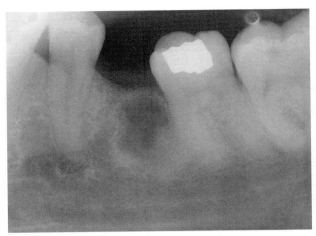

Figure 91   Ossifying fibroma.

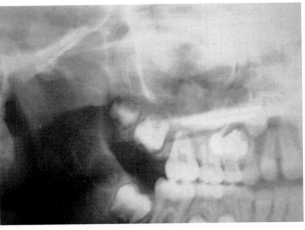

Figure 92   Fibrous dysplasia.

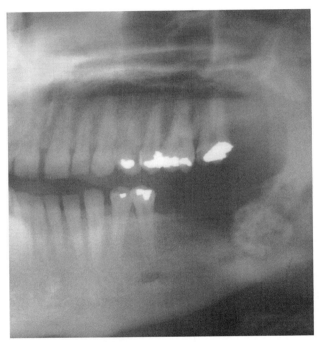

Figure 93   Osteoblastoma.

Benign Nonodontogenic Tumors

Disease	Clinical Features	Radiographic Appearance	Other Features
Ossifying fibroma	Third and fourth decades; body of mandible favored	Well-defined lucency, may have opaque foci	Slow growing and asymptomatic; may be indistinguishable from cementifying fibroma; does not recur; microscopy often similar to that of fibrous dysplasia; uncommon
Fibrous dysplasia	First and second decades; maxilla favored	Poorly defined radiographic mass; diffuse opacification often described as ground glass	Slow growing and asymptomatic; causes cortical expansion; may cease growing after puberty; cosmetic problem treated by recontouring; Variants: *monostotic*—one bone affected; *polyostotic*—more than one bone affected; *Albright's syndrome*—fibrous dysplasia plus café-au-lait macules and endocrine abnormalities (precocious puberty in females); *Jaffe-Lichtenstein syndrome*—multiple bone lesions of fibrous dysplasia and skin pigmentations
Osteoblastoma	Second decade; either jaw	Well-defined, lucent to opaque lesion	Diagnostic feature of pain; determination by microscopy often difficult; may be confused with osteosarcoma; recurrence not expected; rare
Chondroma	Any age; any location, especially anterior maxilla and posterior mandible	Relative lucency; may have opacities	May be difficult to separate microscopically from well-differentiated chondrosarcoma; rare
Osteoma	Any age; either jaw	Well defined	Asymptomatic; may be part of Gardner's syndrome (osteomas, intestinal polyps, cysts and fibrous lesions of skin, supernumerary teeth); rare

Continued

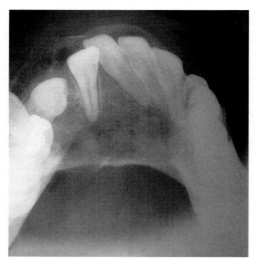

Figure 94   Central giant cell granuloma.

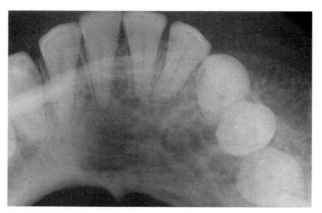

Figure 95   Hemangioma.

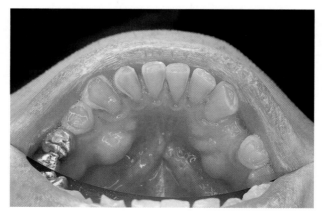

Figure 96   Mandibular tori (exostoses).

Benign Nonodontogenic Tumors *Continued*

Disease	Clinical Features	Radiographic Appearance	Other Features
Central giant cell granuloma	Children and young adults; either jaw	Usually well-defined lucency; may be multilocular or, less frequently, unilocular	May exhibit aggressive behavior; low recurrence rate; asymptomatic; uncommon; rule out hyperparathyroidism
Hemangioma of bone	Young adults; either jaw	Lucent lesion; may resemble honeycomb or be multilocular	Hemorrhage is significant complication with treatment; asymptomatic; rare
Langerhans cell disease	Children and young adults; any bone	Single or multiple lucent lesions; some described as punched out; lesions around root apices sometimes described as resembling floating teeth	Three variants: *Letterer-Siwe syndrome (acute disseminated)*—organs and bone affected, infants, usually fatal; *Hand-Schüller-Christian syndrome (chronic disseminated)*—bone lesions, exophthalmos, diabetes insipidus, and organ lesions, children, fair prognosis; *eosinophilic granuloma (chronic localized)*—bone lesions only, children and adults, good prognosis; surgery, radiation, or chemotherapy; cause unknown
Tori and exostoses	Adults; palate, lingual mandible, and buccal aspect of alveolar bone	May appear as opacity when large	Torus palatinus in 25% of population, torus mandibularis in 10%; cause unknown; little significance
Coronoid hyperplasia	Young adults; coronoid process of mandible	Opaque enlargement	Cause unknown; may affect jaw function

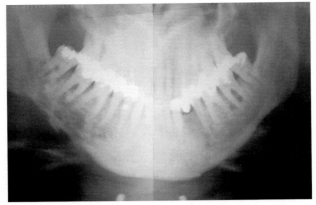

Figure 97   Chronic osteomyelitis in radiated mandible.

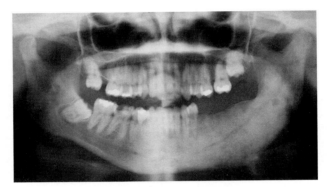

Figure 98   Diffuse sclerosing osteomyelitis.

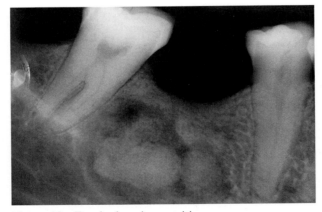

Figure 99   Focal sclerosing osteitis.

Inflammatory Jaw Lesions

Disease	Clinical Features	Radiographic Appearance	Other Features
Acute osteomyelitis	Any age; mandible favored	Little radiographic change early; after 1 to 2 weeks, a diffuse lucency appears	Pain or paresthesia may be present; pus producing if due to *Staphylococcus* infection; uncommon in severe form; most frequently caused by extension of periapical infection
Chronic osteomyelitis	Any age; mandible favored	Focal or diffuse; lucent with sclerotic foci described as moth-eaten pattern; *focal sclerotic type*—well-defined opacification; *diffuse sclerotic type*—diffuse opacification; *Garré's type*—onionskin periosteum	Usually asymptomatic but may be painful; most are related to chronic inflammation in bone of dental origin; many are not treated; nonvital teeth should be extracted or root canals filled; common; *Garré's type* is treated by endodontics or extraction of offending tooth

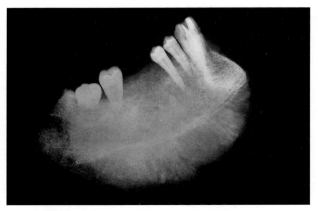

Figure 100   Osteosarcoma.

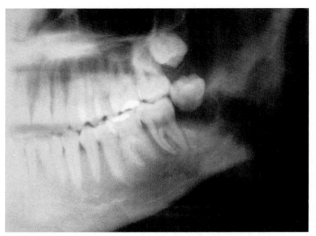

Figure 101   Postradiation chondrosarcoma, third molar area.

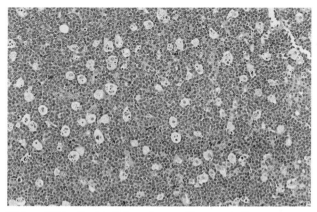

Figure 102   Burkitt's lymphoma ("starry sky" microscopy).

Malignancies of the Jaws

Disease	Clinical Features	Radiographic Appearance	Other Features
Osteosarcoma	Third and fourth decades; mandible or maxilla; juxtacortical subtype arises from periosteum	Poorly defined lucency, often with spicules of opaque material; sunburst pattern may be seen; juxtacortical lesion appears as radiodense mass on periosteum	Swelling, pain, and paresthesia are diagnostic features; patients may have vertical mobility of teeth and uniformly widened periodontal ligament space; prognosis fair to poor, good prognosis for juxtacortical lesions
Chondrosarcoma	Adulthood and old age; maxilla favored slightly	Poorly defined, lucent to moderately opaque	Swelling, pain, or paresthesia may be present; prognosis fair to poor, better if in mandible; often misdiagnosed as benign cartilage lesion; rare
Burkitt's lymphoma	Children; mandible or maxilla	Diffuse lucency	Malignancy of B lymphocytes linked to Epstein-Barr virus; pain or paresthesia may be presenting symptom; prognosis is fair; rare in United States

Continued

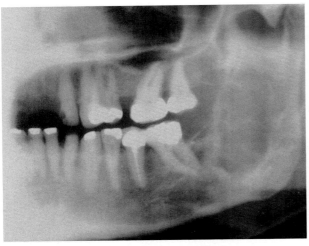

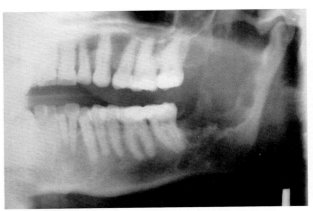

Figure 104   Metastatic breast cancer, mandibular ramus.

Figure 103   Multiple myeloma, mandibular ramus.

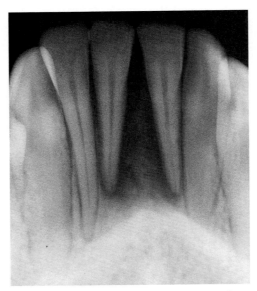

Figure 105   Metastatic osteosarcoma to the anterior mandible.

Malignancies of the Jaws *Continued*

Disease	Clinical Features	Radiographic Appearance	Other Features
Ewing's saroma	Children and young adults; mandible favored	Diffuse lucency; poorly defined; periosteal onionskin reaction may be present; may be multilocular	Swelling, pain, or paresthesia may be present; prognosis is poor; malignant cell is of unknown origin; rare
Multiple myeloma	Adults; mandible favored	Well-defined lucencies described as punched-out lesions; some lesions diffuse	Swelling, pain, or numbness may be presenting complaint; Bence Jones protein in urine of a majority of patients; rare to have only jaw lesions; prognosis is poor; solitary lesions eventually become disseminated
Metastatic carcinoma	Adults; mandible favored; occasionally gingiva	Ill-defined, destructive lucency; may be multilocular; some tumors may have opaque foci (e.g., prostate, breast, lung)	Pain or paresthesia common; origin is most likely from a malignancy of breast, kidney, lung, colon, prostate, or thyroid; uncommon

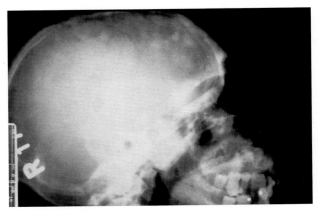

Figure 106   Paget's disease of the cranium.

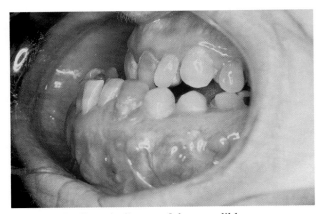

Figure 107   Paget's disease of the mandible.

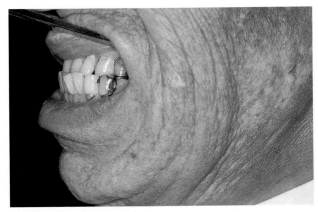

Figure 108   Acromegaly.

Metabolic and Genetic Diseases

Disease	Clinical Features	Radiographic Appearance	Other Features
Paget's disease	Age over 40 years; maxilla favored; bilateral and symmetric; affects entire bone	Diffuse lucent to opaque bone changes; opaque lesions described as cotton wool; hypercementosis, loss of lamina dura, obliteration of periodontal ligament space, and root resorption may be seen	Patients develop pain, deafness, blindness, and headache because of bone changes; initial complaint may be that denture is too tight; diastemas may develop; complications of hemorrhage early, infection and fracture late; alkaline phosphate elevated; cause unknown but affects bone metabolism
Hyperparathyroidism	Any age; mandible favored	Usually well-defined lucency(ies); may be multilocular; a minority of patients show loss of lamina dura	Usually asymptomatic; microscopically identical to central giant cell granuloma; serum calcium elevated; most caused by parathyroid adenoma; rare
Acromegaly	Adults (after closure of epiphyses); mandible; uniform, bilateral	Large jaw; splayed teeth	Excess production of growth hormone after closure of epiphyses (condylar growth becomes active); prognathism, diastemas may appear; rare

Continued

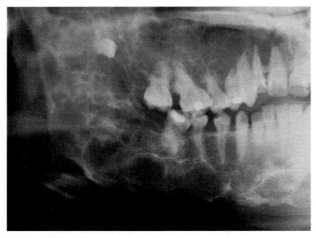

Figure 109   Cherubism.

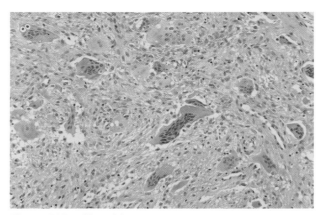

Figure 110   Cherubism.

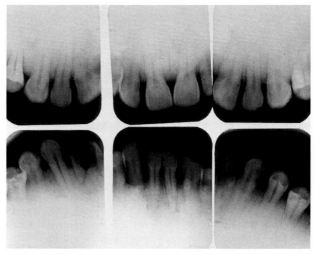

Figure 111   Osteopetrosis.

Metabolic and Genetic Diseases *Continued*

Disease	Clinical Features	Radiographic Appearance	Other Features
Infantile cortical hyperostosis	Infants; mandible and other bones of skeleton	Cortical thickening/sclerosis	Cause unknown; self-limited; treatment is supportive
Phantom bone disease	Young adults; mandible more than maxilla	Gradual lucency of entire bone	Cause unknown; no treatment
Cherubism	Children; mandible favored; uniform, bilateral	Bilateral multilocular lucencies	Autosomal-dominant inheritance pattern; cherublike is face; microscopy similar to that for central giant cell granuloma; process stabilizes after puberty; rare
Osteopetrosis	Children and adults; both jaws (and skull)	Diffuse, homogeneous, and symmetric opacification; may cause arrested root development and delayed eruption	Dominant forms are infantile, recessive (severe), and adult; intermediate form also recessive but has mild presentation; results in inhibition of bone resorption; patients develop anemia, blindness, and deafness; dental complication of infection and fracture; rare

VESICULOBULLOUS DISEASES

Viral Diseases
  Herpes Simplex Infections
  Varicella-Zoster Infections
  Hand-Foot-and-Mouth Disease
  Herpangina
  Measles (Rubeola)
Immunologic Diseases
  Pemphigus Vulgaris
  Mucous Membrane Pemphigoid
  Bullous Pemphigoid
  Dermatitis Herpetiformis
  Linear Immunoglobulin a Disease
Hereditary Diseases
  Epidermolysis Bullosa

VIRAL DISEASES

Oral mucous membranes may be infected by one of several different viruses, each producing a relatively distinct clinical pathologic picture (Table 1-1).

The herpesviruses are a large family of viruses characterized by a DNA core surrounded by a capsid and an envelope. Seven types of herpesviruses are known to be pathogenic for humans, with six of these linked to diseases in the head and neck area.

Herpes Simplex Infections

Herpes simplex virus (HSV) infections are common vesicular eruptions of the skin and mucosa. They occur in two forms—systemic or primary—and may be localized or secondary in nature. Both forms are self-limited, but recurrences of the secondary form are common because the virus can be sequestered within ganglionic tissue in a latent state. Control rather than cure is the usual goal of treatment.

Pathogenesis. Physical contact with an infected individual is the typical route of HSV inoculation for a seronegative individual who has not been previously exposed to the virus or possibly for someone with a low titer of protective antibody to HSV (Figure 1-1). The virus binds to the cell surface epithelium via heparan sulfate, followed by the sequential activation of specific genes during the lytic phase of infection. These genes include immediate early (IE) and early (E) genes coding for regulatory proteins and for DNA replication, and late (L) genes coding for structural proteins. Documentation of the spread of infection through airborne droplets, contaminated water, or contact with inanimate objects is generally lacking. During the primary infection, only a small percentage of individuals show clinical signs and symptoms of infectious systemic disease, whereas a vast majority experience only subclinical disease. This latter group, now seropositive, can be identified through the laboratory detection of circulating antibodies to HSV.

The incubation period after exposure ranges from several days to 2 weeks. In overt primary disease a vesiculoulcerative eruption (primary gingivostomatitis) typically occurs in the oral and perioral tissues. The focus of eruption is expected at the original site of contact.

After resolution of primary herpetic gingivostomatitis, the virus is believed to migrate, through some unknown mechanism, along the periaxon sheath of the trigeminal nerve to the trigeminal ganglion, where it is capable of remaining in a latent or sequestered state. During latency no infectious virus is produced; there is expression of early, but not late, genes; and there is no free virus. No major histocompatibility (MHC) antigens are expressed, so there is no T-cell response during latency.

Reactivation of virus may follow exposure to sunlight ("fever blisters"), exposure to cold ("cold sores"),

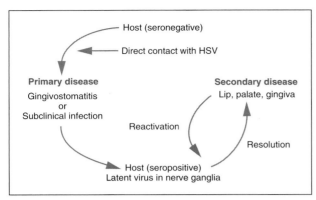

Figure 1-1 Pathogenesis of herpes simplex infections.

TABLE 1-1	Viruses Relevant to Dentistry
Virus Family	**Disease**
Herpesviruses	
HSV1	Primary herpes gingivostomatitis
	Secondary herpes infections
HSV2	Genital herpes
Varicella-zoster	Varicella (chickenpox), zoster (shingles)
Epstein-Barr	Mononucleosis
	Burkitt's lymphoma
	Nasopharyngeal carcinoma
	Hairy leukoplakia
Cytomegalovirus	Salivary gland inclusion disease
HHV6	Roseola infantum
HHV8	Kaposi's sarcoma
Papillomaviruses	Oral papillomas/warts, condyloma acuminatum, focal epithelial hyperplasia, some carcinomas
Coxackieviruses	Herpangina, hand-foot-mouth disease
Measles virus	Measles
Mumps virus	Mumps parotitis

HSV, Herpes simplex virus; *HHV*, human herpesvirus.

trauma, stress, or immunosuppression causing a secondary or recurrent infection.

An immunocompromised host may develop severe secondary disease. HSV-seropositive patients being prepared for bone marrow transplants with chemotherapeutic drugs such as cyclophosphamide (with or without total-body radiation) are at risk for a secondary herpes infection that is particularly severe. Posttransplant chemotherapy also predisposes seropositive patients to severe recurrent oral infections. HSV-seropositive patients infected with human immunodeficiency virus (HIV) may also exhibit intense secondary disease. Uncommonly, HIV-positive patients may have lesions that are coinfected by both HSV and cytomegalovirus. The pathogenesis of dually infected ulcers is unclear. Seronegative patients may rarely be affected with herpetic disease during immunosuppressive transplant states.

The reactivated virus travels by way of the trigeminal nerve to the originally infected epithelial surface, where replication occurs, resulting in a focal vesiculoulcerative eruption. Presumably because the humoral and cell-mediated arms of the immune system have been sensitized to HSV antigens, the lesion is limited in extent, and systemic symptoms usually do not occur. As the secondary lesion resolves, the virus returns to the trigeminal ganglion and evidence of viral particles can no longer be found within the epithelium. It is believed that nearly all secondary lesions develop from reactivated latent virus, although re-infection by different strains of the same subtype is considered a remote possibility.

Most oral-facial herpetic lesions are due to HSV type 1 (HSV1), although a small percentage may be caused by HSV type 2 (HSV2) secondary to oral-genital contact. Lesions caused by either virus are clinically indistinguishable. HSV2 has a predilection for genital mucosa, with infections having a pathogenesis similar to that of HSV1 infections of the head and neck. Latent virus, however, is sequestered in the lumbosacral ganglion. Previous HSV1 infections may provide some protection against HSV2 infection because of antibody cross-reactivity.

Asymptomatic shedding of intact HSV virus particles in saliva can be identified in approximately 2% to 10% of healthy adults in the absence of clinical disease. The level of risk of infection from "shedders" to others has not been measured, although it is probably low and dependent on the quantity of shed viral particles.

There is an association between HSV2 and carcinoma of the cervix. However, the link between HSV1 and oral cancer is less compelling. In experimental studies of oral tissues there is evidence that HSV1 is oncogenic in vitro, provided that cytolysis is inhibited by ultraviolet (UV) light or chemicals. In the hamster cheek pouch model, HSV can induce genetic changes, including chromosome translocations, mutations, and gene amplifications, and in other animal models HSV acts as a cocarcinogen with tobacco and other chemical carcinogens. In patients with oral cancers there is a high prevalence of HSV antibodies and antibodies to the immediate early proteins, but the significance is unclear.

Clinical Features

Primary Herpetic Gingivostomatitis. Primary disease is usually seen in children, although adults who have not been previously exposed to HSV or who fail to mount an appropriate response to a previous infection may be affected. By age 15 about half the population is infected. The vesicular eruption may appear on the skin, vermilion, and oral mucous membranes (Box 1-1; Figure 1-2). Intraorally, lesions may appear on any mucosal surface. This is in contradistinction to the recurrent form of the disease, in which lesions are confined to the hard palate and gingiva. The primary lesions are accompanied by fever, arthralgia, malaise, anorexia, headache, and cervical lymphadenopathy.

After the systemic primary infection runs its course of about 1 week to 10 days, the lesions heal without scar formation. By this time the virus may have migrated to the trigeminal ganglion to reside in a latent form. The number of individuals with primary clinical or subclinical infections in which virus assumes dormancy in nerve tissue is unknown.

Secondary, or Recurrent, Herpes Simplex Infections. Secondary herpes represents the reactivation of latent virus. It is believed that only rarely does reinfection from an exogenous source occur in seropositive individuals. A large majority of the population (up to 90%) have antibodies to HSV, and up to 40% of this group may develop secondary herpes. The pathophysiology of recurrence has been related to either a breakdown in focal immunosurveillance or an alteration in local inflammatory mediators that allows the virus to replicate.

Patients usually have prodromal symptoms of tingling, burning, or pain in the site in which lesions will appear. Within a matter of hours, multiple fragile and short-lived vesicles appear. These become unroofed and coalesce to form maplike superficial ulcers. The lesions heal without scarring in 1 to 2 weeks and rarely become secondarily infected (Box 1-2; Figures 1-3 to 1-6). The number of recurrences is variable and ranges from one per year to as many as one per month. The recurrence rate appears to decline with age with each individual. The secondary lesions typically occur at or near the same site with each recurrence. Regionally, most secondary lesions appear on the vermilion and surrounding skin. This type of disease is usually referred to as *herpes labialis*. Intraoral recurrences are almost always restricted to the hard palate or gingiva.

Immunodeficiency. Secondary herpes in the context of immunosuppression results in significant pain and discomfort, as well as a predisposition to secondary

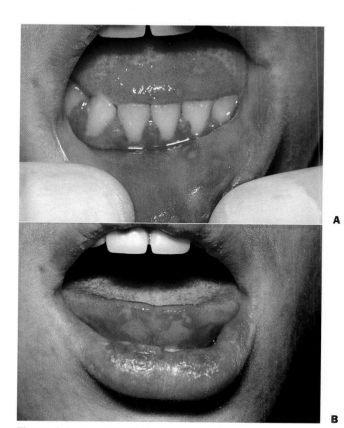

Figure 1-2 A and B, Primary herpes simplex infection.

Box 1-1 Primary Herpes Simplex

CLINICAL FEATURES

Most infections occur during childhood and subclinically
Few primary infections result in clinical disease
Oral and perioral vesicles rupture, forming ulcers
Intraoral lesions on any surface
Systemic signs/symptoms (e.g., fever, malaise)
Self-limited; symptomatic care
Immunocompromised have more severe disease

TREATMENT

Acyclovir and analogs may control virus
Must use early to be effective

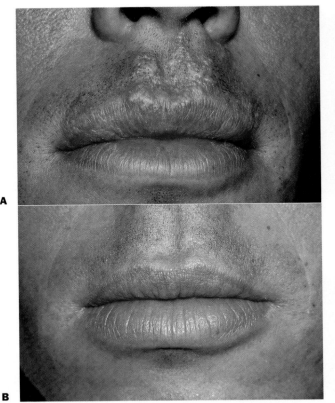

A

B

Figure 1-3   A, Secondary herpes simplex infection. B, Two weeks later.

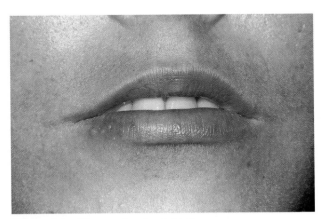

Figure 1-4   Herpes simplex labialis.

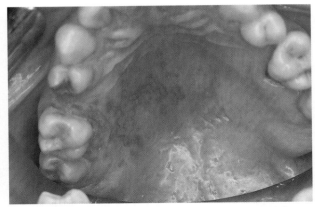

Figure 1-5   **Secondary herpes simplex infection** of the palate.

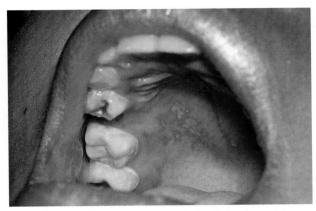

Figure 1-6   **Secondary herpes simplex infection** of the palate.

Herpetic Whitlow. Herpetic whitlow is either a primary or a secondary HSV infection involving the finger(s) (Figure 1-7). Before the universal use of examination gloves, this type of infection typically occurred in dental practitioners who had been in physical contact with infected individuals. In the case of a seronegative clinician, contact could result in a vesiculoulcerative eruption on the digit (rather than in the oral region), along with the signs and symptoms of primary systemic disease. Recurrent lesions, if they occur, would be expected on the finger(s). Herpetic whitlow in a seropositive clinician (e.g., one with a history of HSV infection) is believed to be possible, although less likely because of previous immune stimulation by herpes simplex antigens.

Pain, redness, and swelling are prominent with herpetic whitlow and can be very pronounced. Vesicles

bacterial and fungal infections. In contrast to those occurring in nonimmunocompromised patients, lesions in the immunodeficient patient are atypical in that they can be chronic and destructive. They also are not site restricted orally.

or pustules eventually break and become ulcers. Axillary and/or epitrochlear lymphadenopathy may also be present. The duration of herpetic whitlow is protracted, and may be as long as 4 to 6 weeks.

Histopathology. Microscopically, intraepithelial vesicles containing exudate, inflammatory cells, and characteristic virus-infected epithelial cells are seen (Figure 1-8). The virus-infected keratinocytes contain one or more homogeneous, glassy nuclear inclusions. These cells are also readily found on cytologic preparations. HSV1 cannot be differentiated from HSV2 histologically. After several days, herpes-infected keratinocytes cannot be demonstrated in either biopsy or cytologic preparations. Herpes simplex lesions

in HIV-positive patients may be coinfected with cytomegalovirus. The pathogenesis and significance of this phenomenon are undetermined.

Differential Diagnosis. Primary herpetic gingivostomatitis is usually apparent from clinical features. It can be confirmed by a virus culture (which requires 2 to 4 days for positive identification). Immunologic methods using monoclonal antibodies or DNA in situ hybridization techniques have also become useful for specific virus identification in tissue sections.

The systemic signs and symptoms coupled with the oral ulcers may require differentiation from streptococcal pharyngitis, erythema multiforme, and acute necrotizing ulcerative gingivitis (ANUG, or Vincent's infection). Clinically, streptococcal pharyngitis does not involve the lips or perioral tissues, and vesicles do not precede the ulcers. Oral ulcers of erythema multiforme are larger, usually without a vesicular stage, and are less likely to affect the gingiva. ANUG also commonly affects young adults; however, the oral lesions are

---

Box 1-2 Secondary Herpes Simplex

ETIOLOGY

Reactivation of latent herpes simplex virus type 1
Triggers—sunlight, stress, immunosuppression
Reactivation common; frequency decreases with aging
Prodromal symptoms—tingling and burning

CLINICAL FEATURES

Affects perioral skin, lips, gingiva, palate
Self-limited

TREATMENT

Possible control with acyclovir and analogs
Must administer early
Systemic treatment much more effective than topical treatment

---

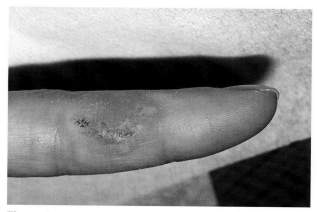

Figure 1-7 Herpetic whitlow.

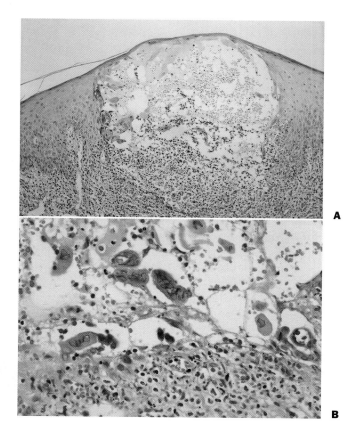

Figure 1-8 **A,** Herpes simplex–induced vesicle. **B,** Virus-infected multinucleated keratinocytes in the wall of a vesicle.

limited to the gingiva and are not preceded by vesicles. Moreover, there is often considerable pain and oral malodor in ANUG.

Secondary herpes is often confused with aphthous stomatitis but can usually be distinguished from it on the basis of clinical features. Multiple lesions, vesicles preceding ulcers, and palatal and gingival location are indicative of herpesvirus infection. In addition, in contrast to herpetic lesions, aphthae usually only on nonkeratinized mucosa, such as the floor of the mouth, alveolar mucosa, and buccal mucosae.

Treatment. One of the most important factors in the treatment of HSV infections is timing. For any drug to be effective, it must be used as soon as possible. No later than 48 hours from the onset of symptoms is generally regarded as the ideal time to start therapeutic measures. A number of virus-specific drugs have been developed. Acyclovir and its analogs have shown the greatest efficacy in the treatment of mucocutaneous infections.

The rationale for the use of topical agents resides in their ability to interrupt viral replication through inhibition of DNA polymerization (acyclovir, penciclovir), or by interference with virus-epithelial interaction and prevention of intracellular access (docosanol). In herpes-infected cells, acyclovir is converted by a virus-induced enzyme (thymidine kinase) and other cellular enzymes to a form that inhibits primarily viral DNA polymerase rather than host cell DNA polymerase. The end result is interruption of viral DNA synthesis and relative sparing of cellular DNA synthesis.

Systemic acyclovir (200- to 400-mg tablets five times per day) is effective in the control of primary genital herpes and, to a lesser degree, primary oral herpes. Supportive therapy (fluids, rest, oral lavage, analgesics, and antipyretics) is an essential component of any primary herpes simplex regimen.

Secondary herpes can be controlled to some degree with systemic acyclovir. Recurrences are not prevented, but the course and severity of the disease are favorably affected. Prophylactic systemic acyclovir is effective in problematic cases and in immunosuppressed patients. In HIV-positive patients with severe disease, aggressive therapy that may include intravenous acyclovir or ganciclovir may be necessary.

Topical acyclovir, although it is only somewhat effective, has been advocated by some for the treatment of secondary herpes. A 5% acyclovir (or analog) ointment applied five times per day when symptoms first appear slightly reduces the duration of herpes lesions and may abort some lesions. It does not prevent recurrence, however, and may be ineffective in some patients.

Varicella-Zoster Infections

Primary varicella-zoster virus (VZV) infections in seronegative individuals are known as *varicella* or chickenpox; secondary or reactivated disease is known as *herpes zoster* or shingles (Box 1-3). Structurally, VZV is very similar to HSV, with a DNA core, a protein capsid, and a lipid envelope. Microscopically, striking similarities can also be noted. The ability of the virus to remain quiescent in sensory ganglia for indefinite periods after a primary infection is common to both. A cutaneous or mucosal vesiculoulcerative eruption following reactivation of latent virus is also typical of both VZV and HSV infections. A number of signs and symptoms, however, appear to be unique to each infection.

Pathogenesis

Varicella. Transmission of varicella is believed to be predominantly through the inhalation of contaminated droplets. The condition is very contagious and is known to spread readily from child to child. Much less commonly, direct contact is an alternative way of acquiring the disease. During the 2-week incubation period, virus proliferates within macrophages, with sub-

---

Box 1-3 Varicella-Zoster

PRIMARY DISEASE (VARICELLA, CHICKENPOX)

Self-limiting
Common in children
Vesicular eruption of trunk and head and neck occurring in crops
Systemic signs/symptoms—fever, malaise, other
Symptomatic treatment

SECONDARY DISEASE (ZOSTER, SHINGLES)

Self-limiting
Adults
Rash, vesicles, ulcers unilateral along dermatome
Postherpetic pain (~15% of cases) can be severe
Immunocompromised and lymphoma patients at risk
Treated with acyclovir and analogs

sequent viremia and dissemination to the skin and other organs. Host defense mechanisms of non-specific interferon production and specific humoral and cell-mediated immune responses are also triggered. Overt clinical disease then appears in most individuals. As the viremia overwhelms body defenses, systemic signs and symptoms develop. Eventually, in a normal host the immune response is able to limit and halt the replication of virus, allowing recovery in 2 to 3 weeks. During the disease process the VZV may progress along sensory nerves to the sensory ganglia, where it can reside in a latent, undetectable form.

Herpes Zoster. Reactivation of latent VZV is uncommon but characteristically follows such occurrences as immunosuppressive states due to malignancy (especially lymphomas and leukemias), drug administration, or HIV infection. Radiation or surgery of the spinal cord or local trauma may also trigger secondary lesions. Prodromal symptoms of pain or paresthesia develop and persist for several days as the virus infects the sensory nerve of a dermatome (usually of the trunk or head and neck). A vesicular skin eruption that becomes pustular and eventually ulcerated follows. The disease lasts several weeks and may be followed by a troublesome postherpetic neuralgia (in approximately 15% of patients) that takes several months to resolve. Local cutaneous hyperpigmentation may also be noted on occasion.

Clinical Features

Varicella. A large majority of the population experiences a primary infection during childhood. Fever, chills, malaise, and headache may accompany a rash that involves primarily the trunk and head and neck. The rash quickly develops into a vesicular eruption that becomes pustular and eventually ulcerates. Successive crops of new lesions appear, owing to repeated waves of viremia. This causes the presence, at any one time, of lesions in all stages of development (Figure 1-9). The infection is self-limiting and lasts several weeks. Oral mucous membranes may be involved in primary disease and usually demonstrate multiple shallow ulcers that are preceded by evanescent vesicles (Figure 1-10). Because of the intense pruritic nature of the skin lesions, secondary bacterial infection is not uncommon and may result in healing with scar formation. Complications, including pneumonitis, encephalitis, and inflammation of other organs, may occur in a very small percentage of cases. If varicella is acquired during pregnancy, fetal abnormalities may occur. When older adults and immunocompromised patients are affected, varicella may be much more severe, protracted, and more likely to produce complications.

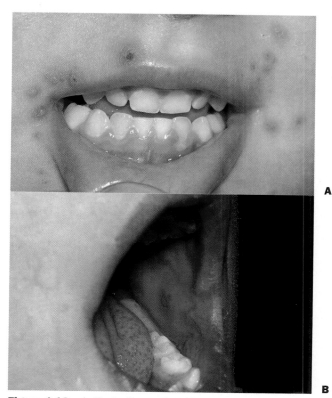

Figure 1-10 A, Varicella, perioral lesions. B, Intraoral lesions.

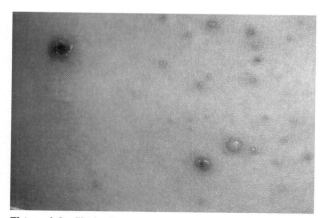

Figure 1-9 Varicella eruption on the trunk of a child.

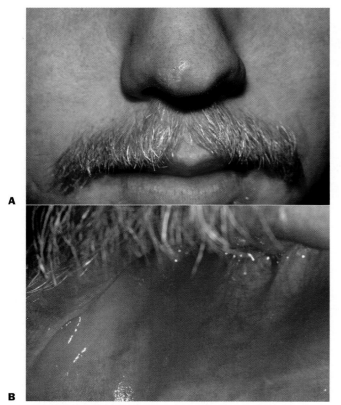

A

B

Figure 1-11   **A, Herpes zoster** of the nose. **B,** Intraoral lesions.

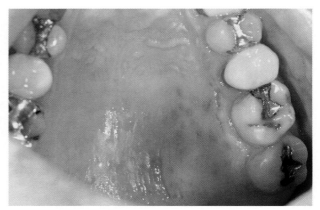

Figure 1-12   **Herpes zoster** of the palate.

Herpes Zoster. Zoster is basically a condition of the older adult population and of individuals who have compromised immune responses. The sensory nerves of the trunk and head and neck are commonly affected. Involvement of the various branches of the trigeminal nerve may result in unilateral oral, facial, or ocular lesions (Figures 1-11 and 1-12). Involvement of facial and auditory nerves produces the *Ramsay Hunt syndrome,* in which there is facial paralysis accompanied by vesicles of the ipsilateral external ear, tinnitus, deafness, and vertigo.

After several days of prodromal symptoms of pain and/or paresthesia in the area of the involved dermatome, a well-delineated unilateral maculopapular rash appears. This may occasionally be accompanied by systemic symptoms as well. The rash quickly becomes vesicular, pustular, and then ulcerative. Remission usually occurs in several weeks. Complications include secondary infection of ulcers, postherpetic neuralgia (which may be refractory to analgesics), motor paralysis, and ocular inflammation when the ophthalmic division of the trigeminal nerve is involved.

Histopathology. The morphology of the VZV and the inflammatory response to its presence in both varicella and herpes zoster are essentially the same as those with HSV. Microscopically, virus-infected epithelial cells show homogeneous nuclei, representing viral products, with margination of chromatin along the nuclear membrane. Multinucleation of infected cells is also typical. Acantholytic vesicles eventually break down and ulcerate. In uncomplicated cases epithelium regenerates from the ulcer margins with little or no scar.

Differential Diagnosis. Varicella is clinically diagnosed by the history of exposure and by the type and distribution of lesions. Other primary viral infections that may show some similarities include primary HSV infection and hand-foot-and-mouth disease.

Herpes zoster is most commonly confused with recurrent HSV infections and may be indistinguishable from them on clinical grounds. The longer duration, greater intensity of prodromal symptoms, unilateral distribution with abrupt ending at the midline, and postherpetic neuralgia all favor a clinical diagnosis of herpes zoster. Diagnosis of equivocal cases can be definitively made through virus antigen typing using laboratory immunologic tests (e.g., immunohistochemistry or DNA in situ hybridization).

Treatment. For varicella, supportive therapy is generally indicated in normal individuals. However, in immunocompromised patients more substantial measures are warranted. Virus-specific drugs that are effective in treating HSV infections have also shown efficacy in the treatment of VZV infections. These include systemically administered acyclovir, vidarabine, and human leukocyte interferon. Corticosteroids are generally contraindicated.

Patients with herpes zoster and intact immune responses have generally been treated empirically. However, it has been shown that oral acyclovir used at high doses (800 mg five times per day for 7 to 10 days) can shorten the disease course and reduce postherpetic pain. Analgesics provide only limited relief from pain. Topically applied virus-specific drugs may have some benefit if used early. Topically applied substance P inhibitor (capsaicin) may provide some relief from postherpetic pain. The use of topical or systemic corticosteroids cannot yet be recommended. In patients with compromised immune responses, systemically administered acyclovir, vidarabine, or interferon is indicated, although success is variable.

Hand-Foot-and-Mouth Disease

Etiology and Pathogenesis. One of the subdivisions of the family of viruses known as picornavirus (literally, small [pico] RNA virus) is the Coxsackie group named after the New York town where the virus was first identified. Certain Coxsackie subtypes cause oral vesicular eruptions: hand-foot-and-mouth (HFM) disease and herpangina.

HFM disease is a highly contagious viral infection that is usually caused by Coxsackie type A16, although serologic types A5, A9, A10, B2, and B5 and enterovirus 71 (another type of picornavirus) have been isolated on occasion. The mode of transfer of virus from one individual to another is through either airborne spread or fecal-oral contamination. With subsequent viremia, the virus exhibits a predilection for mucous membranes of the mouth and cutaneous regions of the hands and feet.

Clinical Features. This viral infection typically occurs in epidemic or endemic proportions and predominantly affects children younger than 5 years of age. After a short incubation period, the condition resolves spontaneously in 1 to 2 weeks.

Signs and symptoms are usually mild to moderate in intensity and include low-grade fever, malaise, lymphadenopathy, and sore mouth. Pain from oral lesions is often a patient's chief complaint. The oral lesions begin as vesicles that quickly rupture to become ulcers that are covered by a yellow fibrinous membrane surrounded by an erythematous halo. The lesions,

which are multiple, can occur anywhere in the mouth, although the palate, tongue, and buccal mucosa are favored sites. Multiple maculopapular lesions, typically on the feet, toes, hands, and fingers, appear concomitantly with or shortly after the oral lesions (Figure 1-13). These lesions progress to a vesicular state and eventually become ulcerated and encrusted.

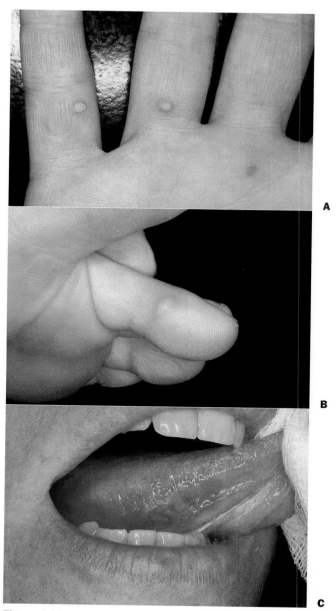

Figure 1-13 **A, B,** and **C, Hand-foot-and-mouth disease.** (Courtesy Dr. Steven K. Young.)

Histopathology. The vesicles of this condition are found within the epithelium because of obligate viral replication in keratinocytes. Eosinophilic inclusions may be seen within some of the infected epithelial cells. As the keratinocytes are destroyed by virus, the vesicle enlarges as it becomes filled with proteinaceous debris and inflammatory cells.

Differential Diagnosis. Because this disease may express itself primarily within the oral cavity, a differential diagnosis should include primary herpes gingivostomatitis and possibly varicella. The relatively mild symptoms, cutaneous distribution, and epidemic spread should help separate this condition from the others. Virus culture or detection of circulating antibodies may be done to confirm the clinical impression.

Treatment. Because of the relatively short duration, the self-limiting nature, and the general lack of virus-specific therapy, treatment for HFM disease is usually symptomatic. Bland mouthrinses such as sodium bicarbonate in warm water may be used to help alleviate oral discomfort.

Herpangina

Etiology and Pathogenesis. Herpangina is an acute viral infection that is caused by another Coxsackie type A virus (types A1–6, A8, A10, A22, B3, and possibly others). It is transmitted by contaminated saliva and occasionally through contaminated feces.

Clinical Features. Herpangina is usually endemic, with outbreaks occurring typically in summer or early autumn. It is more common in children than in adults. Those infected generally complain of malaise, fever, dysphagia, and sore throat after a short incubation period. Intraorally a vesicular eruption appears on the soft palate, faucial pillars, and tonsils (Figure 1-14). A diffuse erythematous pharyngitis is also present.

The signs and symptoms are usually mild to moderate and generally last less than a week. On occasion, the Coxsackievirus responsible for typical herpangina may be responsible for subclinical infections or for mild symptoms without evidence of pharyngeal lesions.

Differential Diagnosis. Diagnosis is usually based on historical and clinical information. The characteristic distribution and short duration of herpangina separate it from other primary viral infections such as herpetic gingivostomatitis, HFM disease, and varicella. The vesic-

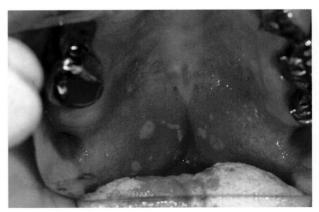

Figure 1-14   Herpangina.

ular eruption, mild symptoms, summer or early autumn presentation, and diffuse pharyngitis also distinguish the condition from streptococcal pharyngitis, and the systemic symptoms distinguish it from aphthous stomatitis. Laboratory confirmation can be made by virus isolation or by detection of serum antibodies.

Treatment. Because herpangina is self-limiting, is mild and of short duration, and causes few complications, treatment usually is not required.

Measles (Rubeola)

Etiology and Pathogenesis. Measles is a highly contagious viral infection caused by a member of the paramyxovirus family of viruses. The virus, known simply as *measles virus*, is a DNA virus and is related structurally and biologically to viruses of the orthomyxovirus family, which cause mumps and influenza. The virus is spread by airborne droplets through the respiratory tract.

German measles, or rubella, is a contagious disease that is caused by an unrelated virus of the togavirus family. It shares some clinical features with measles, such as fever, respiratory symptoms, and rash. These features are, however, very mild and short lived in German measles. In addition, Koplik's spots do not appear in German measles. The significance of the German measles virus lies in its ability to cause congenital defects in a developing fetus. The abnormalities produced are varied and may be severe, especially if the intrauterine infection occurs during the first trimester of pregnancy.

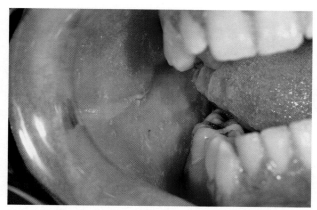

Figure 1-15 **Measles-associated Koplik's spots** in buccal mucosa.

Clinical Features. Measles is predominantly a disease of children, often appearing seasonally in winter and spring. After an incubation period of 7 to 10 days, prodromal symptoms of fever, malaise, coryza, conjunctivitis, photophobia, and cough develop. In 1 to 2 days, pathognomonic small erythematous macules with white necrotic centers appear in the buccal mucosa (Figure 1-15). These lesion spots, known as *Koplik's spots* after the pediatrician who first described them, herald the onset of the characteristic maculopapular skin rash of measles. Koplik's spots generally precede the skin rash by 1 to 2 days. The rash initially affects the head and neck, followed by the trunk and then the extremities. Complications associated with the measles virus include encephalitis and thrombocytopenic purpura. Secondary infection may develop as otitis media or pneumonia.

Histopathology. Infected epithelial cells, which eventually become necrotic, overlie an inflamed connective tissue that contains dilated vascular channels and a focal inflammatory response. Lymphocytes are found in a perivascular distribution. In lymphoid tissues, large characteristic multinucleated macrophages, known as *Warthin-Finkeldey giant cells*, are seen.

Differential Diagnosis. Diagnosis of measles is usually made on the basis of clinical signs and symptoms. Prodromal symptoms, Koplik's spots, and rash should provide sufficient evidence of measles. If necessary, laboratory confirmation can be made through virus culture or serologic tests for anti-bodies to measles virus.

Treatment. There is no specific treatment for measles. Supportive therapy of bed rest, fluids, adequate diet, and analgesics generally suffices.

IMMUNOLOGIC DISEASES

Pemphigus Vulgaris

Pemphigus is an autoimmune mucocutaneous disease characterized by intraepithelial blister formation. This results from a breakdown or loss of intercellular adhesion, thus producing epithelial cell separation known as *acantholysis*. Widespread ulceration following rupture of the blisters leads to painful debilitation, fluid loss, and electrolyte imbalance. Before the use of corticosteroids, death was not an uncommon outcome for patients with pemphigus vulgaris. Four types of pemphigus are recognized: pemphigus vulgaris, pemphigus foliaceus, pemphigus erythematosus, and pemphigus vegetans. These differ in the level of intraepithelial involvement in the disease; pemphigus vulgaris and pemphigus vegetans affect the whole epithelium, and pemphigus foliaceus and pemphigus erythematosus affect the upper prickle cell layer/spinous layer. Only pemphigus vulgaris and pemphigus vegetans involve the oral mucosa. Pemphigus vegetans is very rare and is generally considered a variant of pemphigus vulgaris.

Etiology and Pathogenesis. All forms of the disease retain distinctive presentations both clinically and microscopically but share a common autoimmune etiology. Evident are circulating autoantibodies of the immunoglobulin G (IgG) type that are reactive against components of epithelial desmosome-tonofilament complexes. The specific protein target has been identified as desmoglein 3, one of several proteins in the desmosomal cadherin family (Figure 1-16). The circulating autoantibodies are responsible for the earliest morphologic event: the dissolution or disruption of intercellular junctions and loss of cell-to-cell adhesion. The ease and extent of epithelial cell separation are generally directly proportional to the titer of circulating pemphigus antibody. It is believed that the pemphigus antibody, once bound to the target antigen, activates an epithelial intracellular proteolytic enzyme or group of enzymes that act at the desmosome-tonofilament complex. More recent evidence, however, favors a direct effect of the antibody on the desmoglein

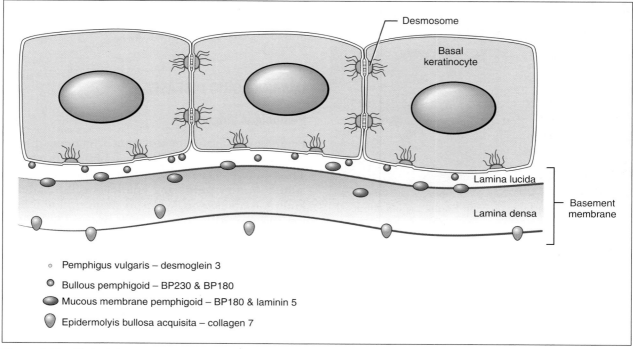

Figure 1-16   Vesiculobullous diseases; antigenic targets.

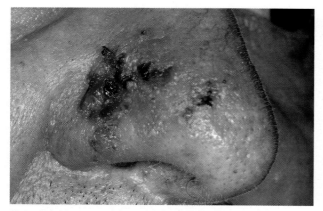

Figure 1-17   Cutaneous pemphigus vulgaris.

Box 1-4 Pemphigus Vulgaris

ETIOLOGY

Autoimmune reaction to intercellular keratinocyte protein (desmoglein 3)
Autoantibodies cause *intraepithelial* blisters

CLINICAL FEATURES

Affects skin and/or mucosa
50% or more of cases begin in the mouth ("first to show, last to go")
Presents as ulcers preceded by vesicles or bullae
Persistent and progressive

TREATMENT

Controlled with immunosuppressives (corticosteroids and azathioprine/cyclophosphamide)
High mortality when untreated (dehydration, electrolyte imbalance, malnutrition, infection)

structure, which increases secondarily—altered and nonfunctional.

Clinical Features. Lesions of pemphigus present as painful ulcers preceded by bullae (Box 1-4; Figure 1-17). The first signs of the disease appear in the oral mucosa in approximately 60% of cases (Figures 1-18 to 1-20). Such lesions may precede the onset of cutaneous lesions by periods of up to 1 year. Bullae rapidly rupture, leaving a red, painful, ulcerated base. Ulcers range in appearance from small aphthouslike lesions to large maplike lesions. Gentle traction on clinically unaffected mucosa may produce stripping of epithelium, a positive Nikolsky's sign. A great deal of discomfort often occurs with confluence and ulceration

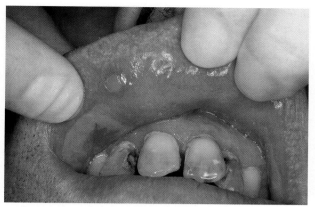

Figure 1-18 **Oral pemphigus vulgaris.**

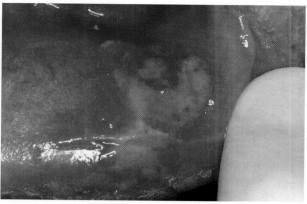

Figure 1-20 **Pemphigus vulgaris** of the lower lip.

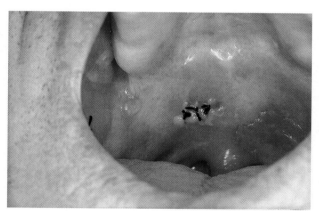

Figure 1-19 **Oral pemphigus vulgaris.** Note tissue slough around black sutures at biopsy site.

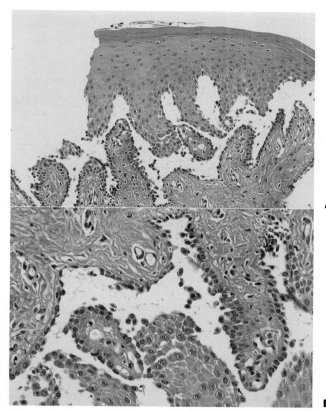

A

B

Figure 1-21 **A** and **B, Oral pemphigus vulgaris** showing intraepithelial separation and Tzanck cells.

of smaller vesicles of the soft palate, buccal mucosa, and floor of the mouth.

The incidence of pemphigus vulgaris is equal in both genders. Genetic and ethnic factors appear to predispose to the development of the disease. An increased incidence has been noted in Ashkenazic Jews and in individuals with certain histocompatibility antigen phenotypes (HLA-DR, HLA-A10, HLA-B, HLA-DQB, HLA-DRB1).

Other autoimmune diseases may occur in association with pemphigus vulgaris, such as myasthenia gravis, lupus erythematosus, rheumatoid arthritis, Hashimoto's thyroiditis, thymoma, and Sjögren's syndrome. A wide range has been noted from childhood to the elderly age-groups, although most cases are noted within the fourth and fifth decades of life.

Histopathology and Immunopathology. Pemphigus vulgaris appears as intraepithelial clefting with keratinocyte acantholysis (Figure 1-21). Loss of desmosomal attachments and retraction of tonofilaments result in free-floating, or acantholytic, *Tzanck cells.* Bullae are suprabasal, and the basal layer remains attached to the basement membrane.

In addition to a standard biopsy, confirmation of pemphigus vulgaris can be made with the use of direct immunofluorescence (DIF) testing (Figures 1-22 and 1-23). DIF testing uses a biopsy specimen in an attempt to demonstrate autoantibody already attached to the tissue. This is preferable to less sensitive indirect immunofluorescence, which uses patient serum to identify circulating antibody. In pemphigus vulgaris, DIF testing of perilesional tissue almost always demonstrates intercellular autoantibodies of the IgG type. C3 and, less commonly, IgA can be detected in the same intercellular fluorescent pattern.

Differential Diagnosis. Clinically, the oral lesions of pemphigus vulgaris must be distinguished from other vesiculobullous diseases, especially mucous membrane pemphigoid, erythema multiforme, and aphthous ulcers. Also, a rare syndrome known as *paraneoplastic pemphigus* may simulate pemphigus vulgaris. Patients with this syndrome have a lymphoma or other malignancy and a mucocutaneous pemphigus-like blistering disorder in which intraepithelial separation (acantholysis) is seen. Unlike pemphigus, the autoantibodies are directed at several antigenic targets, in both epithelium and the basement membrane zone. The underlying malignancy is believed to be responsible for the induction of the autoimmune response.

A diagnosis of *pemphigus vegetans,* a subset of pemphigus vulgaris, may also be entertained in some situations. Although predominantly a skin disease, the vermilion and intraoral mucosa may be involved, often initially. Early acantholytic bullae are followed by epithelial hyperplasia and intraepithelial abscess formation. These pustular "vegetations" contain abundant eosinophils and can have a verrucous appearance. Pemphigus vegetans–type lesions may also be seen during a lull in the general course of pemphigus vulgaris. Spontaneous remissions may occur in pemphigus vegetans, with complete recovery noted— a phenomenon not characteristic of pemphigus vulgaris.

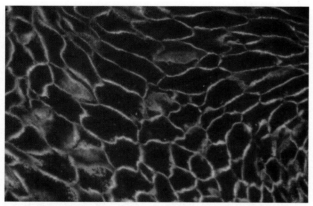

Figure 1-22   **Pemphigus vulgaris;** immunofluorescence pattern. (Courtesy Dr. Troy E. Daniels.)

Treatment and Prognosis. The high morbidity and mortality rates previously associated with pemphigus vulgaris

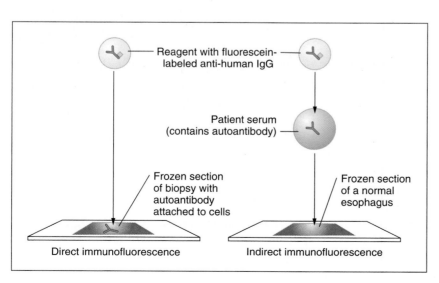

Reagent with fluorescein-labeled anti-human IgG

Patient serum (contains autoantibody)

Frozen section of biopsy with autoantibody attached to cells

Frozen section of a normal esophagus

Direct immunofluorescence

Indirect immunofluorescence

Figure 1-23   Immunofluorescence; laboratory methodology.

Box 1-5 Side Effects of Topical Corticosteroids

Candidiasis
Epithelial atrophy
Telangiectasias
Additional effects on skin—striae, hypopigmentation, acne, folliculitis

Box 1-6 Effects/Side Effects of Systemic Corticosteroids

Antiinflammatory: Therapeutic
Immunosuppression: Therapeutic
Gluconeogenesis: Diabetes, bone/muscle loss
Redistribution of fat: Buffalo hump, hyperlipidemia
Fluid retention: Moon face, weight gain
Vasopressor potentiation: Hypertension worse
Gastric mucosa: Peptic ulcer worse
Adrenal suppression: Adrenal atrophy
Central nervous system effects: Psychologic changes (e.g., euphoria)
Ocular effects: Cataracts, glaucoma

have been radically reduced since the introduction of systemic corticosteroids. The reduction in mortality, however, does carry a degree of iatrogenic morbidity associated with chronic corticosteroid use. Disease control can usually be achieved with an intermediate dose of steroid (prednisone), along with nonsteroid forms of immunosuppression. For more severely affected patients, a high-dose corticosteroid regimen plus other immunosuppressive drugs with or without plasmapheresis may be necessary. Topical corticosteroids may be used intraorally as an adjunct to systemic therapy.

Topical Steroids. Side effects of topical steroids may occur after prolonged or intense dermatologic use (Box 1-5). However, with judicious intraoral use for short periods, it is unlikely that significant systemic effects will occur. Used over a 2- to 4-week period, 15 g of topical steroid should provide sufficient therapeutic effect for most oral ulcers (especially aphthous ulcers) with minimal risk of complication. Because topical steroids can facilitate the overgrowth of *Candida albicans* orally, antifungal therapy may also be needed, especially with use of high-potency corticosteroids.

Systemic Steroids. Because the systemic effects and complications of glucocorticoids are numerous and can often be profound, it is recommended that they be prescribed by an experienced clinician (Box 1-6). Because the adrenals normally secrete most of their daily equivalent of 5 to 7 mg of prednisone in the morning, all the prednisone should be taken early in the morning to simulate the physiologic process, thus minimizing interference with the pituitary-adrenal axis and side effects. It is generally agreed that a slow steroid taper is not necessary if treatment lasts for less than 2 weeks, because adrenal suppression is likely to be minimal.

In patients requiring high-dose, prolonged, or maintenance steroid therapy, an alternate-day regimen may be used after initial therapy and an appropriate clinical response. A short-acting steroid (24 to 36 hours), such as prednisone, is desired because it allows recovery or near-normal functioning of the pituitary-adrenal axis on the "off" (no prednisone) days. In addition, the prednisone tissue effects outlast the adrenocorticotropic hormone (ACTH) suppression.

A combined drug approach that includes alternate-day prednisone plus a steroid-sparing immunosuppressant agent such as azathioprine, mycophenolate, or cyclophosphamide may also be used. The latter regimen helps reduce the complications of high-dose steroid therapy, such as immunosuppression, osteoporosis, hyperglycemia, and hypertension.

The prognosis for patients with pemphigus vulgaris is guarded because of the potential profound side effects of the drugs used for treatment. Once the disease has been brought under control, there is the probable lifelong treatment commitment to low dosage maintenance therapy with these drugs.

Mucous Membrane Pemphigoid

Mucous membrane pemphigoid (MMP) is a chronic blistering or vesiculobullous disease that affects predominantly oral and ocular mucous membranes (Figures 1-24 to 1-27). It is also known as *cicatricial pemphigoid, benign mucous membrane pemphigoid, ocular pemphigus, childhood pemphigoid, mucosal pemphigoid,* and when it affects gingiva exclusively, *gingivosis* and *desquamative gingivitis.*

Etiology and Pathogenesis. MMP is an autoimmune process with an unknown stimulus. Deposits of immunoglob-

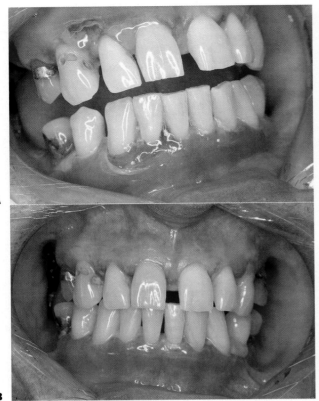

A

B

Figure 1-24   **A, Mucous membrane pemphigoid** of the gingiva. **B,** After control with corticosteroids, mandibular gingiva remains red and friable.

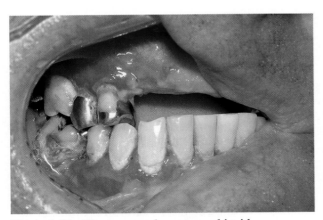

Figure 1-25   Mucous membrane pemphigoid.

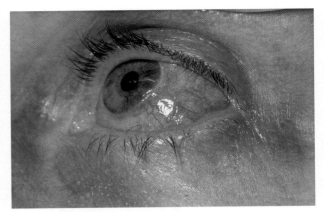

Figure 1-26   Ocular pemphigoid.

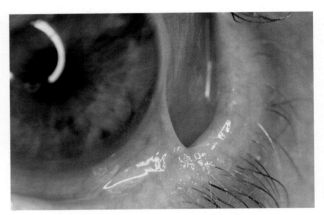

Figure 1-27   **Ocular pemphigoid;** symblepharon resulting from chronicity.

ulins and complement components along the basement zone (on DIF testing) are characteristic. The antigenic targets include laminin 5 (epiligrin) and a 180-kd protein that is also known as *bullous pemphigoid antigen 180 (BP180)*. Circulating autoantibodies against the basement membrane zone antigens in MMP are usually difficult to detect, presumably because of relatively low serum levels.

Clinical Features.   This is a disease of adults and the elderly and tends to affect women more than men. MMP has rarely been reported in children. Oral mucosal lesions typically present as superficial ulcers, sometimes limited to attached gingiva (Box 1-7). Bullae are rarely seen because the blisters are fragile and short lived. Lesions are chronic and persistent, and may heal with a scar (cicatrix)—particularly lesions of the eye. Here there is the risk of scarring of the canthus (symblepharon), inversion of the eyelashes (entropion), and resultant trauma to the cornea (trichiasis). To prevent corneal damage, many patients with ocular pemphigoid will have their eyelashes permanently removed by electrolysis. Extraoral sites in the order of frequency

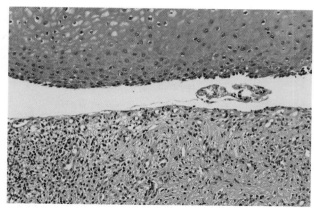

Figure 1-28 **Mucous membrane pemphigoid** showing characteristic subepithelial separation.

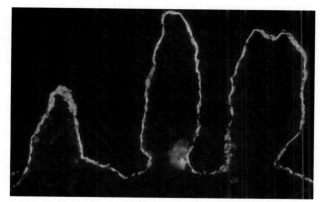

Figure 1-29 **Mucous membrane pemphigoid;** basement membrane immunofluorescent staining. (Courtesy Dr. Troy E. Daniels.)

following oral mucosa are the conjunctiva, larynx, genitalia, esophagus, and skin. Cutaneous lesions are uncommon and usually appear in the head and neck and extremities.

Gingival lesions often present as bright red patches or confluent ulcers extending to unattached gingival mucosa with mild-to-moderate discomfort. Concomitant ulcers may be seen on marginal and attached gingiva.

With chronicity, the pain associated with oral MMP typically diminishes in intensity. Intact epithelium, especially adjacent to ulcers, can often be stripped away with ease, leaving denuded submucosa. This is one of several mucocutaneous diseases in which a positive Nikolsky's sign may be elicited. Because of patient discomfort, routine oral hygiene is often compromised. This results in dental plaque accumulation, which in turn superimposes an additional, but nonspecific, inflammatory response.

Histopathology and Immunopathology. MMP is a subepithelial clefting disorder, and there is no acantholysis. In early stages few lymphocytes are seen, but with time, the infiltrate becomes more dense and mixed (Figures 1-28 and 1-29).

DIF studies of intact oral mucosa demonstrate a linear pattern of homogeneous IgG fluorescence. C3 is commonly found in the same distribution.

Although the fluorescent pattern is not distinguishable from that of cutaneous bullous pemphigoid, the submicroscopic location of the antigenic target (lower part of the lamina lucida) is distinctive. Results of indirect immunofluorescence studies are usually negative, but IgG and, less commonly, IgA have occasionally been demonstrated.

Differential Diagnosis. The clinical differential diagnosis for this vesiculobullous disease must include pemphigus vulgaris (Table 1-2). When the attached gingiva is the exclusive site of involvement, erythematous lichen planus, linear IgA disease, discoid lupus erythematosus, and contact allergy should also be included. Final diagnosis may require DIF confirmation.

TABLE 1-2   Pemphigus Vulgaris vs. Mucous Membrane Pemphigoid

	Pemphigus	Pemphigoid
Tissue antibody	IgG, C3 Circulating auto-IgG	IgG, IgA, C3 No circulating auto IgG
Target protein(s)	Desmoglein 3 (desmosomes)	Laminin 5 and BP180 (basement membrane)
Vesicles	Intraepithelial	Subepithelial
Sites	Oral and skin	Oral and eyes
Treatment	Corticosteroid	Corticosteroid
Prognosis	Fair, significant mortality	Good, significant morbidity

Ig, Immunoglobulin; *C*, complement; *BP*, bullous pemphigoid antigen.

Treatment and Prognosis. Corticosteroids are typically used to control MMP (see treatment of pemphigus vulgaris for corticosteroid effects and side effects). Prednisone is used for moderate to severe disease, and topical steroids for mild disease and maintenance. Very high systemic doses are occasionally required to achieve significant results for some cases of recalcitrant gingival MMP. Because side effects of therapy may outweigh benefits, high-potency topical steroids are often used instead (e.g., clobetasol, betamethasone dipropionate, fluocinonide, desoximetasone). A custom-made, flexible mouth guard may be used to keep the topical medication in place. Scrupulous oral hygiene, including chlorhexidine rinses, further enhances the effectiveness of topical corticosteroids when gingival involvement is marked.

In cases in which standard therapy has failed, other systemic agents have been used with varying success rates. These have included the use of tetracycline and niacinamide, sulfapyridine, sulfones, antibiotics, gold injections, and nutritional supplementation. In severe cases immunosuppressive agents (azathioprine, cyclophosphamide, cyclosporine) may occasionally be added to the prednisone regimen to reduce steroid dose and thus help avoid steroid-associated complications.

Although oral MMP has a relatively benign course, significant debilitation and morbidity lasting for years can occur. Natural history is unpredictable: in some cases a slow spontaneous improvement may be noted, whereas in other cases the course may be especially protracted, with alternating periods of improvement and exacerbation.

Of importance for patients with oral MMP is the possible appearance of ocular disease. If the eyes become affected, definitive early treatment is critical because conjunctival ulceration and scarring can lead to scarring and blindness. Therefore ophthalmologic examination should be part of the treatment plan for patients with oral MMP.

Bullous Pemphigoid

Etiology and Pathogenesis. Bullous pemphigoid and its closely related mucosal counterpart, MMP, appear to share similar etiologic and pathogenetic factors. A difference from MMP is that titers of circulating autoantibodies to basement membrane zone antigens are usually detectable in bullous pemphigoid.

Autoantibodies have been demonstrated against basement membrane zone laminin and so-called bullous pemphigoid antigens 230 (BP230) and 180 (BP180), which are found in hemidesmosomes and in the lamina lucida of basement membrane. Subsequent to binding of circulating autoantibodies to tissue antigens, a series of events occurs, one of which is complement activation. This attracts neutrophils and eosinophils to the basement membrane zone. These cells then release lysosomal proteases, which in turn participate in degradation of the basement membrane attachment complex. The final event is tissue separation at the epithelium–connective tissue interface.

Clinical Features. This bullous disease is seen primarily in the elderly, with the peak incidence in the seventh and eighth decades. Lesions characteristically appear on the skin, although concomitant lesions of mucous membranes occur in approximately one third of patients.

Skin lesions are characterized by a trunk and limb distribution. Although tense vesicles and bullae are typically noted, they are often preceded by or associated with an erythematous papular eruption. Oral mucosal lesions of bullous pemphigoid cannot be distinguished from those of MMP. Bullae and erosions may be noted, especially on the attached gingiva, a commonly affected site. Other areas of involvement may include the soft palate, buccal mucosa, and floor of the mouth.

Histopathology and Immunopathology. Bullae are subepithelial and appear similar to those of MMP. Ultrastructurally, the basement membrane is cleaved at the level of the lamina lucida.

Circulating autoantibody titers neither correlate with nor fluctuate with the level of clinical disease, as is usually the case with pemphigus vulgaris. DIF shows a linear deposition of IgG and C3 along the basement membrane zone. The major bullous pemphigoid antigen is BP230 in size, and the minor antigen is BP180. Both antigens are synthesized by basal keratinocytes.

Treatment. Periods of clinical remission have been noted with bullous pemphigoid. Systemic corticosteroids are generally used to control this disease. Nonsteroidal immunosuppressive agents may also effect control. Antibiotics (tetracycline and erythromycin) and niacinamide have provided some clinical success.

Dermatitis Herpetiformis

Etiology and Pathogenesis. Although no demonstrable circulating autoantibodies are noted in the sera of patients, deposits of IgA are evident in tissue. Cell-mediated immunity may also have a role in the pathogenesis of this disease. In most patients an association is noted between skin disease and gluten-sensitive enteropathy. Improvement of the skin and fat absorption often occurs with a gluten-free diet. Substantiating this relationship is the relapse noted on reintroduction of gluten-containing foods.

Clinical Features. Dermatitis herpetiformis is a chronic disease typically seen in young and middle-aged adults, with a slight male predilection. Periods of exacerbation and remission further characterize this disease. Cutaneous lesions are papular, erythematous, vesicular, and often intensely pruritic. Lesions are usually symmetric in their distribution over the extensor surfaces, especially the elbows, shoulders, sacrum, and buttocks. Of diagnostic significance is the frequent involvement of the scalp and face. Lesions are usually aggregated (herpetiform) but often are individually disposed. In some patients exacerbations may be associated with ingestion of foods or drugs containing iodide compounds. In others a seasonal (summer months) peak may be seen.

In the oral cavity, dermatitis herpetiformis is very rare, with vesicles and bullae having been described

that rupture, leaving superficial nonspecific ulcers with a fibrinous base with erythematous margins. Lesions may involve both keratinized and nonkeratinized mucosa.

Histopathology and Immunopathology. Collections of neutrophils, eosinophils, and fibrin are seen at the papillary tips of the dermis. Subsequent exudation at this location contributes to epidermal separation. A lymphophagocytic infiltrate is seen in perivascular spaces.

The immunologic finding of granular IgA deposits at the tips of the connective tissue papillae is specific for dermatitis herpetiformis. In addition, it is possible to localize the third component of complement (C3) in lesional and perilesional tissue in a distribution similar to that of IgA.

Treatment and Prognosis. Dermatitis herpetiformis is generally treated with dapsone, sulfoxone, and sulfapyridine. Because patients often have an associated enteropathy, a gluten-free diet may also be part of the therapeutic regimen. Elimination of gluten from the diet reduces small bowel pathology within months.

In most instances dermatitis herpetiformis is a lifelong condition, often exhibiting long periods of remission. Many patients, however, may be relegated to long-term dietary restrictions or drug treatment or both.

Linear Immunoglobulin A Disease

Linear IgA disease is a chronic autoimmune disease of the skin that commonly affects mucous membranes, including gingiva. Unlike dermatitis herpetiformis, it is not associated with gluten-sensitive enteropathy (and may not be responsive to dapsone therapy). Skin lesions may be urticarial, annular, targetoid, or bullous. Oral lesions, present in a majority of cases, are ulcerative (preceded by bullae). Ocular lesions, also seen in a majority of cases, are in the form of ulcers. Patients respond to sulfones or corticosteroids.

Microscopically, separation at the basement membrane is seen. Neutrophils and eosinophils often fill the separation (Figure 1-30). With direct immunofluorescence, linear deposits of IgA are found at the epithelium–connective tissue interface. The molecular target is a 120-kd protein.

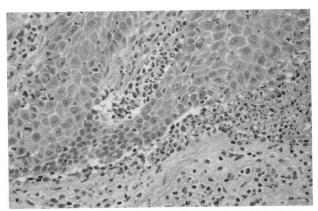

Figure 1-30   **Linear IgA disease** showing subepithelial separation with neutrophils and eosinophils.

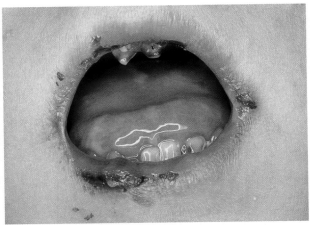

Figure 1-31   **Epidermolysis bullosa** in a child. Note ulcers, constricted opening, and atrophic tongue mucosa.

Although linear IgA disease shares features with dermatitis herpetiformis, cicatricial pemphigoid, and bullous pemphigoid, it cannot be easily subclassified under any one of these well-established entities. Until more is learned about linear IgA disease, it should probably be considered a separate condition.

HEREDITARY DISEASES

Epidermolysis Bullosa

Etiology and Pathogenesis.   *Epidermolysis bullosa* is a general term that encompasses one acquired and several genetic varieties (dystrophic, junctional, simplex) of disease that are basically characterized by the formation of blisters at sites of minor trauma. The several genetic types range from autosomal dominant to autosomal recessive in origin and are further distinguished by various clinical features, histopathology, and ultrastructure. The acquired nonhereditary autoimmune form, known as *epidermolysis acquisita*, is unrelated to the other types and is often precipitated by exposure to specific drugs. In this type, IgG deposits are commonly found in sub–basement membrane tissue and type VII collagen antibodies located below the lamina densa of the basement membrane.

In the hereditary forms of epidermolysis bullosa, circulating antibodies are not evident. Rather, pathogenesis appears to be related to genetic defects in basal cells, hemidesmosomes, or anchoring connective tissue filaments, depending on the disease subtype.

Clinical Features.   The feature common to all subtypes of epidermolysis bullosa is bulla formation from minor trauma, usually over areas of stress such as the elbows and knees (Figure 1-31). Onset of disease is during infancy or early childhood for the hereditary forms and during adulthood for the acquired type. Severity is generally greater with the inherited recessive forms. Blisters may be widespread and severe and may result in scarring and atrophy. Nails may be dystrophic in some forms of this disease.

Oral lesions are particularly common and severe in the recessive forms of this group of diseases and uncommon in the acquired form. Oral manifestations include bullae that heal with scar formation, a constricted oral orifice due to scar contracture, and hypoplastic teeth. These changes are most pronounced in the type known as *recessive dystrophic epidermolysis bullosa*.

Treatment and Prognosis.   The prognosis is dependent on the subtype of epidermolysis bullosa. The range of behavior varies from life threatening in one of the recessive forms, known as *junctional epidermolysis bullosa*, to debilitating in most other forms. Therapy includes avoidance of trauma, supportive measures, and chemotherapeutic agents (none of which is consistently effective). Corticosteroids, vitamin E, phenytoin, retinoids, dapsone, and immunosuppressives have all been suggested as possibly being of some benefit to patients.

BIBLIOGRAPHY

VIRAL DISEASES

Andreoni M, Sarmati L, Nicastri E, et al: Primary human herpesvirus 8 infection in immunocompetent children. JAMA 287:1295-1300, 2002.

Axell T, Liedholm R: Occurrence of recurrent herpes labialis in an adult Swedish population, *Acta Odontol Scand* 48:119-123, 1990.

Eversole R: Viral infections of the head and neck among HIV-seropositive patients, *Oral Surg Oral Med Oral Pathol* 73:155-163, 1992.

Ficarra G, Shillitoe E: HIV-related infections of the oral cavity, *Crit Rev Oral Biol Med* 3:207-231, 1992.

Fiddian A, Ivanyi L: Topical acyclovir in the management of recurrent herpes labialis, *Br J Dermatol* 109:321-326, 1983.

Fiddian A, Yeo J, Stubbings R, et al: Successful treatment of herpes labialis with topical acyclovir, *BMJ* 286:1699-1701, 1983.

Flaitz CM, Nichols CM, Hicks MJ: Herpesviridae-associated persistent mucocutaneous ulcers in acquired immunodeficiency syndrome, *Oral Surg Oral Med Oral Pathol Oral Radiol Endod* 81:433-441, 1996.

Herbert A, Berg J: Oral mucous membrane diseases of childhood, *Semin Dermatol* 11:80-87, 1992.

Pruksananonda P, Hall C, Insel R, et al: Primary human herpesvirus 6 infection in young children, *N Engl J Med* 326:1145-1150, 1992.

Raborn GW, Martel AY, Grace MGA, et al: Oral acyclovir in prevention of herpes labialis, *Oral Surg Oral Med Oral Pathol Oral Radiol Endod* 85:55-59, 1998.

Regezi JA, Eversole LR, Barker BF, et al: Herpes simplex and cytomegalovirus coinfected oral ulcers in HIV-positive patients, *Oral Surg Oral Med Oral Pathol Oral Radiol Endod* 81:55-62, 1996.

Rooney J, Bryson Y, Mannia M, et al: Prevention of ultraviolet light-induced herpes labialis by sunscreen, *Lancet* 338:1419-1422, 1991.

Schubert M, Peterson D, Flournoy N, et al: Oral and pharyngeal herpes simplex virus infection after allogenic bone marrow transplantation: analysis of factors associated with infection, *Oral Surg Oral Med Oral Pathol* 70:286-293, 1990.

Scott DA, Coulter WA, Biagioni PA, et al: Detection of herpes simplex virus type 1 shedding in the oral cavity by polymerase chain reaction and enzyme-linked immunosorbent assay at the prodromal stage of recrudescent herpes labialis, *J Oral Pathol Med* 26:305-309, 1997.

Spruance S, Stewart J, Freeman D: Early application of topical 15% idoxuridine in dimethyl sulfoxide shortens the course of herpes simplex labialis: a multicenter placebo-controlled trial, *J Infect Dis* 161:191-197, 1990.

Spruance S, Stewart J, Rowe N, et al: Treatment of recurrent herpes simplex labialis with oral acyclovir, *J Infect Dis* 161:185-190, 1990.

IMMUNOLOGIC AND HEREDITARY DISEASES

Anhalt G: Pemphigoid: bullous and cicatricial, *Dermatol Clin* 8:701-716, 1990.

Buxton RS, Cowin P, Franke WW, et al: Nomenclature of the desmosomal cadherins, *J Cell Biol* 121:481-483, 1993.

Chan L, Regezi J, Cooper K: Oral manifestations of linear IgA disease, *J Acad Dermatol* 22:362-365, 1990.

Dayan S, Simmons RK, Ahmed AR: Contemporary issues in the diagnosis of oral pemphigoid, *Oral Surg Oral Med Oral Pathol Oral Radiol Endod* 88:424-430, 1999.

Elder MJ, Lightman S, Dart JKG: Role of cyclophosphamide and high dose steroid in ocular cicatricial pemphigoid, *Br J Ophthalmol* 79:264-266, 1995.

Fine JD, Bauer EA, Briggaman RA, et al: Revised clinical and laboratory criteria for subtypes of inherited epidermolysis bullosa, *J Am Acad Dermatol* 24:119-135, 1991.

Fullerton S, Woodley D, Smoller B, et al: Paraneoplastic pemphigus with autoantibody deposition after autologous bone marrow transplantation, *JAMA* 267:1500-1502, 1992.

Helm TN, Camisa C, Valenzuela R, et al: Paraneoplastic pemphigus, *Oral Surg Oral Med Oral Pathol* 75:209-213, 1993.

Jonsson R, Mountz J, Koopman W: Elucidating the pathogenesis of autoimmune disease: recent advances at the molecular level and relevance to oral mucosal disease, *J Oral Pathol Med* 19:341-350, 1990.

Koch PJ, Mahoney MG, Ishikawa H, et al: Targeted disruption of the pemphigus vulgaris antigen (desmoglein 3) gene in mice causes loss of keratinocyte cell adhesion with a phenotype similar to pemphigus vulgaris, *J Cell Biol* 137:1091-1102, 1997.

Marinkovich MP: The molecular genetics of basement membrane diseases, *Arch Dermatol* 129:1557-1565, 1993.

Niimi Y, Zhu X-J, Bystryn JC: Identification of cicatricial pemphigoid antigens, *Arch Dermatol* 128:54-57, 1992.

Otley C, Hall R: Dermatitis herpetiformis, *Dermatol Clin* 8:759-769, 1990.

Porter S, Scully C, Midda M, et al: Adult linear immunoglobulin A disease manifesting as desquamative gingivitis, *Oral Surg Oral Med Oral Pathol* 70:450-453, 1990.

Scully C, Carrozzo M, Gandolfo S, et al: Update on mucous membrane pemphigoid, *Oral Surg Oral Med Oral Pathol Oral Radiol Endod* 88:56-68, 1999.

Vincent SD, Lilly GE, Baker KA: Clinical, historic, and therapeutic features of cicatricial pemphigoid, *Oral Surg Oral Med Oral Pathol* 76:453-459, 1993.

Woodley D: Clearing of epidermolysis bullosa acquisita with cyclosporine, *J Am Acad Dermatol* 22:535-536, 1990.

Wright J, Fine J, Johnson L: Oral soft tissues in hereditary epidermolysis bullosa, *Oral Surg Oral Med Oral Pathol* 71:440-446, 1991.

Zhu X, Niimi Y, Bystryn J: Identification of a 160 kD molecule as a component of the basement membrane zone as a minor bullous pemphigoid antigen, *J Invest Dermatol* 94:817-821, 1990.

ULCERATIVE CONDITIONS

An ulcer is defined simply as loss of epithelium. Ulcers that are preceded by blisters (vesicles or bullae) represent a distinct set of oral conditions, which are discussed in Chapter 1. Ulcerative lesions are commonly encountered in dental patients. Although many oral ulcers have similar clinical appearances, their etiologies encompass many disorders, including reactive, infectious, immunologic, and neoplastic diseases.

REACTIVE LESIONS

Traumatic Ulcerations

Etiology. Ulcers are the most common oral soft tissue lesions. Most are caused by simple mechanical trauma, and a cause-and-effect relationship is usually obvious. Many are a result of accidental trauma and generally appear in regions that are readily trapped between the teeth, such as the lower lip, tongue, and buccal mucosa. A traumatic ulcer in the anterior portion of the tongue of infants with natal teeth is known as *Riga-Fede disease.* Prostheses, most commonly dentures, are frequently associated with traumatic ulcers, which may be acute or chronic.

In unusual circumstances, lesions may be self-induced because of an abnormal habit, and in these circumstances there is some psychologic problem. These so-called *factitial injuries* are often as difficult to diagnose as they are to treat. They may prove to be frustrating clinical problems, especially if there is no clinical suspicion of a self-induced cause. Psychologic counseling may ultimately be required to help resolve the problem.

Traumatic oral ulcers may also be iatrogenic. Naturally, respect for the fragility of oral soft tissues is of paramount importance in the treatment of dental patients. Overzealous tissue manipulation or concentration on treating primarily hard tissues may result in accidental soft tissue injury that is avoidable. Ulcers induced by the removal of adherent cotton rolls, by the negative pressure of a saliva ejector, or by accidental striking of mucosa with rotary instruments are uncommon but entirely preventable.

Chemicals may also cause oral ulcers because of their acidity or alkalinity or because of their ability to act as local irritants or contact allergens. These may be patient induced or iatrogenic. Aspirin burns are still seen, although they are much less common than in the past. When acetylsalicylic acid is placed inappropriately against mucosa in an attempt by the patient to relieve toothache, a mucosal burn or coagulative necrosis occurs. The extent of injury is dependent on the duration and number of aspirin applications. Many over-the-counter medications for toothache, aphthous ulcers, and denture-related injuries have the ability to damage oral mucosa if used injudiciously. Dental cavity medications, especially those containing phenol, may cause iatrogenic oral ulcers. Tooth-etching agents have been associated with chemical burns of mucosa. Endodontic and vital bleaching procedures, which use strong oxidizing agents such as 30% hydrogen peroxide, have also produced burns.

Intraoral ulcers following heat burns are relatively uncommon intraorally. Pizza burns, caused by hot cheese, have been noted on the palate. Iatrogenic heat burns may also be seen after injudicious use of tooth impression material, such as wax, hydrocolloid, or dental compound.

Oral ulcerations are also seen during the course of therapeutic radiation for head and neck cancers. In those malignancies, particularly squamous cell carcinoma, that require large doses of radiation, in the range of 60 to 70 Gy, oral ulcers are invariably seen in tissues within the path of the beam. For malignancies such as lymphoma, in which lower doses in the range of 40 to 50 Gy are tumoricidal, ulcers are likely but are less severe and of shorter duration. Radiation-induced ulcers persist through the course of therapy and for several weeks afterward. If the ulcers are kept clean, spontaneous healing occurs without scar. Similarly, ulcers can occur during the course of chemotherapy. The etiology of both is primarily the treatment-induced reduction in basal cell renewal, resulting in mucosal atrophy and ulceration.

Clinical Features. Acute reactive ulcers of oral mucous membranes exhibit the clinical signs and symptoms of acute inflammation, including variable degrees of pain, redness, and swelling (Box 2-1; Figures 2-1 to 2-7). The ulcers are covered by a yellow-white fibrinous exudate and are surrounded by an erythematous halo.

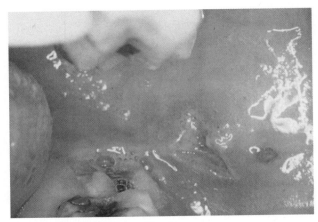

Figure 2-1   Acute traumatic ulcer.

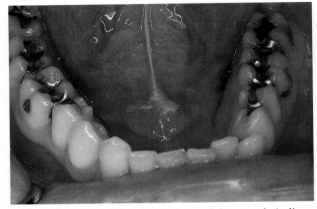

Figure 2-2   **Acute ulcer** of the floor of the mouth (saliva ejector injury).

Box 2-1 Traumatic Ulcers

ACUTE ULCER

Pain
Yellow base, red halo
History of trauma
Heals in 7 to 10 days if cause eliminated

CHRONIC ULCER

Little or no pain
Yellow base, elevated margins (scar)
History of trauma, if remembered
Delayed healing if irritated, especially tongue lesions
Clinical appearance mimics carcinoma and infectious ulcers

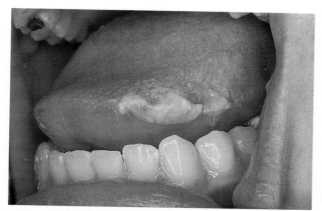

Figure 2-3   Anesthesia-associated acute tongue ulcer.

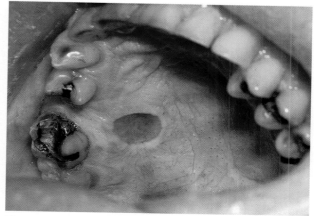

Figure 2-6   **Chronic ulcer** of the palate.

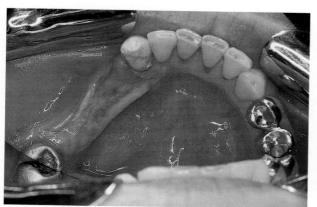

Figure 2-4   **Ulcer** associated with excessive heat from hydrocolloid impression material.

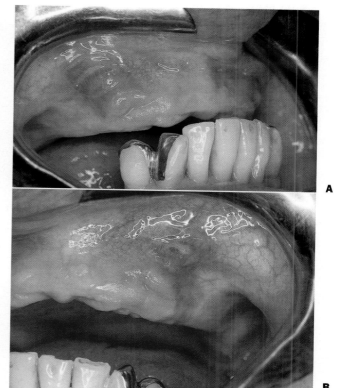

A

B

Figure 2-7   **A** and **B, Ulcers and erythema** caused by a denture flange.

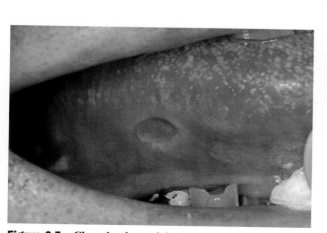

Figure 2-5   Chronic ulcer of the lateral tongue.

Chronic reactive ulcers may cause little or no pain. They are covered by a yellow membrane and are surrounded by elevated margins that may show hyperkeratosis. Induration, often associated with these lesions, is due to scar formation and chronic inflammatory cell infiltration.

A particularly ominous-appearing but benign chronic ulcer known as *traumatic granuloma (traumatic ulcerative granuloma with stromal eosinophilia)* occasionally may be seen in association with deep mucosal injury. This crateriform ulcer may measure 1 to 2 cm in diameter, and healing may take several weeks. It is usually found in the tongue. Another ominous-appearing chronic ulcer, characteristically seen in the hard palate, is known as *necrotizing sialometaplasia*. It is associated with trauma-induced ischemic necrosis of a minor salivary gland and heals spontaneously in several weeks (see Chapter 8).

Histopathology. Acute ulcers show a loss of surface epithelium that is replaced by a fibrin network containing predominantly neutrophils (Figure 2-8). The ulcer base contains dilated capillaries and, with time, granulation tissue. Regeneration of the epithelium begins at the ulcer margins, with proliferating cells moving over the granulation tissue base and under the fibrin clot.

Chronic ulcers have a granulation tissue base, with scar found deeper in the tissue. A mixed inflammatory cell infiltrate is seen throughout. Epithelial regeneration occasionally may not occur because of continued trauma or because of unfavorable local tissue factors. It has been speculated that these factors are related to inappropriate adhesion molecule expression (integrins) and/or inadequate extracellular matrix receptors for the keratinocyte integrins. In traumatic granulomas, tissue injury and inflammation extend into subjacent skeletal muscle. Here a characteristic dense macrophage infiltrate with eosinophils may dominate the histologic picture. The term *granuloma* as used here reflects the large numbers of macrophages that dominate the infiltrate, but this is not a typical granuloma as seen in an infectious process, such as tuberculosis.

Diagnosis. With acute reactive ulcers, the cause-and-effect relationship is usually apparent from the clinical examination and history. When there is a factitial overlay, diagnosis becomes a challenge.

The cause of chronic reactive ulcers may not be as readily apparent. In this circumstance it is important that a differential diagnosis be developed. Conditions

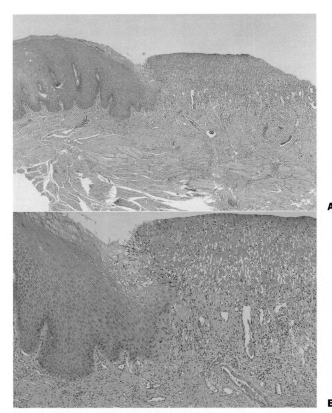

Figure 2-8   **A** and **B**, **Chronic ulcer** showing fibrin covering an inflamed granulation tissue base.

to consider are infection (syphilis, tuberculosis, deep fungal infection) and malignancy. If the lesion is strongly suspected to be of traumatic origin, the cause should be sought. A 2-week observation period is warranted, together with an effort to keep the mouth clean using a bland mouthrinse such as sodium bicarbonate in water. If no change is seen or if the lesion increases in size, a biopsy should be performed.

Treatment. Most reactive ulcers of oral mucous membranes are simply observed. If pain is considerable, topical treatment may be of benefit. This could be in the form of a topical corticosteroid.

BACTERIAL INFECTIONS

Syphilis

Syphilis is a sexually transmitted disease that was virtually incurable until Dr. Paul Ehrlich developed his "magic bullet," arsphenamine, around the turn of

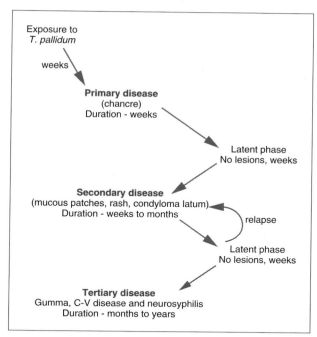

Exposure to
T. pallidum

weeks

Primary disease
(chancre)
Duration - weeks

Latent phase
No lesions, weeks

Secondary disease
(mucous patches, rash, condyloma latum)
Duration - weeks to months

relapse

Latent phase
No lesions, weeks

Tertiary disease
Gumma, C-V disease and neurosyphilis
Duration - months to years

Figure 2-9 Pathogenesis of syphilis (untreated).

Box 2-2 Classification of Syphilis

ACQUIRED

Early
Primary (chancre)
Secondary (oral mucous patches, skin lesions, other organopathy)
Latency

Late
Latency
Tertiary (gumma, cardiovascular diseases, neurosyphilis)

CONGENITAL

Early
Secondary disease
Spirochetemia affecting many organ systems
Stigmata include dental defects, eighth-nerve deafness, ocular keratitis, bone and joint lesions, other organopathy

Late
Latency

the twentieth century. A stunning change in the control of syphilis followed the introduction of penicillin in the early 1940s. By then, approximately 600,000 new cases were reported annually in the United States; during the next 15 years the rate declined to 6000 cases per year. An increase in the number of new cases (>50,000 in 1990), due in part to an association with human immunodeficiency virus (HIV) infection and drug abuse, followed until today, when there seems to be some measure of control of this disease.

Etiology and Pathogenesis. Syphilis is caused by the spirochete *Treponema pallidum* (Figure 2-9). It is acquired by sexual contact with a partner with active lesions, by transfusion of infected blood, or by transplacental inoculation of the fetus by an infected mother.

When the disease is spread through direct contact, a hard ulcer, or *chancre*, forms at the site of spirochete entry (Box 2-2). Later there is development of a painless, nonsuppurative regional lymphadenopathy. The chancre heals spontaneously after several weeks without treatment, leaving the patient with no apparent signs of disease. After a latent period of several weeks, secondary syphilis develops (patients infected via transfusion bypass the primary stage and begin with secondary syphilis). This stage is marked by a spirochetemia with wide dissemination. Fever, flulike symp-

toms, mucocutaneous lesions, and lymphadenopathy are typical. This stage also resolves spontaneously, and the patient enters another latency period. Relapses to secondary syphilis may occur in some patients. In about one third of those who have entered the latency phase and have not been treated, tertiary or, late-stage, syphilis develops. These patients may have central nervous system (CNS) involvement, cardiovascular lesions, or focal necrotic inflammatory lesions, known as *gummas*, of any organ.

Congenital syphilis occurs during the latter half of pregnancy, when the *T. pallidum* organism crosses the placenta from the infected mother. The spirochetemia that develops in the fetus may cause numerous inflammatory and destructive lesions in various fetal organs, or it may cause abortion.

Clinical Features. Primary syphilis results in painless indurated ulcer(s) with rolled margins at the site of inoculation (Box 2-3; Figures 2-10 to 2-14). The lesion does not produce an exudate. The location is usually on the genitalia. Depending on the site of primary infection, lip, oral, and finger lesions also occur and exhibit similar clinical features. Regional lymphadenopathy, typified by firm, painless swelling, is also part of the clinical picture. The lesion heals without therapy in 3 to 12 weeks, with little or no scarring.

Box 2-3 Syphilis

CAUSE

Treponema pallidum, sexually transmitted

CLINICAL FEATURES

Primary phase: Chancre, a chronic ulcer at the site of infection
Secondary phase: Oral mucous patches, condyloma latum, maculopapular rash
Tertiary phase: Gummas (destructive ulcers), central nervous system and cardiovascular diseases
Congenital form: Abnormal shape of molars/incisors, deafness, ocular keratitis, skeletal defects

TREATMENT

Penicillin, tetracyclines

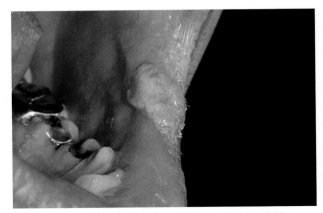

Figure 2-12 **Condyloma latum** of secondary syphilis.

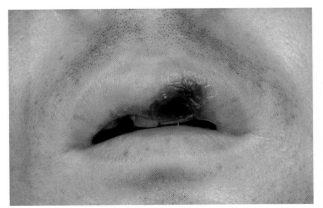

Figure 2-10 **Primary syphilis** (chancre). (From Kerr DA, Ash MM Jr, Millard HD: *Oral diagnosis,* ed 3, St Louis, 1983, Mosby.)

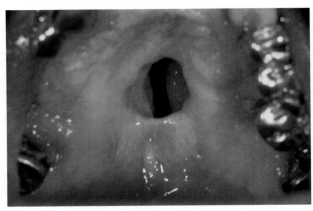

Figure 2-13 **Tertiary syphilis;** palatal fistula resulting from a gumma.

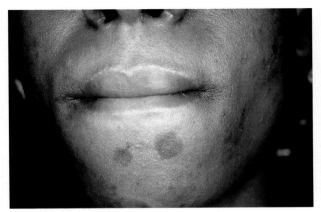

Figure 2-11 **Secondary syphilis;** cutaneous macular lesions.

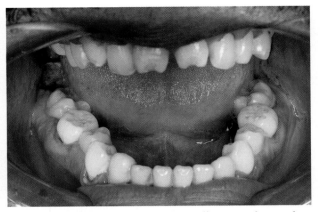

Figure 2-14 **Congenital syphilis;** mulberry molars and notched incisors.

In untreated syphilis, secondary disease begins after about 2 to 10 weeks. The spirochetes are now disseminated widely and are the cause of a reddish brown maculopapular cutaneous rash and mucosal ulcers covered by a mucoid exudate (mucous patches). Elevated broad-based verrucal plaques, known as *condylomata lata,* may also appear on the skin and mucosal surfaces. Inflammatory lesions may potentially occur in any organ during secondary syphilis.

Manifestations of tertiary syphilis take many years to appear and can be profound, since there is a predilection for the cardiovascular system and the CNS. Fortunately, this stage of syphilis has become a rarity because of effective antibiotic treatment.

Manifestations of neural syphilis include general paresis (paralysis) and tabes dorsalis (locomotor ataxia). Inflammatory involvement of the cardiovascular system, especially the aorta, may result in aneurysms. Focal granulomatous lesions (gummas) may involve any organ. Intraorally, the palate is typically affected and can lead to palatal perforation. Development of generalized glossitis with mucosal atrophy has also been well documented in the tertiary stage of this disease. Although patients with so-called syphilitic or luetic glossitis are thought to have an approximately fourfold increased risk of oral squamous cell carcinoma, it is unclear if this is a result of the disease or is due to the carcinogenic agents that were formerly used to treat the condition, such as arsenicals and heavy metals.

The generalized spirochetemia of congenital syphilis may result in numerous clinical manifestations that may affect any organ system in a developing fetus. A mucocutaneous rash may be seen early. When the infectious process involves the vomer, a nasal deformity known as *saddle nose* develops; when periostitis of the tibia occurs, excessive anterior bone growth results in a deformity known as *saber shin.* Other late stigmata of congenital syphilis include conditions known collectively as *Hutchinson's triad:* (1) an inflammatory reaction in the cornea (interstitial keratitis); (2) eighth-nerve deafness; and (3) dental abnormalities consisting of notched or screwdriver-shaped incisors and mulberry molars, presumably occurring because of spirochete infection of the enamel organ of teeth during amelogenesis.

Histopathology. The basic tissue response to *T. pallidum* infections consists of a proliferative endarteritis and infiltration of plasma cells. Endothelial cells proliferate within small arteries and arterioles, producing a concentric layering of cells that results in a narrowed lumen. Plasma cells, along with lymphocytes and macrophages, are typically found in a perivascular distribution. Spirochetes can be demonstrated in the tissues of various lesions of syphilis using silver stains, although they may be scant in tertiary lesions. Gummas may additionally show necrosis and greater numbers of macrophages, resulting in a granulomatous lesion that is similar to other conditions, such as TB.

Differential Diagnosis. Clinically, as well as microscopically, syphilis is said to be the great imitator or mimicker because of its resemblance to many other unrelated conditions. When it presents within the mouth, the chancre may be confused with and must be differentiated from squamous cell carcinoma, chronic traumatic lesions, and other infectious diseases, such as TB and histoplasmosis. The differential diagnosis of secondary syphilis would include many infectious and noninfectious conditions marked by a mucocutaneous eruption. Palatal gummas, although rarely seen, may have a clinical appearance similar to the destructive lesions of T-cell lymphoma.

Definitive diagnosis of syphilis is based on laboratory test confirmation of the clinical impression. Among the several tests available are (1) darkfield examination of scrapings or exudate from active lesions, (2) special silver stain or immunologic preparation of biopsy tissue, and (3) serologic tests for antibodies to *T. pallidum,* such as the Venereal Disease Research Laboratory test (VDRL), rapid plasmin reagin (RPR), and the enzyme-linked immunosorbent assay (ELISA).

Treatment. The drug of choice for treating all stages of syphilis is penicillin. Through the years, *T. pallidum* has remained sensitive to penicillin, as well as to other antibiotics, such as erythromycin and tetracyclines.

Gonorrhea

Etiology. Gonorrhea is one of the most prevalent bacterial diseases in humans. It is caused by the gram-negative diplococcus *Neisseria gonorrhoeae,* which infects columnar epithelium of the lower genital tract, rectum, pharynx, and eyes. Infection is transmitted by direct sexual contact with an infected partner. Containment of the spread of infection in sexual partners is enhanced by the short incubation period of less than 7 days, permitting contact tracing but hampered by the absence of symptoms in many individuals, especially females.

Genital infections may be transmitted to the oral or pharyngeal mucous membranes through orogenital contact. Pharyngeal mucosa is more likely to be infected than oral mucosa because of the type of epithelium and its reduced resistance to trauma. The risk of developing this form of disease is apparently much more likely with fellatio than with cunnilingus. Individuals may have concomitant genital and oral or pharyngeal infections that result from direct exposure to these areas rather than from spread through blood or lymphatics.

Transmission of gonorrhea from an infected patient to dental personnel is regarded as highly unlikely because the organism is very sensitive to drying and requires a break in the skin or mucosa to establish an infection. Gloves, protective eyewear, and a mask should provide adequate protection from accidental transmission.

Clinical Features.   No specific clinical signs have been consistently associated with oral gonorrhea. However, multiple ulcerations and generalized erythema have been described. Symptoms range from none to generalized stomatitis.

In the more common pharyngeal gonococcal infection, presenting signs are usually general erythema with associated ulcers and cervical lymphadenopathy. The chief complaint may be sore throat, although many patients are asymptomatic.

Differential Diagnosis.   Because of the lack of consistent and distinctive oral lesions, other conditions that cause multiple ulcers or generalized erythema should be included in a differential diagnosis. Aphthous ulcers, herpetic ulcers, erythema multiforme, pemphigus, pemphigoid, drug eruptions, and streptococcal infections should be considered. Diagnosis of gonorrhea is traditionally based on demonstration of the organism with Gram's stains or culture on Thayer-Martin medium. Rapid identification of *N. gonorrhoeae* with immunofluorescent antibody techniques and other laboratory tests may also be used to support clinical impressions.

Treatment.   Uncomplicated gonorrhea responds to a single dose of appropriately selected antibiotic. In the West, infections are susceptible to penicillins and treatment is effective using a single dose of 2 to 3.5 g of ampicillin. In the Far East and parts of Africa up to 50% of cases are resistant to penicillins and can be managed with a single 500-mg dose of ciprofloxacin. This regimen is also appropriate for pha-ryngeal gonorrhea, for which ampicillin is generally ineffective.

Tuberculosis

Etiology and Pathogenesis.   Tuberculosis (TB) infects about one third of the world's population and kills approximately 3 million people per year, making it the most important cause of death in the world. In developed countries there was a significant decrease in the incidence of TB as a result of improvements in living conditions, reductions in overcrowding, and antibiotic use. However, the 1980s saw a reemergence of significant numbers of cases of TB, many in association with HIV infection and acquired immunodeficiency syndrome (AIDS) in Europe and Africa. In addition, the issue of multidrug resistance has proved to be an increasing problem in managing the disease.

TB is caused by the aerobic, non–spore-forming bacillus *Mycobacterium tuberculosis* (Figure 2-15). The organism has a thick, waxy coat that does not react with Gram stains but retains the red dyes (Ziehl-Neelsen and Fite techniques). With these stains, the organisms do not decolor with acid-alcohol and are therefore also known as *acid-fast bacilli*. Two major forms of *Mycobacterium* are recognized: *M. tuberculosis* and *M. bovis*. *M. tuberculosis* is an airborne infection that is transmitted by inhalation of infected droplets. *M. bovis* is primarily a disease of cows that is transmitted to humans through infected milk, producing intestinal or tonsillar lesions. Two other closely related forms of *Mycobac-*

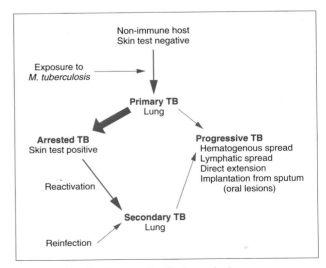

Figure 2-15   Pathogenesis of tuberculosis.

terium are recognized: *M. avium* and *M. intracellulare.* Both are nonvirulent in healthy individuals but cause disseminated disease in immunocompromised individuals, such as those with HIV infection or AIDS.

The spread of *M. tuberculosis* infection is through small airborne droplets, which carry the organism to pulmonary air spaces. Phagocytosis by alveolar macrophages follows, and the battle between bacterial virulence and host resistance begins. The pathogenicity of *M. tuberculosis* is due both to its ability to resist degradation by macrophages and to the development of a type IV hypersensitivity reaction. This latter feature explains the destructiveness of the lesions in the host tissues and the emergence of drug-resistant strains. As the immune system is sensitized by the mycobacterial antigens, a positive tuberculin reactivity develops. The Mantoux and tine skin tests, which use a tubercle bacillus antigen called *purified protein derivative (PPD)*, determine if an individual is hypersensitive to antigen challenge. A positive inflammatory skin reaction indicates that the individual's cell-mediated immune system has been sensitized and signifies previous exposure and subclinical infection. It does not necessarily imply active disease.

A granulomatous inflammatory response to *M. tuberculosis* follows sensitization. In most cases the cell-mediated immune response is able to control the infection, allowing subsequent arrest of the disease. Inflammatory foci may eventually undergo dystrophic calcification, but latent organisms in these foci may become reactivated at a later date. In a small number of cases the disease may progress through airborne, hematogenous, or lymphatic spread, so-called miliary spread.

Oral mucous membranes may become infected through implantation of organisms found in sputum or, less commonly, through hematogenous deposition. Similar seeding of the oral cavity may also follow secondary or reactivated TB.

Clinical Features. Unless the primary infection becomes progressive, an infected patient will probably exhibit no symptoms (Box 2-4; Figure 2-16). Skin testing and chest radiographs may provide the only indicators of infection. In reactivated disease, low-grade signs and symptoms of fever, night sweats, malaise, and weight loss may appear. With progression, cough, hemoptysis, and chest pain (pleural involvement) develop. As other organs become involved through the spread of organisms, a highly varied clinical picture appears and is dependent on the organs involved.

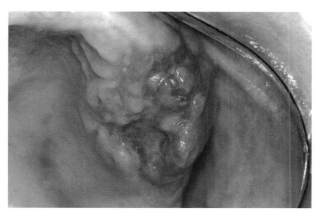

Figure 2-16 **Tuberculosis** of the maxillary alveolar ridge.

Box 2-4 Tuberculosis

ETIOLOGY

Mycobacterium tuberculosis; oral lesions follow lung infections
Risk factors—overcrowding, debilitation, immunocompromise
Important public health disease

CLINICAL FEATURES

Chronic ulcers, nonhealing and indurated, often multiple

HISTOPATHOLOGY

Caseating granulomas (macrophages) with Langhans giant cells

TREATMENT

Prolonged, multidrug therapy required (isoniazid, rifampin, ethambutol)

Oral manifestations that usually follow implantation of *M. tuberculosis* from infected sputum may appear on any mucosal surface. The tongue and the palate are favored locations. The typical lesion is an indurated, chronic, nonhealing ulcer that is usually painful. Bony involvement of the maxilla and mandible may produce tuberculous osteomyelitis. This most likely follows hematogenous spread of the organism. Pharyngeal involvement results in painful ulcers, and laryngeal lesions may cause dysphagia and voice changes.

Histopathology. The basic microscopic lesion of TB is granulomatous inflammation, in which granulomas

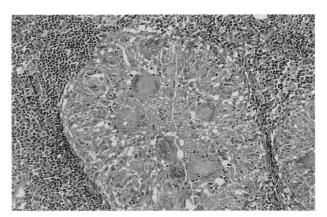

Figure 2-17   **Tuberculosis** granuloma composed of macrophages and multinucleated giant cells.

show central caseous necrosis (Figure 2-17). In tissues *M. tuberculosis* incites a characteristic macrophage response in which focal zones of macrophages become surrounded by lymphocytes and fibroblasts. The macrophages develop an abundant eosinophilic cytoplasm, giving them a superficial resemblance to epithelial cells, in which case they are frequently called *epithelioid cells.* Fusion of macrophages results in the appearance of Langhans giant cells, in which nuclei are distributed around the periphery of the cytoplasm. As the granulomas age, central necrosis occurs, which is usually referred to as *caseous necrosis* because of the gross cheesy texture of these zones.

A Ziehl-Neelsen or Fite stain must be used to confirm the presence of the organism in the granulomas because several infectious and noninfectious conditions may also produce a similar granulomatous reaction. In the absence of acid-fast bacilli, other microscopic considerations would include syphilis, cat-scratch disease, tularemia, histoplasmosis, blastomycosis, coccidioidomycosis, sarcoidosis, and some foreign body reactions, such as those induced by beryllium.

Differential Diagnosis. On the basis of clinical signs and symptoms alone, oral TB cannot be differentiated from several other conditions. A chronic indurated ulcer should prompt the clinician to consider primary syphilis and oral manifestations of deep fungal diseases. Noninfectious processes that should be considered clinically are squamous cell carcinoma and chronic traumatic ulcer. Major aphthae might also be included, although a history of recurrent disease should help separate this condition from the others.

Treatment. First-line drugs likely to be employed for treatment of TB include isoniazid, rifampin, pyrazinamide, and ethambutol. Drug combinations are often used in 6-, 9-, or 12-month treatment regimens but may be extended as long as 2 years. Streptomycin is rarely used for first-line treatment except in multidrug-resistant cases. Oral lesions would be expected to resolve with treatment of the patient's systemic disease. Unfortunately, infection with multidrug-resistant organisms appears to be increasing, and serious public health consequences could result.

Patients who convert from a negative to a positive skin test response may benefit from prophylactic chemotherapy, typically using isoniazid for 1 year. This is dependent both on risk factors involved, such as age and immune status, and on the opinion of the attending physician.

Leprosy

Etiology and Pathogenesis. Leprosy, also known as *Hansen's disease,* is a chronic infectious disease that is caused by the acid-fast bacillus, *Mycobacterium leprae.* Worldwide, 20 million individuals are thought to be infected. It is the most common cause of peripheral neuritis in the world. Because the causative organism is difficult to grow in culture, it has been maintained in the footpads of mice and in the armadillo, which has a low core body temperature. Leprosy is only moderately contagious; transmission of the disease requires frequent direct contact with an infected individual for a long period. Inoculation through the respiratory tract is also believed to be a potential mode of transmission.

Clinical Features. There is a clinical spectrum of disease that ranges from a limited form (tuberculoid leprosy) to a generalized form (lepromatous leprosy); the latter has a more seriously damaging course. Generally, skin and peripheral nerves are affected, since the organism grows best in temperatures less than the core body temperature of 37° C. Cutaneous lesions appear as erythematous plaques or nodules, representing a granulomatous response to the organism. Similar lesions may occur intraorally or intranasally. In time, severe maxillofacial deformities can appear, producing the classic destruction of the anterior maxilla called *facies leprosa.* Damage to peripheral nerves results in anesthesia leading to trauma to the extremities and consequent ulceration, as well as bone resorption.

Histopathology. Microscopically, a granulomatous inflammatory response, in which macrophages and multinucleated giant cells predominate, is usually seen. Infiltration of nerves by mononuclear inflammatory cells is also present. Well-formed granulomas, similar to those present in the tissue lesions of TB, are typically seen in tuberculoid leprosy. Poorly formed granulomas with sheets of macrophages is the pattern more typical of leproid leprosy. Acid-fast bacilli can be found within macrophages and are best demonstrated with the Fite stain. Organisms are most numerous in the lepromatous form of leprosy.

Diagnosis. Important for establishing a diagnosis is a history either of contact with a known infected patient or of living in a known endemic area. Signs and symptoms associated with skin and nerve involvement should provide additional clues to the nature of the disease. The appearance of oral lesions without skin lesions is highly improbable. A biopsy must be performed to confirm diagnosis because there is no laboratory test for leprosy.

Treatment. Current treatment centers on a chemotherapeutic approach in which several drugs are used for a protracted period, typically years. The drugs most commonly used include dapsone, rifampin, clofazimine, and minocycline. The known teratogen thalidomide is useful to manage the complications of leprosy therapy.

Actinomycosis

Etiology and Pathogenesis. Actinomycosis is a chronic bacterial disease that, as the name suggests, exhibits some clinical and microscopic features that are funguslike. It is caused by *Actinomyces israelii,* an anaerobic or microaerophilic, gram-positive bacterium. On rare occasions, other *Actinomyces* species may be involved, or a related aerobic bacterium, *Nocardia asteroides,* may be responsible for a similar clinical picture. *A. israelii* is a normal inhabitant of the oral cavity in a majority of healthy individuals. It is usually found in tonsillar crypts, gingival crevices, carious lesions, and nonvital dental root canals. Actinomycosis is not regarded as a contagious disease, because infection cannot be transmitted from one individual to another. Infections usually appear after trauma, surgery, or previous infection. Tooth extraction, gingival surgery, and oral infections predispose to the development of this condition. Evidence of other important predisposing factors has been slight, although actinomycotic infections have been recorded in osteoradione-

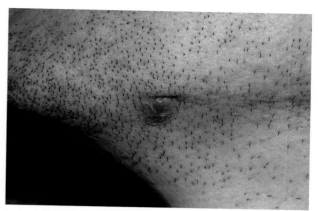

Figure 2-18 **Actinomycosis;** associated mandibular sinus tract.

crosis of the jaws and in patients with serious systemic illness.

Clinical Features. Most infections by *A. israelii* are seen in the thorax, abdomen, and head and neck and are usually preceded by trauma or direct extension of a contiguous infection (Figure 2-18). When it occurs in the head and neck, the condition is usually designated *cervicofacial actinomycosis.* It typically presents as a swelling of the mandible that may simulate a pyogenic infection. The lesion may become indurated and eventually form one or more draining sinuses, leading from the medullary spaces of the mandible to the skin of the neck. The skin lesions are indurated and are described as having a "woody hard" consistency. Less commonly the maxilla may be involved, resulting in an osteomyelitis that may drain through the gingiva. The pus draining from the chronic lesion may contain small yellow granules, known as *sulfur granules,* that represent aggregates of *A. israelii* organisms. Radiographically, this infection presents as a radiolucency with irregular and ill-defined margins.

Histopathology. A granulomatous inflammatory response with central abscess formation is seen in actinomycosis (Figures 2-19 and 2-20). In the center of the abscesses, distinctive colonies of gram-positive organisms may be seen. Radiating from the center of the colonies are numerous filaments with clubbed ends.

Differential Diagnosis. Clinically, actinomycosis may have to be differentiated from osteomyelitis caused by other bacterial or fungal organisms. Infections of the

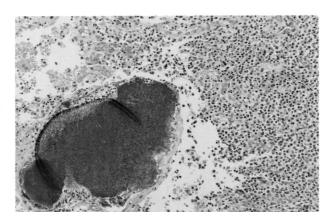

Figure 2-19 **Actinomycosis** colony (sulfur granule) surrounded by pus.

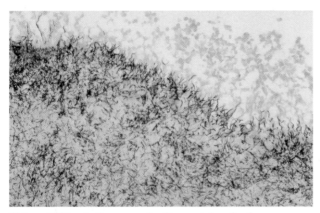

Figure 2-20; Actinomycosis; Gram stain of colony showing peripheral gram-positive filaments.

soft tissue of the neck, such as scrofula, and *Staphylococcus* infections, such as botryomycosis, may also be considered.

Definitive diagnosis is dependent on identification of the actinomycotic organism. This may be done through direct examination of exudate, microscopic evaluation of tissue sections, or microbiologic culture of pathologic material.

Treatment. Long-term, high-dose penicillin is the required antibiotic regimen for actinomycosis. For severe cases intravenous penicillin followed by oral penicillin is a standard regimen. Less severe cases still require protracted courses of oral penicillin. Tetracycline and erythromycin have also been used to effect cures. In addition, drainage of abscesses and surgi-

cal excision of scar and sinus tracts is recommended to aerate tissue and to enhance penetration of antibiotics.

Noma

Noma, also known as *cancrum oris* and *gangrenous stomatitis*, is a devastating disease of malnourished children and is characterized by a destructive process of orofacial tissues. The condition is rare in developed countries but is a relatively common cause of childhood mortality and morbidity in parts of Africa, South America, and Asia.

Etiology and Pathogenesis. Necrosis of tissue occurs as a consequence of invasion by anaerobic bacteria in a host whose systemic health is significantly compromised. It has been proposed that noma results from oral contamination by a heavy infestation of Bacteroidaceae, particularly *Fusobacterium necrophorum* and a consortium of other microorganisms, including *Borrelia vincentii, Staphylococcus aureus,* and *Prevotella intermedia.* These opportunistic pathogens invade oral tissues whose defenses are weakened by malnutrition, acute necrotizing gingivitis, debilitating conditions, trauma, and other oral mucosal ulcers. Other predisposing factors include debilitation due to systemic disease, such as pneumonia or sepsis.

Clinical Features. Noma typically affects children. A related disorder, noma neonatorum, occurs in low-birth-weight infants who also suffer from other debilitating diseases. The initial lesion of noma is a painful ulceration, usually of the gingiva or buccal mucosa, that spreads rapidly and eventually becomes necrotic. Denudation of the involved bone may follow, eventually leading to necrosis and sequestration. Teeth in the affected area may become loose and may exfoliate. Penetration of organisms into the cheek, lip, or palate may also occur, resulting in fetid necrotic lesions.

Treatment. Therapy involves treating the underlying predisposing condition, as well as the infection itself. Therefore fluids, electrolytes, and general nutrition are restored, along with the introduction of antibiotics. Antibiotics of choice include clindamycin, piperacillin, and the aminoglycoside gentamicin. Debridement of necrotic tissue may also be beneficial if destruction is extensive.

FUNGAL INFECTIONS

Deep Fungal Infections

Etiology and Pathogenesis. Deep fungal infections are characterized by primary involvement of the lungs. Infections may potentially disseminate from this focus to involve other organs.

The deep fungal infections having a significant incidence of oral involvement include histoplasmosis, coccidioidomycosis, blastomycosis, and cryptococcosis (Box 2-5; Table 2-1). Oral infections typically follow implantation of infected sputum in oral mucosa. Oral infections may also follow hematogenous spread of fungus from another site such as the lung.

Histoplasmosis is worldwide in distribution, although it is endemic in the midwestern United States. Inhalation of yeast from the dust of dried pigeon droppings is regarded as the most common source of infection. Coccidioidomycosis is endemic in the western United States, especially in the San Joaquin Valley of California, where it is known as *valley fever*. Blastomycosis is usually encountered in North America, especially in the Ohio-Mississippi river basin area. *Cryptococcus* infections may be transmitted through inhalation of avian excrement. *Cryptococcus* infections also may occur in immunocompromised patients.

Clinical Features. The initial signs and symptoms of deep fungal infections are usually related to lung involvement and include cough, fever, night sweats, weight loss, chest pain, and hemoptysis. A skin eruption resembling erythema multiforme occasionally appears concomitantly with coccidioidomycosis infection (Box 2-6; Figure 2-21).

Oral lesions are usually preceded by pulmonary infection. Primary involvement of oral mucous membranes is a highly unlikely route of infection. Swallowed infected sputum may potentially cause oral or

---

Box 2-5 Deep Fungal Infections*

Pathogenesis: Inhalation of spores
Symptoms: Cough, fever, weight loss, other
Primary site: Lung; may be asymptomatic
Oral lesions: Chronic, nonhealing ulcers secondary to lung disease
Microscopy: Granulomatous inflammation with organisms
Treatment: Ketoconazole, fluconazole, itraconazole, amphotericin B

*Histoplasmosis (*Histoplasma capsulatum*), coccidioidomycosis (*Coccidioides immitis*), blastomycosis (*Blastomyces dermatitidis*), cryptococcosis (*Cryptococcus neoformans*).

TABLE 2-1   **Deep Fungal Infections: Morphologic Features**

Organism	Size (μm)	Histology	Appearance
Histoplasmosis	2–5	Yeasts in macrophages	
Coccidioidomycosis	30–60	Endospores in spherules	
Blastomycosis	8–15	Budding yeasts	
Cryptococcosis	2–15	Yeasts with thick capsule	

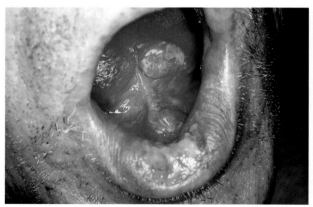

Figure 2-21   **Histoplasmosis**-caused chronic ulcers.

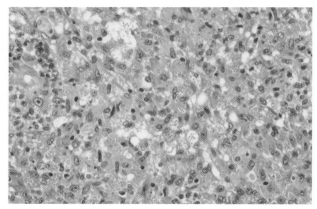

Figure 2-22   **Histoplasmosis** showing macrophages with cytoplasmic microorganisms.

Box 2-6 Chronic Infectious Ulcers

TYPES

Syphilis, tuberculosis, histoplasmosis, other deep fungal infections

CLINICAL FEATURES

Mimic carcinomas and traumatic ulcers
Nonhealing, persistent, often multiple

DIAGNOSIS

Biopsy necessary
Culture may be required

TREATMENT

Appropriate antimicrobial agent

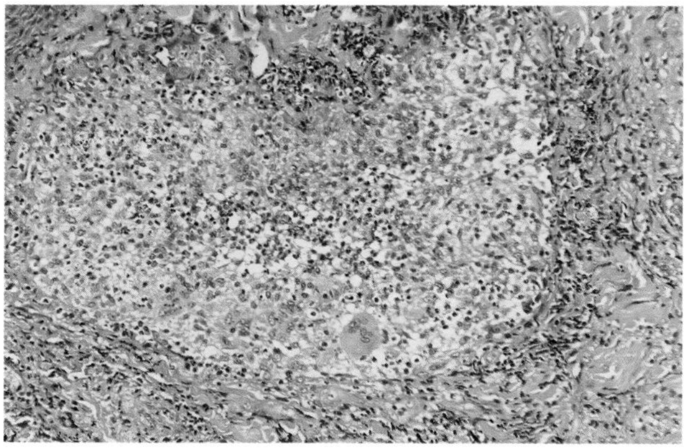

Figure 2-23   **Blastomycosis** showing granuloma (macrophages) with a central abscess.

gastrointestinal lesions. Also, erosion into pulmonary blood vessels by the inflammatory process may result in hematogenous spread to almost any organ. The usual oral lesion is ulcerative. Whether single or multiple, lesions are nonhealing, indurated, and frequently painful. Purulence may be an additional feature of blastomycotic lesions.

Histopathology. The basic inflammatory response in a deep fungal infection is granulomatous. In the presence of these microorganisms, macrophages and multinucleated giant cells dominate the histologic picture (Figures 2-22 and 2-23). Purulence may be a feature of blastomycosis and, less likely, coccidioidomycosis and cryptococcosis. Peculiar to blastomycosis is pseudoepitheliomatous hyperplasia,

associated with superficial infections in which ulceration has not yet occurred.

Differential Diagnosis. Clinically, the chronic, nonhealing oral ulcers caused by deep fungal infections may resemble those of oral squamous cell carcinoma, chronic trauma, oral TB, and primary syphilis. Blastomycosis may also produce a clinical picture that simulates cervicofacial actinomycosis. Culture of organisms from lesions or microscopic identification of organisms in biopsy tissue is required to establish a definitive diagnosis.

Treatment. Treatment of deep mycotic infections is generally with antimicrobials such as ketaconazole, fluconazole, and amphotericin B. Both ketaconazole and fluconazole can be administered orally. Amphotericin B is highly toxic, particularly to the kidneys, and side effects are relatively common. Surgical resection or incision and drainage may occasionally be used to enhance drug effects in treating some necrotic lung infections.

Subcutaneous Fungal Infections: Sporotrichosis

Etiology and Pathogenesis. Some fungal infections affect primarily subcutaneous tissues. One of these, sporotrichosis, is of significance because it may have oral manifestations. It is caused by *Sporothrix schenckii* and results from inoculation of the skin or mucosa by contaminated soil or thorny plants. After an incubation period of several weeks, subcutaneous nodules, which frequently become ulcerated, develop. Systemic involvement is rare but may occur in individuals with defective or suppressed immune responses.

Clinical Features. Lesions appear at the site of inoculation and spread along lymphatic channels. On the skin, red nodules appear, with subsequent breakdown, exudate production, and ulceration. Orally, lesions typically present as nonspecific chronic ulcers. Lymphadenopathy may also be present.

Histopathology. The inflammatory response to *S. schenckii* is granulomatous. Central abscesses may be found in some of the granulomas, and overlying epithelium may exhibit pseudoepitheliomatous hyperplasia. The relatively small, round to oval fungus may be seen in tissue sections.

Diagnosis. Definitive diagnosis is based on culture of infected tissue on Sabouraud agar. Special silver stains may also be used to identify the organism in tissue biopsy specimens.

Treatment. Sporotrichosis is usually treated with a solution of potassium iodide. In cases of toxicity or allergy to iodides, ketoconazole has been used with limited success. Generally, patients respond well to treatment, with little morbidity.

Opportunistic Fungal Infections: Phycomycosis (Mucormycosis) and Aspergillosis

Etiology and Pathogenesis. *Phycomycosis*, also known as *mucormycosis*, is a generic term that includes fungal infections caused by the genera *Mucor* and *Rhizopus*, and occasionally others. Organisms in this family of fungi, which normally are found in bread mold or decaying fruit and vegetables, are opportunistic, infecting humans when systemic health is compro-

mised. Aspergillus is ubiquitous in the environment. Infections typically occur in patients with poorly controlled ketoacidotic diabetes, immunosuppressed transplant recipients, patients with advanced malignancies, patients being treated with steroids or radiation, and patients who are immunosuppressed for any other reason, including HIV infection and AIDS.

The route of infection is through either the gastrointestinal tract or the respiratory tract, and infections may occur anywhere along these routes.

Clinical Features. In the head and neck, lesions are most likely to occur in the nasal cavity, paranasal sinuses, and possibly the oropharynx. Pain and swelling precede ulceration. Tissue necrosis may result in perforation of the palate. Extension into the orbit or brain is a common complication. The fungus has a propensity for arterial wall invasion, which may lead to hematogenous spread, thrombosis, or infarction.

Histopathology. Microscopically, an acute and chronic inflammatory infiltrate is seen in response to the fungus (Figure 2-24). The organism is usually readily identified in hematoxylin and eosin–stained sections in areas of tissue necrosis. Characteristic necrotic vessel walls containing thrombi and fungi may be evident. Microscopically, the fungus consists of large, pale-staining, nonseptate hyphae that tend to branch at right angles.

Differential Diagnosis. It is important for clinicians to recognize that phycomycosis represents one of several opportunistic infections that may affect an immunocompromised host. Necrotic lesions of the nasal and paranasal sinuses should raise the suspicion of this type of infection. Confirmation must be made by identifi-

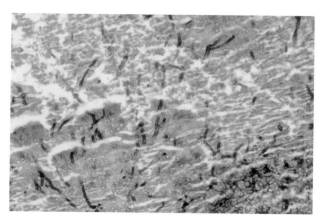

Figure 2-24 Silver stain of *Aspergillus* in a tissue section with green counterstain.

cation of the fungus in biopsy tissue, exudates, or cultures. Because of the severity of underlying disease and the often rapid course that this infection may take, diagnosis of phycomycosis may not be made until after death.

Perforating palatal lesions are generally rare but may be seen in association with other diseases such as gummatous necrosis of tertiary syphilis, midline granuloma (T-cell lymphoma), and Wegener's granulomatosis. Rarely, malignancies of nasal and sinus origin (squamous cell carcinoma and salivary gland adenocarcinoma) may present through the palate. A biopsy is required to differentiate these lesions.

Treatment. Amphotericin B is the drug of choice for treatment of phycomycosis and aspergillosis. Surgical debridement of the upper respiratory tract lesions is also often required. The prognosis is generally dependent on the severity of underlying disease and the institution of appropriate therapy. Death is a relatively frequent consequence of this infection. Generally, lung infections are more likely to be lethal than upper respiratory tract infections.

IMMUNOLOGIC DISEASES

Aphthous Ulcers

Of all the types of nontraumatic ulceration that affect oral mucosa, aphthous ulcers (canker sores) are probably the most common. The incidence ranges from 20% to 60%, depending on the population studied. Prevalence tends to be higher in professional persons, in those in upper socioeconomic groups, and in those who do not smoke.

Etiology. Although the cause of aphthous ulcerations is unknown, several possibilities have been postulated (Box 2-7).

There is considerable evidence that aphthous ulcers are related to a focal immune dysfunction in which T lymphocytes have a significant role. The nature of the initiating stimulus remains a mystery. The causative agent could be endogenous (autoimmune) antigen or exogenous (hyperimmune) antigen, or it could be a nonspecific factor, such as trauma in which chemical mediators may be involved. Neurogenic inflammation could result from an initiating stimulus. Focal release of a neuropeptide, such as substance P, could mediate lymphocytic infiltration and epithelial necrosis, generating an aphthous ulcer. Focal

---

> **Box 2-7 Aphthous Ulcers: Possible causes**
>
> Immunologic disorder—T-cell mediated
> Neurogenic inflammation—neuropeptide (e.g., substance P) induced
> Mucosal healing defect—inhibition by cytokines
> Microbiologic—viral, bacterial
> Nutritional deficiency—vitamin B_{12}, folic acid, iron

TABLE 2-2   Aphthous Ulcers vs. Secondary Herpes Simplex Infection

	Aphthous Ulcers	Herpes Infection
	Immune dysfunction	HSV1
Triggers	Stress, trauma, diet, hormones, depressed immunity	Stress, trauma, ultraviolet light, depressed immunity
Appearance	Little prodrome Nonspecific microscopy No vesicles Single, oval ulcer	Prodromal symptoms Viral cytopathic changes Vesicles precede ulcers Multiple, confluent ulcers
Sites	Nonkeratinized mucosa	Keratinized mucosa
Treatment	Corticosteroids, tetracycline	Antiviral treatment

HSV1, Herpes simplex virus type 1.

---

release of cytokines may effect delayed healing, which typifies the clinical course of these lesions.

Because of the clinical similarity of oral aphthous ulcers to secondary herpes simplex virus (HSV) infections (Table 2-2), a viral cause has been extensively investigated, but this has not been substantiated. Hypersensitivity to bacterial antigens of *Streptococcus sanguis* has been suggested, but this theory has been discarded.

Deficiencies of vitamin B_{12}, folic acid, and iron as measured in serum have been found in only a small percentage of patients with aphthous ulcers. Correction of these deficiencies has produced improvement or cures in this small group. Patients with malabsorption conditions such as *celiac disease* (*gluten-sensitive enteropathy* or *nontropical sprue*) and *Crohn's disease* have been reported as having occasional aphthous-type ulcers. In such cases deficiencies of folic acid and factors related to underlying disease may be part of the cause.

Other causes of aphthous ulcers that have been investigated include hormonal alterations, stress, trauma, and food allergies to substances in nuts, chocolate, and gluten. None of these is seriously regarded as being important in the primary causation of aphthous ulcers, although any of them may have a modifying or triggering role. Although HIV-positive patients may have more severe and protracted aphthouslike ulcers, the role of HIV and other agents is unknown.

Clinical Features. Three forms of aphthous ulcers have been recognized: minor, major, and herpetiform aphthous ulcers (Table 2-3). All are believed to be part of the same disease spectrum, and all are believed to have a common etiology. Differences are essentially clinical and correspond to the degree of severity. All forms present as painful recurrent ulcers. Patients occasionally have prodromal symptoms of tingling or burning before the appearance of the lesions. The ulcers are not preceded by vesicles and characteristically appear on the vestibular and buccal mucosa, tongue, soft palate, fauces, and floor of the mouth. Only rarely do these lesions occur on the attached gingiva and hard palate, thus providing an important clinical sign for the separation of aphthous ulcers from secondary herpetic ulcers. In patients with AIDS, however, aphthouslike ulcers may occur in any mucosal site.

Minor Aphthous Ulcers. Minor aphthous ulcers are the most commonly encountered form. This type usually appears as a single painful, oval ulcer, less than 0.5 cm in diameter, that is covered by a yellow fibrinous membrane and surrounded by an erythematous halo (Figures 2-25 and 2-26). Multiple oral aphthae may occasionally be seen. When the lateral or ventral surfaces of the tongue are affected, pain tends to be out of proportion to the size of the lesion (Figure 2-27). Minor aphthous ulcers generally last 7 to 10 days and heal without scar formation. Recurrences vary from one individual to another. Periods of freedom from disease may range from a matter of weeks to as long as years.

In some patients with recalcitrant aphthae a diagnosis of Crohn's disease may be considered. This gran-

TABLE 2-3 Aphthous Ulcers: Clinical Features

	Minor Aphthae	Major Aphthae	Herpetiform Aphthae
Size	<0.5 cm	>0.5 cm	<0.5 cm
Shape	Oval	Ragged oval, crateriform	Oval
Number	1–5	1–10	10–100
Location	Nonkeratinized mucosa	Nonkeratinized mucosa	Any intraoral site
Treatment	Topical corticosteroids, tetracycline mouthrinse	Topical/systemic/intralesional corticosteroids, immunosuppressives	Topical/systemic corticosteroids, tetracycline mouthrinse

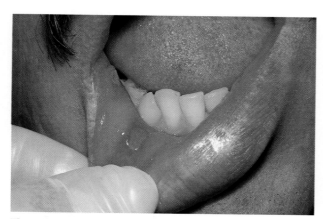

Figure 2-25 Minor aphthous ulcers.

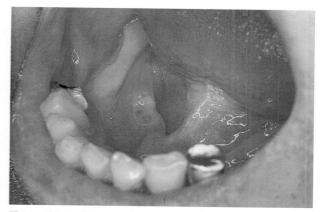

Figure 2-26 Minor aphthous ulcer of the floor of the mouth.

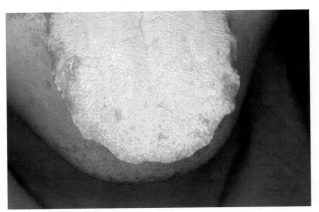

Figure 2-27 **Minor aphthous ulcers** of the lateral tongue.

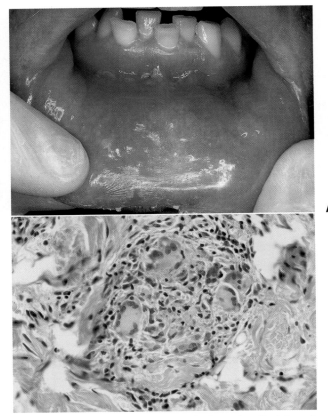

Figure 2-28 **A,** Crohn's-associated ulcers (vestibule) and mucosal nodules of the lower lip. **B,** Biopsy specimen of one of the nodules showing a granuloma with multinucleated giant cells.

ulomatous disease may affect the gastrointestinal tract from mouth to anus. Oral manifestations include mucosal fissures and small, multiple, hyperplastic nodules on the buccal mucosa, producing a cobblestone appearance (Figure 2-28). Biopsy findings of these mucosal nodules show small, noncaseating granulomas characteristic of Crohn's disease. HIV-positive patients may develop minor aphthous ulcers, although proportionately more have major or herpetiform lesions.

Major Aphthous Ulcers. Major aphthous ulcers were previously thought to be a separate entity, and this form was referred to as *periadenitis mucosa necrotica recurrens* or Sutton's disease. It is now regarded as the most severe expression of aphthous stomatitis. Lesions are larger (>0.5 cm) and more painful and persist longer than minor aphthae (Figure 2-29). Because of the depth of inflammation, major aphthous ulcers appear crateriform clinically and heal with scar formation. Lesions may take as long as 6 weeks to heal, and as soon as one ulcer disappears, another one starts. In patients who experience an unremitting course with significant pain and discomfort, systemic health may be compromised because of difficulty in eating and psychologic stress. The predilection for movable oral mucosa is as typical for major aphthous ulcers as it is for minor aphthae. HIV-positive patients may have aphthous lesions in any intraoral site.

Herpetiform Aphthous Ulcers. Herpetiform aphthous ulcers present clinically as recurrent crops of small ulcers (Figure 2-30). Although movable mucosa is predominantly affected, palatal and gingival mucosa may also be involved. Pain may be considerable, and healing generally occurs in 1 to 2 weeks. Unlike herpes infec-

tions, herpetiform aphthous ulcers are not preceded by vesicles and exhibit no virus-infected cells. Other than the clinical feature of crops of oral ulcers, there has been no finding that can link this disease to a viral infection.

Histopathology. Because the diagnosis of these ulcers is usually evident clinically, biopsies are usually unnecessary and are therefore rarely performed. Aphthous ulcers have nonspecific microscopic findings, and there are no histologic features that are diagnostic (Figures 2-31 and 2-32). At no time are virus-infected cells evident. Essentially, the same microscopic changes are found in all forms of aphthous ulcers. Studies have shown that mononuclear cells are found in submucosa and perivascular tissues in the preulcerative stage. These cells are predominantly CD4 lymphocytes, which are soon outnumbered by CD8 lymphocytes as the ulcerative stage develops.

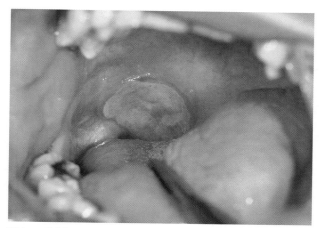

Figure 2-29   Major aphthous ulcer.

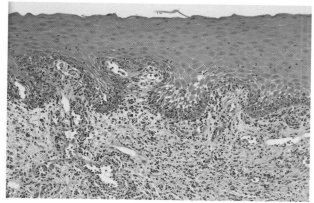

Figure 2-31   **Preaphthous ulceration.** Intense lymphocytic infiltrate and basilar epithelial edema seen in preulcerative stage of an aphthous lesion.

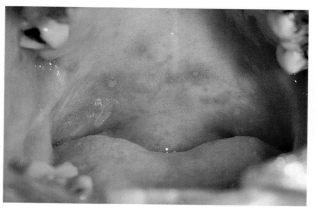

Figure 2-30   **Herpetiform aphthous ulcers.** The patient also had numerous lip and buccal mucosa lesions.

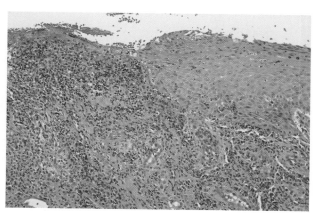

Figure 2-32   **Aphthous ulcer** showing nonspecific changes.

Macrophages and mast cells are common inhabitants of the ulcer.

Differential Diagnosis.   Diagnosis of aphthous ulcers is generally based on the history and clinical appearance (see Table 2-3). The lesions of secondary (recurrent) oral herpes are often confused with aphthous ulcers but can usually be distinguished from them. A history of vesicles preceding ulcers, location on the attached gingiva and hard palate, and crops of lesions indicate herpetic rather than aphthous ulcers. Other painful oral ulcerative conditions that may simulate the various forms of aphthous ulcers include trauma, pemphigus vulgaris, mucous membrane pemphigoid, and neutropenia.

Treatment.   In patients with occasional or few minor aphthous ulcers, usually no treatment is needed apart from a bland mouthrinse such as sodium bicarbonate in warm water to keep the mouth clean. However, when patients are more severely affected, some forms of treatment can provide significant control (but not necessarily a cure) of this disease. Rational treatment would include drugs that can manipulate or regulate immune responses. In this category corticosteroids currently offer the best chance for disease containment. In severely affected patients systemic steroids may be used for immediate control. A low to moderate dose of prednisone for a short period is effective. A typical regimen might be 20 to 40 mg daily for 1 week, followed by another week at half the initial dose. However, for patients with mild to moderate disease, only topical therapy appears justified. Topical steroids, if used judiciously, can be relatively efficacious and safe (see treatment of pemphigus vulgaris

---

Box 2-8 Topical Corticosteroid Preparations*

Clobetasol propionate (Temovate gel/cream)
Clobetasol propionate plus "oral adhesive" (50% Temovate ointment plus 50% Orabase)
Betamethasone dipropionate (Diprosone cream/ointment)
Fluocinonide (Lidex gel)
Betamethasone plus clotrimazole (Lotrisone cream)

*High to intermediate potency.

Box 2-9 Behçet's Syndrome

ETIOLOGY

Immunodysfunction, vasculitis

ORGANS AFFECTED

Nonkeratinized oral mucosa (minor aphthae)
Genitals (ulcers)
Eyes (conjunctivitis, uveitis, retinitis)
Joints (arthritis)
Central nervous system (headache, nerve palsies, inflammation)

TREATMENT

Corticosteroids, other immunosuppressives

---

for corticosteroid effects and side effects). Although nearly all topical compounds have been developed for use on the skin, it has been standard practice to prescribe these agents for use on mucous membranes (Box 2-8). Intralesional injection of triamcinolone may be used for individual or focal problematic lesions.

Antibiotics. Antibiotics have been used in the treatment of aphthous ulcers with fair to good results. Tetracycline suspensions, used topically, often produce excellent results. In addition to their antibacterial effect of keeping the mouth clean, tetracyclines speed the resolution of the ulcers by local inhibition of matrix metalloproteinases. Since tetracyclines readily break down in solution, they must be made up fresh each time they are used. A typical regimen for treating aphthous ulcers consists of emptying a 250-mg capsule of tetracycline in 30 ml (1 fluid ounce) of warm water and then rinsing the mouth for several minutes. This is repeated up to four times a day for 4 days. Results are best if this mouthrinse is used on the first day that the ulcers appear or when they are in a prodromal stage.

Other Drugs. Because of their rather profound side effects, immunosuppressive drugs, such as azathioprine and cyclophosphamide, are generally justified only for the treatment of severely affected patients (to permit reduced prednisone dosages). Recent studies indicate that thalidomide may provide relief to severely affected patients, especially AIDS patients. Two other drugs that have shown some therapeutic efficacy are pentoxifylline and colchicine.

Behçet's Syndrome

Behçet's syndrome is a multisystem disease (gastrointestinal, cardiovascular, ocular, CNS, articular, pulmonary, dermal) in which recurrent oral aphthae are a consistent feature. Although the oral manifestations are usually relatively minor, involvement of other sites, especially the eyes and CNS, can be quite serious.

Etiology. The cause of this condition is basically unknown, although the underlying disease mechanism may likely be an immunodysfunction in which vasculitis is a feature. Behçet's syndrome may have a genetic predisposition as well, particularly in reference to the frequent presence of human leukocyte antigen HLA-B51 within this group. Also, some indirect evidence that has been presented suggests a viral etiology.

Clinical Features. The lesions of this syndrome typically affect the oral cavity, the eyes, and the genitalia (Box 2-9; Figures 2-33 and 2-34). Other regions or systems are less commonly involved. Recurrent arthritis of the wrists, ankles, and knees may be associated. Cardiovascular manifestations are believed to result from vasculitis and thrombosis. CNS manifestations are frequently in the form of headaches, although infarcts have been reported. Pustular erythema nodosum–like skin lesions have also been described. Relapsing polychondritis (e.g., auricular cartilage, nasal cartilage) in association with Behçet's stigmata has been designated as the *MAGIC syndrome* (*m*outh *a*nd *g*enital ulcers with *i*nflamed *c*artilage).

Oral manifestations of this syndrome appear identical to the ulcers of aphthous stomatitis. The ulcers are usually the minor aphthous form and are found in the typical aphthous distribution.

Ocular changes are found in most patients with Behçet's syndrome. Uveitis, conjunctivitis, and

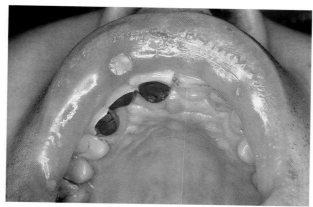

Figure 2-33 **Behçet's syndrome,** oral component (aphthous ulcer).

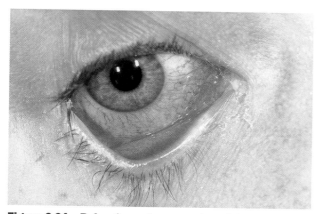

Figure 2-34 **Behçet's syndrome** conjunctivitis.

retinitis are among the more common inflammatory processes.

Genital lesions are ulcerative in nature and may cause significant pain and discomfort. Painful ulcerative lesions may also occur around the anus. Inflammatory bowel disease and neurologic problems have been described in some patients.

Histopathology. T lymphocytes are prominent in the ulcerative lesions of Behçet's syndrome. However, neutrophilic infiltrates in which the cells appear within vessel walls (vasculitis) have also been described. Immunopathologic support of a vascular target in this condition comes from the demonstration of immunoglobulins and complement in the vessel walls.

Diagnosis. The diagnosis of Behçet's syndrome is based on clinical signs and symptoms associated with the

various regions affected. There are no specific findings in biopsy tissue, and there are no supportive laboratory tests.

Treatment. There is no standard therapy for Behçet's syndrome. Systemic steroids are often prescribed and immunosuppressive drugs, such as chlorambucil and azathioprine, may be used instead of or in addition to steroids. Dapsone, cyclosporine, thalidomide, and interferon may have a role in the treatment of these patients.

Reiter's Syndrome

Etiology. Classically, Reiter's syndrome is a triad of nonspecific urethritis, conjunctivitis, and arthritis that follows bacterial dysentery or exposure to a sexually transmissible disease. An abnormal immune response to microbial antigen(s) is now regarded as a likely mechanism for the multiple manifestations of this syndrome. A male with HLA-B27 has a 20% risk for Reiter's disease after an episode of *Shigella* dysentery.

Clinical Features. The onset of Reiter's syndrome is acute, with the simultaneous appearance of urethritis, conjunctivitis, and oligoarthritis affecting large and small joints of the lower limbs. This usually occurs 1 to 3 weeks after a sexual episode or following an attack of dysentery. Other features include fever, weight loss, vasomotor abnormalities in the feet, and skin lesions consisting of faint macules, vesicles, and pustules on the hands and feet. There is bilateral conjunctivitis and, in 10% of cases, acute iritis. The arthritis is self-limiting, and remission occur in 2 to 3 months.

Oral lesions have been described as relatively painless aphthous-type ulcers occurring almost anywhere in the mouth. Tongue lesions resemble geographic tongue.

Highly characteristic of this syndrome is its occurrence predominantly in white men in their third decade. The duration of the disease varies from weeks to months, and recurrences are not uncommon.

Diagnosis. Diagnosis is dependent on recognition of the various signs and symptoms associated with this syndrome. The erythrocyte sedimentation rate (ESR) is elevated in the acute phase of the disease but persists after arthritis resolves. By tissue typing, over 70% of patients will have the HLA-B27 genotype.

Treatment. Nonsteroidal antiinflammatory agents are generally used in the treatment of this disease. Antibiotics have also been added to the treatment regimen, with varied success. Systemic corticosteroids are rarely required.

Erythema Multiforme

Erythema multiforme (EM) is a self-limiting hypersensitivity reaction characterized by target skin lesions and/or ulcerative oral lesions. It has been divided into two subtypes: a minor form, usually associated with an HSV trigger, and a major severe form, triggered by certain systemic drugs.

Etiology and Pathogenesis. The basic cause of EM is unknown, although a hypersensitivity reaction is suspected. Some evidence suggests that the disease mechanism may be related to antigen-antibody complexes that are targeted for small vessels in the skin or mucosa. In about half the cases, precipitating or triggering factors can be identified. These generally fall into the two large categories of infections and drugs. Other factors, such as malignancy, vaccination, autoimmune disease, and radiotherapy, are occasionally cited as possible triggers. Infections frequently reported include HSV infection (due to HSV types 1 and 2), TB, and histoplasmosis. Various types of drugs have precipitated EM, with barbiturates, sulfonamides, and some antiseizure medications such as carbamazepine and phenytoin being among the more frequent offenders. Although these drugs are pharmacologically unrelated, the mechanism by which EM is precipitated EM is related to similar protein folds that expose regions that are antigenically similar.

Clinical Features. EM is usually an acute, self-limited process that affects the skin or mucous membranes or both (Box 2-10). Between 25% and 50% of patients with cutaneous EM have oral manifestations of this disease (Figures 2-35 and 2-36). It may on occasion be chronic, or it may be a recurring acute problem. In recurrent disease, prodromal symptoms may be experienced before any eruption. Young adults are most commonly affected. Individuals often develop EM in the spring or fall and may have such recrudescences chronically. The term *erythema multiforme* was coined to indicate the multiple and varied clinical appearances that are associated with the cutaneous manifestations of this disease. The classic skin lesion of EM is the target or iris lesion. It consists of concentric ery-

---

Box 2-10 Erythema Multiforme

ETIOLOGY

Minor (less severe) form usually triggered by herpes simplex virus
Major form (Stevens-Johnson syndrome) often triggered by drugs
Hypersensitivity reactions to infectious agents, drugs, or idiopathic

CLINICAL FEATURES

Multiple oral ulcers and/or target skin lesions
Self-limiting, but may recur

TREATMENT

Supportive therapy
Corticosteroids occasionally used for severe form

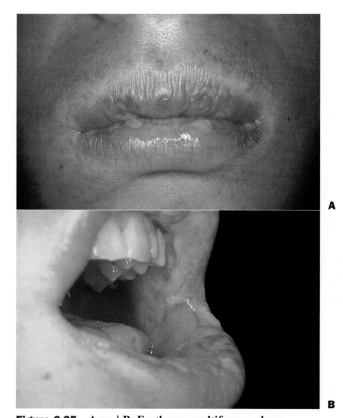

A

B

Figure 2-35   **A** and **B**, Erythema multiforme ulcers.

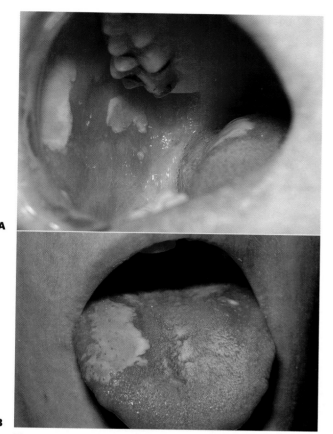

A

B

Figure 2-36 A and B, Erythema multiforme ulcers.

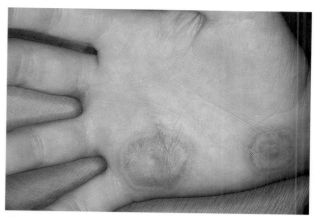

Figure 2-37 **Erythema multiforme** cutaneous target lesions.

thematous rings separated by rings of near-normal color. Typically, the extremities are involved, usually in a symmetric distribution (Figure 2-37). Other types of skin manifestations of EM include macules, papules, vesicles, bullae, and urticarial plaques.

Orally, EM characteristically presents as an ulcerative disease, varying from a few aphthous-type lesions to multiple superficial, widespread ulcers in EM major. Short-lived vesicles or bullae are infrequently seen at the initial presentation. Any area of the mouth may be involved, with the lips, buccal mucosa, palate, and tongue being most frequently affected. Recurrent oral lesions may appear as multiple painful ulcers similar to those of the initial episode or as less symptomatic erythematous patches with limited ulceration.

Symptoms range from mild discomfort to severe pain. Considerable apprehension may also be associated with this condition initially, because of the occa-

sional explosive onset occurring in some patients. Systemic signs and symptoms of headache, slightly elevated temperature, and lymphadenopathy may accompany more intense disease.

At the severe end of the EM spectrum (EM major), intense involvement of the mouth, eyes, skin, genitalia, and occasionally the esophagus and respiratory tract may be seen concurrently. This form of EM major is sometimes called *Stevens-Johnson syndrome*. Characteristically, the lips show crusting ulceration at the vermilion border that may cause exquisite pain. Superficial ulceration, often preceded by bullae, is common to all the sites affected. Ocular inflammation (conjunctivitis and uveitis) may lead to scarring and blindness in some patients.

Histopathology. The microscopic pattern of EM consists of epithelial hyperplasia and spongiosis (Figure 2-38). Basal and parabasal apoptotic keratinocytes are also usually seen. Vesicles occur at the epithelium–connective tissue interface, although intraepithelial vesiculation may be seen. Epithelial necrosis is a frequent finding. Connective tissue changes usually appear as infiltrates of lymphocytes and macrophages in perivascular spaces and in connective tissue papillae.

Immunopathologic studies are nonspecific for EM. The epithelium shows negative staining for immunoglobulins. Vessels have, however, been shown to have IgM, complement, and fibrin deposits in their walls. This latter finding has been used to support an immune complex vasculitis cause for EM. Autoantibodies to desmoplakins 1 and 2 have been identified

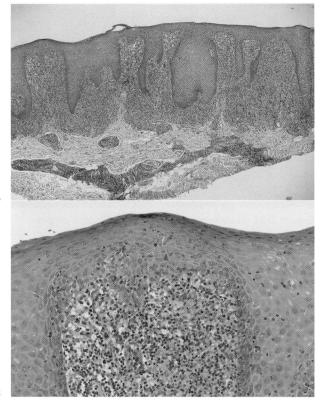

Figure 2-38 **Oral erythema multiforme** biopsy specimen showing epithelial hyperplasia with intense interface and deep perivascular lymphocyte and macrophage infiltrate.

	Erythema Multiforme	**Herpes Infection**
Appearance	Large oral and lip ulcers Skin target lesions	Small oral/perioral ulcers Skin ulcers
Symptoms	Mild to severe	Moderate to severe
Sites	Buccal, tongue, lips, palate, extremities	Gingiva, lips, perioral skin
Age	Young adults	Children
Cause	Hypersensitivity	HSV
Treatment	Symptomatic, steroids	Acyclovir

TABLE 2-4 Erythema Multiforme vs. Primary Herpes Simplex Infection

HSV, Herpes simplex virus.

in a subset of EM major–affected patients, suggesting that both cell-mediated and humoral immune systems may contribute to the pathogenesis of EM.

Differential Diagnosis. When target, or iris, skin lesions are present, clinical diagnosis is usually straightforward. However, in the absence of these or any skin lesions, several possibilities should be considered for the oral expression of this disease. Included would be primary HSV infections (Table 2-4), aphthous ulcers, pemphigus vulgaris, mucous membrane pemphigoid, and erosive lichen planus. The general lack of systemic symptoms; the favored oral location of the lips, buccal mucosa, tongue, and palate (rarely gingiva); the larger ulcers (usually not preceded by blisters); the presence of target skin lesions; and a history of recent drug ingestion or infection should favor a diagnosis of EM.

Treatment. In EM minor, symptomatic treatment, including keeping the mouth clean with bland mouthrinses,

may be all that is necessary. In EM major, topical corticosteroids with antifungals may help control disease. The use of systemic corticosteroids is controversial and is believed by some to be contraindicated. Acyclovir at 400 to 600 mg daily may be effective in preventing recurrences in patients who have an HSV-triggered disease, although the efficacy is not clear. Supportive measures, such as oral irrigation, adequate fluid intake, and use of antipyretics, may provide patients with substantial benefit.

Drug Reactions

Etiology and Pathogenesis. Although the skin is more commonly involved in adverse reactions to drugs, the oral mucosa may occasionally be the target. Virtually any drug has the potential to cause an untoward reaction, but some have a greater ability to do so than others. Also, some patients have a greater tendency than others to react to drugs. Some of the drugs that are more commonly cited as being involved in adverse reactions are listed in Box 2-11.

The pathogenesis of drug reactions may be related to either immunologic or nonimmunologic mechanisms (Box 2-12). The immunologic mechanisms are triggered by an antigenic component (hapten) on the drug molecule, resulting in a hyperimmune response, or drug allergy. The potential for drug allergy is directly dependent on the immunogenicity of the drug, the frequency of exposure, the route of administration (topical more likely than oral), and the innate reactivity of the patient's immune system. Mechanisms involved in drug allergy include immunoglobulin E (IgE)–mediated reactions, cytotoxic reactions (antibody binds to a drug that is already attached to a cell

Box 2-11 Ulcerative and Erythematous Drug Reactions: Representative Causative Drugs

Analgesic
  Aspirin
  Codeine
Antibiotic
  Erythromycin
  Penicillin
  Streptomycin
  Sulfonamides
  Tetracycline
Anticonvulsant
  Barbiturates
  Phenytoin
Antifungal
  Ketoconazole
Antiinflammatory
  Indomethacin
Antimalarial
Cardiovascular
  Methyldopa
  Oxprenolol
Psychotherapeutic
  Meprobamate
  Chlorpromazine
Other
  Retinoids
  Cimetidine
  Gold compounds
  Local anesthetics

Box 2-12 Drug Reactions: Mechanisms

HYPERIMMUNE RESPONSE (ALLERGY)

Related to drug immunogenicity, frequency, route of delivery, patient's immune system
Mediated by:
  Mast cells coated with IgE
  Ab reaction to cell-bound drug
  Deposition of circulating Ag-Ab complexes

NONIMMUNOLOGIC RESPONSE (NOT AB DEPENDENT)

Direct release of inflammatory mediators by mast cells
Overdose, toxicity, side effects

IgE, Immunoglobulin E; *Ab,* antibody; *Ag,* antigen.

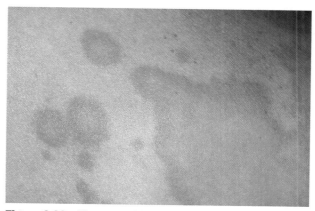

Figure 2-39 Hypersensitivity reaction. Cutaneous urticaria associated with hypersensitivity to metronidazole.

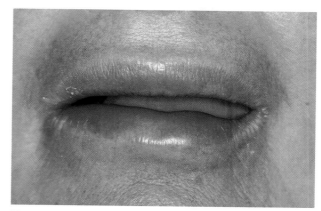

Figure 2-40 Acquired angioedema producing lip swelling.

directly affect mast cells, causing the release of chemical mediators. The reactions may also be a result of overdose, toxicity, or side effects of the drugs.

Clinical Features. Cutaneous manifestations of drug reactions are widely varied. Changes may appear rapidly, as in anaphylaxis, angioedema, and urticaria, or after several days of drug use. Manifestations include urticaria, maculopapular rash, erythema, vesicles, ulcers, and target lesions (EM) (Figures 2-39 to 2-42).

Acquired angioedema is an IgE-mediated allergic reaction that is precipitated by drugs or foods such as nuts and shellfish. These substances may act as sensitizing agents (antigens) that elicit IgE production. On antigenic rechallenge, mast cells bound with IgE in the skin or mucosa release their contents to cause

surface), and circulation of antigen (drug)–antibody complexes.

Drug reactions that are nonimmunologic in nature do not stimulate an immune response and are not antibody dependent. In this type of response, drugs may

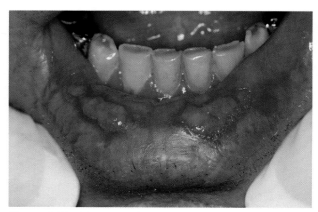

Figure 2-41 **Drug reaction** to captopril.

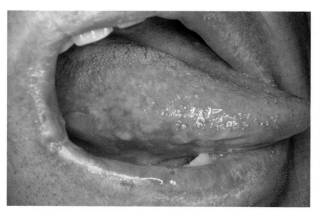

Figure 2-42 **Lichenoid drug reaction.**

the clinical picture of angioedema. *Hereditary angioedema* produces similar clinical changes but through a different mechanism. Individuals who inherit this rare autosomal-dominant trait develop a spontaneous mutation, which results in a deficiency of the inhibitor of the first component of complement C1 esterase. Absent or dysfunctional C1 esterase inhibitor leads ultimately to release of vasoactive peptides and the often serious clinical manifestations that characterize this condition.

Angioedema, by either an acquired or a hereditary pathway, appears as a soft, diffuse, painless swelling, usually of the lips, neck, or face. There is typically no color change. The condition generally subsides after 1 to 2 days and may recur at a later date. Curiously, minor trauma can also precipitate the swelling. Emergency treatment may be required if the process leads to respiratory distress because of glottic or laryngeal involvement. Antihistamines and, in problematic cases, corticosteroids are used to treat this form of allergy.

Oral manifestations of drug reactions may be erythematous, vesicular, or ulcerative in nature. They may also mimic erosive lichen planus, in which case they are known as *lichenoid drug reactions* (Box 2-13). The widespread ulcers typical of EM are often representative of a drug reaction.

Histopathology. The microscopy of drug reactions includes such nonspecific features as spongiosis, apoptotic keratinocytes, lymphoid infiltrates, eosinophils, and ulceration. An interface pattern of mucositis (i.e., a lymphoid infiltrate focused at the epithelium–connective tissue interface) is often seen in mucosal allergic reactions. Although biopsy findings may not be diagnostic, they may be helpful in ruling out other diagnostic considerations.

Diagnosis. Because the clinical and histologic features of drug reactions are highly variable and nonspecific, the diagnosis of drug reaction requires a high index of suspicion and careful history taking. Recent use of a drug is important, although delayed reaction (up to 2 weeks) may occasionally be noted (e.g., with ampicillin). Withdrawal of the suspected drug should result in improvement, and reinstitution of the drug (a procedure that is usually ill advised for the patient's safety) should exacerbate the patient's condition. If rechallenge is performed, minute amounts of the offending drug or a structurally related drug should cause a reaction.

Treatment. The most important measures in the management of drug reactions are identification and withdrawal of the causative agent. If this is impossible or undesirable, alternative drugs may have to be substituted or the eruption may have to be dealt with on an empirical basis. Antihistamines and occasionally corticosteroids may be useful in the management of oral and cutaneous eruptions due to drug reactions.

Contact Allergies

Etiology and Pathogenesis. Contact allergic reactions can be caused by antigenic stimulation by a vast array of foreign substances. The immune response is predominantly T-cell mediated. In the sensitization phase, epithelial Langerhans cells appear to have a major role in the recognition of foreign antigen. These dendritic cells are responsible for processing antigens that enter the epithelium from the external environment. The Langerhans cells subsequently present the appropriate antigenic determinants to T lymphocytes. After antigenic rechallenge, local lymphocytes secrete chemical mediators of inflammation (cytokines) that produce the clinical and histologic changes characteristic of this process.

Clinical Features. Lesions of contact allergy occur directly adjacent to the causative agent. Presentation is varied and includes erythematous, vesicular, and ulcerative lesions (Figures 2-43 and 2-44).

Although contact allergy is frequently seen on the skin, it is relatively uncommon intraorally. Some of the many materials containing agents known to cause oral contact allergic reactions are toothpaste, mouthwash, candy, chewing gum, topical antimicrobials, topical steroids, iodine, essential oils, and denture base material. *Cinnamon* has been specifically identified as an etiologic agent in oral contact stomatitis. Lesions associated with this offender are usually white or even

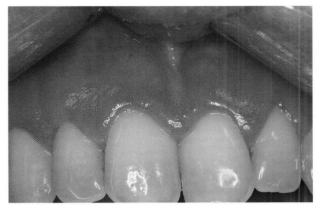

Figure 2-43   **Contact allergy** resulting in erythematous gingiva.

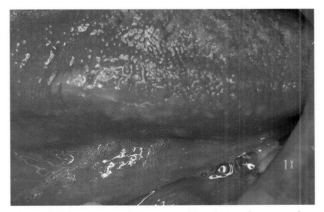

Figure 2-44   **Contact allergy** resulting in erythema and ulcerations of the lateral tongue.

lichenoid, although ulcerative and red lesions may be seen. A related lesion, plasma cell gingivitis, is also a form of contact allergy to cinnamon-containing agents such as toothpastes and chewing gums. The condition primarily affects the attached gingiva as a bright red bilateral band. This lesion is discussed in Chapter 4.

Histopathology. Microscopically, the epithelium and connective tissue show inflammatory changes. Spongiosis and vesiculation may be seen within the epithelium, and perivascular lymphophagocytic infiltrate is found in the immediate supporting connective tissue. Blood vessels may be dilated, and occasionally eosinophils may be seen.

Diagnosis. Careful history taking to establish a cause-and-effect relationship is essential. Biopsy find-

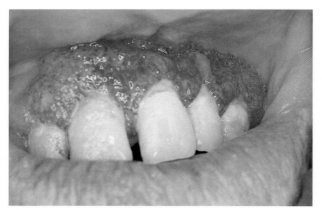

Figure 2-45   **Wegener's granulomatosis**, gingival expression.

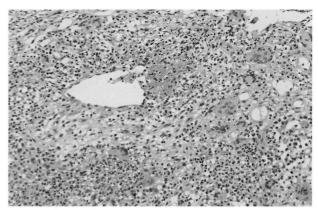

Figure 2-46   **Wegener's granulomatosis**; granulomatous inflammation and necrotizing vasculitis.

ings may be confirmatory. Patch testing of oral mucosa is difficult, and false-negative results may be problematic.

Treatment. Treatment should be directed at elimination of the offending material if it can be identified. In uncomplicated cases lesions should heal in 1 to 2 weeks. Topical steroids may hasten the healing process.

Wegener's Granulomatosis

Etiology. Wegener's granulomatosis is a serious, systemic, inflammatory condition of unknown etiology. Efforts to identify a cause have generally focused on infection and immunologic dysfunction but have been unproductive.

Clinical Features. Classically, the triad of upper respiratory tract, lung, and kidney involvement is seen in this condition. Occasionally, only two of the three sites are affected. Lesions may also present in the oral cavity and skin and, potentially, in any other organ system (Figure 2-45).

This is a rare disease of middle age. Initial presentation is often associated with head and neck manifestations of sinusitis, rhinorrhea, nasal stuffiness, and epistaxis. In a majority of cases nasal or sinus (usually maxillary) ulcerations are present. Necrosis and perforation of the nasal septum or palate are occasionally seen. Intraoral lesions consist of red, hyperplastic, granular lesions on the attached gingiva.

Kidney involvement consists of focal necrotizing glomerulitis. Renal failure is the final outcome of kidney disease. Inflammatory lung lesions, varying in intensity from slight to severe, may eventually lead to respiratory failure.

Histopathology. The basic pathologic process is granulomatous, with characteristic necrotizing vasculitis (Figure 2-46). Necrosis and multinucleated giant cells may be seen in the granulomatous areas. The affected small vessels show a mononuclear infiltrate within their walls in the presence of fibrinoid necrosis. Diagnosis may be made by exclusion of other diseases, particularly midline granuloma (Table 2-5).

Diagnosis. Diagnosis is generally dependent on the finding of granulomatous inflammation and necrotizing vasculitis in biopsy tissue of upper respiratory tract lesions—evidence of involvement of lung and/or kidney lesions. Demonstration of antineutrophil cytoplasmic antibodies (cANCAs) from indirect immunofluorescence on blood adds confirmatory evidence. Antineutrophil perinuclear antibodies (pANCAs) represent antibodies to myeloperoxidases and are usually positive in many forms of vasculitis and polyarteritis and therefore are not specific for Wegener's granulomatosis.

Treatment. Before the development of chemotherapeutic agents, renal failure and death were common outcomes of this disease process. The use of the cytotoxic agent cyclophosphamide combined with corticosteroids has provided afflicted patients with a relatively favorable prognosis. With treatment, remissions occur in approximately 75% of cases.

TABLE 2-5 Wegener's Granulomatosis vs. Midline Granuloma (T-Cell Lymphoma)

	Wegener's Granuloma	Midline Granuloma
Etiology	Unknown? Infectious? Immune dysfunction	Malignancy of T lymphocytes
Organs	Upper airways, lungs, kidneys	Upper airways, palate, gingiva
Pathology	Granulomatous and necrotizing vasculitis	T-cell lymphoma (angiocentric)
Diagnosis	Biopsy, positive antineutrophil cytoplasmic antibodies (cANCAs)	Biopsy, immunologic studies
Treatment	Cyclophosphamide, prednisone	Radiation, chemotherapy

Midline Granuloma

Midline granuloma is a diagnosis made by exclusion of other granulomatous and necrotizing midfacial lesions. Because midline granuloma has many features that overlap with Wegener's granulomatosis, these two conditions were at one time classified together under the rubric *midline lethal granuloma*. Most, if not all cases, represent occult peripheral T-cell lymphomas.

Clinical Features. Midline granuloma is a unifocal destructive process, generally in the midline of the oronasal region (Figure 2-47). Lesions appear clinically as aggressive necrotic ulcers that are progressive and nonhealing. Extension through soft tissue, cartilage, and bone is typical. Perforation of the nasal septum and hard palate may also be seen. Clinically, other diseases that produces destructive lesions of the midline of the nose or palate include Wegener's granulomatosis, infectious disease, and carcinoma.

Histopathology. Microscopically, the process appears as acute and chronic inflammation in partially necrotic tissue. Angiocentric inflammation is a common finding and is typical of many T-cell lymphomas. Because of the almost trivial inflammatory appearance of this condition, several biopsies may be required before lymphoma can be diagnosed. Immunohistochemistry and molecular studies will establish T-cell clonality consistent with lymphoma.

Treatment. The treatment of choice is local radiation. It is relatively effective and has produced a reasonably optimistic prognosis.

Chronic Granulomatous Disease

Chronic granulomatous disease is a rare systemic (X-linked or autosomal recessive) disease caused by defects in the nicotinamide adenine dinucleotide phos-

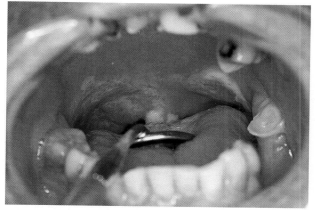

Figure 2-47 **Midline granuloma** presenting as oropharyngeal ulcers.

phate (NADPH) oxidase complex that results in altered neutrophil and macrophage function. These cells, although they have the capacity to phagocytose microorganisms, lack the ability to kill certain bacteria and fungi because of inadequate superoxide and other oxygen metabolites that are toxic to organisms.

Manifestations appear during childhood and, because of the more frequent X-linked inheritance pattern, occur predominantly in males. The process may affect many organs, including the lymph nodes, lung, liver, spleen, bone, and skin, as recurrent or persistent infections. Oral lesions are frequently seen in the form of multiple ulcers that are also recurrent or persistent. Granulomatous disease and abnormal nitroblue tetrazolium neutrophil function test results would support clinical suspicions.

Cyclic Neutropenia

Cyclic neutropenia, a rare blood dyscrasia , is manifested as severe cyclic depletions of neutrophils from the blood and marrow, with a mean cycle, or periodicity, of about 21 days. Both autosomal-dominant and sporadic forms are due to a mutation in the gene coding for neutrophil elastase located at chromosome 19p13.3. Fever, malaise, oral ulcers, cervical lymphadenopathy, and infections may appear during neutropenic episodes. Patients are also prone to exaggeration of periodontal disease. There is no definitive treatment. Early recognition of infections is important in management, as is judicious use of antibiotics.

NEOPLASMS

Squamous Cell Carcinoma

Relative to the incidence of all cancers, oral and oropharyngeal squamous cell carcinomas represent about 3% of cancers in men and 2% of cancers in women. Annually, nearly 30,000 new cases of oral and oropharyngeal cancer are expected to occur in men and women in the United States. The ratio of cases in men and women is now about 2 to 1. Previously this ratio was 3 to 1, and this shift has been attributed to an increase in smoking by women and to their longer life expectancy.

Deaths due to oral and oropharyngeal cancer represent approximately 2% of the total in men and 1% of the total in women. The total number of annual deaths due to oral and pharyngeal cancer is as high as 9500 in the United States.

The trend in survival of patients with this malignancy has been rather disappointing during the past several decades (Figure 2-48). The overall survival rate of all patients with oral cancers is about 50%. The survival rates for blacks have been estimated to be significantly lower. Geographic variations in oral and oropharyngeal carcinoma survival rates exist in the United States and around the world and are most likely attributed to genetic and environmental differences unique to local populations.

In India and some other Asian countries, oral cancer is the most common type of malignancy and may account for more than 50% of all cancer cases. This finding is generally linked to the high prevalence of a unique smokeless tobacco habit. The tobacco, typically mixed with areca (betel) nut, slaked lime, and spices, is known as the quid, or pan, and is held in the buccal vestibule for long periods. This combination of ingredients, which may vary from one locale to another, is more carcinogenic than tobacco used alone.

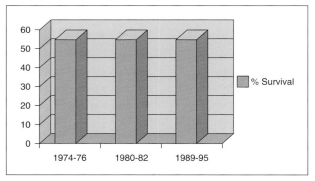

Figure 2-48   Oral cancer 5-year survival rates.

Etiology. Of all factors believed to contribute to the etiology of oral cancer, tobacco is regarded as the most important. All forms of tobacco smoking have been strongly linked to the cause of oral cancer. Cigar and pipe smoking are linked to a greater risk for the development of oral cancer than that with cigarette smoking. "Reverse smoking," the habit of holding the lighted end of the cigarette inside the mouth, as may be the habit in India and some South American countries, is associated with a significantly high risk of oral cancer. This high risk is due to the intensity of tobacco combustion adjacent to palatal and lingual tissues. In any event, the time-dose relationship of carcinogens found in tobacco is of paramount importance in the cause of oral cancer. In addition to an overall increased risk of development of cancer in all regions of the mouth, pipe smokers appear to have a special predilection for squamous cell carcinoma of the lower lip.

The chronic use of smokeless tobacco, whether in the form of snuff (ground and finely cut tobacco) or chewing tobacco (loose-leaf tobacco), is believed to increase the risk of oral cancer, although the risk level is probably quite low. In view of this lower oral cancer risk, some have advocated smokeless tobacco as an alternative to cigarettes, although the rationale for this is suspect when safe, alternative smoking cessation methods exist. In addition, many patients who use smokeless tobacco products also consume cigarettes and alcohol and thereby increase their risk of oral cancer. Moreover, the use of smokeless tobacco also carries with it other health risks such as elevated blood pressure, physiologic dependence, and worsening periodontal disease.

Alcohol, although not believed to be a carcinogen itself, appears to add to the risk of oral cancer development. Identification of alcohol alone as a carcinogenic factor has proved to be somewhat difficult because of the combination of smoking and drinking habits by most patients with oral cancer. However, recent epidemiologic studies suggest that alcohol use alone may increase the risk for oral cancer. The effects of alcohol have been thought to occur through its ability to irritate mucosa and to act as a solvent for carcinogens (especially those in tobacco). Contaminants and additives with carcinogenic potential that are found in alcoholic drinks have also been thought to have a role in oral cancer development. Molecular studies have suggested that the carcinogenic risks associated with alcohol may be related to the effects of an alcohol metabolite, acetaldehyde, through the alteration of keratinocyte gene expression.

Some microorganisms have been implicated in oral cancer. *Candida albicans* has been suggested as a possible causative agent because of its potential to produce a carcinogen, *N*-nitrosobenzylmethylamine. Epstein-Barr virus has been linked to Burkitt's lymphoma and nasopharyngeal carcinoma, but not to oral cancer.

Studies have demonstrated the occasional presence of human papillomavirus (HPV) subtypes 16 and 18 in oral squamous cell carcinomas, suggesting a possible role for this virus in oral cancers. This association is strongest for oropharyngeal squamous cell carcinomas where up to 50% of tumors from this site may contain evidence of HPV. Verrucous carcinoma has also been identified as a lesion possibly related to HPV infection. The mechanism by which HPV is thought to contribute to carcinogenesis is through protein (E6) inhibition of p53, leading to acceleration of the cell cycle and compromised DNA repair.

Although poor nutritional status has been linked to an increased rise of oral cancer, the only convincing nutritional factor that has been associated with oral cancer is iron deficiency of *Plummer-Vinson syndrome (Patterson-Kelly syndrome, sideropenic dysphagia).* Typically affecting middle-aged women, the syndrome includes a painful red tongue, mucosal atrophy, dysphagia due to esophageal webs, and a predisposition to the development of oral squamous cell carcinoma.

Ultraviolet (UV) light is a known carcinogenic agent that is a significant factor in basal cell carcinomas of the skin and squamous cell carcinomas of the skin and lip. The cumulative dose of sunlight and the amount

of protection by natural pigmentation are of great significance in the development of these cancers. In the UV light spectrum, radiation with a wavelength of 2900 to 3200 nm (UVB) is more carcinogenic than light of 3200 to 3400 nm (UVA).

A compromised immune system puts patients at risk for oral cancer. This increased risk has been documented for bone marrow and kidney transplant recipients, who are iatrogenically immunosuppressed. The total-body radiation and high-dose chemotherapy that are used to condition patients for bone marrow transplants also put patients at lifelong risk for solid and lymphoid malignancies. It has long been suspected that AIDS predisposes patients to oral cancer, but evidence is generally lacking.

Chronic irritation is generally regarded as a modifier rather than an initiator of oral cancer. Mechanical trauma from ill-fitting dentures, broken fillings, and other frictional rubs is unlikely to cause oral cancer. If, however, a cancer is started from another cause, these factors will probably hasten the process. Poor oral hygiene is also regarded as having a comparable modifying effect, although many patients with poor oral hygiene also have other more important risk factors for oral cancer, such as tobacco habits and alcohol consumption.

Pathogenesis. Oral cancer, like most other malignancies, arises from the accumulation of a number of discrete genetic events that lead to invasive cancer (Figures 2-49 to 2-51). These changes occur in genes that encode for proteins that control the cell cycle, cell survival, cell motility, and angiogenesis. Each genetic mutation confers a selective growth advantage, permitting clonal expansion of mutant cells with an increased malignant potential. This process is known as clonal evolution. The multistep genetic progression to cancer was first characterized in colonic mucosa, correlating with the sequential evolution of adenomatous polyps to adenocarcinoma. It was shown that a small number of genetic changes were required for acquisition of the malignant phenotype. For example, mutations of the *APC* and *K-ras* genes occur early in tumor progression, whereas alterations of *p53* and *DCC* occur more frequently in advanced tumors.

Conceptually, oral cancers progress through two important biologic stages. The first is loss of cell cycle control through increased proliferation and reduced apoptosis. Clinically, this is most obvious in patients with in situ carcinomas, where an increased number of dividing cells can be seen in all levels of the epithelium. The second stage is increased tumor cell motility, leading to invasion and metastasis. Here, neoplastic epithelial cells penetrate the basement membrane and invade underlying tissues and eventually reach regional lymph nodes.

Both stages are a result of the activation, or up-regulation, of oncogenes and the inactivation, or down-regulation, of tumor suppressor genes (antioncogenes) (Box 2-14). Oncogenes, or proto-oncogenes under normal circumstances, encode proteins that positively regulate critical cell growth functions, such as proliferation, apoptosis, cell motility, internal cell signaling, and angiogenesis. If these genes are altered through one of several mechanisms (e.g., mutation), then there is overexpression of the encoded protein, giving rise to a clone of cells with a growth/motility advantage. Tumor suppressor genes encode proteins that negatively regulate or suppress proliferation. Alteration of these genes (changes in both maternal and paternal alleles are required) essentially "releases the brake" on proliferation for a clone of cells. Tumor suppressor genes are believed to play a more important role in oral cancer development than oncogenes.

Alterations of genes that control the cell cycle seem to be of critical importance in the development of oral

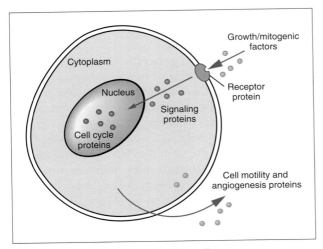

Figure 2-49   Gene expression in oral cancer.

Box 2-14 Oral Cancer Pathogenesis

Oncogenes and tumor suppressor genes:
  Mutation, amplification, or inactivation
Loss of control of:
  Cell cycle (proliferation vs. inhibition, signaling)
  Cell survival (apoptosis vs. antiapoptosis)
  Cell motility

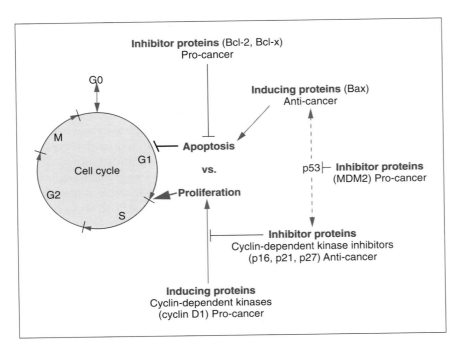

Figure 2-50   Cell cycle regulation; controls at G1-S.

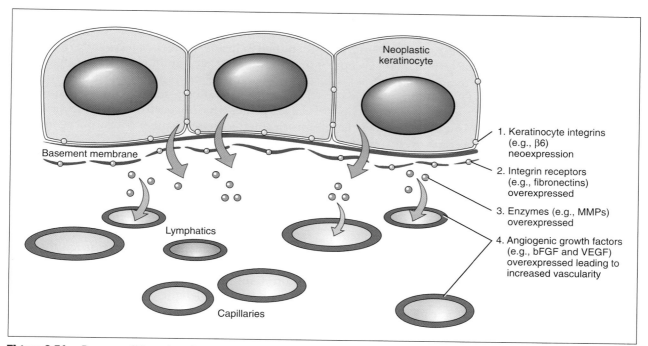

Figure 2-51 Cancer cell invasion through enhanced cell motility and angiogenesis.

1. Keratinocyte integrins (e.g., β6) neoexpression
2. Integrin receptors (e.g., fibronectins) overexpressed
3. Enzymes (e.g., MMPs) overexpressed
4. Angiogenic growth factors (e.g., bFGF and VEGF) overexpressed leading to increased vascularity

cancer. Normally, cell division is divided into four phases: G1 (gap 1), S (DNA synthesis), G2 (gap 2), and M (mitosis). A key event is the progression from the G1 to S phase. Genetic alterations, if unrepaired in the G1 phase, may be carried into the S phase and perpetuated in subsequent cell divisions. The G1-S "checkpoint" is normally regulated by a well-coordinated and complex system of protein interactions whose balance and function are critical to normal cell division. Overexpression of oncogenic proteins or underexpression of antioncogenic proteins can tip the balance in favor of proliferation and neoplastic transformation. For example, *p53* normally is a tumor suppressor gene and a key negative regulator at G1-S of the cell cycle. In about 50% of oral cancers *p53* is mutated and its encoded protein is nonfunctional. Defective p53 protein allows cells to proceed into the S phase of the cell cycle before DNA can be repaired. The result is an accumulation of deleterious genetic defects that contribute to malignant transformation. This key protein may be dysregulated in oral precancer as well and may serve as an indicator of high-risk lesions. The MDM2 protein mediates the degradation of p53 and is frequently overexpressed in oral cancers.

Overexpression of the cyclin D1 protein can be identified in many oral cancers, leading to increased pro-liferation and premature progression through the G1-S checkpoint. Two important groups of intrinsic cell cycle proteins that regulate proliferation are cyclins and their catalytic binding enzymes, the cyclin-dependent kinases. In turn, these proteins are regulated by a class of inhibitory proteins known as cyclin-dependent kinase inhibitors. Reduced expression of the cyclin-dependent kinase inhibitors, $p16^{ink4a}$ and $p27^{kip1}$, is another important feature of oral cancer and is associated with loss of cell cycle control and increased proliferation.

The biologic antithesis of proliferation is apoptosis (programmed cell death). If cells live longer, they may have a biologic advantage that favors the development of neoplasia. Some genes that control apoptosis are altered in cancers (e.g., *BCL-2* gene, which is over-expressed in mantle cell lymphomas as a result of a chromosome translocation). In oral cancers the anti-apoptotic proteins Bcl-2 and Bcl-X are also often over-expressed. Moreover, expression of the proapoptotic protein Bax also has been positively correlated with increased sensitivity to chemotherapeutic agents in head and neck cancers.

Several other oncogenes that function in the regulation of cell growth and for the transport of signals from the cell membrane to the nucleus are also frequently altered in many oral cancers. These include genes that code for *growth factors,* such as int-2 and hst-1 (fibroblast growth factor); *growth factor receptors,* such as erbB1 and erbB2 (epidermal growth factor receptors); *proteins involved in signal transduction,* such as ras (guanosine triphosphate [GTP]–binding proteins); and *nuclear regulatory proteins* such as myc (transcriptional activator proteins). Correlations have now been identified between growth receptor overexpression and patient outcome.

Many oral cancers pass through a premalignant phase (dysplasia or in situ carcinoma), whereas others appear to arise de novo without clinical or microscopic evidence of a preexisting lesion. Invasive carcinomas have developed the ability to penetrate basement membrane and connective tissue, as well as enter the vascular system. These tumors are believed to have developed this biologic advantage through molecular lesions in genes and proteins associated with cell movement and extracellular matrix degradation. Changes in the phenotype of cell adhesion molecules (e.g., cadherins and integrins) release cells from their normal environment and give them the ability to migrate. This, coupled with the enzymatic degradation of basement membrane and connective tissue, provides the necessary components for invasion of the proliferating tumor.

Critical cell adhesions proteins are frequently altered in invasive oral cancer. These include intercellular adhesion molecule (ICAM), e-cadherin, and the neoexpression of beta-6 integrin, a protein that assists keratinocyte motility. Matrix-related proteins produced by tumor cells and possibly by connective tissue elements (e.g., fibroblasts, macrophages) contribute to the breakdown of basement membrane and extracellular matrix proteins. Tenascin, an antiadhesion molecule not evident in normal mucosa, is frequently detected in oral squamous cell carcinomas. Matrix metalloproteinases (MMPs 1, 2, 9, 13) have also been demonstrated in invasive carcinomas and are believed to play a significant role in the degradation of connective tissue elements. In particular, MMPs 3 and 13 are associated with advanced head and neck carcinomas.

For tumors to grow much greater than 1 mm in size, a new blood supply is required (angiogenesis). This occurs through tumor-mediated induction or overexpression of angiogenic proteins (e.g., vascular endothelial growth factor [VEGF], basic fibroblastic growth factor [FGF]) and/or the suppression of pro-

teins that inhibit angiogenesis. VEGF, FGF, and interleukin 8 (IL-8) (proinflammatory cytokine) have been identified in head and neck cancers and are believed to be responsible, at least in part, for the angiogenesis associated with the progression of these tumors. The genetic alteration leading to the overexpression of these proteins has not been determined, but it likely involves interactions with other critical oncogenes and immunosuppressor genes.

Another important feature of cancer cells is an increased replicative life span. Telomeres are DNA-protein complexes found at the end of chromosomes and are required for chromosome stability. Normal cells have a finite life span related to telomere shortening that occurs with each successive cell division. When a critical telomere reduction is reached, the chromosome and subsequently the cell are subject to degradation. Cancer cells often develop a mechanism to maintain telomere length and chromosome integrity and thus long-term viability. This is associated with the production of telomerase, an intranuclear enzyme that is not present in normal adult cells but is found in cancer cells. Most head and neck carcinomas have telomerase activity through neoexpression of the enzyme, giving the neoplastic cell extended life.

Clinical Features

Carcinoma of the Lips. From a biologic viewpoint, carcinomas of the lower lip are separated from carcinomas of the upper lip. Carcinomas of the lower lip are far more common than upper lip lesions (Figures 2-52 and 2-53). UV light and pipe smoking are much more important in the cause of lower lip cancer than in the cause of upper lip cancer. The growth rate is slower for lower lip cancers than for upper lip cancers. The prognosis for lower lip lesions is generally very favorable, with over 90% of patients alive after 5 years. By contrast, the prognosis for upper lip lesions is considerably worse.

Lip carcinomas account for 25% to 30% of all oral cancers. They appear most commonly in patients between 50 and 70 years of age and affect men much more often than women. Some components of lipstick may have sunscreen properties and account, in part, for this finding. Lesions arise on the vermilion and typically appear as a chronic nonhealing ulcer or as an exophytic lesion that is occasionally verrucous in nature. Deep invasion generally appears later in the course of the disease. Metastasis to local submental or

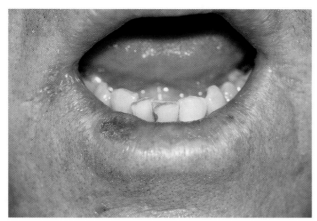

Figure 2-52 **Squamous cell carcinoma** of the lip.

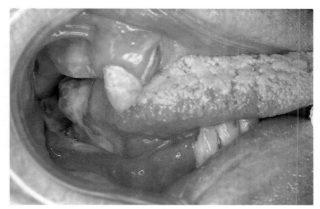

Figure 2-54 **Advanced squamous cell carcinoma** of the posterior-lateral tongue.

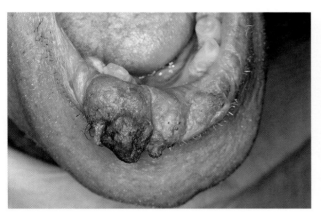

Figure 2-53 **Exophytic squamous cell carcinoma** of the lip.

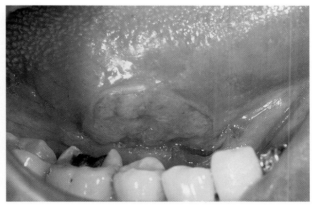

Figure 2-55 **Squamous cell carcinoma** of the lateral tongue in a 34-year-old man.

submandibular lymph nodes is uncommon but is more likely with larger, more poorly differentiated lesions.

Carcinoma of the Tongue. Squamous cell carcinoma of the tongue is the most common intraoral malignancy. Excluding lip lesions, it accounts for between 25% and 40% of oral carcinomas. It has a definite predilection for men in their sixth, seventh, and eighth decades. However, lesions may uncommonly be found in the very young. These lesions often exhibit a particularly aggressive behavior.

Lingual carcinoma is typically asymptomatic. In later stages, as deep invasion occurs, pain or dysphagia may be a prominent patient complaint. Similar to other oral cancers, these present in one of four ways: as an indurated, nonhealing ulcer, as a red lesion, as a white lesion, or as a red-and-white lesion (Figures 2-54 to 2-57). The neoplasm may occasionally have a prominent exophytic, as well as endophytic, growth pattern. A small percentage of leukoplakias of the tongue represent invasive squamous cell carcinoma or eventually become squamous cell carcinoma. Most erythroplakic patches that appear on the tongue are either in situ or invasive squamous cell carcinomas at the time of discovery.

The most common location of cancer of the tongue is the posterior-lateral border, accounting for as many as 45% of tongue lesions. Lesions very uncommonly develop on the dorsum or on the tip of the tongue. Approximately 25% of tongue cancers occur in the posterior one third or base of the tongue. These lesions are more troublesome than the others because of their

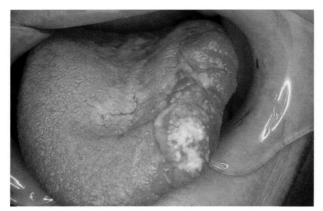

Figure 2-56 **Squamous cell carcinoma** of the lateral tongue.

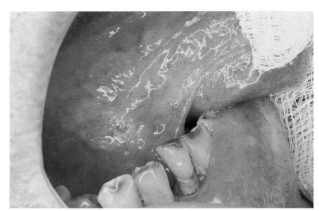

Figure 2-58 **Early squamous cell carcinoma** of the floor of the mouth.

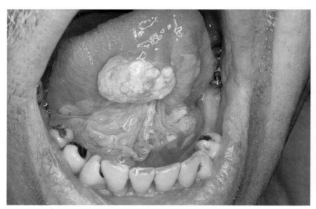

Figure 2-57 **Squamous cell carcinoma** of the ventral surface of the tongue.

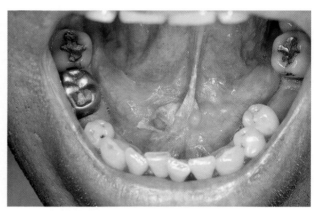

Figure 2-59 **Early squamous cell carcinoma** of the floor of the mouth.

silent progression in an area that is difficult to visualize. Accordingly, these lesions are more often advanced or have metastasized regionally by the time they are discovered, reflecting a significantly poorer prognosis than for lesions of the anterior two thirds.

Metastases from tongue cancer are relatively common at the time of primary treatment. In general, metastatic deposits from squamous cell carcinoma of the tongue are found in the lymph nodes of the neck, usually on the ipsilateral (same) side. The first nodes to become involved are the submandibular or jugulodigastric nodes at the angle of the mandible. Uncommonly, distant metastatic deposits may be seen in the lung or the liver.

Carcinoma of the Floor of the Mouth. The floor of the mouth is the second most common intraoral location

of squamous cell carcinomas, accounting for 15% to 20% of cases. Again, carcinomas in this location occur predominantly in older men, especially those who are chronic alcoholics and smokers. The usual presenting appearance is that of a painless, nonhealing, indurated ulcer (Figure 2-58). It may also appear as a white or red patch (Figure 2-59). The lesion occasionally may widely infiltrate the soft tissues of the floor of the mouth, causing decreased mobility of the tongue (Figures 2-60 and 2-61). Metastasis to submandibular lymph nodes is not uncommon for lesions of the floor of the mouth.

Carcinoma of the Buccal Mucosa and Gingiva. Lesions of the buccal mucosa and lesions of the gingiva each account for approximately 10% of oral squamous cell carcinomas. Men in their seventh decade typify the

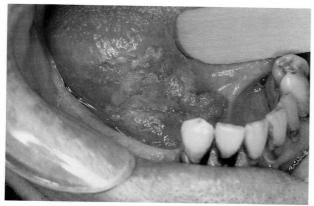

Figure 2-60 **Squamous cell carcinoma** of the floor of the mouth.

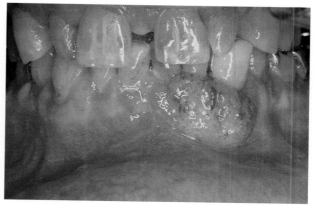

Figure 2-62 **Squamous cell carcinoma** of the gingiva.

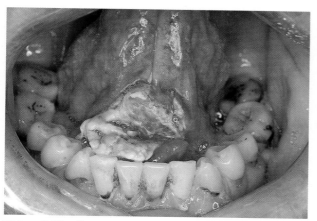

Figure 2-61 **Squamous cell carcinoma** of the floor of the mouth.

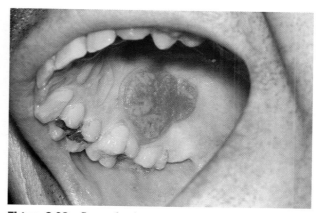

Figure 2-63 **Second primary squamous cell carcinoma** of the palate in a 34-year-old man.

group affected. The presenting clinical appearance varies from a white patch to a nonhealing ulcer to an exophytic lesion (Figure 2-62). In the last-mentioned group is the clinical pathologic entity *verrucous carcinoma*. This subset of squamous cell carcinoma, some associated with the use of smokeless tobacco, presents as a broad-based, wartlike mass. It is slow growing and very well differentiated, rarely metastasizes, and has a very favorable prognosis.

Carcinoma of the Palate. There is some justification for the separation of cancers of the hard palate from those of the soft palate. In the soft palate and contiguous faucial tissues, squamous cell carcinoma is a fairly common occurrence, accounting for 10% to 20% of intraoral lesions. In the hard palate, squamous cell carcinomas are relatively rare. By contrast, salivary

gland adenocarcinomas are relatively common in the palate. However, palatal carcinomas are commonly encountered in countries such as India, where reverse smoking is common.

Palatal squamous cell carcinomas generally present as asymptomatic red or white plaques or as ulcerated and keratotic masses (adenocarcinomas initially appear as nonulcerated masses) (Figure 2-63). Metastasis to cervical nodes or large lesions signify an ominous course (Figure 2-64).

Histopathology. Most oral squamous cell carcinomas are moderately or well-differentiated lesions (Figures 2-65 and 2-66). Keratin pearls and individual cell keratinization are usually evident. Invasion into subjacent structures in the form of small nests of hyperchromatic cells is also typical. In situ carcinoma

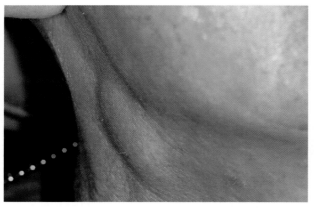

Figure 2-64   **Metastasis of squamous cell carcinoma** of the tongue to a submandibular lymph node.

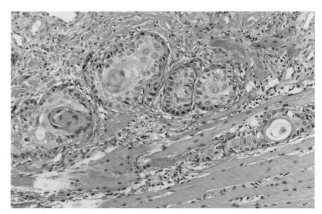

Figure 2-66   **Squamous cell carcinoma** showing tumor nest invading skeletal muscle.

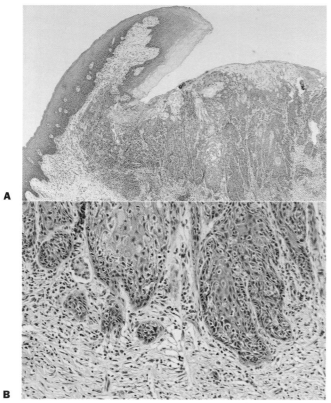

Figure 2-65   A and **B, Squamous cell carcinoma** of the tongue.

extension into salivary excretory ducts can be regarded as a high-risk microscopic indicator of potential recurrence. Considerable variation between tumors is seen relative to the numbers of mitoses, nuclear pleomorphism, and the amount of kera-tinization. In hematoxylin and eosin–stained sections of poorly differentiated lesions, keratin is absent or is seen in minute amounts. It can, however, be identified using immunohistochemical techniques for the demonstration of antigenic determinants on otherwise occult keratin intermediate filaments. A significant inflammatory host response is usually found surrounding the nests of invading tumor cells. Lymphocytes, plasma cells, and macrophages may all be seen in large numbers.

Rarely, an oral squamous cell carcinoma appears as a proliferation of spindle cells that may be mistaken for a sarcoma. This type of tumor, known as *spindle cell carcinoma* or sarcomatoid carcinoma, arises from the surface epithelium, usually of the lips and occasionally of the tongue. Immunohistochemical staining can be used to identify keratin antigens in this lesion when hematoxylin and eosin–stained sections show equivocal findings (Figure 2-67).

Verrucous carcinoma is characterized by very well differentiated epithelial cells that appear more hyperplastic than neoplastic. A key feature is the invasive nature of the lesion in the form of broad, pushing margins. The advancing front is usually surrounded by lymphocytes, plasma cells, and macrophages. Diagnosis based solely on microscopic features is often difficult; it is frequently necessary to consider the lesion in the context of clinical presentation.

Another microscopic variant that has a predilection for the base of the tongue and pharynx is biologically highly malignant and is known as *basaloid-squamous carcinoma*. In these tumors a basaloid pattern of tumor cells is seen adjacent to tumor cells that exhibit squamous differentiation. This tumor

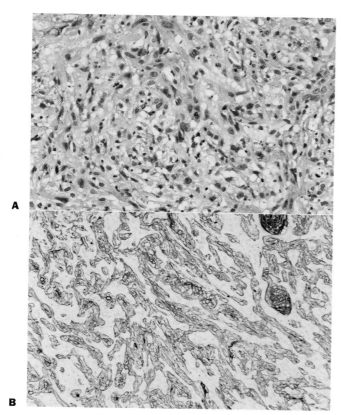

Figure 2-67 **A, Spindle cell squamous cell carcinoma. B,** Immunohistochemical stain for keratins showing positive staining of tumor cells.

may be confused microscopically with basaloid adenoid cystic carcinoma and adenosquamous carcinoma.

Differential Diagnosis. When oral squamous cell carcinomas present in their typical clinical form of chronic, nonhealing ulcers, other ulcerative conditions should be considered. An undiagnosed chronic ulcer must always be considered potentially infectious until biopsy findings prove otherwise. It may be impossible on clinical grounds to separate TB, syphilis, and deep fungal infections expressing oral manifestations from oral cancer. Chronic trauma, including factitial injuries, may also mimic squamous cell carcinoma. Careful history taking is especially important, and biopsy findings confirm the diagnosis. In the palate and contiguous tissues, midline granuloma and necrotizing sialometaplasia would be serious diagnostic considerations.

Surgical Management of Squamous Cell Carcinoma of the Oral Cavity (Eric Carlson, DMD, MD). General clinical experience with patients with squamous cell carcinoma of the oral cavity

shows that they most commonly present with one of the four following clinical scenarios: early disease (T_{1-2}, N_0), locally advanced disease (T_{3-4}, N_0), locally and regionally advanced disease (T_4, N_{1-2}), or nonresectable disease. Treatment of resectable squamous cell carcinoma of the oral cavity is based on the location and stage of the primary tumor. As such, local surgery of the primary tumor, as well as regional surgery of the neck nodes, is considered and individually planned for each patient. Local surgery of the primary tumor must consider the removal of soft tissue and bone, as indicated. The removal of the cancer in soft tissue is referred to as a *wide local excision*, incorporating a 1.0- to 1.5-cm linear margin of clinically normal appearing soft tissue at the periphery of the specimen. A partial glossectomy, or hemiglossectomy, is a specific type of wide local excision indicated for the management of malignant disease of the tongue. The removal of squamous cell carcinoma in bone is referred to as a *resection*, incorporating a 2-cm linear margin of radiographically normal appearing bone at the periphery of the specimen. Mandibular resections are subclassified as *marginal resections* whereby the inferior border of the mandible is preserved, or as *segmental resections* whereby the full height of the mandible is sacrificed, thereby creating a defect in continuity of the mandible. Disarticulation resections are a variant of segmental mandibular resection whereby the tempor mandibular joint is sacrificed. A *composite resection* is a commonly performed ablative surgery for oral squamous cell carcinoma and includes the sacrifice of hard and soft tissue. Typically, composite resections include a monobloc sacrifice of neck nodes, the mandible, and the soft tissues corresponding to the primary tumor in the tongue or floor of mouth, for example (Figure 2-68).

Management of the neck is perhaps one of the most interesting and controversial aspects of the surgical management of oral squamous cell carcinoma. Neck dissections are performed in one of three instances. The first is where palpable cervical lymphadenopathy exists. A neck examination must be performed before an incisional biopsy of a suspicious oral lesion is performed. This examination of the neck is one part of tumor, node, metastasis (TNM) staging and is performed even before a definitive diagnosis of squamous cell carcinoma is established. The N stage is entirely clinically based, and the TNM classification is not modified if computed tomography (CT) scan findings contradict the clinical examination.

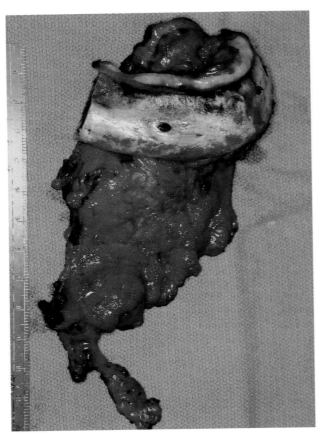

Figure 2-68 Composite resection performed for T_4, N_0, M_0 squamous cell carcinoma of the anterior floor of the mouth. The specimen consists of a monobloc resection of the floor of the mouth, mandible, and ipsilateral neck nodes.

The second indication for neck dissection includes positive lymphadenopathy divulged by special imaging studies (CT or magnetic resonance imaging [MRI]). It is possible that a clinical examination may result in an N_0 classification, whereas the patient's imaging study may reveal enlarged lymph nodes with hypodense (necrotic) centers, likely indicative of metastatic squamous cell carcinoma. This scenario may occur in obese patients whose clinical neck examinations are unreliable. Nonetheless, under such circumstances, the neck staging remains N_0, and a neck dissection is indicated.

The third, and most thought-provoking, indication for neck dissection is the management of the neck when lymphadenopathy is not apparent. *Occult neck disease* is defined as cancer present in lymph nodes in the neck that cannot be palpated clinically. As such,

these neck dissections are performed for N_0 disease. Numerous studies have examined the likelihood of occult neck disease as a function of the anatomic site of the primary cancer, as well as a function of its size and thickness. What is clear from these studies is that early squamous cell carcinoma of the oral tongue (T_{1-2}, N_0) may be associated with occult neck disease in nearly 40% of cases. This is the reason why many surgeons advocate performing a neck dissection for early squamous cell carcinoma of the tongue. Early disease of the floor of the mouth (followed by disease of the buccal mucosa, maxillary gingiva, mandibular gingiva, and lip) carries a quantitatively lower, yet significant, risk of occult neck disease. Therefore prophylactic neck dissections play an important role in the management of many early squamous cell carcinomas of the oral cavity.

Neck dissections may be classified as comprehensive or selective. *Comprehensive neck dissections* include radical neck dissection and modified radical neck dissection. Both are performed when patients present with palpable (N+) cervical lymphadenopathy in the neck. By definition, radical neck dissection removes lymph nodes in oncologic levels I to V of the neck (Figure 2-69), along with the sternocleidomastoid muscle, the internal jugular vein, and the spinal accessory nerve. Owing to the observation that the spinal accessory nerve is rarely involved in the cancer, the more commonly performed modified radical neck dissection (MRND) is described. MRND sacrifices lymph nodes in levels I to V, yet preserves the sternocleidomastoid muscle or internal jugular vein, or commonly, the spinal accessory nerve. Type 1 MRND preserves the spinal accessory nerve while sacrificing all of the afore mentioned structures (Figure 2-70).

Selective neck dissections, most commonly performed for the N_0 neck, sacrifice lymph nodes exclusively. By definition, then, the sternocleidomastoid muscle, internal jugular vein, and spinal accessory nerve are intentionally preserved. Supraomohyoid neck dissection is the most common type of selective neck dissection and removes lymph node levels I to III (Figure 2-71). This neck dissection, therefore, is indicated when managing the N_0 neck with a high likelihood of occult neck disease.

The surgical management of squamous cell carcinoma ultimately is based on decision making for optimal control of local disease while also addressing existing or potential lymph node drainage in the neck. The use of radiation therapy often plays a role in the sole management of squamous cell carcinoma of the

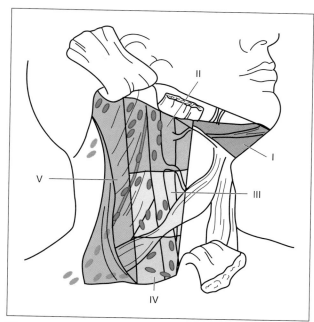

Figure 2-69 The oncologic lymph node levels of the neck. Level I = submental/submandibular nodes; level II = upper jugular nodes; level III = middle jugular nodes; level IV = lower jugular nodes; level V = posterior triangle nodes.

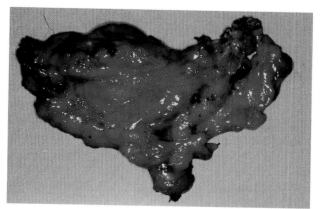

Figure 2-71 Specimen from a supraomohyoid dissection.

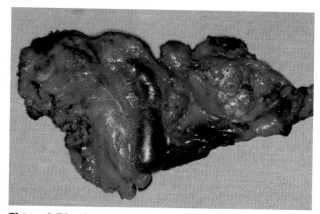

Figure 2-70 Specimen from a type 1 modified radical neck dissection. The internal jugular vein is noted on the medial aspect of the sternocleidomastoid muscle. The spinal accessory innervation of the trapezius muscle remains intact in this type of neck dissection.

oral cavity, with or without chemotherapy, or as an adjunct in the postoperative phase. It is sound practice that the administration of radiation therapy should be planned after a thorough review of the patient's histopathology. General indications for the postoperative administration of radiation therapy include the following:

- Positive soft tissue margin
- More than one positive lymph node without extra-capsular invasion
- One or more lymph nodes with extracapsular invasion
- Bone invasion by the cancer, even with negative bone margins
- Perineural invasion in the specimen
- The presence of comorbid immunosuppressive disease, such as HIV/AIDS

This approach represents a departure from the previously accepted dogma that radiation therapy is administered to most, if not all, postoperative patients. Therefore surgery and radiation therapy are tailored to each patient's specific cancer, rather than treating all patients in a similar fashion. Unfortunately, despite numerous refinements in surgery and radiation therapy, the 5-year survival rate of 50% for all patients with squamous cell carcinoma (including all sites and stages) has not improved in the past 50 years.

Radiotherapy Management of Squamous Cell Carcinoma of the Oral Cavity (John Kim, MD)

Clinical Evaluation and Staging. Patients with biopsy-proven squamous cell carcinoma of the oral cavity should undergo a complete history and physical examination. The clinical examination includes indirect mirror laryngoscopy and/or direct flexible fiberoptic laryngoscopy to rule out synchronous head and neck primary cancers and to assess the airway of patients with large tumors. The primary site and regional lymph nodes are imaged with a CT scan and/or an MRI scan. Positron emission tomography (PET) scanning may help identify occult metastases. PET scanning is not yet widely available, and its role in routine clinical practice is being evaluated. A dental panoramic film is obtained to assess dental status, as well as assess possible mandibular involvement of oral cavity tumors. Other staging investigations include blood work (complete blood count, electrolytes, renal function, liver enzymes, and baseline thyroid function studies for radiotherapy patients) and a chest x-ray film or CT scan of the thorax. Patients with advanced disease may undergo a bone scan and a CT scan or ultrasound examination of the liver.

Patients are staged according to the American Joint Committee on Cancer (AJCC) *Cancer Staging Manual* or the International Union Against Cancer (UICC) Classification of Malignant Tumors. Radiotherapy patients require a pretreatment dental consultation whether they are dentulous or edentulous. The attending dentist should have knowledge of the radiotherapy fields and high-dose radiotherapy volumes. Some patients will require pretreatment dental extractions within the high-dose radiother-apy treatment volumes. Teeth that are loose or periodontally involved, those with large or unrestorable caries or apical pathology, or those that are im-pacted should be extracted before radiation therapy. Any questionable tooth should be extracted and not be given the benefit of the doubt, since osteoradionecrosis poses a serious problem for the patient.

Routine dental procedures should also take place before treatment. Fluoride carrier trays are constructed for dentate patients for the daily application of neutral pH topical fluoride, which continues for the remainder of the patient's life. Patients are also educated on the importance of maintaining meticulous dental hygiene, which is essential to minimize the risks of increased rates of dental caries in xerostomic (dry mouth) patients and osteoradionecrosis of the mandible following radiotherapy.

Primary Radiotherapy. External-beam radiotherapy (EBRT) is delivered with external beams of photons—alone or in combination with external electron beams. Usually, multiple treatment fields (or portals) are employed. The principle of EBRT is to encompass the gross oral cavity (primary) disease and a surrounding tissue margin. This additional margin allows for the inclusion of potential local microscopic spread of

cancer, day-to-day variation of treatment setup, patient movement, organ movement (e.g., swallowing), and buildup of the radiation dose at the edge of the radiation beam (penumbra). Patient movement is minimized with the use of immobilization devices. All patients undergoing head and neck irradiation are immobilized with a neck rest and plastic mask (Figure 2-72) or bite block device. Regional lymph nodes (primary echelon lymph nodes) at risk for harboring microscopic or occult disease are usually included in the radiotherapy fields, even for patients who present with clinical N_0 necks. One study demonstrated a 49% risk of occult nodal metastases in patients with clinical T_{1-3}, N_0 carcinomas of the oral cavity who underwent elective neck dissections. Ipsilateral levels I and II are at highest risk for occult metastases (see description of oncologic node region levels elsewhere in this chapter). Midline lesions are at higher risk for bilateral occult nodal metastases than unilateral lesions. Areas of potential occult disease are usually treated to a lower dose than gross disease. Gross nodal disease is usually treated to the same dose as the primary oral cavity cancer.

Radiotherapy side effects result from irradiation of normal tissues that cannot be excluded from the treatment portal. For all or part of the treatment, some critical normal tissues may be excluded from one or more of the radiation fields by the use of shielding or beam-shaping devices introduced in the radiation beam. Normal structures can also be avoided by using beam geometries that avoid critical structures completely from one or more of the radiation fields. For example, ipsilateral EBRT techniques can be used to avoid the contralateral parotid and preserve salivary function following radiotherapy. CT-based radiotherapy planning systems allow for more accurate identification of gross disease and normal structures (Figure 2-73). Conformal radiotherapy techniques such as three-dimensional planning, stereotactic radiotherapy, and intensity-modulated radiotherapy (IMRT) may offer better tumor coverage and sparing of normal tissues. A full discussion of conformal radiotherapy is beyond the scope of this section.

Brachytherapy is a treatment method that delivers very high but localized radiation doses. It involves the placement of radioactive sources in the tumor bed. A type of brachytherapy called interstitial implant or interstitial radiotherapy (ISRT) can be used to treat oral cavity carcinomas of the floor of the mouth or tongue—alone or in combination with EBRT. This technique requires a general anesthetic. One method

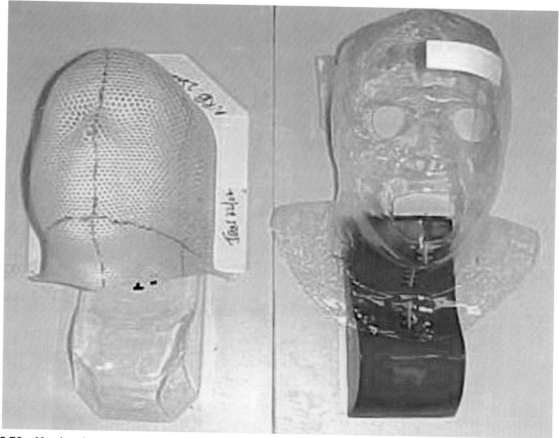

Figure 2-72 Head and neck immobilization: examples of masks with neck rests.

of ISRT involves surgically placing catheters through the tumor bed that can then be loaded with radioactive sources when the patient is transferred to a room with proper radiation protection (afterloading technique). Good 5-year local control rates ranging from 70% to 95% have been achieved for early (T_{1-2}) oral tongue lesions. Some authors advocate the importance of ISRT in the radiotherapy management of tongue lesions. However, there are risks of soft tissue necrosis and osteoradionecrosis of the mandible with this technique, which have been well described. Recommend is primary surgery for these patients because of absence of the risk of osteoradionecrosis of the mandible, good local control rates, good functional outcomes (speech and swallowing), and available surgical expertise. Primary radiotherapy for oral tongue carcinomas is an option for patients who are not candidates for primary surgery.

Some patients will not be eligible for radiotherapy. Previous high-dose head and neck radiotherapy is an absolute contraindication to radiotherapy. Relative contraindications to radiotherapy include bone or cartilage invasion, collagen vascular disorders (particularly scleroderma), previous low-dose radiotherapy, and young age.

Conventional (Standard) Dose Fractionation Schedules. A course of conventional external-beam radiotherapy is fractionated over a protracted period of time, since the dose per fraction is known to directly correlate with late normal tissue toxicity (side effects occurring after completion of radiotherapy). Standard or conventional fraction sizes range from 1.8 to 2.55 Gray (Gy) per fraction. Gross disease is treated to a total dose of 51 to 70 Gy. A common North American dose fractionation schedule delivers a total of 66 to 70 Gy in 2 Gy per fraction over 6.5 to 7 weeks, not including weekends, to gross disease, and 50 Gy in 2 Gy per fraction delivered daily over 5 weeks to a site of potential occult microscopic disease.

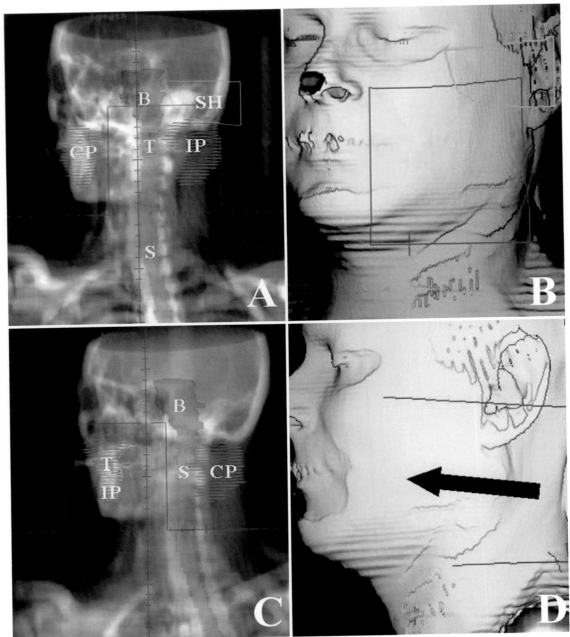

Figure 2-73   Radiotherapy plan (CT based) for a patient with an early squamous cell carcinoma of the left retromolar trigone. The two treatment portals (anterior oblique and posterior oblique) that encompass the primary lesion and the first-echelon regional lymph nodes are illustrated. *T,* Tumor; *B,* brainstem; *S,* spinal cord; *IP,* ipsilateral left parotid; *CP,* contralateral right parotid; *SH,* normal tissue shield. **A,** Anterior oblique portal outlined on a digitally reconstructed radiograph. Note that the contralateral parotid is outside of the treatment field. **B,** Anterior oblique portal outlined on a three-dimensional reconstruction of the patient. **C,** Posterior oblique portal outlined on a digitally reconstructed radiograph. Note that the contralateral parotid and spinal cord are outside of the radiotherapy field. **D,** Radiation beam orientation for posterior oblique portal on a three-dimensional reconstruction of the patient.

Nonconventional Fractionation Schedules. Hyperfractionation is a dose escalation strategy used to spare late normal tissue toxicity by decreasing the dose per fraction. The total radiotherapy dose can be increased while not increasing late toxicity. Multiple doses per day are employed so that the overall duration of treatment is not increased. Acceleration is the delivery of multiple courses of near-conventional fraction sizes, but in an overall shorter treatment period. This strategy is used to overcome the potential effects of cancer cell repopulation. The first report of a randomized clinical trial has demonstrated the benefit of hyperfractionation and an acceleration variant, known as concomitant boost, as compared with standard fractionation in head and neck squamous cell carcinoma, including locally advanced (stage III and IV) carcinomas. There was a significant improvement in local-regional control for the hyperfractionation and concomitant boost schedules as compared with the standard fractionation schedule. Two-year local-regional control rates were 54.4% (p = 0.045), 54.5% (p = 0.05), and 46%, respectively. There was a trend toward increased disease-free survival for the hyperfractionation and accelerated (concomitant boost) schedules. Others have reported improved results with nonconventional fractionation schedules.

Concurrent Chemotherapy. Individual clinical trials have produced conflicting results regarding the benefit of adding chemotherapy to radiotherapy. Despite this, recent metaanalyses of many randomized clinical trials of radiotherapy combined with neoadjuvant (before irradiation), concurrent (during irradiation), or adjuvant (after irradiation) chemotherapy have shown the most promising results for concurrent chemotherapy. An improvement in overall survival has been demonstrated for locally advanced head and neck carcinomas. Platinum-based regimens are most commonly used in the treatment of head and neck squamous cell carcinomas. Optimal doses and scheduling of chemotherapy regimens are undetermined. There are no published randomized clinical trials comparing concurrent chemotherapy with altered fractionation schedules in patents with locally advanced head and neck squamous cell carcinomas. Patients with oral cavity carcinomas comprise a minority of the studied population of head and neck cancer patients managed with either approach. Both treatment approaches may be considered for individual patients with locally advanced carcinomas of the oral cavity, particularly those who are not candidates for surgery. Both treatment strategies are associated with increased side effects.

Combined Surgery and Radiotherapy. Patients with advanced primary or regional nodal (>3 cm) disease who are treated with single-modality therapy with either conventional radiotherapy fractionation or surgery have poor local-regional control rates. Combined surgery and radiotherapy may improve local-regional control for patients who are candidates for both treatments. Planned combined therapy offers the benefit of a coordinated multidisciplinary approach between the surgeon and the radiation oncologist. An example of planned combined therapy is the integration of a neck dissection following radiotherapy for lymph nodes greater than 3 cm when the primary lesion is treated with radiation. Lymph nodes greater than 3 cm are suboptimally treated with conventional radiotherapy alone.

Adjuvant Radiotherapy. Patients treated with primary surgery may require postoperative radiotherapy. Adjuvant radiotherapy is recommended on the basis of operative or pathologic findings of the surgically removed primary lesion or regional lymph nodes. Postoperative radiotherapy is indicated for positive or close surgical resection margins, multiple positive lymph nodes, or extracapsular lymph node extension. Postoperative radiotherapy is also considered for intraoperative tumor rupture or cut-through, intraoperative revision of initially positive margins, the presence of perineural invasion, and when there has been a preoperative incisional biopsy of the neck. Patients with large nodes (>3 cm) and advanced primary lesions with cortical bone, skin, or muscle involvement may be managed with planned combined therapy (see Combined Surgery and Radiotherapy). Preoperative radiotherapy indications are similar to those for postoperative radiotherapy.

Palliative Radiotherapy. Patients who are not candidates for curative therapies either because of very advanced incurable cancers, significant comorbid illnesses, or patient refusal of surgery may be candidates for palliative radiotherapy. The objective of treatment should be to alleviate symptoms such as pain, obstruction, or bleeding.

Therapeutic Radiation Complications. Along with the therapeutic effects of radiation are side effects that are dose dependent (Box 2-15). Some of these are reversible, whereas others are not (Figures 2-74 to 2-77). Radiation-induced mucositis and ulcers and the

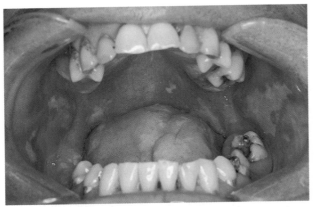

Figure 2-74   Radiation mucositis. Note erythema and multiple mucosal ulcers.

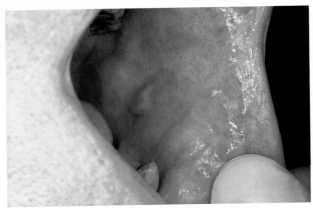

Figure 2-76   Postradiation telangiectasias in buccal mucosa.

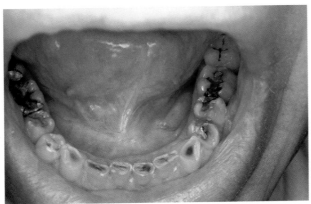

Figure 2-75   Postradiation scar in the floor of the mouth, the site of the patient's primary squamous cell carcinoma.

Box 2-15 Therapeutic Radiation Side Effects

TEMPORARY

Mucosal ulcers/mucositis
Pain
Taste alterations
Candidiasis
Dermatitis
Erythema
Focal alopecia

PERMANENT

Xerostomia
Cervical caries
Osteoradionecrosis
Telangiectasias
Epithelial atrophy
Focal alopecia
Focal hyperpigmentation

---

accompanying pain, xerostomia, loss of taste, and dysgeusia are common side effects. Radiation mucositis is a reversible condition that begins 1 to 2 weeks after the start of therapy and ends several weeks after the termination of therapy. Oral candidiasis often accompanies the mucositis. Use of antifungals, chlorhexidine rinses, or salt-soda rinses helps reduce morbidity.

Permanent damage to salivary gland tissue situated in the beam path may produce significant levels of xerostomia. Some recovery is often noted, especially at lower radiation levels. Xerostomia is frequently a patient's chief complaint during the postradiation period. The frequent use of water or artificial saliva is of minimal benefit to these patients. Pilocarpine, used during the course of radiation, may provide some protective measure of salivary function. With the dryness

also comes the potential for the development of cervical, or so-called radiation, caries. This problem can be minimized with regular follow-up dental care and scrupulous oral hygiene. Custom-fitted soft trays are made for the fully or partially dentate patient to permit the nightly application of neutral pH fluoride directly to the teeth. This treatment is initiated at the start of cancer treatment and continues for the remainder of the patient's life. It has been shown to significantly reduce the incidence of cervical caries and thereby the need for future dental extractions.

Skin in the path of the radiation beam also suffers some damage. Alopecia is temporary at lower

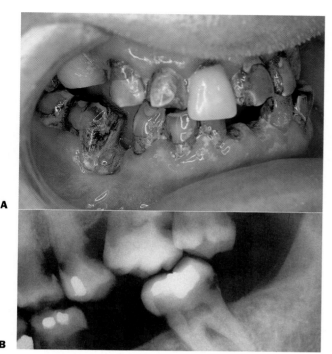

A

B

Figure 2-77 A and B, **Radiation-associated cervical caries**.

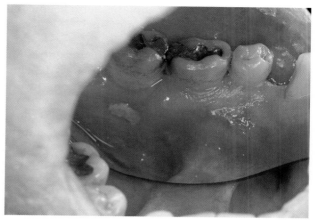

Figure 2-78 **Osteoradionecrosis** of the lingual mandible precipitated by trauma.

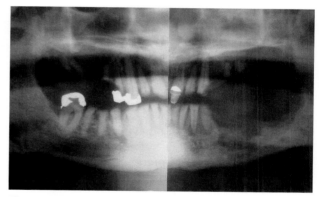

Figure 2-79 **Osteoradionecrosis** of the mandible.

radiation levels but permanent at the higher levels required in the treatment of squamous cell carcinoma. Skin erythema is temporary, but the telangiectasias and atrophy that follow are permanent. Cutaneous pigmentation in the line of therapy is also a late complication, and it, too, may be permanent.

A more insidious problem lies in the damage that radiation causes to bone, which may result in osteonecrosis (Figures 2-78 and 2-79). Radiation apparently has deleterious effects on osteocytes, osteoblasts, and endothelial cells, causing reduced capacity of bone to recover from injury. Injury may come in the form of trauma (such as extractions), advancing periodontal disease, and periapical inflammation associated with nonvital teeth. Once osteonecrosis occurs, varying amounts of bone (usually in the mandible) are lost. This may be an area as small as a few millimeters in size to as large as half the jaw or more. The most important factor responsible for osteonecrosis is the amount of radiation directed through bone on the path to the tumor. Oral health is also of considerable significance. Poor nutrition and chronic alcoholism appear to be influential in the progression of this complication. Conservative surgical removal of necrotic bone may assist in the healing

process. Also, if available, the use of a hyperbaric oxygen chamber may provide the patients with a healing advantage.

Because osteonecrosis is a danger that is always present after radiation, tooth extractions should be avoided after therapy. If absolutely necessary, tooth removal should be performed as atraumatically as possible, using antibiotic coverage. It is preferable to commit to a treatment plan that schedules tooth removal before radiation therapy begins. Initial soft tissue healing before therapy is begun reduces the risk of nonhealing of the extraction sites. Prosthetic devices such as dentures and partial dentures, if carefully constructed and monitored, can be worn without difficulty. Xerostomia does not seem to cause difficulty in the wearing of these prostheses. Continued careful surveillance of the patient's oral health, during and after radiation therapy, helps keep complications to an acceptable minimum.

Prognosis. Similar to other cancers, the prognosis for patients with oral squamous cell carcinoma is dependent on both the histologic subtype (grade) and the clinical extent (stage) of the tumor. Of the two, the clinical stage is significantly more important. Other, more abstract factors that may influence the clinical course include the patient's age, gender, general health, immune system status, and mental attitude.

The grading of a tumor is the microscopic determination of the level of differentiation of the tumor cells. Well-differentiated lesions generally have a less aggressive biologic course than poorly differentiated lesions. Of all squamous cell carcinoma histologic subtypes, the most well differentiated lesion, verrucous carcinoma, has the most favorable prognosis. The less-differentiated lesions have a correspondingly poorer prognosis.

The most important indicator of prognosis is the clinical stage of the disease. Once metastasis to cervical nodes has occurred, the 5-year survival rate is reduced by approximately half. The overall 5-year survival rate for oral squamous cell carcinoma ranges from 45% to 50%. If the neoplasm is small and localized, the 5-year cure rate may be as high as 60% to 70% (lower lip lesions may rate as high as 90%). However, if cervical metastases are present at the time of diagnosis, the survival figures drop precipitously to about 25%.

The TNM system mentioned earlier for the clinical staging of oral squamous cell carcinoma was devised to provide clinical uniformity. T is a measure of the primary tumor size, N is an estimation of the regional lymph node metastasis, and M is a determination of distant metastases (Box 2-16; Figure 2-80). Use of this system allows more meaningful comparison of data from different institutions and helps guide therapeutic decisions. As the clinical stage advances from I to IV, the prognosis worsens (Table 2-6).

Another factor that comes into play in the overall prognosis of oral cancer is the increased risk for the development of a second primary lesion. The risk of a second primary lesion in the head and neck region or upper airways is about 5% per year for the first 7 years following the initial tumor. The mechanism for this finding is not entirely known. It was thought for several decades that the mucosa lining the entire mouth and upper aerodigestive tract was exposed to similar carcinogens from tobacco and alcohol and was in effect "condemned mucosa." This so-called field canceriza-

TABLE 2-6　TNM Clinical Staging of Oral Squamous Cell Carcinoma

Stage	TNM Designation
I	T_1, N_0, M_0
II	T_2, N_0, M_0
III	T_3, N_0, M_0
	T_{1-3}, N_1, M_0
IV	T_4, N_0, M_0
	T_4, N_1, M_0
	T_{any}, N_{2-3}, M_0
	T_{any}, N_{any}, M_1

Box 2-16 TNM Clinical Staging System for Oral Squamous Cell Carcinoma

T—TUMOR

T_1—tumor < 2 cm
T_2—tumor 2 to 4 cm
T_3—tumor > 4 cm
T_4—tumor invades deep subjacent structures

N—NODES

N_0—no palpable nodes
N_1—single ipsilateral node ≤ 3 cm
N_{2A}—single ipsilateral node 3 to 6 cm
N_{2B}—multiple ipsilateral nodes ≤ 6 cm
N_{2C}—contralateral or bilateral nodes ≤ 6 cm
N_3—node > 6 cm

M—METASTASIS

M_0—no distant metastasis
M_1—distant metastasis

---

tion theory was used to explain the relatively high incidence of new primary tumors in patients who had oral or oropharyngeal cancer. Recently the field cancerization theory has been called into question with the finding that many second primary lesions, including some at unusual anatomic sites in the head and neck and lungs of patients with a history of oral cancer, are genetically very similar, if not identical, to the original tumor. This suggests that these second tumors may not in fact represent a new malignancy but, rather, a metastasis or recurrence of the original tumor elsewhere. Since many of the second tumors develop in sites not normally connected anatomically to the primary tumor by known lymphatic pathways, it has been proposed that there is intraepithelial migration of malignant cells. It is not yet clear which scenario is correct or if indeed both mechanisms occur in dif-

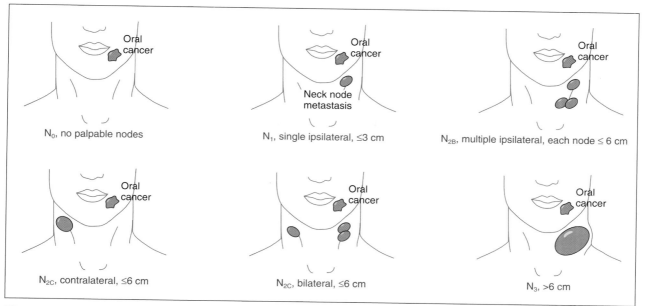

Figure 2-80 Lymph nodes in TNM staging (N_{2A}, single ipsilateral node 3 to 6 cm).

ferent settings. It is perhaps more likely that in some patients secondary lesions do represent new primary tumors, but in others the secondary tumors may represent recurrent or metastatic disease.

Carcinoma of the Maxillary Sinus

Etiology. Malignancies of the paranasal sinuses occur most commonly in the maxillary sinus. The cause is unknown, although squamous metaplasia of sinus epithelium associated with chronic sinusitis and oral antral fistulas is believed by some investigators to be a predisposing factor.

Clinical Features. This is a disease of older age, affecting predominantly patients older than age 40. Men are generally afflicted more than women. Past history in these patients frequently includes symptoms of sinusitis. As the neoplasm progresses, a dull ache in the area occurs, with eventual development of overt pain. Specific signs and symptoms referable to oral structures are common, especially when the neoplasm has its origin in the sinus floor. As the neoplasm extends toward the apices of the maxillary posterior teeth, referred pain may occur. Toothache, which actually represents neoplastic involvement of the superior alveolar nerve, is not an uncommon symptom in patients with maxillary sinus malignancies. In ruling out dental disease by history and clinical tests, it is imperative that the dental practitioner be aware that sinus neo-plasms may present through the alveolus. Without this suspicion, unfortunate delays in definitive treatment may occur. Other clinical signs of invasion of the alveolar process include recently acquired malocclusion, displacement of teeth, and vertical mobility of teeth (teeth undermined by neoplasm). Failure of a socket to heal after an extraction may be indicative of tumor involvement. Paresthesia should always be viewed as an ominous sign and should cause the clinician to consider intraosseous malignancy. Occasional maxillary sinus cancers may present as a palatal ulcer and mass representing extension through the bone and soft tissue of the palate (Figures 2-81 and 2-82).

Histopathology. Of the malignancies that originate in the maxillary sinus, squamous cell carcinoma is the most common histologic type. These lesions are generally less differentiated than those occurring in oral mucous membranes. Infrequently, adenocarcinomas arising presumably from mucous glands in the sinus lining may be seen.

Diagnosis. From a clinical standpoint, when oral signs and symptoms appear to be related to antral carcinoma, a dental origin must be ruled out. This is best accomplished by the dental practitioner because of familiarity with normal tooth-jaw relationships and experience in interpretation of vitality tests. Other clinical considerations related to malignancies in the age-group in which antral carcinomas occur

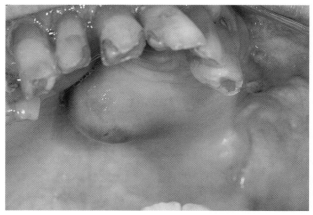

Figure 2-81   **Carcinoma of the maxillary sinus** presenting through the palate.

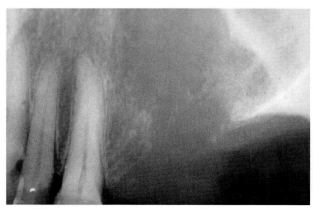

Figure 2-82   **Carcinoma of the maxillary sinus** producing ill-defined maxillary radiolucency.

are metastatic disease and plasma cell myeloma. Osteosarcoma and other, less common sarcomas that are usually found in a younger age-group might also be included. Palatal involvement should also cause the clinician to consider adenocarcinoma of minor salivary gland origin, lymphoma, and squamous cell carcinoma.

Treatment and Prognosis.   Maxillary sinus carcinomas are generally treated with surgery or radiation or both. A combination of the two seems to be somewhat more effective than either modality alone. Radiation is often completed first, with surgical resection following. Chemotherapy used in conjunction with radiation has been somewhat successful.

In any event, the prognosis is only fair at best. Cure is directly dependent on the clinical stage of the disease at the time of initial treatment. Compared with oral lesions, sinus lesions are discovered in a more advanced stage because of delays in seeking treatment and delays in making a definitive diagnosis. The anatomy of the area also influences the prognosis. The 5-year survival rate is about 25%. If the disease is discovered early, the likelihood of survival increases.

BIBLIOGRAPHY

INFECTIOUS DISEASES

Centers for Disease Control: Summaries of notifiable diseases in the United States, *MMWR* 39:10, 1991.

Enwonwu CO, Falkler WA, Idibge EO, et al: Noma (cancrum oris): questions and answers, *Oral Dis* 5:144-149, 1999.

Frieden TR, Sterling T, Pablos-Mendez A, et al: The emergence of drug-resistant tuberculosis in New York City, *N Engl J Med* 328:521-532, 1993.

Gobel M, Iseman MD, Madsen LA: Treatment of 171 patients with pulmonary tuberculosis resistant to isoniazid and rifampin, *N Engl J Med* 328:527-532, 1993.

Morbidity and mortality report, Centers for Disease Control: Congenital syphilis—New York City, 1986-1988, *Arch Dermatol* 126:288-289, 1990.

IMMUNOLOGIC DISEASES

Alpsoy E, Yilmaz E, Basaran E: Interferon therapy for Behçet's disease, *J Am Acad Dermatol* 31:617-619, 1994.

Aslanzadeh J, Heim K, Espy M, et al: Detection of HSV-specific DNA in biopsy tissue of patients with erythema multiforme by polymerase chain reaction, *Br J Dermatol* 126:19-23, 1992.

Devaney K, Travis W, Hoffman G, et al: Interpretation of head and neck biopsies in Wegener's granulomatosis, *Am J Surg Pathol* 14:555-564, 1990.

Hamuryudan V, Yurdakul S, Serdaroglu S, et al: Topical alpha interferon in the treatment of oral ulcers in Behçet's syndrome: a preliminary report, *Clin Exp Rheumatol* 8:51-54, 1990.

Hoffman G, Kerr G, Leavitt R, et al: Wegener's granulomatosis: an analysis of 158 patients, *Ann Intern Med* 116:488-498, 1992.

Kallenberg CG: Antineutrophil cytoplasmic antibodies (ANCA) and vasculitis, *Clin Rheumatol* 9(suppl):132-135, 1990.

Khandwala A, VanInwegen RG, Alfano MC: 5% amlexanox oral paste, a new treatment for recurrent minor aphthous ulcers. I. Clinical demonstration of acceleration of wound healing and resolution of pain, *Oral Surg Oral Med Oral Pathol Oral Radiol Endod* 83:222-230, 1997.

Landesberg R, Fallon M, Insel R: Alterations of T helper/inducer and T suppressor/inducer cells in patients with recurrent aphthous ulcers, *Oral Surg Oral Med Oral Pathol* 69:205-208, 1990.

Lo Muzio L, della Valle A, Mignogna MD, et al: The treatment of oral aphthous ulceration or erosive lichen planus with topical clobetasol propionate in three preparations: a clinical and pilot study on 54 patients, *J Oral Pathol Med* 30:611-617, 2001.

Lozada-Nur F, Miranda C, Maliksi R: Double-blind clinical trial of 0.05% clobetasol proprionate ointment in orabase and 0.05% fluocinonide ointment in orabase in the treatment of patients with oral vesiculoerosive diseases, *Oral Surg Oral Med Oral Pathol* 77:598-604, 1994.

MacPhail L, Greenspan D, Feigal D, et al: Recurrent aphthous ulcers in association with HIV infection, *Oral Surg Oral Med Oral Pathol* 71:678-683, 1991.

Miller R, Gould A, Bernstein M: Cinnamon-induced stomatitis venenata, *Oral Surg Oral Med Oral Pathol* 73:708-716, 1992.

O'Duffy J: Behçet's syndrome, *N Engl J Med* 323:326-327, 1990.

Orme R, Nordlund J, Barich L, et al: The MAGIC syndrome (mouth and genital ulcers with inflamed cartilage), *Arch Dermatol* 126: 940-944, 1990.

Pedersen A: Recurrent aphthous ulceration: virologic and immunologic aspects, *APMIS Suppl* 37:1-37, 1993.

Phelan J, Eisig S, Freedman P, et al: Major aphthous-like ulcers in patients with AIDS, *Oral Surg Oral Med Oral Pathol* 71:68-72, 1991.

Plemons J, Rees T, Zachariah N: Absorption of a topical steroid and evaluation of adrenal suppression in patients with erosive lichen planus, *Oral Surg Oral Med Oral Pathol* 69:688-693, 1990.

Ship JA: Recurrent aphthous stomatitis: an update, *Oral Surg Oral Med Oral Pathol Oral Radiol Endod* 81:141-147, 1996.

NEOPLASMS

Bartek J, Lukas J, Bartkova J: Perspective: defects in cell cycle control and cancer, *J Pathol* 187:95-99, 1999.

Bartkova J, Kukas J, Muller H, et al: Abnormal patterns of D-type cyclin expression and G1 regulation in human head and neck cancer, *Cancer Res* 55:949-956, 1995.

Bourhis J, Pignon JP: Meta-analyses in head and neck squamous cell carcinoma: what is the role of chemotherapy? *Hematol Oncol Clin North Am* 13:769-775, 1999.

Brennan JA, Boyle JO, Koch WM, et al: Association between cigarette smoking and mutation of the p53 gene in squamous cell carcinoma of the head and neck, *N Engl J Med* 332:712-717, 1995.

Chu PG, Weiss LM: Keratin expression in human tissues and neoplasms, *Histopathology* 40:403-439, 2002.

Curran S, Murray GI: Matrix metalloproteinases in tumor invasion and metastasis, *J Pathol* 189:300-308, 1999.

Curtis RE, Rowlings PA, Deeg HJ, et al: *N Engl J Med* 336:897-904, 1997.

Daley TD, Lovas JG, Peters E, et al: Salivary gland duct involvement in oral epithelial dysplasia and squamous cell carcinoma, *Oral Surg Oral Med Oral Pathol Oral Radiol Endod* 81:186-192, 1996.

Downey MG, Going JJ, Stuart RC, et al: Expression of telomerase RNA in esophageal and oral cancer, *J Oral Pathol Med* 30:577-581, 2001.

Ferlito A, Shaha AR, Rinaldo A: The incidence of lymph node micrometastases in patients pathologically staged N0 in cancer or oral cavity and oropharynx, *Oral Oncol* 38:3-5, 2002.

Ferretti G, Raybould T, Brown A, et al: Chlorhexidine prophylaxis for chemotherapy and radiotherapy-induced stomatitis: a randomized double-blind trial, *Oral Surg Oral Med Oral Pathol* 69:331-338, 1990.

Field JK: Oncogenes and tumor suppressor genes in squamous cell carcinoma of the head and neck, *Eur J Cancer B Oral Oncol* 28B:667-676, 1992.

Flaitz CM, Nichols CM, Adler-Storthz K, et al: Intraoral squamous cell carcinoma in human immunodeficiency virus infection, *Oral Surg Oral Med Oral Pathol Oral Radiol Endod* 80:55-62, 1995.

Franceschi S, Gloghini A, Maestro R, et al: Analysis of the p53 gene in relation to tobacco and alcohol in cancers of the upper aero-digestive tract, *Int J Cancer* 60:872-876, 1995.

Fu KK, Pajak TF, Trotti A, et al: A Radiation Therapy Oncology Group (RTOG) phase III randomized study to compare hyper-fractionation and two variants of accelerated fractionation to standard fractionation radiotherapy for head and neck squamous cell carcinomas: first report of RTOG 9003, *Int J Radiat Oncol Biol Phys* 48:7-16, 2000.

Fujita M, Hirokawa Y, Kashiwado K, et al: An analysis of mandibular bone complications in radiotherapy for T1 and T2 carcinoma of the oral tongue, *Int J Radiat Oncol Biol Phys* 34:333-339, 1996.

Ghali GE, Li BDL, Minnard EA: Management of the neck relative to oral malignancy, *Selected Readings in Oral and Maxillofacial Surgery* 6:1-36, 2000.

Gopalakrisnan R, Weghorst CM, Lehman TA, et al: Mutated and wild-type p53 expression and HPV integration in proliferative verrucous leukoplakia and oral squamous cell carcinoma, *Oral Surg Oral Med Oral Pathol Oral Radiol Endod* 83:471-477, 1997.

Gstaiger M, Jordan RCK, Lim MS, et al: The F-box protein Skp2 is the product of an oncogene and is overexpressed in human cancers, *Proc Natl Acad Sci USA* 98:5043-5048, 2001.

Holley SL, Parkes G, Matthhias C, et al: Cyclin D1 polymorphism and expression in patients with squamous cell carcinoma of the head and neck, *Am J Pathol* 159:1917-1924, 2001.

Horiot JC, Bontemps P, van den Bogaert W, et al: Accelerated fractionation (AF) compared to conventional fractionation (CF) improves loco-regional control in the radiotherapy of advanced head and neck cancers: results of the EORTC 22851 randomized trial, *Radiother Oncol* 44:111-121, 1997.

Inoue T, Inoue T, Yoshida K, et al: Phase III trial of high-vs. low-dose-rate interstitial radiotherapy for early mobile tongue cancer, *Int J Radiat Oncol Biol Phys* 51:171-175, 2001.

Johansson N, Airola K, Grenman R, et al: Expression of collagenase-3 (matrix metalloproteinase-13) in squamous cell carcinomas of the head and neck, *Am J Pathol* 151:499-508, 1997.

Jones J, Watt FM, Speight PM: Changes in the expression of alpha-V integrins in oral squamous cell carcinomas, *J Oral Pathol Med* 26:63-68, 1997.

Jordan RCK, Bradley G, Slingerland J: Reduced levels of the cell cycle inhibitor p27[kip1] in epithelial dysplasia and carcinoma of the oral cavity, *Am J Pathol* 152:585-590, 1998.

Ke LD, Adler-Storthz K, Clayman GL, et al: Differential expression of epidermal growth factor receptor in human head and neck cancers, *Head Neck* 20:320-327, 1998.

Kropveld A, van Mansfeld AD, Nabben N, et al: Discordance of p53 status in matched primary tumors and metastases in head and neck squamous cell carcinoma patients, *Eur J Cancer B Oral Oncol* 32B:388-393, 1996.

Lazarus P, Stern J, Zwiebel N, et al: Relationship between p53 mutation incidence in oral cavity squamous cell carcinomas and patient tobacco use, *Carcinogenesis* 17:733-739, 1996.

Leong PP, Rezai B, Koch WM, et al: Distinguishing second primary tumors from lung metastases in patients with head and neck squamous cell carcinoma, *J Natl Cancer Inst* 90(13):972-977, 1998.

Matsuura K, Hirokawa Y, Fujita M, et al: Treatment results of stage I and II oral tongue cancer with interstitial brachytherapy: maximum tumor thickness is prognostic of nodal metastasis, *Int J Radiat Oncol Biol Phys* 40:535-539, 1998.

Mazeron JJ, Grimard L, Benk V: Curietherapy versus external irradiation combined with curietherapy in stage II squamous cell carcinomas of mobile tongue and floor of mouth, *Recent Results in Cancer Res* 134:101-110, 1994.

McDonald JS, Jones H, Pavelic LJ, et al: Immunohistochemical detection of the H-ras, K-ras, and N-ras oncogenes in squamous cell carcinoma of the head and neck, *J Oral Pathol Med* 23:342-346, 1994.

Medina JE: A rational classification of neck dissections, *Otolaryngol Head Neck Surg* 100:169-176, 1989.

Michalides R, Van Veelen N, Hart A, et al: Overexpression of cyclin D1 correlates with recurrence in a group of forty-seven operable squamous cell carcinomas of the head and neck, *Cancer Res* 55:975-978, 1995.

O'Shaughnessy JA, Kelloff GJ, Gordon GB, et al: Treatment and prevention of intraepithelial neoplasia: an important target for accelerated new agent development, *Clin Cancer Res* 8:314-346, 2002.

Ostwald C, Muller P, Barten M, et al: Human papillomavirus in oral squamous cell carcinomas and normal oral mucosa, *J Oral Pathol Med* 23:220-225, 1994.

Pena JC, Thompson CB, Recant W, et al: Bcl-xl and Bcl-2 expression in squamous cell carcinoma of the head and neck, *Cancer* 85:164-170, 1999.

Ramos D, Chen BL, Regezi J, et al: Tenascin-C matrix assembly in oral squamous cell carcinoma, *Int J Cancer* 75:680-687, 1998.

Regezi JA, Dekker NP, McMillan A, et al: p53, p21, Rb, and MDM2 proteins in tongue cancers in tongue carcinoma from patients <35 years versus >75 years, *Oral Oncol* 35:379-383, 1999.

Riethdorf S, Friedrich RE, Ostwald C, et al: P53 gene mutations and HPV infection in primary head and neck squamous cell carcinomas do not correlate with overall survival: a long-term follow-up study, *J Oral Pathol Med* 26:315-321, 1997.

Robbins KT, Medina JE, Wolfe GT, et al: Standardizing neck dissection terminology: official report of the academy's committee for head and neck surgery and oncology, *Arch Otolaryngol Head Neck Surg* 117:601-605, 1991.

Rose BR, Thompson CH, Tattersall MH, et al: Squamous carcinoma of the head and neck: molecular mechanisms and potential biomarkers, *Aust NZ J Surg* 70:601-606, 2000.

Rowley H: The molecular genetics of head and neck cancer, *J Laryngol Otol* 112:607-612, 1998.

Sankaranarayanan R: Oral cancer in India: an epidemiologic and clinical review, *Oral Surg Oral Med Oral Pathol* 69:325-330, 1990.

Saunders J: The genetic basis of head and neck carcinoma, *Am J Surg* 174:459-461, 1997.

Schoelch ML, Le QT, Silverman S Jr, et al: Apoptosis-associated proteins and the development of oral squamous cell carcinoma, *Oral Oncol* 35:77-85, 1999.

Schoelch ML, Regezi JA, Dekker NP, et al: Cell cycle proteins and the development of oral squamous cell carcinoma, *Oral Oncol* 35:333-342, 1999.

Scully C: Viruses and oral squamous cell carcinoma, *Eur J Cancer B Oral Oncol* 28B:57-59, 1992.

Shah JP, Andersen PE: Evolving role of modifications in neck dissection for oral squamous carcinoma, *Br J Oral Maxillofac Surg* 33:3-8, 1995.

Shahnavaz SA, Bradley G, Regezi JA, et al: Patterns of CDKN2A gene loss in sequential oral epithelial dysplasias and carcinomas, *Cancer Res* 61:2371-2375, 2001.

Shahnavaz SA, Regezi JA, Bradley G, et al: p53 gene mutations in sequential oral epithelial dysplasias and carcinomas, *J Pathol* 190:417-422, 2000.

Shin DM, Kim J Ro JY, et al: Activation of p53 gene expression in premalignant lesions during head and neck tumorigenesis, *Cancer Res* 54:321-326, 1994.

Stuschke M, Thames HD: Hyperfractionated radiotherapy of human tumors: overview of the randomized clinical trials, *Int J Radiat Oncol Biol Phys* 37:259-267, 1997.

Sugerman PB, Joseph BK, Savage NW: Review article: the role of oncogenes, tumor suppressor genes and growth factors in oral squamous cell carcinoma: a case of apoptosis versus proliferation, *Oral Dis* 1:172-188, 1995.

Sumida T, Sogawa K, Sugita A, et al: Detection of telomerase activity in oral lesions, *J Oral Pathol Med* 27:111-115, 1998.

Tanaka N, Ogi K, Odajima T, et al: pRb/p21 protein expression is correlated with clinicopathologic findings in patients with oral squamous cell carcinoma, *Cancer* 92:2117-2125, 2001.

Timmons SR, Nwankwo JO, Domann FE: Acetaldehyde activates Jun/AP-1 expression and DNA binding activity in human oral keratinocytes. *Oral Oncol* 38:281-290, 2002.

Tsai CH, Yang CC, Chou LSS, et al: The correlation between alteration of p16 gene and clinical status in oral squamous cell carcinoma, *J Oral Pathol Med* 30:527-531, 2001.

Valdez IH, Wolff A, Atkinson JC, et al: Use of pilocarpine during head and neck radiation therapy to reduce xerostomia and salivary dysfunction, *Cancer* 71:1848-1851, 1993.

Watts S, Brewer E, Fry T: Human papillomavirus DNA types in squamous cell carcinomas of the head and neck, *Oral Surg Oral Med Oral Pathol* 71:701-707, 1991.

Wilson GD, Richman PI, Dische S, et al: p53 status of head and neck cancer: relation to biological characteristics and outcome of radiotherapy, *Br J Cancer* 71:1248-1252, 1995.

Xia W, Lau YK, Zhang HZ, et al: Strong correlation between c-erbB-2 overexpression and overall survival of patients with oral squamous cell carcinoma, *Clin Cancer Res* 3:3-9, 1997.

Yeudall WA: Human papillomaviruses and oral neoplasia, *Eur J Cancer B Oral Oncol* 28B:61-66, 1992.

WHITE LESIONS

Hereditary Conditions
   Leukoedema
   White Sponge Nevus
   Hereditary Benign Intraepithelial Dyskeratosis
   Follicular Keratosis
Reactive Lesions
   Focal (Frictional) Hyperkeratosis
   White Lesions Associated With Smokeless Tobacco
   Nicotine Stomatitis
   Hairy Leukoplakia
   Hairy Tongue
   Dentifrice-associated Slough
Preneoplastic and Neoplastic Lesions
   Actinic Cheilitis
   Idiopathic Leukoplakia
Other White Lesions
   Geographic Tongue
   Lichen Planus
   Lupus Erythematosus
Nonepithelial White-Yellow Lesions
   Candidiasis
   Mucosal Burns
   Submucous Fibrosis
   Fordyce's Granules
   Ectopic Lymphoid Tissue
   Gingival Cysts
   Parulis
   Lipoma

Lesions of the oral mucosa, which are white in color, result from a thickened layer of keratin, epithelial hyperplasia, intracellular epithelial edema, and/or reduced vascularity of subjacent connective tissue. White or yellow-white lesions may also be due to fibrin exudate covering an ulcer, submucosal deposits, surface debris, or fungal colonies.

HEREDITARY CONDITIONS

Leukoedema

Leukoedema is a generalized opacification of the buccal mucosa that is regarded as a variation of normal. It can be identified in the majority of the population.

Etiology and Pathogenesis. To date, the cause of leukoedema has not been established. Factors such as smoking, alcohol ingestion, bacterial infection, salivary conditions, and electrochemical interactions have been implicated, but none are proven causes.

Clinical Features. Leukoedema is usually discovered as an incidental finding. It is asymptomatic and symmetrically distributed in the buccal mucosa. It appears as a gray-white, diffuse, filmy, or milky surface (Figure 3-1). In more exaggerated cases a whitish cast with surface textural changes, including wrinkling or corrugation, may be seen. With stretching of the buccal mucosa, the opaque changes dissipate. It is more apparent in nonwhites, especially African-Americans.

Histopathology. In leukoedema the epithelium is parakeratotic and acanthotic, with marked intracellular edema of spinous cells. The enlarged epithelial cells have small, pyknotic nuclei in optically clear cytoplasm.

Differential Diagnosis. White sponge nevus, hereditary benign intraepithelial dyskeratosis, and the response to chronic cheek biting and lichen planus may show clinical similarities to leukoedema. The overall thickness of these lesions, their persistence on stretching, and specific microscopic features are distinctive.

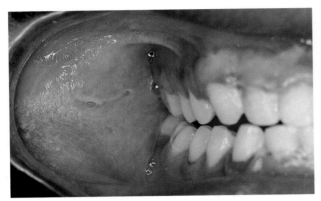

Figure 3-1   Leukoedema.

Treatment and Prognosis. No treatment is necessary because the changes are innocuous and there is no malignant potential.

White Sponge Nevus

White sponge nevus (WSN) is an autosomal-dominant condition that appears to be due to keratin 4 and/or 13 point mutations. It affects oral mucosa bilaterally, and no treatment is required.

Clinical Features. WSN presents as an asymptomatic, folded, white lesion that may affect several mucosal sites (Figure 3-2). Lesions tend to be thickened and have a spongy consistency. The presentation intraorally is almost always bilateral and symmetric and usually appears early in life, typically before puberty. The characteristic clinical manifestations of this particular form of keratosis are usually best observed on the buccal mucosa, although other areas such as the tongue and vestibular mucosa may also be involved. The conjunctival mucosa is usually spared, but mucosa of the esophagus, anus, vulva, and vagina may be affected.

Histopathology. Microscopically, the epithelium is greatly thickened, with marked spongiosis, acanthosis, and parakeratosis (Figure 3-3). Within the stratum spinosum, marked hydropic or clear cell change may be noted, often beginning in the parabasal region and extending very close to the surface. Perinuclear eosinophilic condensation of cytoplasm is characteristic of prickle cells in WSN. It is often possible to see columns of parakeratin extending from the spinous layer to the surface.

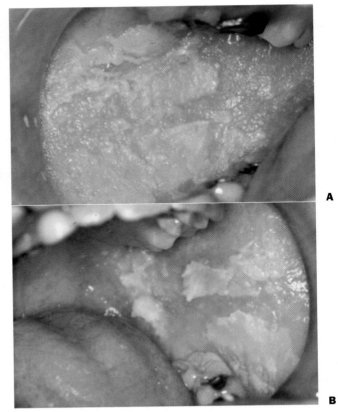

A

B

Figure 3-2   **A** and **B,** White sponge nevus.

Differential Diagnosis. The differential diagnosis includes hereditary benign epithelial dyskeratosis, lichen planus, lichenoid drug reaction, lupus erythematosus, cheek chewing, and possibly candidiasis (Table 3-1). Once tissue diagnosis is confirmed, no additional biopsies are necessary.

Treatment. There is no treatment necessary for this condition, since it is asymptomatic and benign.

Hereditary Benign Intraepithelial Dyskeratosis

Etiology. Hereditary benign intraepithelial dyskeratosis (HBID), also known as *Witkop's disease,* is a rare, hereditary condition (autosomal dominant). It was noted within a triracial isolate of white, Indian, and African-American composition in Halifax County, North Carolina. The initial cohort of 75 patients was traced to a single common female ancestor who lived nearly 130 years earlier. Using genetic linkage and molecular analysis, one group has localized the HBID gene to telomeric region of chromosome

4q35. The precise gene that causes the condition has not been characterized.

Clinical Features. HBID presentation includes early onset (usually within the first year of life) of bulbar conjunctivitis and oral white lesions. Preceding the bulbar

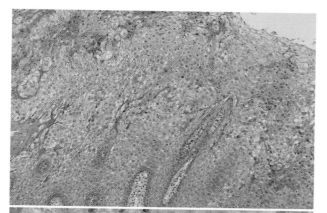

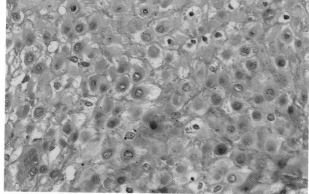

Figure 3-3 **A,** White sponge nevus showing edema and keratosis. **B,** High magnification of epithelium showing characteristic perinuclear condensation of keratin.

conjunctivitis are foamy gelatinous plaques that represent the ocular counterpart of the oral mucosal lesions.

Oral lesions consist of soft, asymptomatic, white folds and plaques of spongy mucosa. Areas characteristically involved include the buccal and labial mucosa and labial commissures, as well as the floor of the mouth and lateral surfaces of the tongue, gingiva, and palate. The dorsum of the tongue is usually spared. Oral lesions are generally detected within the first year of life, with a gradual increase in intensity until midadolescence.

In some patients ocular lesions may vary seasonally, with spontaneous shedding of conjunctival plaques. Patients may complain of photophobia, especially in early life. Blindness, secondary to corneal vascularization, has been reported.

Histopathology. Similarities between oral and conjunctival lesions are noted microscopically. Epithelial hyperplasia and acanthosis are present with intracellular edema. Enlarged hyaline keratinocytes are the dyskeratotic elements and are present in the superficial half of the epithelium. Normal cellular features are noted within the lower spinous and basal layers. Inflammatory cell infiltration within the lamina propria is minimal, and the epithelium–connective tissue junction is well defined.

Treatment. No treatment is necessary, because this condition is self-limiting and benign. It appears to pose no risk of malignant transformation.

Follicular Keratosis

Etiology and Pathogenesis. Follicular keratosis *(Darier's disease, Darier-White disease)* is an autosomal-dominant disorder. Many cases also appear sporadically as new mutations. Screening of candidate genes has led to

TABLE 3-1 **Bilateral Buccal Mucosa White Lesions: Differential Diagnosis**

Disease	Features/Action
White sponge nevus and HBID	Hereditary; does not disappear when stretched; biopsy to confirm; HBID may also involve conjunctiva
Lichen planus	Look for white reticulations (striae) and skin lesions; biopsy
Lichenoid drug reaction	Look for white lesions in context of new drug history
Cheek chewing	White shaggy lesions along occlusal plane
Lupus erythematosus	Delicate radiating striae; biopsy
Candidiasis	Look for predisposing factors; can rub off; responds to antifungal therapy

HBID, Hereditary benign intraepithelial dyskeratosis.

the discovery that mutations in ATP2A2, a gene that encodes the sarcoplasmic/endoplasmic reticulum calcium-adenosinetriphosphatase (Ca^{2+}-ATPase) isoform 2, cause this condition. It has been proposed that abnormalities in this calcium pump function interfere with cell growth and differentiation of calcium-dependent processes.

Clinical Features. The onset occurs between the ages of 6 and 20 years. The disease has a predilection for the skin, but 13% of patients have oral lesions. Skin manifestations are characterized by small, skin-colored papular lesions symmetrically distributed over the face, trunk, and intertriginous areas. The papules eventually coalesce and feel greasy because of excessive keratin production. The coalesced areas subsequently form patches of vegetating to verrucous growths that have a tendency to become infected and malodorous. Lesions may also occur unilaterally or in a zosteriform pattern. Thickening of the palms and soles (hyperkeratosis palmaris et plantaris) by excessive keratotic tissue is not uncommon. Fingernail changes may include fragility, splintering, and subungual keratosis. Nail changes are often helpful in establishing a diagnosis.

The extent of the oral lesions may parallel the extent of skin involvement. Favored oral mucosal sites include the attached gingiva and hard palate. The lesions typically appear as small, whitish papules, producing an overall cobblestone appearance. Papules range from 2 to 3 mm in diameter and may become coalescent. Extension beyond the oral cavity into the oropharynx and pharynx may occur.

Histopathology. Oral lesions closely resemble the cutaneous lesions. Features include (1) suprabasal lacunae (clefts) formation containing acantholytic epithelial cells, (2) basal layer proliferation immediately below and adjacent to the lacunae or clefts, (3) formation of vertical clefts that show a lining of parakeratotic and dyskeratotic cells, and (4) the presence of specific benign dyskeratotic cells—*corps ronds* and *grains*. Corps ronds are large, keratinized squamous cells with round, uniformly basophilic nuclei and intensely eosinophilic cytoplasm. Grains are smaller parakeratotic cells with pyknotic, hyperchromatic nuclei.

Treatment and Prognosis. Vitamin A analogs or retinoids have been used effectively, but long-term therapy is tolerated poorly. The disease is chronic and slowly progressive; remissions may be noted in some patients.

REACTIVE LESIONS

Focal (Frictional) Hyperkeratosis

Etiology. Focal (frictional) hyperkeratosis is a white lesion that is related to chronic rubbing or friction against an oral mucosal surface. This results in a presumably protective hyperkeratotic white lesion that is analogous to a callus on the skin.

Clinical Features. Friction-induced hyperkeratoses occur in areas that are commonly traumatized, such as the lips, lateral margins of the tongue, buccal mucosa along the occlusal line, and edentulous ridges (Figures 3-4 to 3-7). Chronic cheek or lip chewing may result in opacification (keratinization) of the area affected. Chewing on edentulous alveolar ridges produces the same effect.

Histopathology. As the name indicates, the primary microscopic change is hyperkeratosis (Figure 3-8). A few chronic inflammatory cells may be seen in the subjacent connective tissue.

Diagnosis. Careful history taking and examination should indicate the nature of this lesion. If the practitioner is clinically confident of a traumatic cause, no biopsy may be required. Patients should be advised to discontinue the causative habit, or the offending tooth or denture should be smoothed. The lesion should resolve or at least be reduced in intensity with time,

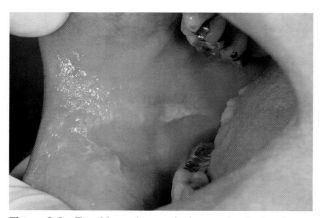

Figure 3-4   **Focal hyperkeratosis** due to cheek chewing.

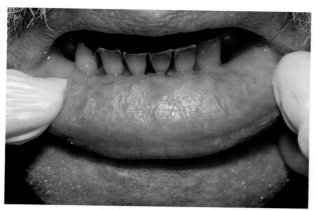

Figure 3-5 **Focal hyperkeratosis** due to chronic rubbing of the lip against teeth.

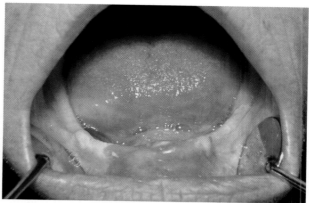

Figure 3-7 **Focal hyperkeratosis** and erythema associated with an ill-fitting lower denture.

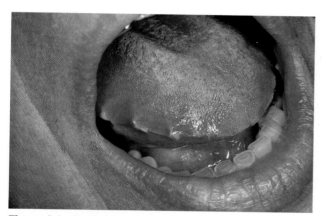

Figure 3-6 **Focal hyperkeratosis** related to tongue-thrusting habit.

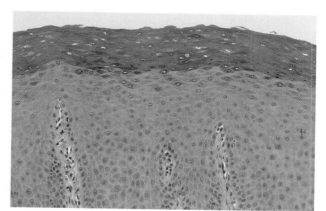

Figure 3-8 **Focal hyperkeratosis** biopsy specimen. Note that the epithelial maturation pattern is otherwise normal.

TABLE 3-2 **Solitary White Lesion: Differential Diagnosis**

Disease	Features/Action
Frictional keratosis	Look for cause (e.g., ill-fitting denture, trauma); biopsy
Dysplasia, in situ carcinoma, squamous cell carcinoma	Assess risk factors; biopsy
Burn	History of aspirin or other agent application at site of lesion—discontinue use
Lupus erythematosus	Delicate radiating striae; biopsy
Hairy leukoplakia	Lateral borders of tongue; look for irregular surface architecture; often bilateral; biopsy

confirming the clinical diagnosis. Resolution of the lesion would also allow unmasking of any underlying lesion that may not be related to trauma (Table 3-2). If there is any doubt about the clinical diagnosis, a biopsy should be taken.

Treatment. Observation is generally all that is required for simple frictional hyperkeratotic lesions. Control of the habit causing the lesion should result in clinical improvement. There is no malignant potential.

White Lesions Associated With Smokeless Tobacco

There are marked geographic and gender differences in tobacco use. In the United States there is a relatively high prevalence of smokeless tobacco users in the southern and western states. Usage by men in New York and Rhode Island is less than 1% of the population, but in West Virginia it exceeds 20%. Among teenagers, whites are the predominant users of smokeless tobacco, with males making up nearly all of this group. Smokeless tobacco is also used in Sweden, and in regions such as the Indian subcontinent and Southeast Asia, usage is even more common and the materials more destructive in Southeast Asia. The tobacco preparations are generally of a higher (alkaline) pH and are often mixed with other ingredients, including shredded areca (betel) nut, and also containing lime, camphor, and spices.

The general increase in smokeless tobacco consumption has been related to both peer pressure and increased media advertising, which often glamorizes the use of smokeless tobacco, or snuff dipping. In addition, individuals who have been intense smokers or those who wish to avoid smoking may gravitate to this alternative. The clinical results of long-term exposure to smokeless tobacco include the development of oral mucosal white patches with a slightly increased malignant potential, dependence, alterations of taste, acceleration of periodontal disease, and significant amounts of dental abrasion.

Etiology. A causal relationship has been documented between smokeless tobacco and white tissue changes. Although all forms of smokeless tobacco may potentially cause alterations in the oral mucosa, snuff (particulate, finely divided, or shredded tobacco) appears to be much more likely to cause oral lesions than chewing tobacco. Oral mucosa responds to the topically induced effects of tobacco with inflammation and keratosis. Dysplastic changes may follow, with a low-potential risk of malignant change. Smokeless tobacco–induced alterations in tissues are thought to be a response to tobacco constituents and perhaps other agents that are added for flavoring or moisture retention. Carcinogens, such as nitrosonornicotine, an organic component of chewing tobacco and snuff, have been identified in smokeless tobacco. The pH of snuff, which ranges between 8.2 and 9.3, may be another factor that contributes to the alteration of mucosa.

Duration of exposure to smokeless tobacco that is necessary to produce mucosal damage is measured in terms of years. It has been demonstrated that leukoplakia can be predicted with the use of three tins of tobacco per week or duration of the habit for more than 2 years.

Clinical Features. White lesions associated with smokeless tobacco develop in the immediate area where the tobacco is habitually placed (Figures 3-9 and 3-10). The most common area of involvement is the mucobuccal fold of the mandible in either the incisor or the molar region. The mucosa develops a granular to wrinkled appearance. In advanced cases a heavy, folded character may be seen. Less often, an erythroplakic or red component may be admixed with the white keratotic component. The lesions are generally painless and asymptomatic, and their discovery is often incidental to routine oral examination.

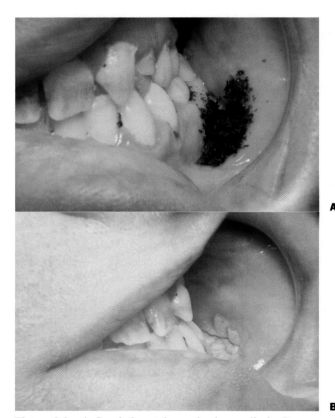

Figure 3-9   **A,** Smokeless tobacco in the vestibule. **B,** Keratotic pouch induced by tobacco contact.

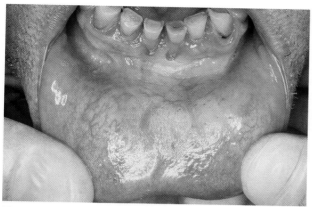

Figure 3-10 **Snuff dipper's pouch.** Note incisal edge abrasion wear and periodontal disease.

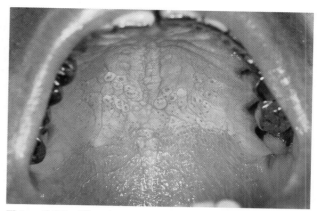

Figure 3-12 **Nicotine stomatitis.**

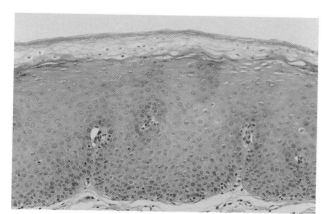

Figure 3-11 **Smokeless tobacco lesion** biopsy specimen showing acanthosis and edematous parakeratosis.

Histopathology. Slight-to-moderate parakeratosis, often in the form of spires or chevrons, is noted over the surface of the affected mucosa (Figure 3-11). Superficial epithelium may demonstrate vacuolization or edema. A slight to moderate chronic inflammatory cell infiltrate is typically present. Epithelial dysplasia may occasionally develop in these lesions, especially in long-time users. On occasion, a diffuse zone of basophilic stromal alteration may be seen, usually adjacent to inflamed minor salivary glands.

Treatment and Prognosis. With discontinuation of tobacco use, some lesions may disappear after several weeks. It would be prudent to perform a biopsy on persistent lesions. A long period of exposure to smokeless tobacco increases the risk of transformation to ver-

rucous or squamous cell carcinoma, although this risk is probably low.

Nicotine Stomatitis

Etiology. Nicotine stomatitis is a common tobacco-related form of keratosis. It is typically associated with pipe and cigar smoking, with a positive correlation between intensity of smoking and severity of the condition. The importance of the direct topical effect of smoke can be appreciated in instances in which the hard palate is covered by a removable prosthesis, resulting in sparing of the mucosa beneath the appliance and hyperkeratosis of exposed areas. The combination of tobacco carcinogens and heat is markedly intensified in *reverse smoking* (lit end positioned inside the mouth), adding a significant risk for malignant conversion.

Clinical Features. The palatal mucosa initially responds with an erythematous change followed by keratinization. Subsequent to the opacification or keratinization of the palate, red dots surrounded by white keratotic rings appear (Figures 3-12 and 3-13). The dots represent inflammation of the salivary gland excretory ducts.

Histopathology. Nicotine stomatitis is characterized by epithelial hyperplasia and hyperkeratosis (Figure 3-14). The minor salivary glands in the area show inflammatory change, and excretory ducts may show squamous metaplasia.

Treatment and Prognosis. This condition rarely evolves into malignancy except in individuals who *reverse smoke.*

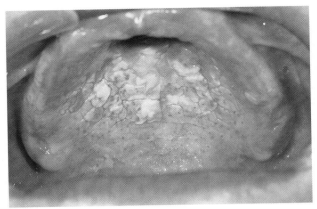

Figure 3-13   Nicotine stomatitis.

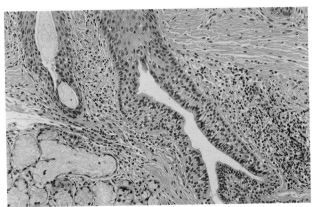

Figure 3-14   **Nicotine stomatitis** biopsy specimen showing salivary duct metaplasia and inflammation.

Although the risk of carcinoma development in the palate is minimal, nicotine stomatitis is a marker of heavy tobacco use and hence may indicate an increased risk of epithelial dysplasia and neoplasia elsewhere in the oral cavity, oropharynx, and upper respiratory tract. Nicotine stomatitis should therefore be viewed as a potential indicator of significant epithelial change at sites other than the hard palate.

Hairy Leukoplakia

Etiology and Pathogenesis. In 1984 an unusual white lesion was first described along the lateral margins of the tongue, predominantly in male homosexuals. Evidence indicates that this particular form of leukoplakia, known as *hairy leukoplakia*, represents an opportunistic infection that is related to the presence of Epstein-Barr virus (EBV) and that is found almost exclusively in

---

Box 3-1 Oral Manifestations of AIDS

INFECTIONS

Viral: Herpes simplex, herpes zoster, hairy leukoplakia, cytomegalovirus, warts
Bacterial: Tuberculosis bacillary angiomatosis
Fungal: Candidiasis, histoplasmosis

NEOPLASMS

Kaposi's sarcoma (HHV8)
Lymphomas, high grade

OTHER

Aphthous ulcers
Xerostomia
Gingivitis and periodontal disease

AIDS, Acquired immunodeficiency syndrome; *HHV8*, human herpesvirus 8.

---

human immunodeficiency virus (HIV)–infected individuals. In a small percentage of cases hairy leukoplakia may be seen in patients with other forms of immunosuppression, in particular, those associated with organ transplantation (medically induced immunosuppression). A few cases have been reported in patients who are taking corticosteroids, and a few in patients who are otherwise healthy.

The prevalence of hairy leukoplakia in HIV-infected patients has been declining as a result of new chemotherapeutic regimens for HIV. Of importance is that this lesion has been associated with subsequent or concomitant development of the clinical and laboratory features of acquired immunodeficiency syndrome (AIDS) in as many as 80% of cases. There is a positive correlation with depletion of peripheral CD4 cells and the presence of hairy leukoplakia. Several other oral conditions have also been described as having a greater-than-expected frequency in patients with AIDS (Box 3-1).

The presence of EBV in hairy leukoplakia, as well as in the normal epithelium of patients with AIDS, has been confirmed. Through the use of molecular methods, viral particles have been localized within the nuclei and cytoplasm of the oral epithelial cells of hairy leukoplakia. Studies further indicate that this particular virus replicates within the oral hairy leukoplakia lesion. It is not understood why the lateral surface of the tongue is the favored site.

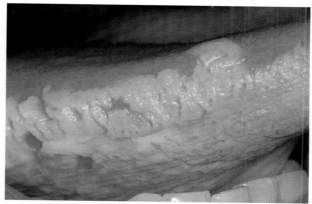

Figure 3-16 **Hairy leukoplakia** of the lateral and ventral tongue.

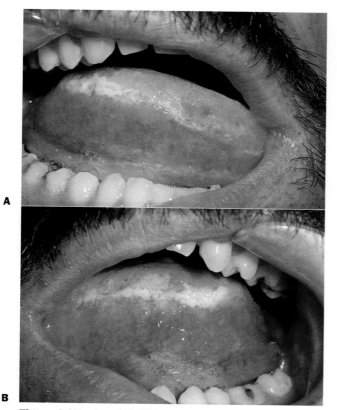

Figure 3-15 **A** and **B, Hairy leukoplakia,** bilateral.

Clinical Features. Hairy leukoplakia presents as a well-demarcated white lesion that varies in architecture from a flat, plaquelike, to papillary/filiform or corrugated lesion (Figures 3-15 and 3-16). It may be unilateral or bilateral. The vast majority of cases has been located along the lateral margins of the tongue, with occasional extension onto the dorsal surface. Rarely, hairy leukoplakia may be seen on the buccal mucosa, the floor of the mouth, or the palate. Lesions have not been seen in the vaginal or anal mucosa.

In general, there are no associated symptoms, although an associated infection with *Candida albicans* might call attention to the presence of this condition. In more severe cases the patient may become visually aware of the lesion.

Histopathology. The characteristic microscopic feature of hairy leukoplakia is found in the nuclei of upper level keratinocytes (Figure 3-17). Viral inclusions or peripheral displacement of chromatin with a resultant smudgy nucleus is evident. This is seen in the context of a markedly hyperparakeratotic surface, often with the formation of keratotic surface irregularities and ridges. *C. albicans* hyphae are often seen extending into the superficial epithelial cell layers. Beneath the surface, within the spinous cell layer, cells show ballooning degeneration and perinuclear clearing. There is a general paucity of subepithelial inflammatory cells, and Langerhans cells are scant.

Immunopathologic studies have demonstrated the presence of EBV within the cells, showing nuclear inclusions and basophilic homogenization. Further confirmation has been accomplished by ultrastructural demonstration of intranuclear virions of EBV.

Differential Diagnosis. The clinical differential diagnosis of hairy leukoplakia includes idiopathic leukoplakia, frictional hyperkeratosis (tongue chewing), and leukoplakia associated with tobacco use. Other entities that might be considered are lichen planus, lupus erythematosus, and hyperplastic candidiasis.

Treatment and Prognosis. There is no specific treatment for hairy leukoplakia. For patients whose immune status is unknown and in whom biopsy findings indicate hairy leukoplakia, investigation for HIV infection or other causes of immunosuppression should be undertaken. Some discretion is required because a small percentage of patients with hairy leukoplakia that are is not associated with AIDS.

For cosmetic reasons, patients may request treatment of their lesions. Responses to acyclovir, ganciclovir, tretinoin, and podophyllum have been reported, with a return of lesions often noted on discontinuation of therapy.

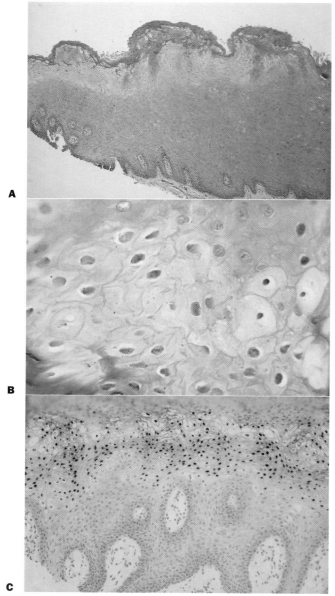

A

B

C

Figure 3-17 **A,** Hairy leukoplakia showing acanthosis, parakeratosis, and edema. **B,** Upper level keratinocytes showing nuclear viral inclusions. **C,** In situ hybridization for EBV showing positive nuclear signal.

Approximately 10% of individuals with diagnosed hairy leukoplakia have AIDS at the time of diagnosis, and an additional 20% develop this disease in the following year. The probability of AIDS developing in individuals with HIV-associated hairy leukoplakia is approximately 50% within 1.5 years; within 2.5 years the probability is 80%.

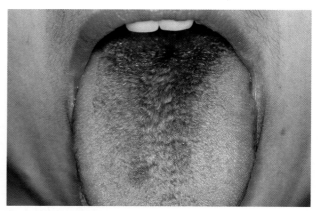

Figure 3-18 Hairy tongue.

Hairy Tongue

Hairy tongue is a clinical term referring to a condition of filiform papillae overgrowth on the dorsal surface of the tongue.

Etiology. There are numerous initiating or predisposing factors for hairy tongue. Broad-spectrum antibiotics, such as penicillin, and systemic corticosteroids are often identified in the clinical history of patients with this condition. In addition, oxygenating mouthrinses containing hydrogen peroxide, sodium perborate, and carbamide peroxide have been cited as possible etiologic agents in this condition. Hairy tongue may also be seen in individuals who are intense smokers and in individuals who have undergone radiotherapy to the head and neck region for malignant disease. The basic problem is believed to be related to an alteration in microbial flora, with attendant proliferation of fungi and chromogenic bacteria, and papillae overgrowth.

Clinical Features. The clinical alteration translates to hyperplasia of the filiform papillae, with concomitant retardation of the normal rate of desquamation. The result is a thick, matted surface that serves to trap bacteria, fungi, cellular debris, and foreign material (Figure 3-18).

Hairy tongue is predominantly a cosmetic problem, since symptoms are generally minimal. However, when extensive elongation of the papillae occurs, a gagging or a tickling sensation may be felt. The color may range from white to tan to deep brown or black, depending on diet, oral hygiene, and the composition of the bacteria inhabiting the papillary surface.

Histopathology. Microscopic examination of a biopsy specimen confirms the presence of elongated filiform papillae, with surface contamination by clusters of microorganisms and fungi. The underlying lamina propria is generally mildly inflamed.

Diagnosis. Because the clinical features of this lesion are usually quite characteristic, confirmation by biopsy is not necessary. Cytologic or culture studies are of little value.

Treatment and Prognosis. Identification of a possible etiologic factor, such as antibiotics or oxygenating mouthrinses, is helpful. Discontinuing one of these agents should result in improvement within a few weeks. In others there may be benefit to brushing the dorsum of the tongue with a slurry of sodium bicarbonate (baking soda) in water. In cases of individuals who have undergone radiotherapy, with resultant xerostomia and altered bacterial flora, management is more difficult. Brushing the tongue and maintaining fastidious oral hygiene should be of some benefit (application of a 1% solution of podophyllum resin with thorough rinsing has also been described as a useful treatment). It is important to emphasize to patients that this process is entirely benign and self-limiting and that the tongue should return to normal after institution of physical debridement and proper oral hygiene.

Dentifrice-associated Slough

Dentifrice-associated slough is a relatively common phenomenon that has been associated with the use of several different brands of toothpaste. It is believed to be a superficial chemical burn or reaction to a component in the dentifrice, possibly the detergent or flavoring compounds. Clinically, it appears as a superficial whitish slough of the buccal mucosa, typically detected by the patient as oral peeling (Figure 3-19). The condition is painless and is not known to progress to anything significant. The problem resolves with a switch to another, blander toothpaste.

PRENEOPLASTIC AND NEOPLASTIC LESIONS

Actinic Cheilitis

Actinic, or solar, cheilitis represents accelerated tissue degeneration of the vermilion of the lips, especially the lower lip, secondary to chronic exposure to sunlight. This condition occurs almost exclusively in whites and is especially prevalent in those with fair skin.

Etiology and Pathogenesis. The wavelengths of light most responsible for actinic cheilitis and, in general, other degenerative actinically related skin conditions are usually considered to be those between 2900 and 3200 nm (ultraviolet B [UVB]). This radiant energy affects not only the epithelium but also the supporting connective tissue.

Clinical Features. The affected vermilion of the lips takes on an atrophic, pale to silvery gray, glossy appearance, often with fissuring and wrinkling at right angles to the cutaneous-vermilion junction (Figure 3-20). Slightly firm, bilateral swelling of the lower lip is also common. In advanced cases the junction is irregular or totally effaced, with a degree of epidermization of the vermilion. Mottled areas of hyperpigmentation and

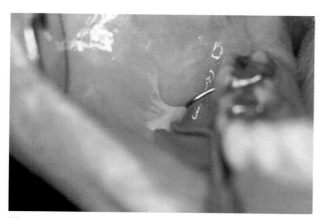
Figure 3-19 Dentifrice-associated slough.

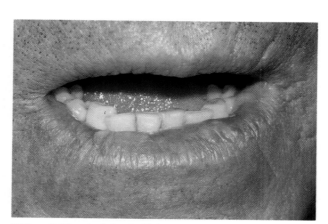
Figure 3-20 Actinic cheilitis.

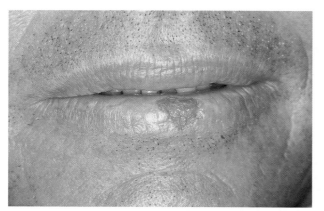

Figure 3-21   **Actinic cheilitis** with chronic ulcer.

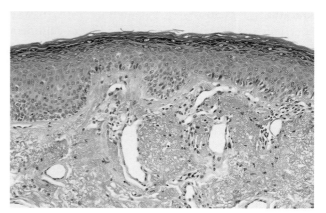

Figure 3-22   **Actinic cheilitis** showing hyperkeratosis, basophilic change of collagen, and telangiectasias.

keratosis are often noted, as well as superficial scaling, cracking, erosion, ulceration, and crusting (Figure 3-21).

Histopathology. The overlying epithelium is typically atrophic and hyperkeratotic (Figure 3-22). Basophilic change of submucosa (elastin replacement of collagen) and telangiectasia are also seen.

Treatment. Because of the positive relationship between exposure to UV light and carcinoma, lip protection is indicated. The use of lip balm containing the sunscreen agent para-aminobenzoic acid (PABA) or its derivatives is indicated during periods of sun exposure in high-risk patients. Sun-blocking opaque agents also boost the effectiveness of the balm.

Chronic sun damage mandates periodic examination and a biopsy if ulceration persists or if there is induration. If atypical changes are noted within the epithelium, a vermilionectomy may be performed in association with mucosal advancement to replace the damaged vermilion. This operation is associated with some morbidity, primarily in relation to lip paresthesia, therefore prompting some to advocate wedge excision for suspicious lesions. Acceptable results are also obtainable with the use of laser surgery or cryosurgery, as well as with topical 5-fluorouracil.

Idiopathic Leukoplakia

Leukoplakia is a clinical term indicating a white patch or plaque of oral mucosa that cannot be rubbed off and cannot be characterized clinically as any other disease. This excludes lesions such as lichen planus, candidiasis, leukoedema, white sponge nevus, and

obvious frictional keratosis. Leukoplakias may have similar clinical appearances but have a considerable degree of microscopic heterogeneity. Because leukoplakias may range microscopically from benign hyperkeratosis to invasive squamous cell carcinomas, a biopsy is mandatory to establish a definitive diagnosis.

Etiology and Pathogenesis. Many cases of leukoplakia are etiologically related to the use of tobacco in smoked or smokeless forms and may regress after discontinuation of tobacco use. Other factors, such as alcohol abuse, trauma, and *C. albicans* infection, may have a role in the etiology of leukoplakia. Nutritional factors have also been cited as important, especially relative to iron deficiency anemia and development of sideropenic dysphagia (Plummer-Vinson or Paterson-Kelly syndrome).

Rates of transformation to squamous cell carcinoma have varied from study to study as a result of differences in the underlying pathology and differences in the use of putative carcinogens such as tobacco. Geographic differences in the transformation rate, as well as in the prevalence and location of oral leukoplakias, are likely related to the differences in tobacco habits in various parts of the world. In U.S. populations the majority of oral leukoplakias are benign and probably never become malignant. Approximately 5% of leukoplakias are malignant at the time of first biopsy, and approximately 5% of the remainder undergo subsequent malignant transformation. From 10% to 15% of the dysplasias that present as clinical leukoplakias will develop into squamous cell carcinoma (Figures 3-23 and 3-24).

There are wide ranges of risk of transformation from one anatomic site to another, such as the floor of the mouth, where transformation rates are comparatively high, although paradoxically many show only minimal amounts of epithelial dysplasia.

Clinical Features. Leukoplakia is a condition associated with a middle-aged and older population. The vast majority of cases occur after the age of 40 years. Over time there has also been a shift in gender predilection, with near parity in the incidence of leukoplakia, apparently as a result of the change in smoking habits of women.

Predominant sites of occurrence have changed through the years (Box 3-2). At one time, the tongue was the most common site for leukoplakia, but this area has given way to the mandibular mucosa and the buccal mucosa, which account for almost half of the leukoplakias (Figures 3-25 to 3-28). The palate, maxillary ridge, and lower lip are somewhat less often involved, and the floor of the mouth and retromolar sites are less often involved.

The relative risk of neoplastic transformation varies from one region to another. Although the floor of the mouth accounts for a relatively small percentage (10%) of leukoplakias, a large percentage are found to be dysplastic, carcinoma in situ, or invasive carcinoma when examined microscopically. Leukoplakia of the lips and tongue also exhibits a relatively high percentage of dysplastic or neoplastic change. In contrast to these sites, the retromolar area exhibits these changes in only about 10% of cases.

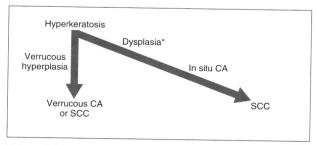

Figure 3-23   Idiopathic leukoplakia pathogenesis. *Malignant transformation 10%-15%.

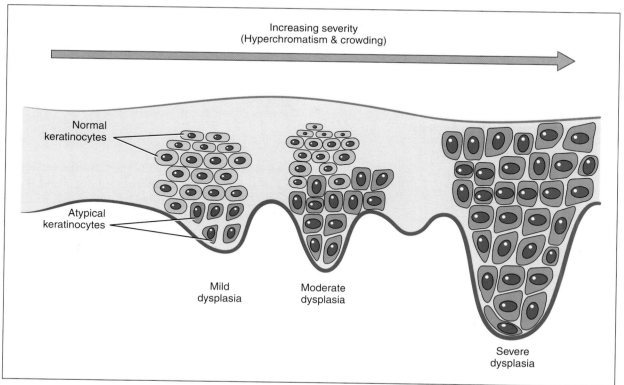

Figure 3-24   Progression of dysplasia.

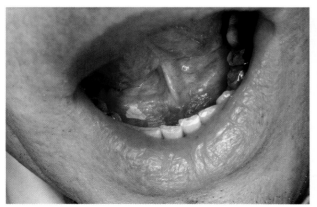

Figure 3-25 **Idiopathic leukoplakia** of the floor of the mouth. The microscopic diagnosis was hyperkeratosis.

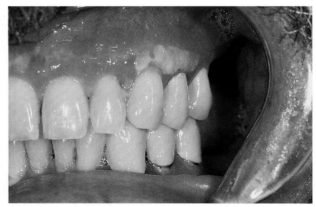

Figure 3-26 **Idiopathic leukoplakia** of the gingiva. The microscopic diagnosis was hyperkeratosis.

Box 3-2 Idiopathic Leukoplakia

RISK FACTORS

Tobacco, alcohol, nutrition, unknown

SITES OF OCCURRENCE

Vestibule, buccal > palate, alveolar ridge, lip > tongue, floor

HIGH-RISK SITES FOR MALIGNANT TRANSFORMATION

Floor > tongue > lip > palate > buccal > vestibule > retromolar

AGE

Usually over 40 years

MICROSCOPIC DIAGNOSES AT FIRST DIAGNOSIS

Hyperkeratosis—80%
Dysplasia—12%
In situ carcinoma—3%
Squamous cell carcinoma—5%

TRANSFORMATION RATES

All idiopathic leukoplakias—5% to 15%
All dysplasias—10% to 15%

>, More frequently affected.

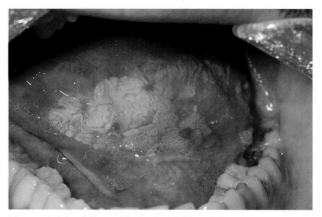

Figure 3-27 **Idiopathic leukoplakia** of the lateral tongue. The microscopic diagnosis was dysplasia.

On visual examination, leukoplakia may vary from a barely evident, vague whiteness on a base of uninflamed, normal-appearing tissue to a definitive white, thickened, leathery, fissured, verrucous (wartlike) lesion. Red zones may also be seen in some leukoplakias, prompting use of the term *speckled leuko-* *plakia (erythroleukoplakia).* On palpation, some lesions may be soft, smooth, or finely granular. Other lesions may be roughened, nodular, or indurated.

Proliferative verrucous leukoplakia has been segregated from other leukoplakias. This type of leukoplakia begins as simple keratosis and eventually becomes verrucous in nature. Lesions tend to be persistent, multifocal, and sometimes aggressive. Recurrence is common. The cause is unknown, although some may be associated with human papillomavirus and some with tobacco use. The diagnosis is determined clinicopathologically and is usually made retrospectively. Malignant transformation to verrucous or squamous cell carcinoma is seen in more than 15% of cases.

Histopathology. Histologic changes range from hyperkeratosis, dysplasia, and carcinoma in situ to invasive squamous cell carcinoma (Figures 3-29 to 3-31). The term *dysplasia* indicates abnormal epithelium and disordered growth, whereas *atypia* refers to abnormal nuclear features (Box 3-3). Increasing degrees of dysplasia are designated as mild, moderate, and severe and are subjectively determined microscopically. Specific microscopic characteristics of dysplasia include (1) drop-shaped epithelial ridges, (2) basal cell crowding, (3) irregular stratification, (4) increased and abnormal mitotic figures, (5) premature keratinization, (6) nuclear pleomorphism and hyperchromatism, and (7) an increased nuclear-cytoplasmic ratio.

It is generally accepted that the more severe the epithelial changes, the more likely a lesion is to evolve into cancer. However, there is no way microscopically to predict which dysplasias, mild to severe, will progress to squamous cell carcinoma. When the entire thickness of epithelium is involved with these changes in a so-called top-to-bottom pattern, the term *carcinoma in situ* may be used. Designation of carcinoma in situ may also be used when cellular atypia is particularly severe, even though the changes may not be evident from basement membrane to surface. Carcinoma in situ is not regarded as a reversible lesion, although it may take many years for invasion to occur. A majority of squamous cell carcinomas of the upper aerodigestive tract, including the oral cavity, are preceded by epithelial dysplasia. Conceptually, invasive carcinoma begins when a microfocus of epithelial cell invades the lamina propria 1 to 2 mm beyond the basal lamina. At this early stage, the risk of regional metastasis is low.

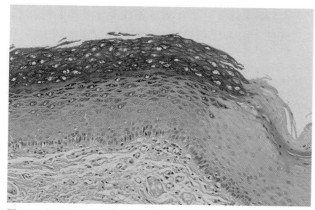

Figure 3-28 **Idiopathic leukoplakia** of the lateral tongue. The microscopic diagnosis was squamous cell carcinoma.

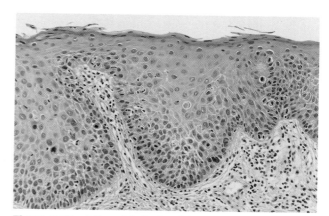

Figure 3-30 **Idiopathic leukoplakia** diagnosed as moderate dysplasia.

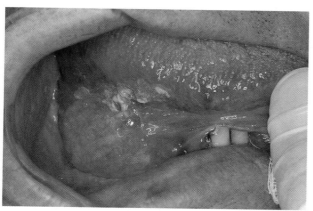

Figure 3-29 **Idiopathic leukoplakia** diagnosed as hyperkeratosis.

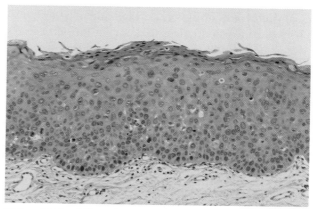

Figure 3-31 **Idiopathic leukoplakia** diagnosed as severe dysplasia.

Box 3-3 Dysplasia: Microscopic Features

EPITHELIAL ARCHITECTURE

Drop-shaped rete pegs
Basal cell crowding
Irregular stratification
Reduced intercellular adhesion

CYTOLOGIC ATYPIA

Pleomorphic nuclei—hyperchromatic, smudgy, angular
Increased nuclear-cytoplasmic ratios
Increased and abnormal mitoses

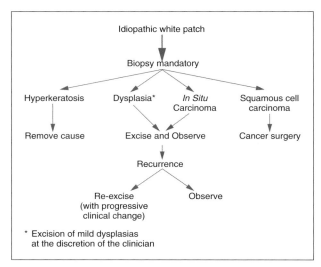

Figure 3-32　**Idiopathic leukoplakia:** diagnosis and management.

Differential Diagnosis. The first step in developing a differential diagnosis for a white patch (leukoplakia) on the oral mucosa is to determine whether the lesion can be removed with a gauze square or tongue blade. If the lesion can be removed, it represents a pseudomembrane, fungus colony, or debris. If there is evidence of bilateral buccal mucosa disease, hereditary conditions, cheek chewing, lichen planus, and lupus erythematosus should be considered. Concomitant cutaneous lesions would give weight to the latter two. If either chronic trauma or tobacco use is elicited in the patient's history, frictional or tobacco-associated hyperkeratoses should be considered, respectively. Elimination of a suspected cause should result in some clinical improvement. Also included in a differential diagnosis for tongue leukoplakia would be hairy leukoplakia and geographic tongue.

If the lesion in question is not removable and is not clinically diagnostic, it should be considered an idiopathic leukoplakia and a biopsy should be performed. For extensive lesions, multiple biopsies may be necessary to avoid sample error. The clinically most suspicious areas (red, ulcerated, or indurated areas) should be included in the area to be biopsied.

Treatment and Prognosis. In the absence of dysplastic or atypical epithelial changes, periodic examinations and rebiopsy of new suspicious areas are recommended. If a lesion is mildly dysplastic, some clinical judgment should be exercised in patient management. Potential etiologic factors should be considered. Removal of mildly dysplastic lesions is in the patient's best interest if there is no apparent causative factor and the lesion is small (Figure 3-32). If considerable morbidity would result because of the lesion's size or location, follow-up surveillance is acceptable.

If leukoplakia is diagnosed as moderate to severe dysplasia, removal becomes obligatory. Various surgical methods such as scalpel excision, cryosurgery, electrosurgery, and laser surgery seem to be equally effective in ablating these lesions. For large lesions, grafting procedures may be necessary after surgery. It is important to note that many idiopathic leukoplakias may recur after complete removal. It is impossible to predict which lesions will return and which will not.

OTHER WHITE LESIONS

Geographic Tongue

Etiology. Geographic tongue, also known as *erythema migrans* and *benign migratory glossitis*, is a condition of unknown cause. In a few patients emotional stress may enhance the process. Geographic tongue has been associated, probably coincidentally, with several different conditions, including psoriasis, seborrheic dermatitis, Reiter's syndrome, and atopy.

Clinical Features. Geographic tongue is seen in approximately 2% of the U.S. population and affects women slightly more often than men. Children may occasionally be affected. It is characterized initially by the presence of atrophic patches surrounded by elevated keratotic margins. The desquamated areas appear red and may be slightly tender (Figures 3-33 to 3-36). When followed over a period of days or weeks, the pattern changes, appearing to move across the dorsum of the tongue. There is a strong association between geographic tongue and *fissured (plicated) tongue*. The significance of this association is unknown, although symptoms may be more common when fissured tongue is present, presumably because of secondary fungal infection in the base of the fissures.

Rarely, similar alterations have been described in the floor of the mouth, buccal mucosa, and gingiva. The red atrophic lesions and white keratotic margins mimic the lingual counterparts.

Although most patients with geographic tongue are asymptomatic, occasionally patients complain of irritation or tenderness, especially in relation to the consumption of spicy foods and alcoholic beverages. The severity of symptoms varies with time and is often an indicator of the intensity of lesional activity. Lesions periodically disappear and recur for no apparent reason.

Histopathology. Filiform papillae are atrophic, and the margins of the lesion demonstrate hyperkeratosis and acanthosis (Figure 3-37). Closer to the central portion of the lesion, corresponding to the circinate erythematous areas, there is loss of keratin, with intraepithelial neutrophils and lymphocytes. Leukocytes are often noted within a microabscess near the surface. An inflammatory cell infiltrate within the underlying lamina propria, consisting chiefly of neutrophils, lymphocytes, and plasma cells, is seen. Although the histologic picture is reminiscent of psoriasis, a clinical link between geographic tongue and cutaneous psoriasis has not been substantiated and is likely coincidental.

Differential Diagnosis. Based on clinical appearance, geographic tongue is usually diagnostic. Only rarely might a biopsy be required for a definitive diagnosis. In equivocal cases, clinical differential diagnosis might

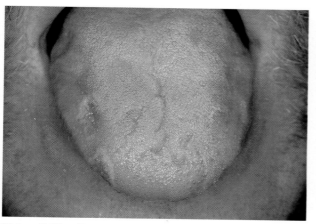

Figure 3-33 Geographic tongue.

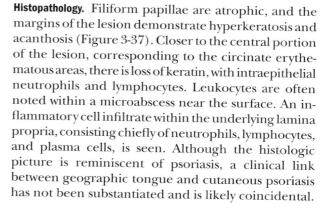

Figure 3-35 Geographic tongue.

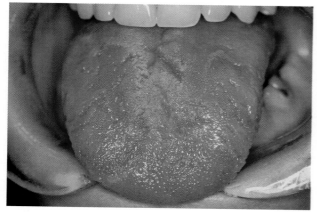

Figure 3-34 Geographic tongue.

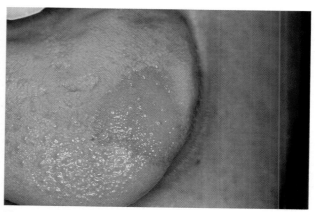

Figure 3-36 Geographic tongue.

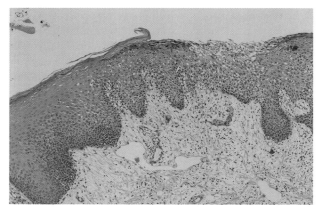

Figure 3-37   **Geographic tongue** biopsy specimen showing hyperkeratotic epithelium adjacent to edematous and inflamed epithelium.

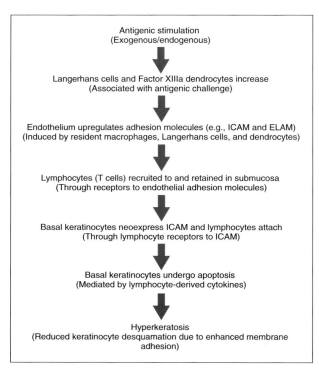

Figure 3-38   **Lichen planus:** hypothetical molecular events.

include candidiasis, leukoplakia, lichen planus, and lupus erythematosus.

Treatment and Prognosis. Because of the self-limiting and usually asymptomatic nature of this condition, treatment is not required. However, when symptoms occur, treatment is empirical. Considerable benefit may be gained by keeping the mouth clean using a mouthrinse composed of sodium bicarbonate in water. Topical steroids, especially ones containing an antifungal agent, may be helpful in reducing symptoms. Reassuring patients that this condition is totally benign and does not portend more serious disease helps relieve anxiety.

Lichen Planus

Lichen planus is a chronic mucocutaneous disease of unknown cause. It is relatively common, affecting between 0.2% and 2% of the population. In oral mucosa it typically presents as bilateral white lesions, occasionally with associated ulcers. The importance of this disease relates to its degree of frequency of occurrence, its occasional similarity to other mucosal diseases, and its occasionally painful nature.

Etiology and Pathogenesis. Although the cause of lichen planus is unknown, it is generally considered to be an immunologically mediated process that microscopically resembles a hypersensitivity reaction (Figure 3-38). It is characterized by an intense T-cell infiltrate (CD4 and especially CD8 cells) localized to the epithelium—connective tissue interface. Other immuneregulating cells (macrophages, factor XIIIa–positive

dendrocytes, Langerhans cells) are seen in increased numbers in lichen planus tissue. The disease mechanism appears to involve several steps that could be described as follows: an initiating factor/event, focal release of regulatory cytokines, up-regulation of vascular adhesion molecules, recruitment and retention of T lymphocytes, and cytotoxicity of basal keratinocytes mediated by the T lymphocytes.

The factor that initiates lichen planus is unknown. It is apparent, however, that recruitment and retention of lymphocytes is a requisite process. From what is known of leukocyte kinetics in tissue, attraction of lymphocytes to a particular site would require cytokine-mediated up-regulation of adhesion molecules on endothelial cells and concomitant expression of receptor molecules by circulating lymphocytes. In oral lichen planus there is in fact increased expression of several vascular adhesion molecules (known by acronyms ELAM-1, ICAM-1, VCAM-1) and infiltrating lymphocytes that express reciprocal receptors (known as L-selectin, LFA-1, and VLA4), supporting the hypothesis that there is activation of a lymphocyte homing mechanism in lichen planus. Some of the cytokines that are believed to be responsible for the up-regulated adhesion molecules are tumor necrosis factor (TNF-α), interleukin-1, and interferon-γ. The source of these cytokines is thought to be from resident macrophages, factor XIIIa–positive dendrocytes, Langerhans cells, and the lymphocytes themselves.

The overlying keratinocytes in lichen planus have a significant role in disease pathogenesis. They may be another source of chemoattractive and proinflammatory cytokines mentioned earlier, and more important, they appear to be the immunologic target of the recruited lymphocytes. This latter role seems to be enhanced through keratinocyte expression of the adhesion molecule ICAM-1, which would be attractive to lymphocytes with corresponding receptor molecules (LFA-1). This could set up a favorable relationship between T cells and keratinocytes for cytotoxicity. The T cells appear to mediate basal cell death through the triggering of apoptosis.

Clinical Features. Lichen planus is a disease of middle age that affects men and women in nearly equal numbers (Box 3-4). Children are rarely affected. The severity of the disease commonly parallels the patient's level of stress. An association between lichen planus and hepatitis C infection has been suggested. There appears to be no relationship between lichen planus and either hypertension or diabetes mellitus, as previously proposed. Many of these cases likely represent lichenoid drug reactions to the medications used to manage these conditions, which may mimic lichen planus clinically.

Several types of lichen planus within the oral cavity have been described. The most common type is the *reticular form,* which is characterized by numerous interlacing white keratotic lines or striae (so-called Wickham's striae) that produce an annular or lacy pattern. The buccal mucosa is the site most commonly involved (Figures 3-39 to 3-44). The striae, although occurring typically in a symmetric pattern on the buccal mucosa bilaterally, may also be noted on the tongue and less commonly on the gingiva and the lips. Almost any mucosal tissue may demonstrate manifestations of lichen planus. This form generally presents with minimal clinical symptoms and is often an incidental discovery.

The *plaque form* of lichen planus tends to resemble leukoplakia clinically but has a multifocal distribution. Such plaques generally range from slightly elevated to smooth and flat. The primary sites for this variant are the dorsum of the tongue and the buccal mucosa.

Box 3-4 Lichen Planus

CAUSE

Unknown; basal keratinocyte destruction by T lymphocytes

CLINICAL FEATURES

Adults; relatively common (0.2% to 1% of population); persistent
White keratotic striae are characteristic
Types—reticular, erosive (ulcerative), plaque, papular, erythematous (atrophic)
Pain—erosive form (occasionally erythematous form)

POSSIBLE RISK OF CARCINOMA TRANSFORMATION

May be slightly increased with erosive form (0.4% to 2.5% of cases)

PATHOLOGY

An interface mucositis with hyperkeratosis

TREATMENT

Observation, topical and systemic corticosteroids, or other immunosuppressive agents

---

The *erythematous* or *atrophic form* of lichen planus appears as red patches with very fine white striae. It may be seen in conjunction with reticular or erosive variants. The proportion of keratinized areas to atrophic areas varies from one area to another. The attached gingiva, commonly involved in this form of lichen planus, exhibits a patchy distribution, often in four quadrants. Patients may complain of burning, sensitivity, and generalized discomfort.

In the *erosive form* of lichen planus the central area of the lesion is ulcerated. A fibrinous plaque or pseudomembrane covers the ulcer. The process is a rather dynamic one, with changing patterns of involvement noted from week to week. Careful examination usually demonstrates keratotic striae, peripheral to the site of erosion, and erythema.

A rarely encountered form of lichen planus is the *bullous variant.* The bullae range from a few millimeters to centimeters in diameter. Such bullae are generally short lived and, on rupturing, leave a painful ulcer. Lesions are usually seen on the buccal mucosa, especially in the posterior and inferior regions adjacent to the second and third molars. Lesions are less common on the tongue, gingiva, and inner aspect of the lips. Reticular or striated keratotic

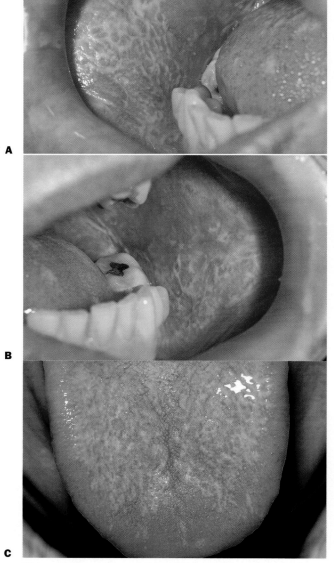

Figure 3-39   **A, B, and C, Oral lichen planus,** reticular form.

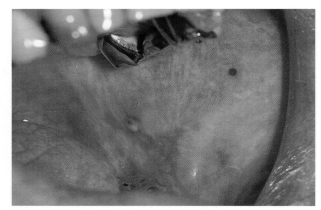

Figure 3-40   **Oral lichen planus,** erosive form.

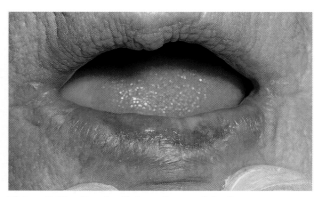

Figure 3-41   **Erosive lichen planus** of the lip.

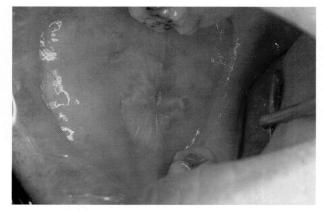

Figure 3-42   **Oral lichen planus,** plaque form.

areas should be seen with this variant of lichen planus.

On the skin, lichen planus is characterized by the presence of small, violaceous, polygonal, flat-topped, pruritic papules on the flexor surfaces. Other clinical varieties include hypertrophic, atrophic, bullous, follicular, and linear forms. Cutaneous lesions have been reported in 20% to 60% of patients presenting with oral lichen planus. Although the oral changes are rel-

atively persistent over time, corresponding skin lesions tend to wax and wane and exhibit a relatively short natural history (1 to 2 years).

Histopathology. The microscopic criteria for lichen planus include hyperkeratosis, basal layer vac-

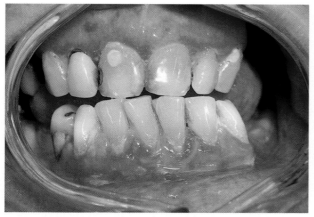

Figure 3-43 **Erythematous lichen planus** of the gingiva.

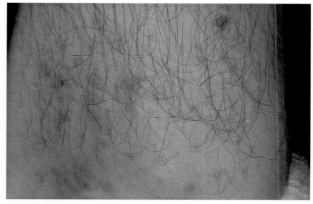

Figure 3-44 **Cutaneous lichen planus** of the ankle.

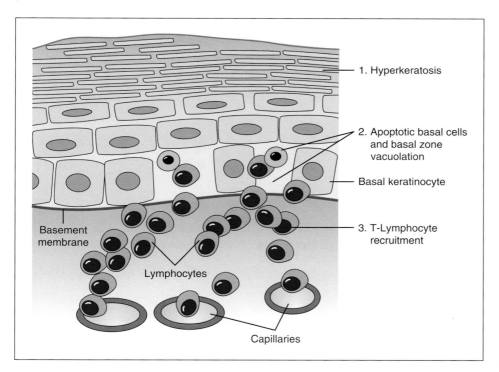

1. Hyperkeratosis

2. Apoptotic basal cells and basal zone vacuolation

Basal keratinocyte

3. T-Lymphocyte recruitment

Basement membrane

Lymphocytes

Capillaries

Figure 3-45 **Lichen planus:** diagnostic features.

uolization with apoptotic keratinocytes, and a lymphophagocytic infiltrate at the epithelium–connective tissue interface (Figures 3-45 to 3-48). With time, the epithelium undergoes gradual remodeling, resulting in reduced thickness and occasionally a sawtooth rete ridge pattern. Within the epithelium are increased numbers of Langerhans cells (as demonstrated with immunohistochemistry), presumably processing and presenting antigens to the subjacent T lymphocytes. Discrete eosinophilic ovoid bodies rep-

resenting the apoptotic keratinocytes are noted at the basal zone. These colloid, or Civatte, bodies are seen in other conditions such as drug reactions, contact hypersensitivity, lupus erythematosus, and some nonspecific inflammatory reactions.

Direct immunofluorescence demonstrates the presence of fibrinogen in the basement membrane zone in 90% to 100% of cases. Althoughimmunoglobulins and complement factors may be found as well, they are far less common than fibrinogen deposits.

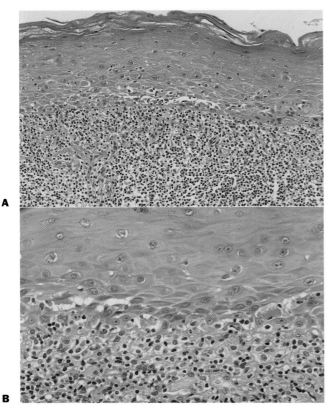

A

B

Figure 3-46   **Lichen planus** biopsy specimen showing hyperkeratosis, interface lymphocytic infiltrate, and basilar vacuolization with apoptosis.

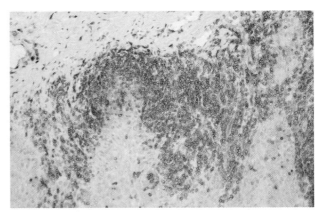

Figure 3-47   **Lichen planus.** Immunohistochemical stain for CD3 antigen demonstrating that infiltrate is predominantly T lymphocytes.

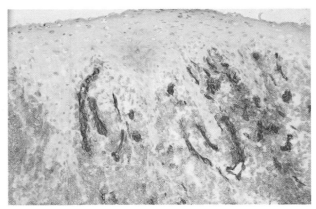

Figure 3-48   **Lichen planus.** Immunohistochemical stain for PECAM antigen showing adhesion molecule overexpression on capillaries *(dark red)* and lymphocytes.

Differential Diagnosis. Other diseases with a multifocal bilateral presentation that should be included in a clinical differential diagnosis are lichenoid drug reaction, lupus erythematosus, white sponge nevus, hairy leukoplakia, cheek chewing, graft-versus-host disease, and candidiasis. Idiopathic leukoplakia and squamous cell carcinoma might be considered when lesions are plaquelike. Erosive or atrophic lichen planus affecting the attached gingiva must be differentiated from cicatricial pemphigoid, pemphigus vulgaris, chronic lupus erythematosus, contact hypersensitivity, and chronic candidiasis.

Treatment and Prognosis. Although lichen planus cannot generally be cured, some drugs can provide satisfactory control. Corticosteroids are the single most useful group of drugs in the management of lichen planus. The rationale for their use is their ability to modulate inflammation and the immune response. Topical application and local injection of steroids have been successfully used in controlling but not curing

this disease. In circumstances in which symptoms are severe, systemic steroids may be used for initial management. The addition of antifungal therapy to a corticosteroid regimen typically enhances clinical results. This is likely a result of elimination of secondary *C. albicans* growth in lichen planus–involved tissue. Antifungals also prevent the overgrowth of *C. albicans* that may be associated with corticosteroid use. Application of topical tacrolimus has shown promising results in the treatment of symptomatic oral lichen planus in preliminary studies.

Because of their antikeratinizing and immunomodulating effects, systemic and topical vitamin A analogs (retinoids) have been used in the management of lichen planus. Reversal of white striae can be achieved with topical retinoids, although the effects may be only temporary. Systemic retinoids have been used in cases of severe lichen planus with various degrees of success. The benefits of systemic therapy must be carefully weighed against the rather significant side effects—cheilitis, elevation of serum liver enzyme and triglyceride levels, and teratogenicity. In cases with significant tissue involvement, more than one drug may be indicated. Various combinations of systemic steroids, topical steroids, and retinoids may be used with some success. Some cases of oral lichen planus may also respond to systemic hydroxychloroquine.

Clinical overdiagnosis of lichen planus, coincidental occurrence of lichen planus and oral cancer, and microscopic confusion with dysplasias that have lichenoid features have contributed to the controversy of malignant potential of this disease. Nonetheless, it appears that there is a *bona fide* risk of oral squamous cell carcinoma developing in oral lichen planus, but this risk is low and probably lower than reported rates. If malignant transformation occurs, it is more likely to be associated with the erosive and atrophic forms of the disease. Because lichen planus is a chronic condition, patients should be observed periodically and should be offered education about the clinical course, rationale of therapy, and possible risk of malignant transformation.

Lupus Erythematosus

Lupus erythematosus (LE) may be seen in one of two well-recognized forms—systemic (acute) lupus erythematosus (SLE) and discoid (chronic) lupus erythematosus (DLE)—both of which may have oral manifestations. A third form, known as *subacute*

lupus, has also been described. In the spectrum of LE, SLE is of particular importance because of the profound impact it has on many organs. DLE is the less aggressive form, affecting predominantly the skin and rarely progressing to the systemic form. It may, however, be of great cosmetic significance because of its predilection for the face. Subacute cutaneous LE, described as lying intermediate between SLE and DLE, results in skin lesions of mild to moderate severity. It is marked by mild systemic involvement and the appearance of some abnormal autoantibodies.

Etiology and Pathogenesis. LE is believed to be an autoimmune disease involving both the humoral and the cell-mediated arms of the immune system.

Autoantibodies directed against various cellular antigens in both the nucleus and the cytoplasm have been identified. These antibodies may be found in the serum or in tissue, bound to antigens. Circulating antibodies are responsible for the positive reactions noted in the antinuclear antibody (ANA) and LE cell tests that are performed to help confirm the diagnosis of lupus. Also circulating in serum are antigen-antibody complexes that mediate disease in many organ systems.

Clinical Features

Discoid Lupus Erythematosus. DLE is characteristically seen in middle age, especially in women. Lesions commonly appear solely on the skin, most commonly on the face and scalp (Table 3-3; Figures 3-49 to 3-52). Oral and vermilion lesions are also commonly seen, but usually in the company of cutaneous lesions. On the skin, lesions appear as disk-shaped erythematous plaques with hyperpigmented margins. As the lesion

TABLE 3-3 **Lupus Erythematosus**

	Discoid	Systemic
Organs	Skin and oral only	Skin, oral, heart, kidneys, joints
Symptoms	No	Fever, malaise, weight loss
Serology	No detectable antibodies	Positive ANA, anti-DNA antibodies
Histopathology	Basal cell loss, lymphocytes at interface and perivascular, keratosis	Similar to discoid
DIF	Granular/linear basement membrane deposits of IgG and C3	Similar to discoid

ANA, Antinuclear antibody; *LE,* lupus erythematosus; *DIF,* direct immunofluorescence; *IgG,* immunoglobulin G; *C,* complement.

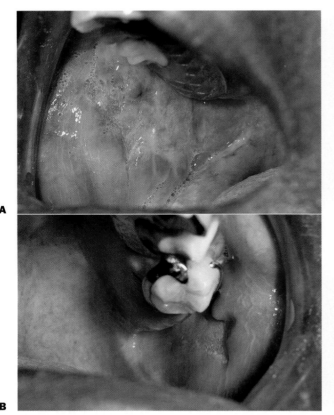

A

B

Figure 3-49 **A and B, Discoid (chronic) lupus erythematosus.**

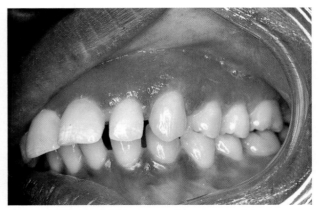

Figure 3-50 **Discoid lupus erythematosus** of the maxillary gingiva.

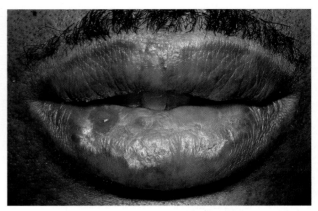

Figure 3-51 **Discoid lupus erythematosus** of the lip.

expands peripherally, the center heals, with the formation of scar and loss of pigment. Involvement of hair follicles results in permanent hair loss (alopecia).

Mucous membrane lesions appear in about 25% of patients with cutaneous DLE. The buccal mucosa, gingiva, and vermilion are most commonly affected. Lesions may be erythematous or ulcerative with delicate white, keratotic striae radiating from the periphery. The diagnosis of oral lesions may not be evident on the basis of clinical appearance. Progression of DLE to SLE is very unlikely, although the potential does exist.

Systemic Lupus Erythematosus. In SLE, skin and mucosal lesions are relatively mild, and patients' complaints are dominated by multiple organ involvement (Figure 3-53). Numerous autoantibodies directed against nuclear and cytoplasmic antigens are found in SLE-affected patients. These antibodies, when complexed to their corresponding antigens either in serum

or in the target organ, can cause lesions in nearly any tissue, resulting in a wide variety of clinical signs and symptoms.

Involvement of the skin results in an erythematous rash, classically seen over the malar processes and bridge of the nose. This "butterfly" distribution is usually associated with SLE. Other areas of the face, trunk, and hands may also be involved. The lesions are nonscarring and may flare as systemic involvement progresses.

Oral lesions of SLE are generally similar to those seen in DLE. Ulceration, erythema, and keratosis may be seen. In addition to the vermilion, the buccal mucosa, gingiva, and palate are often involved.

Systemic symptoms of SLE may initially consist of fever, weight loss, and malaise. Typically, with disease progression many organ systems become involved. The

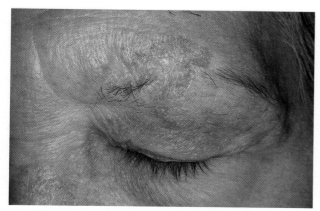

Figure 3-52 **Discoid lupus erythematosus** of the face.

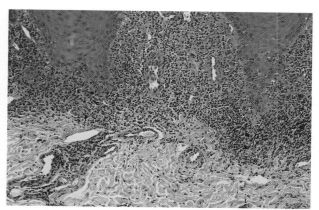

Figure 3-54 **Oral discoid lupus erythematosus** showing interface and perivascular lymphocytic infiltrate.

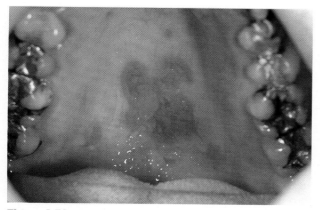

Figure 3-53 **Systemic lupus erythematosus,** oral lesion.

joints, kidneys, heart, and lungs are most commonly affected, although many other organs may express manifestations of this disease. Kidney lesions (glomerulonephritis) showing a range of forms and severity are, however, the most important, because they are most commonly responsible for the death of SLE-affected patients.

Serologic tests for autoantibodies yield positive results in patients with SLE. The ANA test is regarded as a reliable and relatively specific test for SLE. Among the antibodies that may cause a positive ANA test result are anti–single-stranded DNA, anti–double-stranded DNA, and antinuclear ribonuclear protein. Specific tests for these and other autoantibodies of SLE are also available. Another serologic test for SLE is the LE cell test, although it is less sensitive and less specific than the ANA test. Antibodies to Ro (SS-A)

and La (SS-B) cytoplasmic antigens may also be present in SLE.

Histopathology. In DLE, basal cell destruction, hyperkeratosis, epithelial atrophy, lymphocytic infiltration (subepithelial and perivascular distribution), and vascular dilation with edema of the submucosa are seen (Figure 3-54). It appears that the basal keratinocytes are a primary target in mucous membranes. Because this is also the case for lichen planus, the two diseases may, on occasion, be difficult to separate by routine microscopic studies.

In SLE, oral lesions are microscopically similar to lesions of DLE, although inflammatory cell infiltrates are less intense and more diffuse. Other organs, when involved in SLE, show vasculitis, mononuclear infiltrates, and fibrinoid necrosis. Direct immunofluorescent testing of skin and mucosal lesions shows granular-linear deposits of immunoglobulins (IgG, IgM, IgA), complement (C3), and fibrinogen along the basement membrane zone in a majority of patients.

Differential Diagnosis. Clinically, lesions of oral LE most often resemble erosive lichen planus but tend to be less symmetrically distributed. The keratotic striae of LE are also much more delicate and subtle than Wickham's striae of lichen planus and show characteristic radiation from a central focus. Erythematous gingival lupus may be confused with mucous membrane pemphigoid, erythematous lichen planus, erythematous candidiasis, and contact hypersensitivity.

Treatment. DLE is usually treated with topical corticosteroids. High-potency ointments can be used intraorally. In refractory cases antimalarials or sulfones may be used.

Systemic steroids may be used in the treatment of SLE. The prednisone dose is generally dependent on the severity of the disease, and prednisone may be combined with immunosuppressive agents for their therapeutic and steroid-sparing effects. Antimalarials and nonsteroidal antiinflammatory drugs may also help control this disease.

NONEPITHELIAL WHITE-YELLOW LESIONS

Candidiasis

Candidiasis is a common opportunistic oral mycotic infection that develops in the presence of one of several predisposing conditions. Clinical presentation is variable and is dependent on whether the condition is acute or chronic (Box 3-5).

Etiology and Pathogenesis. Candidiasis is caused by *C. albicans* and much less commonly by other species of *Candida: C. parapsilosis, C. tropicalis, C. glabrata, C. krusei, C. pseudotropicalis,* and *C. guilliermondi. C. albicans* is a commensal organism residing in the oral cavity in a majority of healthy persons. Transformation, or escape from a state of commensalism to that of a pathogen, relates to local and systemic factors. The organism is a unicellular yeast of the Cryptococcaceae family and may exist in three distinct biologic and morphologic forms: the vegetative or yeast form of oval cells (blastospores), measuring 1.5 to 5 μm in diameter; the elongated cellular form (pseudohyphae); and the chlamydospore form, which consists of cell bodies measuring 7 to 17 μm in diameter, with a thick, refractile, enclosing wall. As evidenced by its frequency in the general population, *C. albicans* is of weak pathogenicity, thereby reflecting the necessity for local or systemic predisposing factors to produce a disease state (Box 3-6).

Infection with this organism is usually superficial, affecting the outer aspects of the involved oral mucosa or skin. In severely debilitated and immunocompromised patients, such as patients with AIDS, infection may extend into the alimentary tract (candidal esophagitis), bronchopulmonary tract, or other organ systems. The opportunistic nature of this organism is observed in the frequency of mild forms of the disease secondary to short-term use of systemic antibiotic therapy for minor bacterial infections.

Clinical Features. The most common form of candidiasis is acute pseudomembranous, also known as *thrush* (Box 3-7). Young infants and the elderly are commonly affected. Estimates of disease frequency range up to 5% of neonates, 5% of cancer patients, and 10% of institutionalized, debilitated elderly patients. This infection is common in patients being treated with radiation or chemotherapy for leukemia and solid tumors, with up to half of those in the former group and 70% in the latter group affected. Recalcitrant candidiasis has been recognized in patients who have HIV infections and AIDS.

Oral lesions of *acute candidiasis (thrush)* are characteristically white, soft plaques that sometimes grow centrifugally and merge (Figures 3-55 to 3-61). Plaques are composed of fungal organisms, keratotic

---

Box 3-5 Candidiasis

SYNONYMS

Thrush, angular cheilitis, median rhomboid glossitis, denture sore mouth, yeast infection, candidal leukoplakia, antibiotic stomatitis, moniliasis

CAUSE

Candida albicans and other *Candida* species in oral flora
Predisposing factors required
Opportunistic overgrowth

TYPES

Acute, chronic, mucocutaneous

Box 3-6 Candidiasis: Predisposing Factors

Immunodeficiency
   Immunologic immaturity of infancy
   Acquired immunosuppression
Endocrine disturbances
   Diabetes mellitus
   Hypoparathyroidism
   Pregnancy
   Hypoadrenalism
Corticosteroid therapy, topical or systemic
Systemic antibiotic therapy
Malignancies and their therapies
Xerostomia
Poor oral hygiene

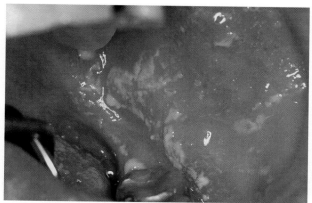

Figure 3-55   **Candidiasis,** pseudomembranous type.

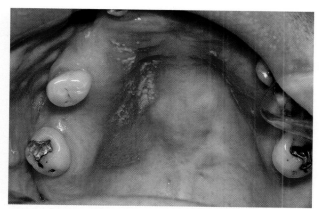

Figure 3-57   **Candidiasis,** pseudomembranous type.

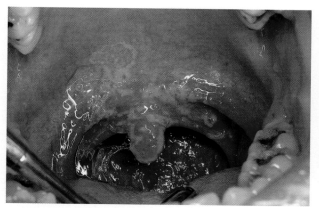

Figure 3-56   **Candidiasis,** pseudomembranous type.

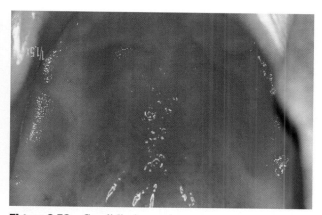

Figure 3-58   **Candidiasis,** erythematous type.

debris, inflammatory cells, desquamated epithelial cells, bacteria, and fibrin. Wiping away the plaques or pseudomembranes with a gauze sponge leaves a painful erythematous, eroded, or ulcerated surface. Although lesions of thrush may develop at any location, favored sites include the buccal mucosa and mucobuccal folds, the oropharynx, and the lateral aspects of the tongue. In most instances in which the pseudomembrane has not been disturbed, the associated symptoms are minimal. In severe cases patients may complain of tenderness, burning, and dysphagia.

Persistence of acute pseudomembranous candidiasis may eventually result in loss of the pseudomembrane, with presentation as a more generalized red lesion, known as *acute erythematous candidiasis*. Along the dorsum of the tongue, patches of depapillation and dekeratinization may be noted. In the past, this particular form of candidiasis was known as *antibiotic stomatitis* or *antibiotic glossitis* because of its common relationship to antibiotic treatment of acute infections. Broad-spectrum antibiotics or concurrent administration of multiple narrow-spectrum antibiotics may produce this secondary infection to a much greater degree than do single narrow-spectrum antibiotics. Withdrawal of the offending antibiotic, if possible, and institution of appropriate oral hygiene lead to improvement. In contrast to the acute pseudomembranous form, oral symptoms of the acute atrophic form are quite marked because of numerous erosions and intense inflammation.

Chronic erythematous candidiasis is a commonly seen form occurring in as many as 65% of geriatric individuals who wear complete maxillary dentures (denture sore mouth). Expression of this form of candidiasis depends on the conditioning of the oral

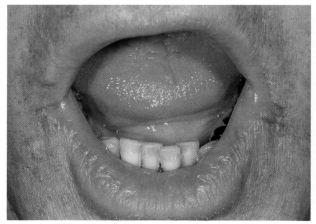

Figure 3-59   **Candidiasis,** angular cheilitis form.

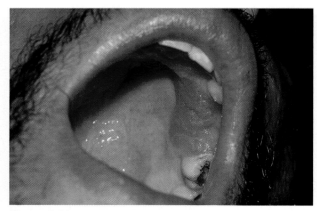

Figure 3-61   **Candidiasis,** hyperplastic type.

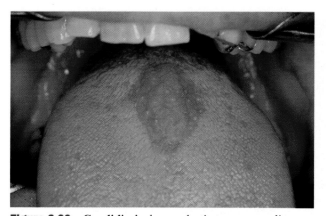

Figure 3-60   **Candidiasis,** hyperplastic type or median rhomboid glossitis.

Box 3-7 Candidiasis: Classification

ACUTE

Pseudomembraneous (white colonies)
Erythematous (red mucosa)

CHRONIC

Erythematous (red mucosa)
Hyperplastic (white keratotic plaque)

MUCOCUTANEOUS

Localized (oral, face, scalp, nails)
Familial
Syndrome associated

---

mucosa by a covering prosthesis. There is a distinct predilection for the palatal mucosa as compared with the mandibular alveolar arch. Chronic low-grade trauma secondary to poor prosthesis fit, less than ideal occlusal relationships, and failure to remove the appliance at night all contribute to the development of this condition. The clinical appearance is that of a bright red, somewhat velvety to pebbly surface, with relatively little keratinization.

Also seen in individuals with denture-related chronic atrophic candidiasis is *angular cheilitis.* This condition is especially prevalent in individuals who have deep folds at the commissures secondary to overclosure. In such circumstances small accumulations of saliva gather in the skin folds at the commissural angles and are subsequently colonized by yeast organisms (and often by *Staphylococcus aureus*). Clinically, the lesions are moderately painful, fissured, eroded, and encrusted. Angular cheilitis may also occur in individuals who habitually lick their lips and deposit small amounts of saliva in the commissural angles.

A circumoral type of atrophic candidiasis may be noted in those with severe lip-licking habits with extension of the process onto the surrounding skin. The skin is fissured and demonstrates a degree of brown discoloration on a slightly erythematous base. This condition is to be distinguished from *perioral dermatitis,* which characteristically shows less crusting and a circumferential zone of uninvolved skin immediately adjacent to the cutaneous-vermilion junction.

Chronic candidal infections are also capable of producing a hyperplastic tissue response (*chronic hyperplastic candidiasis*). When occurring in the retrocommissural area, the lesion resembles speckled leukoplakia and, in some classifications, is known as *candidal leukoplakia*. It occurs in adults with no apparent predisposition to infection by *C. albicans,* and it is believed by some clinicians to represent a premalignant lesion.

Hyperplastic candidiasis may involve the dorsum of the tongue in a pattern referred to as *median rhomboid glossitis*. It is usually asymptomatic and is generally discovered on routine oral examination. The lesion is found anterior to the circumvallate papillae and has an oval or rhomboid outline. It may have a smooth, nodular, or fissured surface and may range in color from white to a more characteristic red. A similar-appearing red lesion may also be present on the adjacent hard palate ("kissing lesion"). Whether on the tongue or on the palate, the condition may occasionally be mildly painful, although most cases are asymptomatic. In the past, this particular condition was believed to be a developmental anomaly, presumably secondary to persistence of the tuberculum impar of the developing tongue. Since it is never seen in children, it more likely a hyperplastic form of candidiasis. Microscopically, epithelial hyperplasia is evident in the form of bulbous rete ridges. *C. albicans* hyphae can usually be found in the upper levels of the epithelium. A thick band of hyalinized connective tissue separates the epithelium from deeper structures.

Nodular papillary lesions of the hard palatal mucosa predominantly seen beneath maxillary complete dentures are thought to represent, at least in part, a response to chronic fungus infection. The *papillary hyperplasia* is composed of individual nodules that are ovoid to spherical and form excrescences measuring 2 to 3 mm in diameter on an erythematous background.

Mucocutaneous candidiasis is a rather diverse group of conditions. The localized form of mucocutaneous candidiasis is characterized by long-standing and persistent candidiasis of the oral mucosa, nails, skin, and vaginal mucosa. This form of candidiasis is often resistant to treatment, with only temporary remission following the use of standard antifungal therapy. This form begins early in life, usually within the first 2 decades. The disease begins as a pseudomembranous type of candidiasis and is soon followed by nail and cutaneous involvement.

A familial form of mucocutaneous candidiasis, believed to be transmitted in an autosomal-recessive fashion, occurs in nearly 50% of patients with an associated endocrinopathy. The endocrinopathy usually consists of hypoparathyroidism, Addison's disease, and occasionally hypothyroidism or diabetes mellitus. Other forms of familial mucocutaneous candidiasis have associated defects in iron metabolism and cell-mediated immunity.

A rare triad of chronic mucocutaneous candidiasis, myositis, and thymoma has been described. The role of the thymus relates to a deficiency in T cell–mediated immunologic function, hence providing an opportunity for the proliferation of *Candida*.

A final form of candidiasis, both acute and chronic, is becoming increasingly evident within the immunosuppressed population of patients, in particular those infected with HIV. This form of candidiasis was originally described in 1981 and is now well recognized as being one of the more important opportunistic infections that afflict this group of patients. The significantly depleted cell-mediated arm of the immune system is believed to be responsible for allowing the development of severe candidiasis in these patients.

Histopathology. In acute candidiasis, fungal hyphae are seen penetrating the upper layers of the epithelium at acute angles (Figure 3-62). Neutrophilic infiltration of the epithelium with superficial microabscess formation is also typically seen. Fungal forms may be enhanced in tissue sections by staining with methenamine silver or periodic acid–Schiff (PAS) reagent. The predominant fungal forms growing in this particular form of the disease are pseudohyphae.

Epithelial hyperplasia is a rather characteristic feature of chronic candidiasis. However, organisms may be sparse, making histologic demonstration sometimes difficult. Although chronic candidiasis may give rise to oral leukoplakia, there is no clear evidence that chronic candidiasis is in and of itself a precancerous state.

Clinical laboratory tests for this organism involve removal of a portion of the candidal plaque, which is then smeared on a microscope slide and macerated with 20% potassium hydroxide or stained with PAS. The slide is subsequently examined for typical hyphae. Also, culture identification and quantification of organisms may be done on Sabouraud broth, blood agar, or cornmeal agar.

Differential Diagnosis. Candidal white lesions should be differentiated from slough associated with chemical burns, traumatic ulcerations, mucous patches of syphilis, and white keratotic lesions. Red lesions of candidiasis should be differentiated from drug reactions, erosive lichen planus, and discoid lupus erythematosus.

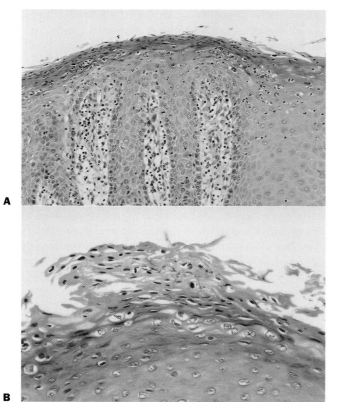

A

B

Figure 3-62 **Oral candidiasis. A,** Psoriasiform pattern. **B,** High magnification of fungal hyphae in keratin layer.

Treatment and Prognosis. Attending to predisposing factors is an important component of management of patients with candidiasis. The majority of infections may be simply treated with topical applications of nystatin suspension, although this may be prove to be ineffective, since contact time with the lesion is short (Box 3-8). Nystatin cream or ointment is often effective when applied directly to the affected tissue on gauze pads and for denture-associated candidiasis when applied directly to the denture-bearing surface itself. In both circumstances prolonged contact time with the lesion proves to be an effective delivery strategy. Clotrimazole can be conveniently administered in troche form. Topical applications of either nystatin or clotrimazole should be continued for at least 1 week beyond the disappearance of clinical manifestations of the disease. It is important to note that antifungals designed specifically for oral use contain considerable amounts of sugar, making them undesirable for the treatment of candidiasis in dentulous patients with xerostomia. Sugar-free antifungal vaginal suppositories, dissolved

---

Box 3-8 Candidiasis: Treatment

TOPICAL

Nystatin—oral suspension* and pastille*; powder and ointment for denture
Clotrimazole—oral troches,* vaginal tablets (dissolved in mouth)

SYSTEMIC

Fluconazole, ketoconazole

*Contains sugar; do not use with dentate patients with xerostomia.

---

in the mouth, are an excellent treatment alternative to avoid the complication of dental caries.

For hyperplastic candidiasis, topical and systemic antifungal therapy may be ineffective at completely removing the lesions, particularly those that occur on the buccal mucosa, near the commissures. In these circumstances surgical management may be necessary to complement antifungal medications.

In cases of chronic mucocutaneous candidiasis or oral candidiasis associated with immunosuppression, topical agents may not be effective. In such instances systemic administration of medications such as ketoconazole, fluconazole, or itraconazole may be necessary. All are available in oral form. Caution must be exercised, however, because these drugs may be hepatotoxic.

The prognosis for acute and most other forms of chronic candidiasis is excellent. The underlying defect in most types of mucocutaneous candidiasis, however, militates against cure, although intermittent improvement may be noted after the use of systemic antifungal agents.

Mucosal Burns

Etiology. The most common form of superficial burn of the oral mucosa is associated with topical applications of chemicals, such as aspirin or caustic agents. Topical abuse of drugs, accidental placement of phosphoric acid–etching solutions or gel by a dentist, or overly fastidious use of alcohol-containing mouthrinses may produce similar effects.

Clinical Features. In cases of short-term exposure to agents capable of inducing tissue necrosis, a localized

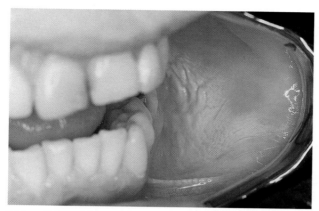

Figure 3-63 **Mucosal burn** (necrosis) due to prolonged aspirin contact.

mild erythema may occur (Figure 3-63). As the concentration and contact time of the offending agent increase, surface coagulative necrosis is more likely to occur, resulting in the formation of a white slough, or membrane. With gentle traction the surface slough peels from the denuded connective tissue, producing pain.

Thermal burns are commonly noted on the hard palatal mucosa and are generally associated with hot, sticky foods. Hot liquids are more likely to burn the tongue or the soft palate. Such lesions are generally erythematous rather than white (necrosis), as is seen with chemical burns.

Another form of burn that is potentially quite serious is the electrical burn. In particular, children who chew through electrical cords receive rather characteristic initial burns that are often symmetric. The result of these accidents is significant tissue damage, often followed by scarring. The surface of these lesions tends to be characterized by a thickened slough that extends deep into the connective tissue.

Histopathology. In cases of chemical and thermal burns in which an obvious clinical slough has developed, the epithelial component shows coagulative necrosis through its entire thickness. A fibrinous exudate is also evident. The underlying connective tissue is intensely inflamed. Electrical burns are more destructive, showing deep extension of necrosis, often into muscle.

Treatment. Management of chemical, thermal, or electrical burns is quite varied. For patients with thermal or chemical burns, local symptomatic therapy aimed at keeping the mouth clean, such as sodium bicarbonate mouthrinses with or without the use of systemic

analgesics, is appropriate. Alcohol-based commercial mouthrinses should be discouraged because of their drying effect on the oral mucosa. For patients with electrical burns, management may be much more difficult. The services of a pediatric dentist or oral and maxillofacial surgeon may be necessary in more severe cases. Pressure stents may be required over the damaged areas to prevent early contracture of the wounds. After healing, further definitive surgical or reconstructive treatment may be necessary because of extensive scar formation.

Submucous Fibrosis

Etiology. Several factors contributing to submucous fibrosis include general nutritional or vitamin deficiencies and hypersensitivity to various dietary constituents. The primary factor appears to be habitual chewing of the areca (betel) nut. It appears that the condition is due to impaired degradation of normal collagen by fibroblasts rather than excess production. Also, chronic consumption of chili peppers or chronic and prolonged deficiency of iron and B complex vitamins, especially folic acid, increases the hypersensitivity to many potential irritants (areca nut, dietary spices, and tobacco), with an attendant inflammatory reaction and fibrosis.

Clinical Features. Rarely seen in North America, submucous fibrosis is relatively common in Southeast Asia, India, and neighboring countries. The condition is seen typically between the ages of 20 and 40.

Oral submucous fibrosis presents as a whitish yellow change that has a chronic, insidious biologic course. It is characteristically seen in the oral cavity, but on occasion it may extend into the pharynx and the esophagus. Submucous fibrosis may occasionally be preceded by or be associated with vesicle formation. In time, the affected mucosa, especially the soft palate and the buccal mucosa, loses its resilience and elasticity. Fibrous bands are readily palpable in the soft palate and buccal mucosa. The clinical result is significant trismus and considerable difficulty in eating. The process then progresses from the lamina propria to the underlying musculature.

Histopathology. Microscopically, the principal feature is atrophy of the epithelium and subjacent fibrosis (Figure 3-64). Epithelial dysplasia may occasionally be evident. The lamina propria is poorly vascularized and hyalinized; fibroblasts are few. A diffuse mild to moderate inflammatory infiltrate is present. Type I colla-

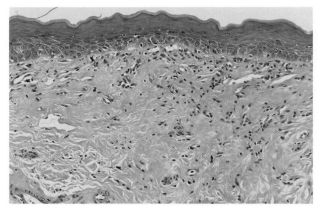

Figure 3-64   **Submuous fibrosis** showing epithelial atrophy over fibrotic submucosa.

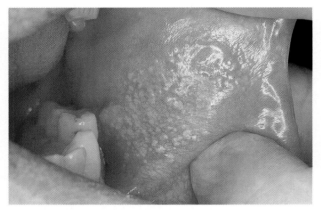

Figure 3-65   **Fordyce's granules.**

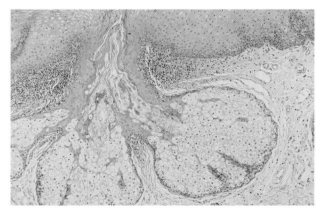

Figure 3-66   **Fordyce's granules** showing sebaceous gland lobules.

gen predominates in submucosa, whereas type III collagen tends to localize at the epithelium–connective tissue interface, and around blood vessels, salivary glands, and muscle.

Treatment and Prognosis.   Eliminating causative agents is part of the management of submucous fibrosis. Therapeutic measures include local injections of chymotrypsin, hyaluronidase, and dexamethasone, with surgical excision of fibrous bands and submucosal placement of vascularized free flap grafts. All methods of treatment, however, have proved to be of only modest help in this essentially irreversible condition.

The primary importance of submucous fibrosis relates to its premalignant nature. The development of squamous cell carcinoma has been noted in as many as one third of patients with submucous fibrosis.

Fordyce's Granules

Fordyce's granules represent ectopic sebaceous glands or sebaceous choristomas (normal tissue in an abnormal location). This condition is regarded as developmental and can be considered a variation of normal.

Fordyce's granules are multiple, often seen in aggregates or in confluent arrangements (Figures 3-65 to 3-66). The sites of predilection include the buccal mucosa and the vermilion of the upper lip. The lesions generally are symmetrically distributed. They tend to become obvious after puberty, with maximal expression occurring between 20 and 30 years of age. The lesions are asymptomatic and are often discov-

ered incidentally by the patient or by the practitioner during a routine oral examination. A large proportion of the population is affected by this particular condition; it is seen in over 80% of individuals.

Microscopically, lobules of sebaceous glands are aggregated around or adjacent to excretory ducts. The heterotopic glands are well formed and appear functional.

No treatment is indicated for this particular condition, because the glands are normal in character and do not cause any untoward effects.

Ectopic Lymphoid Tissue

Ectopic lymphoid tissue may be found in numerous oral locations. Found in the posterolateral aspect of the tongue, it is known as *lingual tonsil.* Aggregates of

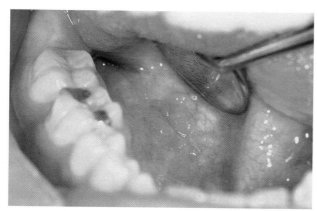

Figure 3-67 **Ectopic lymphoid** tissue in the floor of the mouth.

lymphoid tissue are commonly seen in the soft palate, floor of the mouth, and tonsillar pillars (Figure 3-67).

Lymphoid tissue appears yellow or yellow-white clinically and typically produces small, dome-shaped elevations. The tissue appears uninflamed, and the patient is unaware of its presence. Crypts in the lymphoid tissue may on occasion become obstructed, causing "cystic" dilation of the area. These lesions may then be called *lymphoepithelial cysts*. In a strict sense, however, lymphoepithelial cysts are believed to be derived from cystic changes of embryonically entrapped epithelium within lymphoid tissue.

Generally, lymphoid tissue can be diagnosed on the basis of clinical features alone. Because this is basically normal tissue, no biopsy is necessary.

Gingival Cysts

Gingival cysts of odontogenic origin occur in adults, as well as infants *(Bohn's nodules)*. In infants the relative frequency is highest in the neonatal phase. They occur along the alveolar ridges and involute spontaneously or rupture and exfoliate. Another eponym, *Epstein's pearls*, has been commonly used to designate nonodontogenic neonatal cysts that occur along the palatal midline (fusion of palatine shelves).

Etiology and Pathogenesis. Neonatal gingival cysts are thought to arise from dental lamina remnants. Fetal tissues between 10 and 12 weeks of age show small amounts of keratin within elements of the dental lamina. Toward the end of the twelfth week of gestation, disruption of the dental lamina is evident, with many fragments exhibiting central cystification and keratin accumulation. Gingival cysts are generally numerous in the fetus and infant, increasing in number until the twenty-second week of gestation.

Midline palatal cysts, or Epstein's pearls, are thought to result from epithelial entrapment within the midline of palatal fusion. Small epithelial inclusions within the line of fusion produce microcysts that contain keratin and rupture early in life.

The origin of the gingival cyst of the adult is probably from remnants of the dental lamina (rests of Serres) within the gingival submucosa. Cystic changes of these rests may occasionally result in a multilocular lesion. An alternative theory of pathogenesis relates to the traumatic implantation of surface epithelium into gingival connective tissue.

Clinical Features. Gingival cysts in a neonate present as off-white nodules approximately 2 mm in diameter. Cysts ranging in number from one to many are evident along the alveolar crests. Midline palatal cysts, on the other hand, present along the midpalatal raphe toward the junction of the hard and soft palate.

The gingival cyst of adults occurs chiefly during the fifth and sixth decades. It appears more commonly in the mandible than in the maxilla. There is a great deal of similarity between the gingival cyst in the adult and the lateral periodontal cyst, including the site of predilection, age of occurrence, clinical behavior, and overall morphology. It presents as a painless growth in the attached gingiva, often within the interdental papilla. Only rarely are lesions found in the lingual gingiva. Premolar and bicuspid regions of the mandible are favored locations.

Histopathology. The neonatal gingival cyst is lined by bland stratified squamous epithelium and is filled with keratinaceous debris. The gingival cyst of adults is lined by a thin layer of cuboidal or flattened epithelium with focal thickenings that often show clear cell change.

Treatment. No treatment is indicated for gingival or palatal cysts of the newborn, because they spontaneously rupture early in life. Treatment of gingival cysts of the adult is surgical excision.

Parulis

A parulis, or "gum boil," represents a focus of pus in the gingiva. It is derived from an acute infection, either at the base of an occluded periodontal pocket or at the apex of a nonvital tooth. The path of least resistance most often leads to gingival submucosa. The lesion appears as a yellow-white gingival tumescence with an associated erythema (Figure 3-68). Pain is typical, but once the pus escapes to the surface, symptoms are temporarily relieved. Treatment of the underlying condition (periodontal pocket or nonvital tooth) is required to achieve resolution of the gingival abscess.

Lipoma

Lipoma presents as a yellow or yellow-white uninflamed submucosal mass of adipose tissue. It is included in this section for completeness. Discussion is found in Chapter 7.

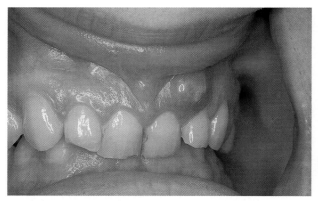

Figure 3-68 Parulis (gingival abscess) associated with periapical abscess.

BIBLIOGRAPHY

HEREDITARY CONDITIONS

Burge SM, Millard PR, Wojnarowska F, et al: Darier's disease: a focal abnormality of cell adhesion, *J Cutan Pathol* 17:160-169, 1990.

Feinstein A, Friedman J, Schewach-Miller M: Pachyonychia congenita, *J Am Acad Dermatol* 19:705-711, 1988.

Lim J, Ng S: Oral tetracycline rinse improves symptoms of white sponge nevus, *J Am Acad Dermatol* 26:1003-1005, 1992.

Nichols GE, Cooper PH, Underwood PB, et al: White sponge nevus, *Obstet Gynecol* 76:545-548, 1990.

Richard G, De Laurenzi V, Didona B, et al: Keratin 13 point mutation underlies the hereditary mucosal epithelial disorder white sponge nevus, *Nat Genet* 11:453-455, 1995.

Rugg E, McLean WH, Allison WE, et al: A mutation in the mucosal keratin K4 is associated with oral white sponge nevus, *Nat Genet* 11:450-452, 1995.

REACTIVE LESIONS

Daniels TE, Hansen LS, Greenspan JS, et al: Histopathology of smokeless tobacco lesions in professional baseball players, *Oral Surg Oral Med Oral Pathol* 73:720-725, 1992.

Grady P, Greene J, Daniels TE, et al: Oral mucosal lesions found in smokeless tobacco users, *J Am Dent Assoc* 121:117-123, 1990.

Robertson PB, Walsh M, Greene J, et al: Periodontal effects associated with the use of smokeless tobacco, *J Periodontol* 61:438-443, 1990.

Walsh PM, Epstein JB: The oral effects of smokeless tobacco, *J Can Dent Assoc* 66(1):22-25, 2000.

PRENEOPLASTIC AND NEOPLASTIC LESIONS

Batsakis JG, Suarez P, el-Naggar AK: Proliferative verrucous leukoplakia and its related lesions, *Oral Oncol* 35(4):354-359, 1999.

O'Shaughnessy JA, Kelloff GJ, Gordon GB, et al: Treatment and prevention of intraepithelial neoplasia: an important target for accelerated new agent development. *Clin Cancer Res* 8:314-346, 2002.

Rojas AI, Ahmed AR: Adhesion receptors in health and disease, *Crit Rev Oral Biol Med* 10:337-358, 1999.

van der Meij EH, Schepman KP, Smeele LE, et al: A review of the recent literature regarding malignant transformation of oral lichen planus, *Oral Surg Oral Med Oral Pathol Oral Radiol Endod* 88:307-310, 1999.

Zakrzewska JM, Lopes V, Speight P, et al: Proliferative verrucous leukoplakia, *Oral Surg Oral Med Oral Pathol Oral Radiol Endod* 82:396-401, 1996.

OTHER WHITE LESIONS

Barker J, Mitra R, Griffiths C, et al: Keratinocytes as initiators of inflammation, *Lancet* 337:211-214, 1991.

Barnard NA, Scully C, Eveson JW, et al: Oral cancer development in patients with oral lichen planus, *J Oral Pathol Med* 22:421-424, 1993.

Boehncke W, Kellner I, Konter U, et al: Differential expression of adhesion molecules on infiltrating cells in inflammatory dermatoses, *J Am Acad Dermatol* 26:907-913, 1992.

Boisnic S, Francis C, Branchet MC, et al: Immunohistochemical study of oral lesions of lichen planus: diagnostic and pathophysiologic aspects, *Oral Surg Oral Med Oral Pathol* 70:462-465, 1990.

Bolewska J, Holmstrup P, Moller-Madsen B, et al: Amalgam-associated mercury accumulations in normal oral mucosa, oral mucosal lesions of lichen planus and contact lesions associated with amalgam, *J Oral Pathol Med* 19:39-42, 1990.

Dekker NP, Lozada-Nur F, Lagenauer LA, et al: Apoptosis-associated markers in oral lichen planus, *J Oral Pathol Med* 26:170-175, 1997.

Ficarra G, Flaitz CM, Gaglioti D, et al: White lichenoid lesions of the buccal mucosa in patients with HIV infection, *Oral Surg Oral Med Oral Pathol* 76:460-466, 1993.

Gandolfo S, Carbone M, Carrozzo M, et al: Oral lichen planus and hepatitis C virus (HCV) infection: is there a relationship? A report of 10 cases, *J Oral Pathol Med* 23:119-122, 1994.

Greenspan JS, Greenspan D, Palefsky JM: Oral hairy leukoplakia after a decade, *Epstein-Barr Virus Report* 2:123-128, 1995.

Holmstrup P, Scholtz AW, Westergaard J: Effect of dental plaque control on gingival lichen planus, *Oral Surg Oral Med Oral Pathol* 69:585-590, 1990.

Hong WK: Chemoprevention in oral premalignant lesions, *Cancer Bull* 38:145-148, 1986.

Hong WK, Lippman SM, Itri LM, et al: Prevention of second primary tumors with isotretinoin in squamous cell carcinoma of the head and neck, *N Engl J Med* 323:795-801, 1990.

Jarvinen J, Kullaa-Mikkonen A, Kotilainen R: Some local and systemic factors related to tongue inflammation, *Proc Finn Dent Soc* 85:197-209, 1990.

Kaliakatsou F, Hodgson TA, Lewsey JD, et al: Management of recalcitrant ulcerative oral lichen planus with topical tacrolimus, *J Am Acad Dermatol* 46:35-41, 2002.

Lozada-Nur F, Robinson J, Regezi JA: Oral hairy leukoplakia in immunosuppressed patients, *Oral Surg Oral Med Oral Pathol* 78:599-602, 1994.

Nakamura S, Hiroki A, Shinohara M, et al: Oral involvement in chronic graft-versus-host disease after allogenic bone marrow transplantation, *Oral Surg Oral Med Oral Pathol Oral Radiol Endod* 82:556-563, 1996.

McCreary CE, McCartan BE: Clinical management of oral lichen planus, *Br J Oral Maxillofac Surg* 37(5):338-343, 1999.

Patton DF, Shirley P, Raab-Traub N, et al: Defective viral DNA in Epstein-Barr virus-associated oral hairy leukoplakia, *J Virol* 64:397-400, 1990.

Podzamczer D, Bolao F, Gudiol F: Oral hairy leukoplakia and zidovudine therapy, *Arch Intern Med* 150:689, 1990.

Porter SR, Kirby A, Olsen I, et al: Immunologic aspects of dermal and oral lichen planus, *Oral Surg Oral Med Oral Pathol Oral Radiol Endod* 83:358-366, 1997.

Ramirez-Amador V, Dekker NP, Lozada-Nur F, et al: Altered interface adhesion molecules in oral lichen planus, *Oral Dis* 2:188-192, 1996.

Regezi JA, Daniels TE, Saeb F, et al: Increased submucosal factor XIIIa-positive dendrocytes in oral lichen planus, *J Oral Pathol Med* 23:114-118, 1994.

Regezi JA, Dekker NP, MacPhail LA, et al: Vascular adhesion molecules in oral lichen planus, *Oral Surg Oral Med Oral Pathol Oral Radiol Endod* 81:682-690, 1996.

Rozycki TW, Rogers RS, Pittelkow MR, et al: Topical tachrolimus in the treatment of symptomatic oral lichen planus, *J Am Acad Dermatol* 46:27-34, 2002.

Salonen L, Axell T, Hellden L: Occurrence of oral mucosal lesions, the influence of tobacco habits and an estimate of treatment time in an adult Swedish population, *J Oral Pathol Med* 19:170-176, 1990.

Shiohara T, Moriya N, Nagashima M: Induction and control of lichenoid tissue reactions, *Springer Semin Immunopathol* 13:369-385, 1992.

Silverman S Jr, Gorsky M, Lozada F: Oral leukoplakia and malignant transformation, *Cancer* 53:563-568, 1984.

Sinor PN, Gupta PC, Murti PR, et al: A case-control study of oral submucous fibrosis with special reference to the etiologic role of areca nut, *J Oral Pathol Med* 19:94-98, 1990.

Sniiders PJ, Schulten EA, Mullink H, et al: Detection of human papillomavirus and Epstein-Barr virus DNA sequences in oral mucosa of HIV-infected patients by the polymerase chain reaction, *Am J Pathol* 137:659-666, 1990.

Sugerman PB, Savage NW, Seymour GJ, et al: Is there a role for tumor necrosis factor-alpha in oral lichen planus? *J Oral Pathol Med* 25:21-24, 1996.

Van Wyk CW, Seedat HA, Phillips VM: Collagen in submucous fibrosis: an electron microscopic study, *J Oral Pathol Med* 19:182-187, 1990.

Vincent SD, Fotos PG, Baker KA, et al: Oral lichen planus: the clinical, historical and therapeutic features of 100 cases, *Oral Surg Oral Med Oral Pathol* 70:165-171, 1990.

Walton LJ, Thornhill MH, Macey MG, et al: Cutaneous lymphocyte-associated antigen (CLA) and alpha e beta 7 integrins are expressed by mononuclear cells in skin and oral lichen planus, *J Oral Pathol Med* 26:402-407, 1997.

Workshop on Oral Healthcare in HIV Disease, *Oral Surg Oral Med Oral Pathol* 73:137-247, 1992.

NONEPITHELIAL WHITE-YELLOW LESIONS

Greenspan D: Treatment of oral candidiasis in HIV infection, *Oral Surg Oral Med Oral Pathol* 78:211-215, 1994.

RED-BLUE LESIONS

INTRAVASCULAR LESIONS

CONGENITAL VASCULAR ANOMALIES

Congenital Hemangiomas and Congenital Vascular Malformations

Etiology. The terms *(congenital) hemangioma* and *(congenital) vascular malformation* have been used as generic designations for many vascular proliferations, and they have also been used interchangeably. Congenital hemangiomas and congenital vascular malformations appear at or around the time of birth. Because of the confusion surrounding the basic origin of many of these lesions, classification of clinical and microscopic varieties has been difficult. None of the numerous proposed classifications has had uniform acceptance, although there is merit in separating benign neoplasms from vascular malformations because of different clinical and behavioral characteristics (Table 4-1). The term congenital hemangioma is used to identify benign congenital neoplasms of proliferating endothelial cells. Congenital vascular malformations include lesions resulting from abnormal vessel morphogenesis. Separation of vascular lesions into one of these two groups can be of considerable significance relative to the treatment of patients. Unfortunately, in actual practice, some difficulty may be encountered in classifying lesions in this way because of overlapping clinical and histologic features.

In any event, congenital hemangiomas have traditionally been subdivided into two microscopic types—capillary and cavernous—that essentially reflect differences in vessel diameter. Vascular malformations may exhibit similar features but may also show vascular channels that represent arteries and veins.

Clinical Features. Congenital hemangioma, also known as *strawberry nevus,* usually presents around the time of birth but may not be apparent until early childhood (Figure 4-1). This lesion may exhibit a rapid growth phase that is followed several years later by an involution phase. In contrast, congenital vascular malformations are generally persistent lesions that grow with the individual and do not involute (Figures 4-2 to 4-4). They may represent arteriovenous shunts and exhibit a bruit or thrill on auscultation. Both types

TABLE 4-1   **Congenital Vascular Lesions**

	Hemangioma	Vascular Malformation
Description	Abnormal endothelial cell proliferation	Abnormal blood vessel development
Elements	Results in increased number of capillaries	A mix of arteries, veins, capillaries (includes AV shunt)
Growth	Rapid congenital growth	Grows with patient
Boundaries	Often circumscribed; rarely affects bone	Poorly circumscribed; may affect bone
Thrill and bruit	No associated thrill or bruit	May produce thrill and bruit
Involution	Usually undergoes spontaneous involution	Does not involute
Resection	Persistent lesions resectable	Difficult to resect; surgical hemorrhage
Recurrence	Recurrences uncommon	Recurrences common

AV, Arteriovenous.

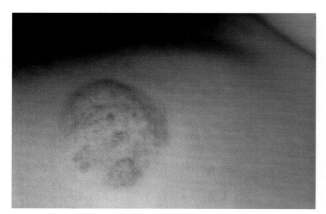

Figure 4-1   Congenital hemangioma.

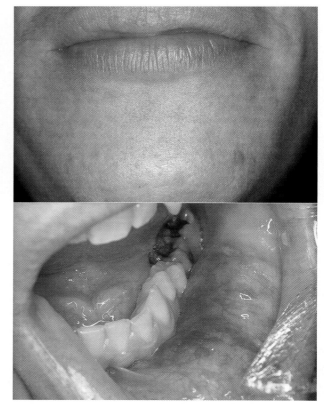

A

B

Figure 4-2   **A** and **B, Oral vascular malformation** causing slight facial asymmetry.

of lesions may range in color from red to blue, depending on the degree of congestion and their depth in tissue. When they are compressed, blanching occurs as blood is pressed peripherally from the central vascular spaces. This simple clinical test (diascopy) can be used to separate these lesions from hemorrhagic lesions in soft tissue (ecchymoses), where the blood is extravascular and cannot be displaced by pressure. Congenital hemangiomas and congenital vascular malformations may be flat, nodular, or bosselated. Other clinical signs include the presence of a bruit or thrill, features associated predominantly with congenital vascular malformations. Lesions are most commonly found on the lips, tongue, and buccal mucosa. Lesions that affect bone are probably congenital vascular malformations rather than congenital hemangiomas.

Vascular malformations are also a component of the rare condition termed *blue rubber bleb nevus syndrome (Bean's syndrome)* where multiple small and large cavernous hemangiomas are present on the skin and throughout the gastrointestinal tract including the mouth. The condition is usually diagnosed in childhood or young adulthood. The significance of this syndrome is its recognition because many of those afflicted may suffer overt life-threatening gastrointestinal bleeding or occult blood loss with severe anemia and iron deficiency.

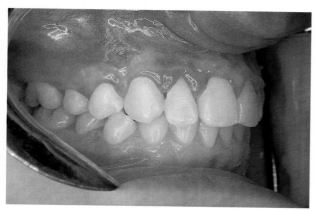

Figure 4-3 **Vascular malformation** of the maxillary mucosa.

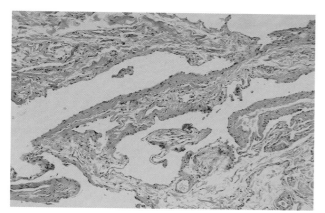

Figure 4-4 **Vascular malformation** composed of large tortuous channels lined by endothelium.

Encephalotrigeminal Angiomatosis (Sturge-Weber Syndrome)

Encephalotrigeminal angiomatosis, or *Sturge-Weber syndrome,* is a condition that includes vascular malformations. In this syndrome, venous malformations involve the leptomeninges of the cerebral cortex, usually with similar vascular malformations of the face. The associated facial lesion, also known as *port-wine stain* or *nevus flammeus,* involves the skin innervated by one or more branches of the trigeminal nerve. Port-wine stains may also occur as isolated lesions of the skin without the other stigmata of encephalotrigeminal angiomatosis. The vascular defect of encephalotrigeminal angiomatosis may extend intra-orally to involve the buccal mucosa and the gingiva. Ocular lesions may also appear.

Neurologic effects of encephalotrigeminal angiomatosis may include mental retardation, hemiparesis, and seizure disorders. Patients may be taking phenytoin (Dilantin) for control of the latter problem, with possible secondary development of drug-induced generalized gingival hyperplasia. Calcification of the intracranial vascular lesion may provide radiologic evidence of the process in the leptomeninges.

A differential diagnosis would include *angioosteohypertrophy syndrome,* which is characterized by vascular malformations of the face (port-wine stains), varices, and hypertrophy of bone. The bony abnormality usually affects long bones but may also involve the mandible or maxilla, resulting in asymmetry, malocclusion, and an altered eruption pattern.

Hereditary Hemorrhagic Telangiectasia (Rendu-Osler-Weber Syndrome)

Hereditary hemorrhagic telangiectasia, or *Rendu-Osler-Weber syndrome,* is a rare condition transmitted in an autosomal-dominant manner. It features abnormal vascular dilations of terminal vessels in skin, mucous membranes, and occasionally viscera (Figure 4-5). The telangiectatic vessels in this condition appear clinically as red macules or papules, typically on the face, chest, and oral mucosa. Lesions appear early in life, persist throughout adulthood, and often increase in number.

Intranasal lesions are responsible for epistaxis, the most common presenting sign of hereditary hemorrhagic telangiectasia. Bleeding from oral lesions is also a common occurrence in affected patients. Control of bleeding may on occasion be a difficult problem. Chronic low-level bleeding may also result in anemia.

Diagnosis of hereditary hemorrhagic telangiectasia is based on clinical findings, hemorrhagic history, and family history. Another condition that might be considered in a differential diagnosis is *CREST syndrome.* This includes *c*alcinosis cutis, *R*aynaud's phenomenon, *e*sophageal dysfunction, *s*clerodactyly, and *t*elangiectasia.

Histopathology. Congenital hemangiomas have been classified microscopically as *capillary hemangiomas* or *cavernous hemangiomas,* depending on whether the microscopic size of the capillaries is small or large, respectively. The vascular spaces are lined by endothelium without muscular support. Clinically, no significant difference is noted between capillary and cavernous hemangiomas.

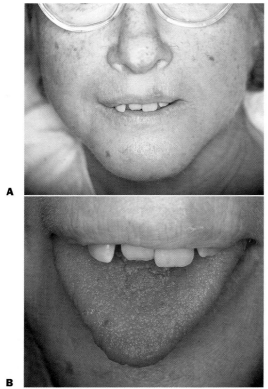

A

B

Figure 4-5 **A** and **B, Rendu-Osler-Weber syndrome.** Note numerous telangiectasias on the skin and tongue. The patient also has a secondary/recurrent herpetic lesion on her upper lip.

Congenital vascular malformations may consist not only of capillaries but also of venous, arteriolar, and lymphatic channels. Direct arteriovenous communications are typical. Lesions may be of purely one type of vessel, or they may be combinations of two or more.

Diagnosis. As a generic group, the diagnosis of congenital vascular lesions is usually self-evident on clinical examination. When they affect the mandible or the maxilla, a radiolucent lesion with a honeycomb pattern and distinct margins is expected. Differentiation between congenital hemangiomas and congenital vascular malformations can be difficult and occasionally impossible. A complete history, a clinical examination, and angiography or magnetic resonance imaging should be definitive.

Treatment. Spontaneous involution during early childhood is likely for congenital hemangiomas. If these lesions persist into the later years of childhood, invo-

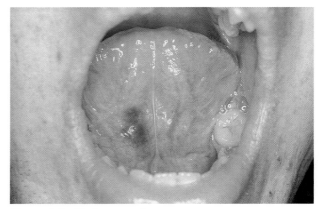

Figure 4-6 **Varix,** ventral tongue.

lution is improbable and definitive treatment may be required. Congenital vascular malformations generally do not involute, and they require intervention if eradication is the goal. Because the margins of these lesions are often ill defined, total elimination may not be practical or possible.

Treatment of vascular lesions continues to center around a careful surgical approach. Adjuncts include selective arterial embolization and sclerosant therapy. Laser therapy is now a valid form of primary treatment of selected vascular lesions.

REACTIVE LESIONS

Varix and Other Acquired Vascular Malformations

A *venous varix*, or varicosity, is a type of acquired vascular malformation that represents focal dilation of a single vein. It is a relatively trivial but common vascular malformation when it appears in the oral mucosa (Figures 4-6 to 4-8). Varices involving the ventral aspect of the tongue are common developmental abnormalities. Varices are also common on the lower lip in older adults, representing vessel wall weakness secondary to chronic sun exposure. Varices are typically blue and blanch with compression. Thrombosis, which is insignificant in these lesions, occasionally occurs, giving them a firm texture. No treatment is required for a venous varix unless it is frequently traumatized or is cosmetically objectionable.

Other *acquired vascular malformations* represent a more complex network or proliferation of thin-walled vessels than simple varices. These are relatively

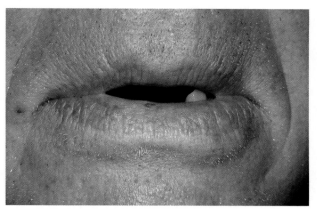

Figure 4-7 **Thrombosed varix** of the lower lip.

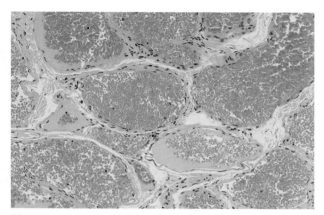

Figure 4-9 **Acquired vascular malformation.**

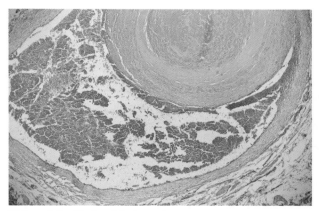

Figure 4-8 **Varix** with thrombus.

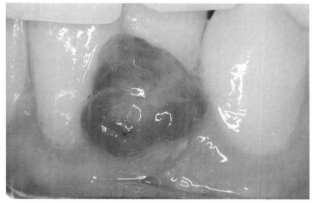

Figure 4-10 **Pyogenic granuloma.**

common, are seen in adults, and are of undetermined cause (Figure 4-9). Some may be related to vessel trauma and subsequent abnormal repair. These lesions present as red-blue discrete and asymptomatic tumescences that can be relatively easily excised.

Pyogenic Granuloma

Etiology. Pyogenic granuloma represents an exuberant connective tissue proliferation to a known stimulus or injury. It appears as a red mass because it is composed predominantly of hyperplastic granulation tissue in which capillaries are very prominent. The term *pyogenic granuloma* is a misnomer in that it is not pus producing, and it does not represent granulomatous inflammation (Table 4-2).

Clinical Features. Pyogenic granulomas are commonly seen on the gingiva, where they are presumably caused by calculus or foreign material within the gingival crevice (Figures 4-10 to 4-12). Hormonal changes of puberty and pregnancy may modify the gingival reparative response to injury, producing what was once called a "pregnancy tumor." Under these circumstances, multiple gingival lesions or generalized gingival hyperplasia may be seen. Pyogenic granulomas are uncommonly seen elsewhere in the mouth but may appear in areas of frequent trauma, such as the lower lip, the buccal mucosa, and the tongue.

Pyogenic granulomas are typically red. Occasionally they may become ulcerated because of secondary trauma. The ulcerated lesions may then become covered by a yellow, fibrinous membrane. They may be pedunculated or broad based and may range in size from a few millimeters to several centimeters. These lesions may be seen at any age and tend to occur more commonly in females than in males.

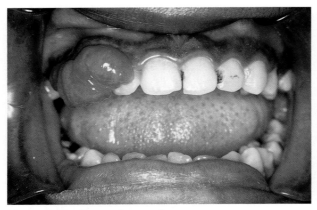

Figure 4-11 Pyogenic granuloma.

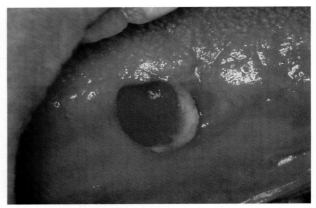

Figure 4-12 Pyogenic granuloma of the lateral tongue.

TABLE 4-2 Gingival Reactive Hyperplasias		
Granuloma	**Pyogenic Granuloma**	**Peripheral Giant Cell**
Etiology	Initiated by trauma or irritation Modified by hormones, drugs	Probably trauma or irritation Not related to hormones or drugs
Location	Predominantly gingiva, but any traumatized soft tissue	Exclusively gingiva Usually anterior to first molars
Histopathology	Hyperplastic granulation tissue Misnomer—neither pus producing nor granulomatous	Hyperplasia of fibroblasts with multinucleated giant cells Not granulomatous inflammation
Treatment	Excision to periosteum or periodontal membrane	Excision to periosteum or periodontal membrane
Recurrence	Some recurrences; no malignant potential	Some recurrences; no malignant potential

Histopathology. Microscopically, pyogenic granulomas are composed of lobular masses of hyperplastic granulation tissue (Figure 4-13). Some scarring may be noted in some of these lesions, suggesting that occasionally there may be maturation of the connective tissue repair process. Variable numbers of chronic inflammatory cells may be seen. Neutrophils are present in the superficial zone of ulcerated pyogenic granulomas.

Differential Diagnosis. Clinically, this lesion is similar to peripheral giant cell granuloma, which also presents as a red gingival mass. A peripheral odontogenic or ossifying fibroma may be another consideration, although these tend to be much lighter in color. Rarely, metastatic cancer may present as a red gingival mass. Biopsy findings are definitive in establishing the diagnosis.

Treatment. Pyogenic granulomas should be surgically excised; this includes the connective tissue from which the lesion arises, as well as removal of local etiologic factors (plaque, calculus, foreign material, source of trauma). Recurrence is occasional and is believed to result from incomplete excision, failure to remove etiologic factors, or reinjury of the area. The end of pregnancy often brings considerable shrinkage of pregnancy-associated pyogenic granulomas, but residual lesion may need to be excised.

Peripheral Giant Cell Granuloma

Etiology. Peripheral giant cell granuloma is a relatively uncommon and unusual hyperplastic connective tissue response to injury of gingival tissues. It is one of the "reactive hyperplasias" commonly seen in oral mucous membranes, representing an exuberant reparative pro-

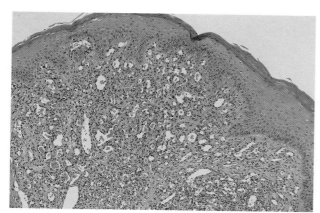

Figure 4-13 **Pyogenic granuloma** showing abundant capillaries.

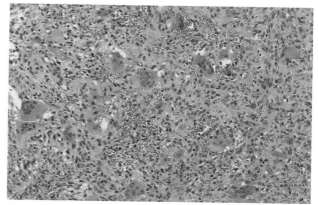

Figure 4-15 **Peripheral giant cell granuloma** showing fibroblastic matrix and abundant multinucleated giant cells.

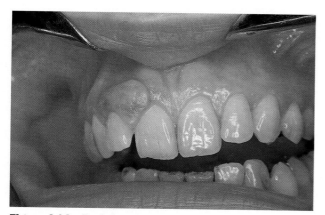

Figure 4-14 **Peripheral giant cell granuloma.**

cess. The feature that sets this lesion apart from the others is the appearance of multinucleated giant cells, but the reason for their presence remains unknown.

Clinical Features. Peripheral giant cell granulomas are seen exclusively in gingiva, usually between the first permanent molars and the incisors (Figure 4-14). They presumably arise from periodontal ligament or periosteum and cause, on occasion, resorption of alveolar bone. When this process occurs on the edentulous ridge, a superficial, cup-shaped radiolucency may be seen. Peripheral giant cell granulomas typically present as red to blue, broad-based masses. Secondary ulceration due to trauma may give the lesions a focal yellow zone as a result of the formation of a fibrin clot over the ulcer. These lesions, most of which are about 1 cm in diameter, may occur at any age and tend to be seen more commonly in females than in males.

Histopathology. Fibroblasts are the basic element of peripheral giant cell granulomas (Figure 4-15). Scattered throughout the fibroblasts are abundant multinucleated giant cells believed to be related to osteoclasts. The giant cells appear to be nonfunctional in the usual sense of phagocytosis and bone resorption.

Islands of metaplastic bone occasionally may be seen in these lesions. This finding has no clinical significance. Chronic inflammatory cells are present, and neutrophils are found in ulcer bases.

Differential Diagnosis. Generally, this lesion is clinically indistinguishable from a pyogenic granuloma. Although a peripheral giant cell granuloma is more likely to cause bone resorption than is a pyogenic granuloma, the differences are otherwise minimal. A biopsy provides definitive diagnostic results. Microscopically, a peripheral giant cell granuloma is identical to its central or intraosseous counterpart, the central giant cell granuloma.

Treatment. Surgical excision is the preferred treatment for peripheral giant cell granulomas. Removal of local factors or irritants is also required. Recurrences, which are occasionally seen, are believed to be related to lack of inclusion of periosteum or periodontal ligament in the excised specimen.

Scarlet Fever

The characteristic effects of scarlet fever, a systemic bacterial infection, are the result of an erythrogenic toxin that causes capillary damage and that is produced by some strains of group A streptococci. Other strains of group A streptococci that are unable to elaborate the toxin can cause pharyngitis and all the attendant features of infection, but without the red skin rash and oral signs of scarlet fever. Spread of all group A streptococcal infections is generally via droplets from contact with an infected individual or, less likely, a carrier. Crowded living conditions promote the spread of streptococcal infections.

Clinically, children are typically affected after an incubation period of several days. In addition to the usual symptoms of all group A streptococcal infections—pharyngitis, tonsillitis, fever, lymphadenopathy, malaise, and headache—the child also exhibits a red skin rash that starts on the chest and spreads to other surfaces. The face is flushed except for a zone of circumoral pallor. The palate may show inflammatory changes, and the tongue may become covered with a white coat in which fungiform papillae are enlarged and reddened (strawberry tongue). Later, the coat is lost, leaving a beefy red tongue (red strawberry tongue or raspberry tongue). In untreated and uncomplicated cases the disease subsides in a matter of days.

Penicillin is the drug of choice for the treatment of group A streptococcal infections. Erythromycin should be used in patients allergic to penicillin. The rationale for antibiotic treatment of this short-lived, self-limited disease is the prevention of complications, particularly rheumatic fever and glomerulonephritis.

NEOPLASMS

Erythroplakia

Etiology. *Erythroplakia* is a clinical term that refers to a red patch on oral mucous membranes. It does not indicate a particular microscopic diagnosis, although after a biopsy most are found to be severe dysplasia or carcinoma. The causes of this lesion are believed to be similar to those responsible for oral cancer. Therefore tobacco probably has a significant role in the induction of many of these lesions. Alcohol, nutritional defects, and other factors may also have modifying roles.

Clinical Features. Erythroplakia is seen much less commonly than its white counterpart, leukoplakia. It should, however, be viewed as a more serious lesion because of the significantly higher percentage of malignancies associated with it (Box 4-1). The lesion appears as a red patch with well-defined margins (Figures 4-16 and 4-17). Common sites of involvement

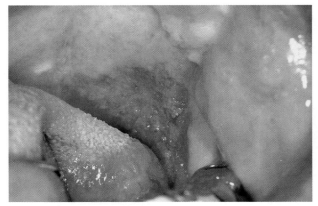

Figure 4-16 **Erythroplakia** of the soft palate.

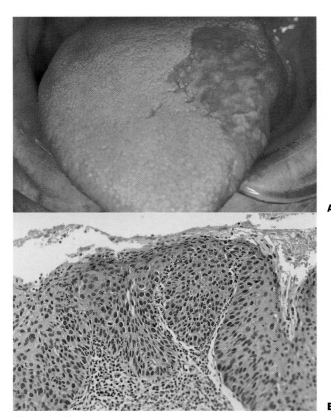

A

B

Figure 4-17 **A, Erythroplakia** of the tongue. **B,** Biopsy specimen showing carcinoma in situ.

include the floor of the mouth, the tongue, and the retromolar mucosa. Individuals between 50 and 70 years of age are usually affected, and there appears to be no gender predilection. Focal white areas representing keratosis may also be seen in some lesions (ery-

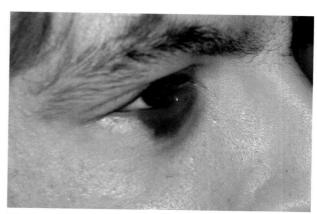

Figure 4-18 Kaposi's sarcoma.

---

throleukoplakia). Erythroplakia is usually supple to the touch unless the lesion is invasive, in which case there may be induration.

Histopathology. Approximately 40% of erythroplakias show severe dysplastic change, and about 50% are squamous cell carcinoma. A relative reduction in keratin production and a relative increase in vascularity account for the clinical color of these lesions.

There is a histologic variant of carcinoma in situ that exhibits changes analogous to the skin lesion termed *Bowen's disease*. Microscopic features that separate this bowenoid change from the usual carcinoma in situ include marked disordered growth, multinucleated keratinocytes, large hyperchromatic keratinocyte nuclei, and atypical individual cell keratinization.

Differential Diagnosis. A differential diagnosis should include Kaposi's sarcoma, ecchymosis, contact allergic reaction, vascular malformation, and psoriasis. The clinical history and examination should distinguish most of these lesions. A biopsy provides a definitive answer.

Treatment. The treatment of choice for erythroplakia is surgical excision. It is generally more important to excise widely than to excise deeply in dysplastic and in situ lesions, because of their superficial nature and the fact that dysplastic cells usually extend beyond the clinically evident lesion. However, because the epithelial changes may extend along the salivary gland excretory ducts in the area, the deep surgical margin should not be too shallow. Several histologic sections may be necessary to assess adequately the involvement of salivary ducts.

It is generally accepted that severely dysplastic and in situ lesions eventually become invasive. The time required for this event can range from months to years. Follow-up examinations are critical for patients with these lesions, because of the potential field effect caused by etiologic agents.

Kaposi's Sarcoma

Etiology. Kaposi's sarcoma is a proliferation of endothelial cell origin, although dermal/submucosal dendrocytes, macrophages, lymphocytes, and probably mast cells may have a role in the genesis of these lesions. A relatively recently discovered herpesvirus known as human herpesvirus 8 (HHV8) or Kaposi's sarcoma herpesvirus (KSHV) has been identified in all forms of Kaposi's sarcoma lesions, as well as in acquired immunodeficiency syndrome (AIDS)–associated body cavity lymphomas and in multicentric *Castleman's disease*. This virus is believed to have a significant role in the induction and/or maintenance of Kaposi's sarcoma through perturbation of focally released cytokines and growth factors.

Clinical Features. Three different clinical patterns of Kaposi's sarcoma have been described (Figures 4-18 to 4-21). It was initially described by Kaposi in 1872 as a rare skin lesion, predominantly in older men living in the Mediterranean basin (Table 4-3). In this classic form it appears as multifocal reddish brown nodules primarily in the skin of the lower extremities, although any organ may be affected. Oral lesions are rare in this type. This classic form has a rather long indolent course and only a fair prognosis.

The second pattern of Kaposi's sarcoma was identified in Africa, where it is considered endemic. It is typically seen in the extremities of blacks. The most commonly affected organ is the skin. Oral lesions are

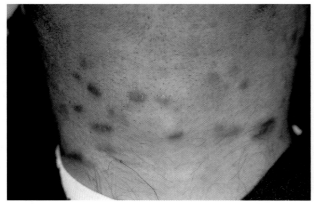

Figure 4-19   **Kaposi's sarcoma** of the neck.

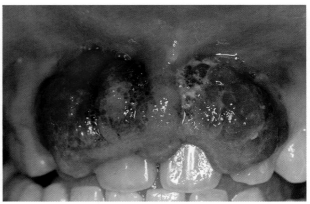

Figure 4-21   **Advanced Kaposi's sarcoma** of the gingiva.

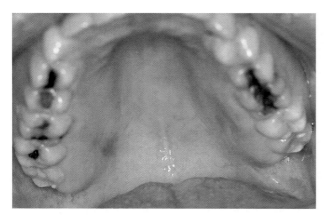

Figure 4-20   **Kaposi's sarcoma** presenting as a dark macule in the right posterior palate.

Box 4-2 Kaposi's Sarcoma: Key Features

Initiation by HHV8 control of endothelial cells
Perpetuation by cytokines and growth factors released by macrophages, lymphocytes, and other cells
Incidence—immunodeficiency type markedly reduced following use of new drugs to treat AIDS
High-risk oral sites—palate and gingiva
Early lesions—blue macule(s)
   Differential—ecchymosis, vascular malformation, erythroplakia, melanoma, blue nevus, amalgam tattoo
Advanced lesions—nodular red-blue mass
Treatment—intralesional chemotherapy, radiation, and surgery (debulking) have produced modest results

HHV8, Human herpesvirus 8; *AIDS*, acquired immunodeficiency syndrome.

TABLE 4-3   **Kaposi's Sarcoma**

	Classic Type	Endemic Type	Immunodeficiency Type
Etiology	HHV8	HHV8	HHV8
Geography	Mediterranean basin	Africa	AIDS and transplant patients
Prevalence	Rare	Endemic	Uncommon
Age	Older men	Children and adults	Young adults
Sites	Skin, lower extremities	Skin, extremities	Skin, mucosa, internal organs
Course	Indolent but progressive	Prolonged	Aggressive
Prognosis	Fair prognosis	Fair prognosis	Poor prognosis

HHV8, Human herpesvirus 8; *AIDS*, acquired immunodeficiency syndrome.

rarely seen. The clinical course is prolonged, and the overall prognosis is also only fair.

The third pattern of Kaposi's sarcoma has been seen in patients with immunodeficiency states, including organ transplants and especially AIDS (Box 4-2). This type differs from the other two forms in several ways. Skin lesions are not limited to the extremities, and they may be multifocal. Oral and lymph node lesions are relatively common. Visceral organs may also be involved, and a younger age-group is affected. The clin-

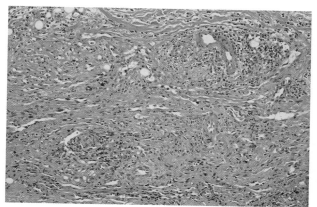

Figure 4-22 **Early Kaposi's sarcoma** showing a subtle increase in the number of capillaries and extravasated red cells.

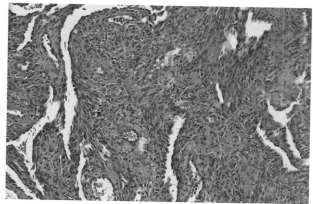

Figure 4-23 **Advanced Kaposi's sarcoma** showing spindle cell proliferation and bizarre capillaries.

ical course is relatively rapid and aggressive, and the prognosis is correspondingly poor.

Kaposi's sarcoma, once occurring in about one third of patients with AIDS, is now seen with considerably less frequency—a shift that appears to be related to antiretroviral drug therapy. About half of AIDS-affected patients with cutaneous Kaposi's sarcoma develop oral lesions. Of significance is that oral lesions may be the initial site of involvement or the only site. Kaposi's sarcoma has been described in most oral regions, although the palate, gingiva, and tongue seem to be the most commonly affected sites. Clinical presentation of oral Kaposi's sarcoma ranges from early, rather trivial-appearing, flat lesions to late, nodular, exophytic lesions. Lesions may be single or multifocal. The color is usually red to blue. AIDS-affected patients with oral Kaposi's sarcoma may have other oral problems concomitantly, such as candidiasis, hairy leukoplakia, advancing periodontal disease, and xerostomia.

Histopathology. Early lesions of Kaposi's sarcoma may be rather subtle, being composed of hypercellular foci containing bland-appearing spindle cells, ill-defined vascular channels, and extravasated red blood cells (RBCs) (Figures 4-22 to 4-24). Later, they may superficially resemble pyogenic granulomas. Atypical vascular channels, extravasated RBCs, hemosiderin, and inflammatory cells are characteristic of advanced Kaposi's sarcoma. Macrophages, factor XIIIa–positive dendrocytes, lymphocytes, and mast cells are also seen in oral Kaposi's sarcoma (early and late stages).

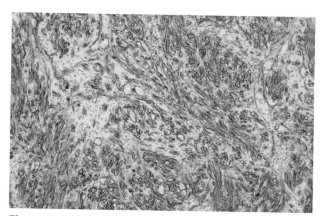

Figure 4-24 **Kaposi's sarcoma.** Positive immunohistochemical stain for CD34 of Kaposi's sarcoma, confirming spindle cells as endothelial cells.

Differential Diagnosis. Clinical considerations include hemangioma, erythroplakia, melanoma, and pyogenic granuloma. Another remarkable look-alike, known as *bacillary angiomatosis*, mimics Kaposi's sarcoma both clinically and microscopically. The causative organism is *Bartonella henselae* or *Bartonella quintana*. Cats are reservoirs for this organism, and fleas may be vectors. Microscopically, neutrophils and bacterial colonies are seen. This condition is cured with erythromycin or tetracycline therapy. Bacillary angiomatosis is uncommon in the skin and very rare in oral mucous membranes.

Treatment. Various forms of treatment have been used for Kaposi's sarcoma, but none has been uniformly successful. Surgery has been useful on localized lesions, and low-dose radiation and intralesional chemotherapy have been gaining favor. For larger and multifocal lesions, systemic chemotherapeutic regimens are being used. Improvement in the underlying immunosuppression may also help to reduce the size and number of the lesions.

METABOLIC-ENDOCRINE CONDITIONS

Vitamin B Deficiencies

Etiology. In various areas of the world, especially those with poor socioeconomic conditions, vitamin B deficiencies may be relatively common because of inadequate dietary intake. In the United States, deficiencies of the B vitamins are relatively uncommon.

Vitamin B deficiencies may involve one or several of the water-soluble B complex vitamins. Decreased intake through malnutrition associated with alcoholism, starvation, or fad diets may lead to clinically apparent disease. Decreased absorption because of gastrointestinal disease (e.g., malabsorption syndromes) or increased utilization because of increased demand (e.g., hyperparathyroidism) may also account for deficiencies.

Most of the vitamins classified under the B complex (biotin, nicotinamide, pantothenic acid, and thiamine) are involved in intracellular metabolism of carbohydrates, fats, and proteins. Others (vitamin B_{12} and folic acid) are involved in erythrocyte development. Deficiencies of individual vitamins may produce distinctive clinical pictures. Significant oral changes have been well documented in deficiencies of riboflavin (ariboflavinosis), niacin (pellagra), folic acid (one of the megaloblastic anemias), and vitamin B_{12} (pernicious anemia) (see the following section).

Clinical Features. In general, the oral changes associated with vitamin B deficiencies consist of cheilitis and glossitis. The lips may exhibit cracking and fissuring that are exaggerated at the corners of the mouth, in which case it is called *angular cheilitis*. The tongue becomes reddened, with atrophy of papillae, and patients complain of pain and burning (Figure 4-25).

In addition to these oral changes, riboflavin deficiency results in keratitis of the eyes and a scaly dermatitis focused on the nasolabial area and genitalia. Niacin deficiency is associated with extraoral problems as well. The "four *D*'s" of niacin deficiency are dermatitis, diarrhea, dementia, and death. The most striking and consistent feature is a symmetrically distributed dermatitis that eventually shows marked

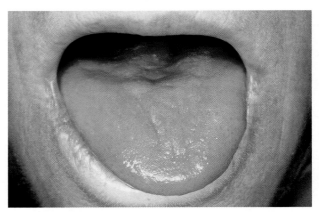

Figure 4-25 **Vitamin B deficiency.** Note angular cheilitis and atrophic red tongue.

thickening and pigmentary changes. Dementia is in the form of disorientation and forgetfulness. The glossitis in this deficiency may be severe and may extend to other mucosal surfaces.

Folic acid deficiency results in a megaloblastic (enlarged RBC precursors) bone marrow, a macrocytic (enlarged circulating erythrocytes) anemia, and gastrointestinal abnormalities, including diarrhea and the general oral lesions described previously. Vitamin B_{12} deficiency shares many of the signs and symptoms of folic acid deficiency. These are detailed in the following sections on anemia.

Diagnosis and Treatment. Diagnosis of B complex deficiencies is based on the history, clinical findings, and laboratory data. Replacement therapy should be curative.

Pernicious Anemia

Etiology. Pernicious anemia is essentially a deficiency of vitamin B_{12} (erythrocyte-maturing factor or extrinsic factor), which is necessary for DNA synthesis, especially in rapidly dividing cells, such as those found in bone marrow and the gastrointestinal tract. Pernicious anemia results from the inability to transport vitamin B_{12} across intestinal mucosa because of a relative lack of a gastric substance (intrinsic factor). This intrinsic factor is normally complexed to vitamin B_{12}, making the vitamin available to mucosal cells for absorption. An autoimmune response directed against the intrinsic factor producing parietal cells in the gastric mucosa is believed to be the probable mechanism responsible for pernicious anemia. The end result is atrophic gastritis, achlorhydria, neurologic changes, megaloblastic bone marrow, and macrocytic anemia. In addition, significant oral manifestations may be seen.

Clinical Features. Pernicious anemia affects adults of either gender. The clinical signs of anemia—weakness, pallor, shortness of breath, difficulty in breathing, and increased fatigue on exertion—may be present. Also, in more severe cases, central nervous system manifestations (headache, dizziness, and tinnitus) and gastrointestinal manifestations (nausea, diarrhea, and stomatitis) may be present.

Specific oral complaints center around the tongue. Pain and burning are typical symptoms. The tongue appears more red because of atrophy of the papillae. The resultant smooth, red appearance has been referred to as *Hunter's glossitis* or *Moeller's glossitis*.

Diagnosis. The clinical picture of pernicious anemia can be only presumptive of this disease. Diagnosis is based on laboratory demonstration of a megaloblastic, macrocytic anemia.

Treatment. Parenteral administration of vitamin B_{12} is curative for this condition. An increased risk of the development of gastric carcinoma is associated with the chronic atrophic gastritis that may occur in pernicious anemia.

Iron Deficiency Anemia

Etiology. Iron deficiency anemia is a rather common anemia caused by iron deficiency. The deficiency may be due to inadequate dietary intake; impaired absorption due to a gastrointestinal malady; chronic blood loss due to such problems as excessive menstrual flow, gastrointestinal bleeding, or aspirin ingestion; and increased demand as experienced during childhood and pregnancy.

Clinical Features. This is a relatively prevalent form of anemia that affects predominantly women. In addition to the clinical signs and symptoms associated with anemias in general, iron deficiency anemia may also result in brittle nails and hair and koilonychia (spoon-shaped nails). The tongue may become red, painful, and smooth. Angular cheilitis may also be seen.

In addition to iron deficiency, the Plummer-Vinson (Paterson-Kelly) syndrome includes dysphagia, atrophy of the upper alimentary tract, and a predisposition to the development of oral cancer.

Diagnosis. Laboratory blood studies show a slight to moderately reduced hematocrit and reduced hemoglobin level. The RBCs are microcytic and hypochromic. The serum iron level is also low, but the total iron binding capacity (TIBC) is elevated.

Treatment. Recognition of the underlying cause of iron deficiency anemia is necessary to treat this condition effectively. Dietary iron supplements are required to elevate hemoglobin levels and replenish iron stores.

Burning Mouth Syndrome

Patients with burning mouth, or burning tongue, syndrome usually exhibit no clinically detectable lesions, although symptoms of pain and burning can be intense. This relatively common "nonlesion" clinical problem is included in this section because the symptoms associated with burning mouth also appear in patients with vitamin B deficiency, pernicious anemia, iron deficiency anemia, or chronic atrophic candidiasis. This is a particularly frustrating problem for both patient and clinician, because there is usually no clear-cut cause once the above-stated conditions are ruled out, and no uniformly successful treatment is present.

Etiology. The etiology of burning mouth syndrome is varied and often difficult to decipher clinically. The symptoms of pain and burning appear to be the result of one of many possible causes (Table 4-4). The following factors have been cited as having possible etiologic significance:

- Microorganisms—especially fungi (*Candida albicans*) and possibly bacteria (staphylococci, streptococci, anaerobes)

TABLE 4-4 **Burning Mouth (Tongue) Syndrome**

Potential Causes	Potentially Helpful Regimens
Idiopathic	Empathy
Candida albicans	Antifungals
Xerostomia—drugs, anxiety, Sjögren's syndrome	Oral lubricants—Moi-Stir, MouthKote, Salivart, Sialor
Nutritional deficiency—B vitamins, iron, zinc	Dietary supplement—vitamins, minerals
Abnormal tongue habit	Topical corticosteroids
Depression, anxiety	Tricyclic antidepressants
Pernicious anemia Diabetes mellitus Hormone imbalance	Medical referral—internist, psychiatrist, gynecologist

---

Box 4-3 Drugs That Cause Xerostomia (Dry Mouth)

Anticholinergics
Antidepressants
Antihistamines
Antihypertensives
Antihypoglycemics
Antiparkinsonians
Beta-blockers
Diuretics
NSAIDs

NSAIDs, Nonsteroidal antiinflammatory drugs.

Box 4-4 Conditions/Factors That Cause Altered Taste

Acute necrotizing gingivitis
Corda tympani injury
Drugs, especially antibiotics
Endocrinopathies
Heavy metal intoxication
Psychologic disorders
Zinc deficiency
Idiopathic causes

- Xerostomia associated with Sjögren's syndrome, anxiety, or drugs (Box 4-3)
- Nutritional deficiencies associated primarily with B vitamin complex or iron, and possibly zinc
- Anemias, namely pernicious anemia and iron deficiency anemia
- Hormone imbalance, especially hypoestrogenemia associated with postmenopausal changes
- Neuropsychiatric abnormalities, such as depression, anxiety, cancer phobia, and other psychogenic problems
- Diabetes mellitus
- Mechanical trauma, such as an oral habit, chronic denture irritation, or sharp teeth
- Idiopathic causes

In some patients, more than one of these factors may be contributing to the problem of burning mouth syndrome. In many others, no specific cause can be identified. Other potential etiologic factors that might be explored are those related to dysgeusia (altered taste), an occasional clinical feature of burning mouth syndrome (Box 4-4). Dysgeusia is associated with an equally long list of factors that include zinc deficiency, drugs (especially antibiotics), endocrine abnormalities, acute necrotizing ulcerative gingivitis (ANUG), heavy-metal intoxication, chorda tympani injury, and psychogenic and idiopathic causes.

The mechanism by which such a varied group of factors causes symptoms of burning mouth syndrome is completely enigmatic. No common thread or underlying defect seems to tie these factors together. It is apparent that burning mouth syndrome occurs in a diverse, complex group of patients. Determination of the cause is a difficult and challenging clinical problem that requires careful, extensive history taking and, often, laboratory support.

Clinical Features. This is a condition that typically affects middle-aged women. Men are affected but generally at a later age than women. Burning mouth syndrome is rare in children and teenagers, very uncommon in young adults, and relatively common in adults older than 40 years of age.

Symptoms of pain and burning may be accompanied by altered taste and xerostomia. Occasionally a patient may attribute the initiation of the malady to recent dental work, such as placement of a new bridge or extraction of a tooth. Symptoms are often described as severe and ever present, or, more typically, as worsening late in the day and evening. Any and all mucosal regions may be affected, although the tongue is by far the most commonly involved site.

Highly characteristic of the complaint of an intensely burning mouth or tongue is a completely normal-appearing oral mucosa. Tissue is intact and has the same color as the surrounding tissue, with normal distribution of tongue papillae.

Some laboratory studies that may prove useful are cultures for *C. albicans,* serum tests for Sjögren's syndrome antibodies (SS-A, SS-B), a complete blood count, serum iron, total iron-binding capacity, and serum B_{12} and folic acid levels. Whether any or all of these tests should be performed is a consideration to be made on an individual basis, dependent on the clinical history and clinical suspicion.

Histopathology. Because no typical clinical lesion is associated with burning mouth syndrome and because symptoms are more generalized than focal, a biopsy is generally not indicated. When an occasional arbitrary site in the area of chief complaint is chosen for biopsy, tissue appears within normal limits in hematoxylin and eosin–stained sections. Special stains may reveal the presence of a few *C. albicans* hyphae.

Diagnosis. Diagnosis is based on a detailed history, non-diagnostic clinical examination, laboratory studies, and exclusion of all other possible oral problems. Making the clinical diagnosis of burning mouth syndrome is generally not the difficult aspect of these cases. Rather, it is determining the subtle factor(s) that led to the symptoms that is difficult if not impossible.

Treatment. If a nutritional deficit is the cause, replacement therapy is curative. If a patient wears a prosthetic device, careful inspection of its fit and tissue base should be done. Relining or remaking the device may help eliminate chronic irritation. If results of fungal cultures are positive, topical nystatin or clotrimazole therapy should produce satisfactory clinical results. If drugs may be involved, consultation with the patient's physician for an alternative drug may prove beneficial.

Because most patients do not fall neatly into one of these categories in which an identified problem can be rectified, treatment becomes difficult. Hormonal changes, neurologic problems, and idiopathic disease are as difficult to identify as they are to treat. A sensitive, empathic approach should be used when treating patients with this problem. Clinicians should be supportive and offer an explanation of the various facets and frustrations of burning mouth syndrome. No great optimism or easy solution should be offered, because patients may ultimately have to accept the disease and learn to live with the problem.

Other referrals may be useful, if only to exhaust all possibilities and reassure patients. The need for psychologic counseling is often difficult to broach with these patients, but it may be necessary after all logical avenues of investigation have been explored.

Empirical treatment is often the approach most clinicians are forced to use for patients with burning mouth syndrome. Even though there may be no evidence of candidiasis, nystatin or clotrimazole may cause a lessening of symptoms. A solution of tetracycline–nystatin–diphenhydramine hydrochloride (Benadryl) or similar remedy may likewise make patients more comfortable. Topical steroids, such as betamethasone (with or without antifungal agent), applied to the area of chief complaint may also be of some benefit. Generally, viscous lidocaine provides only temporary relief of pain, and saliva substitutes are of minimal value in patients suffering from associated (or stated) xerostomia.

Low-dose tricyclic antidepressants may help some patients. However, they should not be used if xerostomia is a presenting sign, because these drugs may exaggerate this problem. Although they have been incompletely evaluated in the clinical setting, substance P inhibitors (e.g., capsaicin) show some promise. The benzodiazepine clonazepam given in low doses has also been suggested for therapy, but its value and mechanism of effect in this condition are unproven. Some benefit may likewise be obtained with the use of gabapentin, although the mechanism to explain its clinical effect is lacking.

IMMUNOLOGIC ABNORMALITIES

Plasma Cell Gingivitis

Etiology. Plasma cell gingivitis was first given the name *plasma cell gingivostomatitis* because of the prominent plasma cell infiltrate in the tissues affected and because of its undetermined origin. This condition was subsequently named *allergic gingivostomatitis* because many cases were linked to chewing gum, which was believed to be eliciting an allergic reaction. When gum was removed from the diet of affected patients, tissues reverted to normal in a matter of weeks. Although similar clinical lesions were noted in patients who did not chew gum, clinical and microscopic evidence still supports an allergic or hypersensitivity reaction. A possible explanation of the appearance of disease in non–gum chewers might be that the disease is a reaction to an ingredient in chewing gum, such as mint or cinnamon flavorings, that might also be found in other foods.

This peculiar condition is of historical interest because it was relatively prevalent at one time but is rarely encountered today. In the early 1970s numerous cases, all nearly identical, were seen throughout the United States. Within a few years the phenomenon all but disappeared. Clinicians speculated that formulas or sources of the offending ingredient(s) were changed, making the product nonallergenic.

Clinical Features. This condition affects adults and occasionally children of either gender. Burning mouth, tongue, or lips is the usual complaint of patients with plasma cell gingivitis. The onset is rather sudden, and the discomfort may wax and wane. This condition should not be classified with burning mouth syndrome, because distinctive clinical changes are present. The attached gingiva is fiery red but not ulcerated; the tongue mucosa is atrophic and red; and the commissures are reddened, cracked, and fissured (Figures 4-26 and 4-27). Patients have no cervical lymphadenopathy and no systemic complaints.

Histopathology. The affected epithelium is spongiotic and is infiltrated by various types of inflammatory cells. Langerhans cells are also prominent, and apoptotic keratinocytes may occasionally be seen. The lamina propria displays prominent capillaries and is infiltrated by plasma cells of normal morphology.

Treatment. Most patients respond rather quickly to the cessation of gum chewing. In non–gum chewers and those gum chewers who do not respond to the elimination of gum, careful dietary history taking is indicated in an attempt to identify an allergic source.

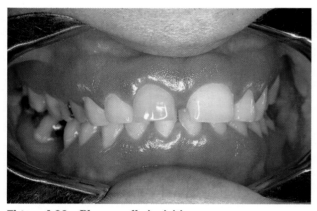

Figure 4-26   Plasma cell gingivitis.

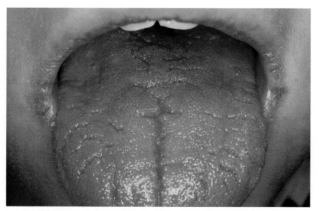

Figure 4-27   Plasma cell gingivitis showing angular cheilitis and fissured red tongue.

Drug Reactions and Contact Allergies

Allergic reactions to drugs taken systemically or used topically often affect the skin but may also affect oral mucous membranes. A wide variety of agents are known to have this capacity, especially in patients who have a predisposition to the development of allergies.

The clinical appearance of allergic response in the skin ranges from red, erythematous lesions to an urticarial rash to a vesiculoulcerative eruption. The same types of changes may appear in oral mucosa. In less intense and less destructive reactions, the mucosa exhibits a generalized redness. When the tongue is the primary target, the pattern may be similar to the changes of vitamin B deficiency and anemia. (A detailed discussion on this subject can be found in Chapter 2.)

EXTRAVASCULAR LESIONS

Petechiae and Ecchymoses

Etiology. Soft tissue hemorrhages in the form of petechiae (pinpoint size) or ecchymoses (larger than pinpoint size) appear intraorally, generally because of trauma or blood disease (dyscrasia) (Box 4-5). Traumatic injury, if blood vessels are significantly damaged, can result in leakage of blood into surrounding connective tissue, producing red to purple lesions. The types of injury are many and, among other things, are related to cheek biting, coughing, fellatio, trauma from prosthetic appliances, injudicious hygiene procedures, and iatrogenic dental injuries.

In patients with blood dyscrasias the presenting sign of minor trauma may also be oral red to purple petechiae or ecchymoses. Dental practitioners can therefore have a significant role in the recognition of this abnormality. After ruling out a traumatic etiology, clinicians should refer patients to an internist or hematologist.

All the various types of leukemia have the potential to produce one or more of the intraoral lesions listed in Box 4-6. In actual practice, monocytic leukemia is most often associated with oral manifestations, myelocytic leukemia (granulocyte series) is next, and lymphocytic leukemia (lymphocytes) is least likely to be associated with oral signs. Acute forms of the leukemias are also more likely than chronic forms to be associated with oral lesions.

Box 4-5 Blood Dyscrasias That May Have Oral Manifestations

Leukemia—monocytic > myelocytic > lymphocytic
Agranulocytosis
Cyclic neutropenia
Infectious mononucleosis
Thrombocytopenic purpura (ITP and TTP)
Hemophilia A and B
Macroglobulinemia
Von Willebrand's disease
Multiple myeloma
Polycythema vera
Sickle cell anemia
Thalassemia
Porphyria

>, More commonly than; *ITP*, idiopathic thrombocytopenic purpura; *TTP*, thrombotic thrombocytopenic purpura.

Box 4-6 Blood Dyscrasias: Oral Manifestations

Mucosal petechiae and ecchymoses—reduced platelets and/or clotting factors
Gingival enlargement
Leukemic infiltrates
Inflammation and hyperplasia (poor oral hygiene)
Excessive bleeding with minor trauma, gingivitis—reduced numbers of platelets and/or clotting factors
Refractory gingivitis
Leukemic infiltrates
Reduced numbers of platelets and/or clotting factors
Loose teeth—leukemic infiltrates in periodontal ligament
Mucosal ulcers—cyclic neutropenia; ulcer mechanism undetermined

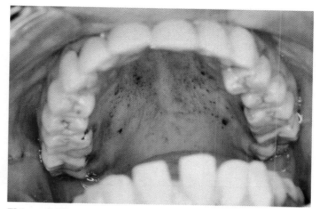

Figure 4-28   **Petechiae** associated with idiopathic thrombocytopenic purpura.

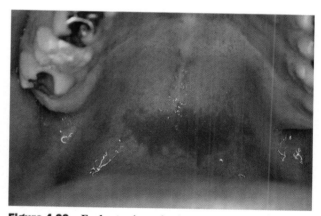

Figure 4-29   **Ecchymosis** at the junction of the hard and soft palate (trauma induced).

Platelet and clotting defects make up another large group of blood dyscrasias that may be responsible for petechiae, ecchymoses, and other intraoral manifestations. Platelet problems may be qualitative or quantitative in nature. They may also be of unknown origin (idiopathic thrombocytopenic purpura), or they may appear secondary to a wide variety of systemic factors, such as drug ingestion, infection, and immunologic disease. Hemophilia and related disorders in which clotting factors are deficient or defective are predominantly hereditary and are characteristically associated with prolonged bleeding and occasional ecchymoses.

Clinical Features. The color of these lesions varies from red to blue to purple, depending on the age of the lesion and the degree of degradation of the extravasated blood. Soft tissue hemorrhagic lesions usually appear in areas accessible to trauma, such as the buccal mucosa, lateral tongue surface, lips, and junction of the hard and soft palate (Figures 4-28 and 4-29). In those injuries that are related to uncomplicated trauma, a cause-and-effect relationship can usually be established after a history has been taken.

The lesions that develop secondary to blood dyscrasias may follow trivial or otherwise insignificant trauma. In addition to petechiae and ecchymoses, other clinical oral signs of blood dyscrasias include gingival enlargement (especially with monocytic leukemia), gingivitis, "spontaneous" gingival hemorrhage, prolonged bleeding after oral surgery, loose teeth, and mucosal ulcers.

Diagnosis. The inability to otherwise explain the appearance of any of these clinical signs should cause clinicians to suspect one of the blood dyscrasias.

Gingivitis that is refractory to standard therapy should be viewed as a potential dyscrasia. The concomitant presence of lymphadenopathy, weight loss, weakness, fever, joint pain, and headache should add to the suspicion of serious systemic disease. Clinicians in this situation should see that patients are evaluated by an internist or hematologist.

BIBLIOGRAPHY

Chang Y, Cesarman E, Pessin MS, et al: Identification of herpesvirus-like DNA sequences in AIDS-associated Kaposi's sarcoma, *Science* 266:1865-1869, 1994.

Dictor M, Rambech E, Way D, et al: Human herpesvirus 8 (Kaposi's sarcoma–associated herpesvirus) DNA in Kaposi's sarcoma lesions, AIDS Kaposi's sarcoma cell lines, endothelial Kaposi's sarcoma simulators, and the skin of immunosuppressed patients, *Am J Pathol* 148:2009-2016, 1996.

Dutree-Meulenberg R, Kozel M, van Jost T: Burning mouth syndrome: a possible role for local contact sensitivity, *J Am Acad Dermatol* 26:935-940, 1992.

Ensoli B, Gendelman R, Markham P, et al: Synergy between basic fibroblast growth factor and HIV-1 tat protein in induction of Kaposi's sarcoma, *Nature* 371:674-680, 1994.

Epstein J, Scully C: HIV infection: clinical features and treatment of thirty-three homosexual men with Kaposi's sarcoma, *Oral Surg Oral Med Oral Pathol* 71:38-41, 1991.

Forbosco A, Criscuolo M, Coukos G: Efficacy of hormone replacement therapy in postmenopausal women with oral discomfort, *Oral Surg Oral Med Oral Pathol* 73:570-574, 1992.

Gordon SC, Daley TD: Foreign body gingivitis: identification of foreign material by energy-dispersive x-ray microanalysis, *Oral Surg Oral Med Oral Pathol Oral Radiol Endod* 83:571-576, 1997.

Gordon SC, Daley TD: Foreign body gingivitis: clinical and microscopic features of 61 cases, *Oral Surg Oral Med Oral Pathol Oral Radiol Endod* 83:562-570, 1997.

Gorsky M, Silverman S, Chinn H: Clinical characteristics and management outcome in the burning mouth syndrome, *Oral Surg Oral Med Oral Pathol* 72:192-195, 1991.

Guttmacher AE, Marchuk DA, White RI: Hereditary hemorrhagic telangiectasia, *N Engl J Med* 333:918-924, 1995.

Karlis V, Glickman RS, Stern R, et al: Hereditary angioedema, *Oral Surg Oral Med Oral Pathol Oral Radiol Endod* 83:462-464, 1997.

Koehler JE, Glaser CA, Tappero JW: *Rochalimaea henselae* infection: a zoonosis with the domestic cat as reservoir, *JAMA* 271:531-535, 1994.

Koehler JE, Quinn FD, Berger TG, et al: Isolation of *Rochalimaea* species from cutaneous and osseous lesions of bacillary angiomatosis, *N Engl J Med* 327:1625-1631, 1992.

Maragon P, Ivanyi L: Serum zinc levels in patients with burning mouth syndrome, *Oral Surg Oral Med Oral Pathol* 71:447-450, 1991.

Miles SA: Pathogenesis of AIDS-related Kaposi's sarcoma: evidence of a viral etiology, *Hematol Oncol Clin North Am* 10:1011-1021, 1996.

Morris CB, Gendelamn R, Marrogi AJ, et al: Immunohistochemical detection of Bcl-2 in AIDS-associated and classical Kaposi's sarcoma, *Am J Pathol* 148:1055-1063, 1996.

Porter SR, Di Alberti L, Kumar N: Human herpes virus 8 (Kaposi's sarcoma herpesvirus), *Oral Oncol* 34:5-14, 1998.

Qu Z, Liebler JM, Powers MR, et al: Mast cells are a major source of basic fibroblast growth factor in chronic inflammation and cutaneous hemangioma, *Am J Pathol* 147:564-573, 1995.

Shovlin CL: Molecular defects in rare bleeding disorders: hereditary hemorrhagic telangiectasia, *Thromb Haemost* 78:145-160, 1997.

Tourne LPM, Fricton JR: Burning mouth syndrome: critical review and proposed management, *Oral Surg Oral Med Oral Pathol* 74:158-167, 1992.

PIGMENTED LESIONS

MELANOCYTIC LESIONS

Melanin-producing cells (melanocytes) have their embryologic origin in the neural crest. These cells migrate to epithelial surfaces and reside among basal cells. They have numerous dendritic processes that extend to adjacent keratinocytes. Organelles representing packaged granules of pigment known as melanosomes are produced by these melanocytes. These melanosomes are not ordinarily retained within the cell itself but, rather, are delivered to the surrounding keratinocytes and occasionally to subjacent macrophages. Light, hormones, and genetic constitution influence the amount of pigment produced.

Melanocytes are found throughout the oral mucosa but go unnoticed because of their relatively low level of pigment production (Figure 5-1). They appear clear with nonstaining cytoplasm on routine histologic preparation. When focally or generally active in pigment production or proliferation, they may be responsible for several different entities in the oral mucous membranes, ranging from physiologic pigmentation to malignant neoplasia.

A relative of the melanocyte, the nevus cell, is responsible for pigmented nevi. Nevus cells, although morphologically different from melanocytes, possess the same enzyme, tyrosinase, which is responsible for conversion of tyrosine to melanin in the melanosome organelle.

Oral melanin pigmentations range from brown to black to blue, depending on the amount of melanin produced and the depth of the pigment relative to the surface. Generally, superficial pigmentation is brown, whereas more deeply located pigmentation is black to blue. Darkening of a preexisting lesion that has not been stimulated by known factors suggests that pigment cells are producing more melanin and/or invading deeper tissue.

Physiologic (Ethnic) Pigmentation

Clinical Features. Physiologic pigmentation is symmetric and persistent and does not alter normal architecture, such as gingival stippling (Figure 5-2). This pigmentation may be seen in persons of any age and is without gender predilection. Often the degree of intraoral pigmentation may not correspond to the degree of cutaneous coloration. Physiologic pigmentation may be found in any location, although the gingiva is the most commonly affected intraoral tissue. A related type of pigmentation, called *postinflammatory pigmentation*, is occasionally seen after mucosal reaction to injury (Figure 5-3). Occasionally in cases of lichen planus, areas surrounding active disease may eventually show mucosal pigmentation.

Histopathology. Physiologic pigmentation is due not to increased numbers of melanocytes but, rather, to increased melanin production. The melanin is found in surrounding basal keratinocytes and subjacent connective tissue macrophages.

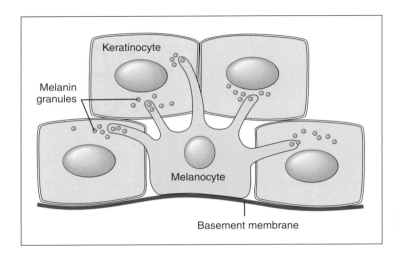

Figure 5-1   Melanocyte-keratinocyte unit. Note dendritic processes of melanocyte and melanin transfer to keratinocytes.

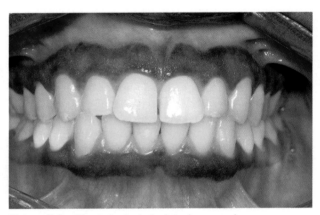

Figure 5-2   Physiologic (ethnic) pigmentation.

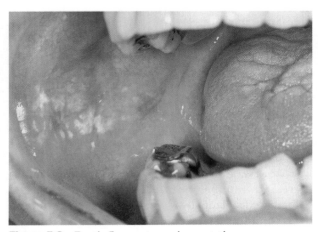

Figure 5-3   Postinflammatory pigmentation.

Differential Diagnosis. A clinical differential diagnosis would include smoking-associated melanosis, Peutz-Jeghers syndrome, Addison's disease, and melanoma. Although physiologic pigmentation is usually clinically diagnostic, a biopsy may be justified if clinical features are atypical.

Smoking-associated Melanosis

Etiology and Pathogenesis. Abnormal melanin pigmentation of oral mucosa has been linked to cigarette smoking and has been designated smoking-associated melanosis or smoker's melanosis. The pathogenesis is believed to be related to a component in tobacco smoke that stimulates melanocytes. Female sex hormones are also believed to be modifiers in this type of pigmentation, because women (especially those taking birth control pills) are more commonly affected than men.

Clinical Features. The anterior labial gingiva is the region most typically affected. Palate and buccal mucosa pigmentation has been associated with pipe smoking. The use of smokeless tobacco has not been linked to oral melanosis. In smoking-associated melanosis the intensity of pigmentation is time and dose related (Figure 5-4).

Histopathology. Melanocytes show increased melanin production, as evidenced by pigmentation of adjacent basal keratinocytes. The microscopic appearance is essentially similar to that seen in physiologic pigmentation and melanotic macules.

Differential Diagnosis. Other entities to consider before a definitive diagnosis is established are physiologic

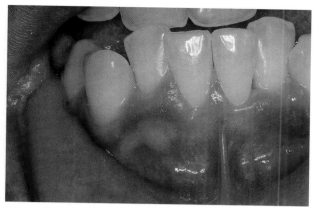

Figure 5-4 Smoking-associated melanosis.

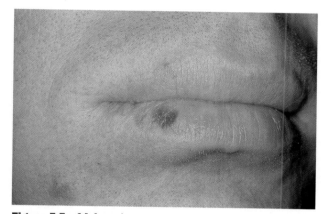

Figure 5-5 Melanotic macule.

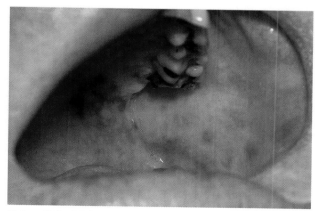

Figure 5-6 Melanotic macules.

pigmentation, Peutz-Jeghers syndrome, Addison's disease, and melanoma.

Treatment. With cessation of smoking, improvement is expected over the course of months to years. Smoker's melanosis, per se, appears to be of little significance. It may, however, potentially mask other lesions or may be cosmetically objectionable.

Oral Melanotic Macule

Clinical Features. Oral melanotic macule (or focal melanosis) is a focal pigmented lesion that may represent (1) an intraoral freckle, (2) postinflammatory pigmentation, or (3) the macules associated with Peutz-Jeghers syndrome or Addison's disease (Box 5-1).

Melanotic macules have been described as occurring predominantly on the vermilion of the lips and gingiva, although they may appear on any mucosal surface. They are asymptomatic and have no malignant potential.

When melanotic macules (freckles) are seen in excess in an oral and perioral distribution, *Peutz-Jeghers syndrome* and *Addison's disease* should be considered (Box 5-2; Figures 5-5 to 5-8). Peutz-Jeghers syndrome

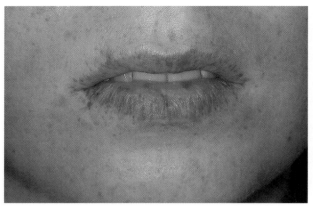

Figure 5-7   Perioral melanotic macules of Peutz-Jeghers syndrome.

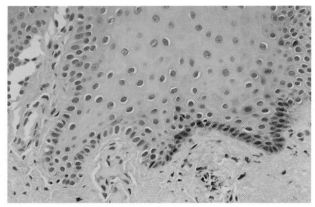

Figure 5-9   **Melanotic macule** showing melanin in basal keratinocytes.

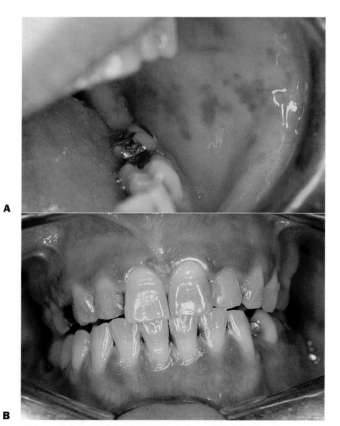

A

B

Figure 5-8   **Addison's disease. A** and **B,** Melanotic macules.

is a condition that is inherited in an autosomal-dominant pattern. In addition to ephelides or melanotic macules, intestinal polyposis is present. These polyps are regarded as hamartomas without, or with very limited, neoplastic potential. They are usually

found in the small intestine (jejunum) and may produce signs and symptoms of abdominal pain, rectal bleeding, and diarrhea.

Addison's disease, primary adrenocortical insufficiency, may result from adrenal gland infection (tuberculosis), autoimmune disease, or idiopathic causes. With reduced cortisol production by the adrenals, pituitary adrenocorticotropic hormone (ACTH) and melanocyte-stimulating hormone (MSH) increase as part of a negative feedback mechanism. Overproduction of both ACTH and MSH results in stimulation of melanocytes, leading to diffuse pigmentation of the skin. Oral freckles and larger melanotic macules occur with the generalized pigmentation. Other presenting signs and symptoms of this syndrome include weakness, weight loss, nausea, vomiting, and hypotension.

Pigmented macules have been described in association with two other rare syndromes. One includes soft tissue myxomas and endocrinopathies *(myxoma syndrome)*. Oral, cutaneous, and cardiac myxomas may be seen in this autosomal-dominant syndrome. The other, known as *Laugier-Hunziker syndrome* or *phenomenon,* is a rare acquired pigmentary disorder that presents as lip, oral, or finger macules, and subungual melanocytic streaks.

Histopathology. Microscopically, melanotic macules are characterized by melanin accumulation in basal keratinocytes and normal numbers of melanocytes (Figure 5-9). Melanophagocytosis is also typically seen.

Differential Diagnosis. These oral pigmentations must be differentiated from early superficial melanomas. They may be confused with blue nevi (palate) or amalgam tattoos. If they are numerous, Peutz-Jeghers syn-

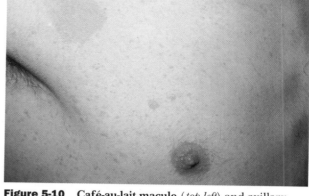

Figure 5-10   Café-au-lait macule (*top left*) and axillary freckling in patient with neurofibromatosis.

drome, Addison's disease, and Laugier-Hunziker syndrome may be possible clinical considerations (Box 5-3).

Treatment. A biopsy may be required to establish a definitive diagnosis of this lesion. Otherwise, no treatment is indicated.

Café-au-Lait Macules

Café-au-lait macules are discrete melanin-pigmented patches of skin that have irregular margins and a brown coloration. They are noted at birth or soon thereafter and may also be seen in normal children. No treatment is required, but they may be indicative of a syndrome of greater significance (Box 5-4).

Individuals with six or more large (>1.5 cm in diameter) café-au-lait macules should be suspected of possibly having neurofibromatosis (NF) (Figure 5-10). There are two forms of this autosomal-dominant disorder, affecting 100,000 people in the United States: neurofibromatosis 1 (NF1; previously called *von Recklinghausen's* disease) and neurofibromatosis 2 (NF2;

formerly known as *acoustic neurofibromatosis*). Although there are some overlapping features, the two conditions are distinct clinically and genetically. NF1 is a relatively common disorder affecting 1 in 3000 individuals. Approximately 50% of cases are inherited, and the remainder represent spontaneous new mutations. The condition is characterized by numerous neurofibromas of the skin, oral mucosa, nerves, central nervous system, and occasionally the jaw. Axillary freckling (Crowe's sign) accompanied by the presence of six or more of these macules is regarded as pathognomonic for NF1. The genetic abnormality is in the neurofibromin gene located on chromosome 17q11.2. This tumor suppressor gene encodes for neurofibromin protein, which down-regulates the function of the p21^{ras} protein. NF2 is characterized by bilateral acoustic neuromas, one or more plexiform neurofibromas, and Lisch nodules. The condition is caused by a mutation in the *NF2* tumor suppressor gene located on chromosome 22q12, which encodes for the merlin protein, which shows structural similarities to a series of cytoskeletal proteins. The normal function of merlin is not known.

Café-au-lait macules may also be associated with Albright's syndrome (polyostotic fibrous dysplasia, endocrine dysfunction, precocious puberty, café-au-lait macules). This sporadic disorder is considered to be strongly associated with mutation of the Gs, alpha gene. Variants have been associated with primary biliary cirrhosis and alopecia. The café-au-lait macules of Albright's syndrome tend to be large and unilateral and have irregular borders.

Microscopically, café-au-lait macules are not particularly remarkable. They generally show excess amounts of melanin in basal keratinocytes and subja-

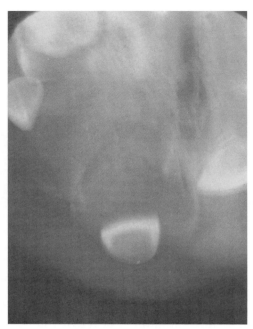

Figure 5-11 Pigmented **neuroectodermal tumor of infancy** as a radiolucency in the anterior maxilla.

cent macrophages. Melanocytes are normal in appearance and may be slightly increased in number.

Pigmented Neuroectodermal Tumor of Infancy

Etiology. Pigmented neuroectodermal tumor of infancy is a rare, benign neoplasm that is composed of relatively primitive pigment-producing cells. Like melanocytes and nevus cells, these cells have their origin in the neural crest.

Clinical Features. This lesion is found in infants usually younger than 6 months of age and occurs typically in the maxilla, although the mandible and the skull have been involved (Figure 5-11). This lesion usually presents as a nonulcerated and occasionally darkly pigmented mass. The latter feature is due to melanin production by tumor cells. Radiographs show an ill-defined lucency that may contain developing teeth.

Histopathology. This neoplasm exhibits an alveolar pattern (i.e., nests of tumor cells with small amounts of intervening connective tissue) (Figure 5-12). The variably sized nests of round to oval cells are found within a well-defined connective tissue margin. Cells located centrally within the neoplastic nests are dense and compact, resembling neuroendocrine

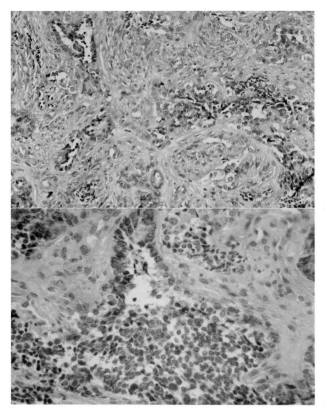

A

B

Figure 5-12 Pigmented **neuroectodermal tumor of infancy. A** and **B,** Nests of round cells with peripheral pigmented cells.

cells; peripheral cells are larger and often contain melanin.

Differential Diagnosis. Few other lesions present in this age-group and in this characteristic location. Malignancies of early childhood, such as neuroblastoma, rhabdomyosarcoma, or "histiocytic" tumors, might be considered. Odontogenic cysts and tumors would not be seriously considered in a differential diagnosis.

Treatment and Prognosis. This lesion has been treated with surgical excision with good results. A few cases of local recurrence have been recorded, and in at least one documented case, metastasis has followed local excision.

Nevomelanocytic Nevus

Etiology. *Nevus* is a general term that may refer to any congenital lesion of various cell types or tissue types.

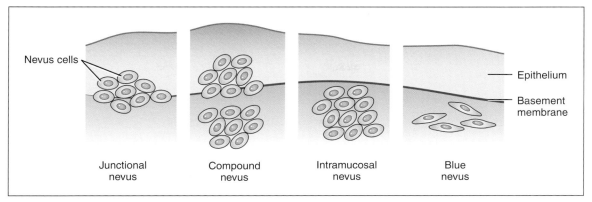

Figure 5-13 Nevocellular nevus subtypes.

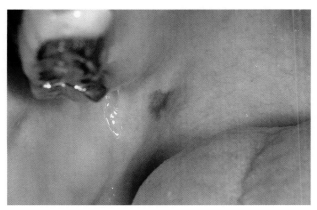

Figure 5-14 Intramucosal nevus.

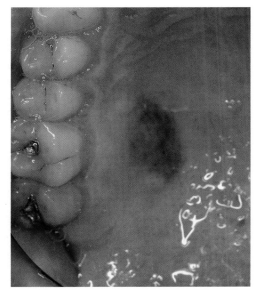

Figure 5-15 Blue nevus.

Generally, however, *nevus* (or mole) used without a modifier refers to a pigmented lesion composed of nevus or melanocytic cells. It is sometimes called, more specifically, *nevomelanocytic nevus, nevocellular nevus, melanocytic nevus,* or *pigmented nevus.*

Nevomelanocytic nevi are collections of nevus cells that are round or polygonal and are typically seen in a nested pattern (Figure 5-13). They may be found in epithelium or supporting connective tissue, or both. The origin of nevus cells has been postulated to be from cells that migrate from the neural crest to the epithelium and dermis (submucosa), or to be from altered resident melanocytes.

Clinical Features. Nevomelanocytic nevi of the skin are common acquired papular lesions that usually appear shortly after birth and throughout childhood. Intraoral nevomelanocytic nevi are relatively rare lesions that may occur at any age. Most oral lesions present as small (<0.5 cm) elevated papules or nodules that are often nonpigmented (20%). The palate is the most commonly affected site. Less common sites are the buccal mucosa, labial mucosa, gingiva, alveolar ridge, and vermilion (Box 5-5; Figures 5-14 and 5-15).

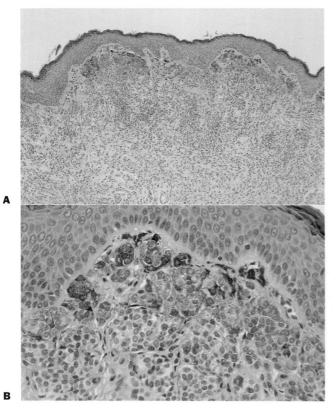

A

B

Figure 5-16   **Intramucosal nevus. A** and **B,** Confluent nests of pigmented nevus cells in submucosa.

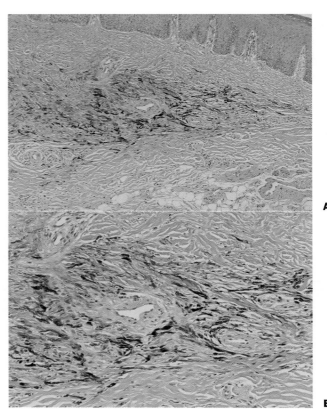

A

B

Figure 5-17   **Blue nevus. A** and **B,** Collection of pigmented spindled nevus cells in submucosa.

Histopathology. Microscopically, several subtypes are recognized (Figures 5-16 and 5-17). Classification is dependent on the location of nevus cells. When cells are located in the epithelium–connective tissue junction, the lesion is called a *junctional nevus;* when cells are located in connective tissue, the lesion is called an *intradermal nevus* or *intramucosal nevus;* and when cells are located in a combination of zones, the lesion is called a *compound nevus.* A fourth type of nevus, in which cells are spindle shaped and found deep in the connective tissue, is known as *blue nevus.* Malignant transformation of an oral benign nevomelanocytic nevus is highly improbable. There are a number of observations that support this statement, including the fact that malignant features are never seen in oral nevi, oral melanomas rarely, if ever contain preexisting nevi histologically, and there are almost no reports of the malignant counterpart of the relatively common oral blue nevus. Because oral nevomelanocytic nevi can mimic melanoma clinically, all undiagnosed pigmented lesions should undergo a biopsy.

In the oral cavity, intramucosal nevi are the most common variety seen, and blue nevi are the second most common. Compound and junctional nevi occur relatively rarely in the oral mucosa. The so-called *dysplastic nevus* that is commonly seen in skin has not been observed in oral mucous membranes.

Differential Diagnosis. Other clinical considerations that should be included along with any type of oral nevomelanocytic nevus are melanotic macule, amalgam tattoo, and melanoma. Lesions of vascular origin might also be considered. These include hematoma, Kaposi's sarcoma, varix, and hemangioma. Diascopy (compression under glass) could be used to rule out the last two lesions, in which the blood is contained within a well-defined vascular system.

Treatment. Because of the infrequency with which oral nevi occur and because of their ability to clinically mimic melanoma, all suspected oral nevi should be excised. Since their size is generally less than 1 cm, excisional biopsy is usually indicated.

Melanoma

Cutaneous Melanoma. Melanomas of the skin have been increasing in frequency during the past several years and now represent approximately 2% of all cancers (excluding carcinomas of the skin). Overall, the cancer-related death rate due to melanoma of the skin is about 1% to 2%. Cutaneous melanoma is more common in locations closer to the equator where UV exposure is greater, and is much more common in whites than in blacks and Asians. Predisposing factors for skin lesions include extensive sun exposure, particularly in childhood, fair natural pigmentation, and precursor lesions, such as congenital nevomelanocytic nevi and dysplastic nevi.

On the skin there are several melanoma subtypes, including nodular melanoma, superficial spreading melanoma, acral-lentiginous melanoma, and lentigo maligna melanoma, each having distinctive microscopic, clinical, and behavioral features. The differences in clinical progression and histology relate, in large part, to recognition that all melanomas have two distinct phases of variable duration: a radial or horizontal growth phase during which malignant melanocytes spread laterally along the epidermal-dermal interface and a vertical growth phase during which there is penetration of the dermis and subcutaneous tissues by malignant melanocytes. In nodular melanoma the radial growth phase is generally very short, but in other types this phase is longer.

Oral Melanoma. Melanomas of oral mucosa are fortunately rare. There is no racial predilection. However, blacks and Asians appear to be proportionately more commonly affected with this neoplasm in the oral mucosa than are whites.

Intraorally, preexisting melanosis was reported to appear before the development of some melanomas. This pigmentary defect, however, very likely represents an early growth phase of these lesions and not benign melanosis. There appear to be two biologic subtypes of oral melanoma: *invasive melanoma* and *in situ melanoma* (Figures 5-18 to 5-24). The former type of oral melanoma shows an invasive or vertical growth pattern without significant lateral spread. The latter type features a junctional growth phase that may last months to years before entering a vertical growth phase. A third term, *atypical melanocytic proliferation*, has been used in relation to microscopically difficult oral pigmentations. This designation indicates the presence of unusual numbers of melanocytes with abnormal morphology at the epithelium–connective tissue inter-

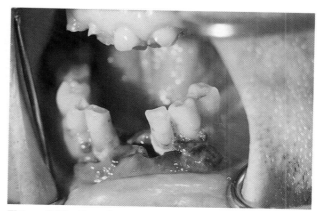

Figure 5-18 Invasive melanoma.

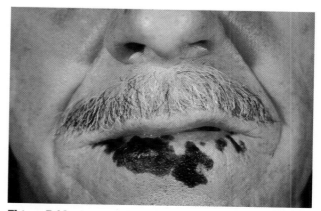

Figure 5-19 In situ melanoma of 8 years' duration.

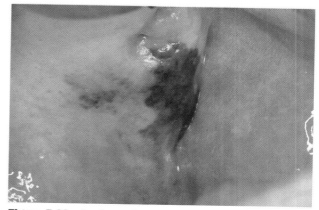

Figure 5-20 In situ melanoma showing lateral spread.

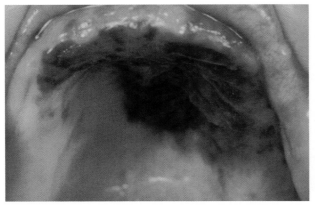

Figure 5-21   **Invasive melanoma** with a several-year history of preceding lateral spread.

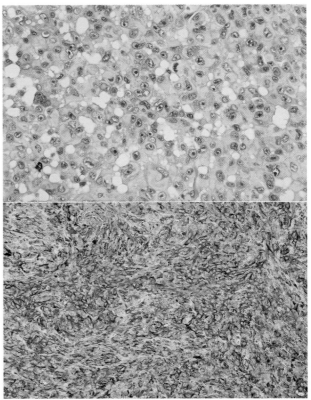

Figure 5-23   **A, Amelanotic melanoma. B,** Positive (*brown*) immunohistochemical stain (HMB-45), helping confirm melanocytic origin.

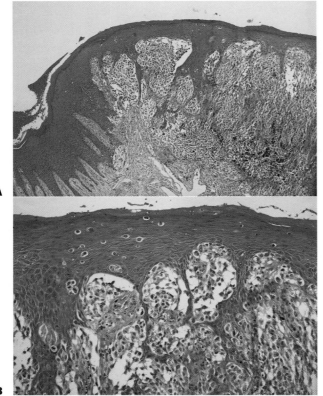

Figure 5-22   **Invasive melanoma. A** and **B,** Note that malignant cells are also invading overlying epithelium (**B**).

face. The changes are not severe enough to justify the diagnosis of melanoma. Lesions designated as "atypical melanocytic proliferation" should be regarded as high-risk lesions and rebiopsied or followed indefinitely.

Melanomas of oral mucosa are much less common than their cutaneous counterparts (Box 5-6). These lesions are found in adults; children are rarely affected. They have a strong predilection for the palate and gingiva. Pigmentation patterns that suggest melanoma include different mixtures of color—such as brown, black, blue, and red—asymmetry, and irregular margins.

Differential Diagnosis.   Intraorally, differential considerations include nevus, amalgam tattoo, physiologic pigmentation, melanotic macule, and Kaposi's sarcoma. The history, symmetry, and uniformity of pigmentation are all of significant value in differentiating these lesions. Because melanomas may initially have a relatively innocuous appearance, a biopsy should be done on any questionable pigmentation.

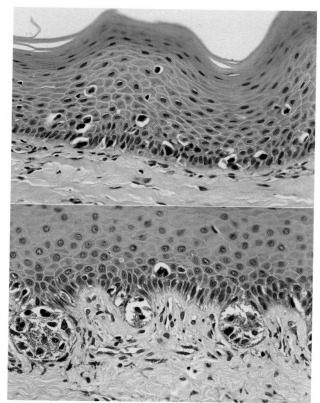

Figure 5-24   **In situ melanoma. A** and **B**, Lateral and intraepithelial spread of malignant cells. Small junctional tumor nests are evident in **B**.

Box 5-6 Oral Melanoma

Palate and gingiva are high-risk sites
   Early lesion—pigmented macule
   Advanced lesion (ABCs)—*asymmetry, borders irregular, color variable, satellite lesions*
No known risk factors
Biologic subtypes
   In situ melanoma
      Prolonged preinvasive junctional phase
      Poor prognosis—delayed diagnosis and undertreatment
   Invasive melanoma
      Connective tissue invasion without junctional phase
      Poor prognosis

Treatment and Prognosis. Surgery remains the primary mode of treatment for melanomas. Chemotherapy is often used, and immunotherapy is occasionally used as an adjunct. Radiotherapy has not been fully explored as a primary treatment method, but it may have a supportive role in disease management. Treatment failures of mucosal melanomas are most commonly linked to incomplete excision, resulting in local recurrence and distant metastasis. Regional lymph node metastases are often detected by a sentinel node biopsy, and this finding affects the choice and extent of therapy. The need for wide surgical excision of in situ melanomas with a radial growth pattern is apparent from the microscopic appearance of this phenomenon.

The prognosis is based on both the histologic subtype and the depth of tumor invasion. The latter feature is a well-established prognosticator for skin lesions that has been applied to oral melanomas. Oral lesions have been found to be of considerably greater thickness (and consequently to be more advanced) than skin lesions at the time of biopsy. After 5 years the survival rate for patients with cutaneous melanomas is about 65%, whereas the survival rate for patients with oral lesions is about 20%. Unfortunately, the survival rate for patients with the oral lesions continues to decline after the traditional measure of 5 years. The overall poor prognosis of oral lesions as compared with skin lesions may therefore be partly related to late recognition of the oral lesions. Another factor is probably the more confining and difficult treatment area of the oral cavity, often precluding the ability to achieve wide margins. Oral lesions may also be inherently biologically more aggressive than skin lesions. Until more lesions are subclassified and measured for depth of invasion, these questions will go unanswered.

NONMELANOCYTIC LESIONS

Amalgam Tattoo (Focal Argyrosis)

Etiology. Amalgam tattoo, or focal argyrosis, is an iatrogenic lesion that follows traumatic soft tissue implantation of amalgam particles or a passive transfer by chronic friction of mucosa against an amalgam restoration. This usually follows tooth extraction, preparation of teeth having old amalgam fillings for gold-casting restorations, or the polishing of old restorations (producing an aerosol of amalgam that becomes impregnated in the tissues).

Clinical Features. This is the most common pigmentation of oral mucous membranes (Figures 5-25 to 5-27). These lesions would be expected in the soft tissues contiguous with teeth restored with amalgam alloy. Therefore the most commonly affected sites are

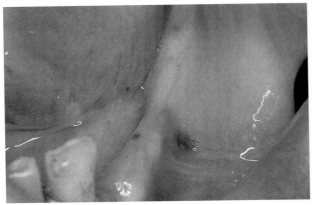

Figure 5-25 Amalgam tattoo.

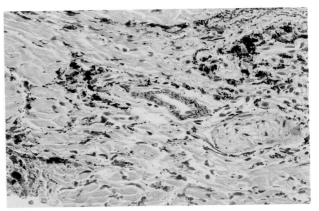

Figure 5-28 **Amalgam tattoo** showing pigment along collagen bundles and around vessels.

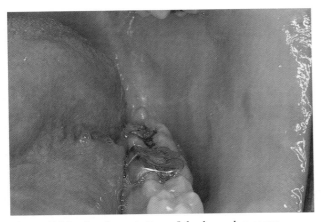

Figure 5-26 **Amalgam tattoo** of the buccal mucosa.

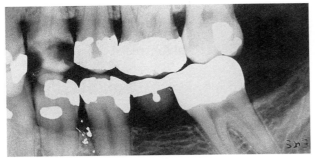

Figure 5-27 **Amalgam tattoo** of the gingiva as detected in a bite-wing radiograph.

sufficient size, they may be detected on soft tissue radiographs.

Histopathology. Microscopically, amalgam particles have an affinity for collagen fibers and elastic fibers of blood vessels, typically staining them a black or golden brown color (Figure 5-28). Few lymphocytes and macrophages are found, except in cases in which particles are relatively large. Multinucleated foreign-body giant cells containing amalgam particles may also be seen.

Differential Diagnosis. The significance of the amalgam tattoo lies in its clinical similarity to melanin-producing lesions. In a gingival or a palatal location, separation from nevi and, more important, early melanoma is mandatory because these are the most common areas for the latter lesions as well. Radiographs, the history, and an even, persistent gray appearance would all help to separate amalgam tattoo from melanoma. Any questionable lesions should undergo a biopsy.

Drug-induced Pigmentations

Tetracycline-associated pigmentation may be found after the treatment of acne with prolonged high doses of *minocycline* (Figure 5-29). Diffuse skin pigmentation may be seen in sun-exposed areas, apparently as a result of increased melanin production, or focal pigment deposits may be seen in the legs and periorbital skin, apparently as a result of drug complexes in melanocytes. Pigmentation of the gingiva and palate may be due to deposits in bone and tooth roots.

Other exogenous drugs that may produce pigmentation of oral tissues include *amino-quinolines* (e.g.,

the gingiva, buccal mucosa, palate, and tongue. Because amalgam is relatively well tolerated by soft tissues, clinical signs of inflammation are rarely seen. The lesions are macular and gray and do not change appreciably with time. If the amalgam particles are of

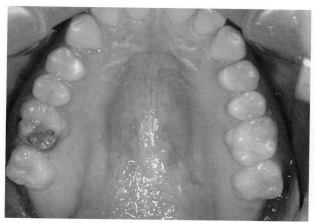

Figure 5-29 **Minocycline pigmentation** of the palate.

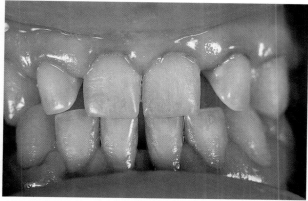

Figure 5-31 **Lead pigmentation** of the gingival margins.

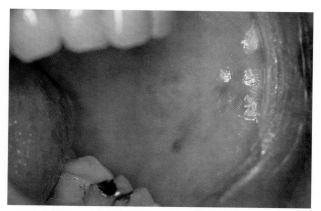

Figure 5-30 **Cyclophosphamide-induced pigmentation** of the buccal mucosa.

chloroquine), *cyclophosphamide, amiodarone,* and *zidovudine (azidothymidine [AZT])* (Figure 5-30). AZT, which is often used in the treatment of acquired immunodeficiency syndrome (AIDS), may cause nail pigmentation in addition to mucosal pigmentation.

Heavy Metal Pigmentations

Etiology. Some heavy metals (arsenic, bismuth, platinum, lead, mercury) may be responsible for oral pigmentation. This phenomenon occurs predominantly after occupational exposure to vapors of these metals. Historically, arsenic and bismuth compounds were used to treat diseases such as syphilis, lichen planus, and other dermatoses, providing another method for oral heavy-metal deposition. *Cis*-platinum, the salt of the heavy metal, has antineoplastic

activity and is used to treat some malignancies. The side effect of a gingival platinum line has been described within this context.

Clinical Features. These heavy metals may be deposited in both skin and oral mucosa (especially in the gingiva). The characteristic color is gray to black, and the distribution is linear when found along the gingival margin (Figure 5-31). Bismuth and lead staining of gingival tissues is known as a bismuth line and a lead line, respectively. This staining is proportional to the amount of gingival inflammation and appears to be a result of the reaction of the heavy metal with bacterially produced hydrogen sulfide in the inflammatory zones.

Significance. The metallic deposits in oral mucosa, per se, are relatively insignificant. The underlying cause must be investigated because of the detrimental effects of systemic toxicity. For dental personnel, chronic mercury vapor exposure is now recognized as a significant occupational hazard if dental amalgam is handled carelessly and without proper precautions. Dental patients, however, are apparently at no risk, because of the relatively short exposure periods that they experience with routine office visits. Toxicity from the restorations themselves is also apparently negligible.

If, in the dental office, the atmospheric air has elevated mercury vapor levels, dental personnel may show elevated body levels of mercury as measured in the hair, nails, saliva, and urine. *Chronic mercury intoxication* may produce symptoms of tremors, loss of appetite, nausea, depression, headache, fatigue, weakness, and insomnia. Hazards due to mercury can be eliminated in the dental office if precautions are observed. The most common recommendations include (1) storage of mercury in sealed containers, (2) coverage of mercury spills with sulfur dust to prevent vaporization, (3) use of hard, seamless floor surfaces instead of carpeting, (4) working in well-ventilated spaces with frequent air filter changes, (5) storage of amalgam scraps under water in a sealed container, (6) use of well-sealed amalgam capsules, and (7) use of water spray and suction when grinding amalgam.

BIBLIOGRAPHY

Barker B, Carpenter WM, Daniels TE, et al: Oral mucosal melanomas: the WESTOP Banff workshop proceedings, *Oral Surg Oral Med Oral Pathol Oral Radiol Endod* 83:672-679, 1997.

Batsakis JG, Suarez P, El-Naggar A: Mucosal melanomas of the head and neck, *Ann Otol Rhinol Laryngol* 107:626-629, 1998.

Buchner A, Merrell P, Hansen L, et al: Melanocytic hyperplasia of the oral mucosa, *Oral Surg Oral Med Oral Pathol* 71:58-62, 1991.

Fitzpatrick J: New histopathologic findings in drug eruptions, *Dermatol Clin* 10:19-36, 1992.

Gerbig AW, Hunziker T: Idiopathic lenticular mucocutaneous pigmentation or Laugier-Hunziker syndrome with atypical features, *Arch Dermatol* 132:844-845, 1996.

Greenberg R, Berger T: Nail and mucocutaneous hyperpigmentation of azidothymidine therapy, *J Am Acad Dermatol* 22:327-330, 1990.

Gupta G, Williams RE, Mackie RM: The labial melanotic macule: a review of 9 cases, *Br J Dermatol* 136:772-775, 1997.

Hicks MJ, Flaitz CM: Oral mucosal melanoma: epidemiology and pathobiology, *Oral Oncol* 36(2):152-169, 2000.

Marghoob AA, Koenig K, Bittencourt FV, et al: Breslow thickness and Clark level in melanoma, *Cancer* 88:589-595, 2000.

Odell EW, Hodgson RP, Haskell R: Oral presentation of minocycline-induced black bone disease, *Oral Surg Oral Med Oral Pathol Oral Radiol Endod* 79:459-461, 1995.

Patton LL, Brahim JS, Baker AR: Metastatic malignant melanoma of the oral cavity: a retrospective study, *Oral Surg Oral Med Oral Pathol* 78:51-56, 1994.

Rees T: Oral effects of drug abuse, *Crit Rev Oral Biol Med* 3:163-184, 1992.

Rustgi AK: Hereditary gastrointestinal polyposis and nonpoly-posis syndromes, *N Engl J Med* 331:1694-1702, 1994.

Slootweg P: Heterologous tissue elements in melanotic neuroectodermal tumor of infancy, *J Oral Pathol Med* 21:90-92, 1992.

Tadini G, D'Orso M, Cusini M, et al: Oral mucosa pigmentation: a new side effect of azidothymidine therapy in patients with acquired immunodeficiency syndrome, *Arch Dermatol* 127:267-268, 1991.

Tanaka N, Amagasa T, Iwaki H, et al: Oral malignant melanoma in Japan, *Oral Surg Oral Med Oral Pathol* 78:81-90, 1994.

Veraldi S, Cavicchini S, Benelli C, et al: Laugier-Hunziker syndrome: a clinical, histopathologic, and ultrastructural study of four cases and review of the literature, *J Am Acad Dermatol* 25:632-636, 1991.

Weyers W, Euler M, Diaz-Cascajo C, et al: Classification of cutaneous malignant melanoma, *Cancer* 86:288-299, 1999.

VERRUCAL-PAPILLARY LESIONS

Reactive/Infectious Lesions

    Squamous Papilloma/Oral Wart

    Papillary Hyperplasia

    Condyloma Latum

    Condyloma Acuminatum

    Focal Epithelial Hyperplasia

Neoplasms

    Keratoacanthoma

    Verrucous Carcinoma

Idiopathic Lesions

    Pyostomatitis Vegetans

    Verruciform Xanthoma

REACTIVE/INFECTIOUS LESIONS

Squamous Papilloma/Oral Wart

Oral squamous papilloma is a generic term that is used to include papillary and verrucous growths composed of benign epithelium and minor amounts of supporting connective tissue.

Oral squamous papilloma (including the vermilion portion of the lip) is the most common papillary lesion of the oral mucosa and makes up approximately 2.5% of all oral lesions. Whether all intraoral squamous papillomas are related etiologically to classic cutaneous verruca vulgaris (warts) is unknown. However, many oral squamous papillomas have been shown to be associated with the same human papillomavirus (HPV) subtype that causes cutaneous warts. Other oral papillomas have been associated with different HPV subtypes. Whether all oral papillomas are of viral origin is also open to question. It has been shown that the class of HPVs is very large (more than 100 subtypes) and that individually these viruses are associated with

many conditions of squamous epithelium. For example, HPV subtypes 2 and 4 have been demonstrated within cutaneous warts by DNA hybridization techniques; flat warts of the skin have been associated with HPV subtypes 3 and 10. HPV subtype 11 has been found within papillomas of the sinonasal tract and the oral cavity. HPV subtypes 16 and 18 have been related to neoplastic changes of cervical squamous epithelium (Table 6-1).

Etiology. HPV, the putative etiologic agent of papillomas of the upper aerodigestive tract, is a member of the papovavirus group. It is a DNA virus containing a single molecule of double-stranded DNA. The viruses themselves are nonenveloped icosahedral particles ranging from 45 to 55 nm in diameter with 72 capsomeres in a skewed arrangement. Various species are antigenically distinct, sharing some common antigenic determinants. Replication of HPV occurs within the nuclei of epithelial cells as a result of stimulation of host DNA synthesis. The viral genome is expressed in both early and late stages, with the host histone proteins being incorporated into the virions. If progeny production is blocked, persistent infection may result. However, if intact viruses are produced, new infective particles can be released with or without cell death.

Clinical Features. Oral squamous papillomas may be found on the vermilion portion of the lips and any intraoral mucosal site, with predilection for the hard and soft palate and the uvula (Box 6-1; Figures 6-1 to 6-3). The latter three sites account for approximately one third of all lesions. The lesions generally measure less than 1 cm in greatest dimension and appear as pink to white exophytic granular or cauliflower-like surface alterations. The lesions generally are solitary in their presentation, although several lesions may be noted on occasion. The lesions are generally asymptomatic.

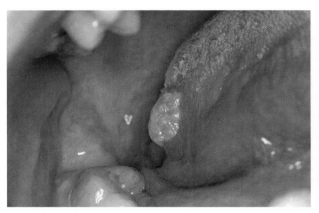

Figure 6-1 **Papilloma**, lateral tongue.

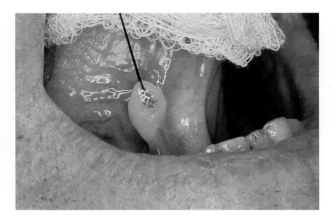

Figure 6-2 **Papilloma**, floor of mouth.

TABLE 6-1 **Lesions Caused by Human Papillomavirus Subtypes**

Lesion	HPV Subtype
Oral papilloma/wart	2, 6, 11, 57
Focal epithelial hyperplasia	13, 32
Dysplastic wart (HIV)	16, 18, others
Verrucous carcinoma	possibly 16, 18
Verruca vulgaris, skin	2, 4, 40
Flat wart	3, 10
Condyloma acuminatum	6, 11
Laryngeal papilloma	11
Conjunctival papilloma	11

HPV, Human papillomavirus; *HIV*, human immunodeficiency virus.

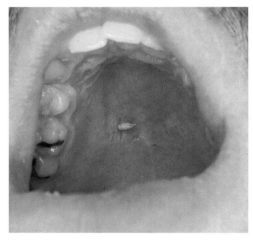

Figure 6-3 **Oral wart,** palate.

Box 6-1 Papilloma

Common oral epithelial proliferation
Most caused by HPV
   Nononcogenic subtypes (HPV subtypes 2, 6, 11, 57)
   "Oral wart" (verruca vulgaris) is a synonym for papilloma
Very low level of infectivity
Little significance
Recurrence/multiple lesions in immunosuppressed patients (e.g., HIV-positive patients, transplant recipients)

HPV, Human papillomavirus; *HIV*, human immunodeficiency virus.

Histopathology. Oral squamous papillomas represent an exaggerated growth of normal squamous epithelium (Figures 6-4 to 6-6). Extensions of epithelium, supported by a well-vascularized connective tissue stroma, project from the surface of the epithelium. The histologic architecture may mimic the pattern of the cuta-neous wart. Upper level epithelial cells demonstrate nuclei that are pyknotic and crenated, often surrounded by an edematous or optically clear zone, forming the so-called "koilocytic" cell. This cell is thought to be indicative of a virally altered state.

Dysplastic Oral Warts. Some oral papillomas in patients with acquired immunodeficiency syndrome (AIDS) exhibit microscopic changes that are dysplastic in appearance (Box 6-2; Figure 6-7). The degree of dysplasia ranges from mild to severe. The outcome, or natural history, of these dysplastic warts is unknown, although invasive carcinoma has yet to be reported despite several years of follow-up. A wide variety of HPV subtypes, including 16 and 18, can be demonstrated in these lesions.

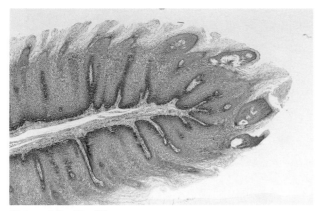

Figure 6-4 Papilloma.

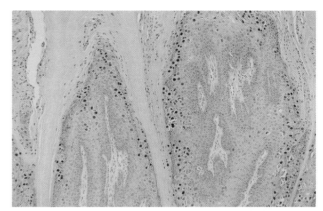

Figure 6-6 **Oral wart.** Immunohistochemical stain for common human papillomavirus in an oral wart. Positive, brown-staining nuclei are seen in upper level keratinocytes.

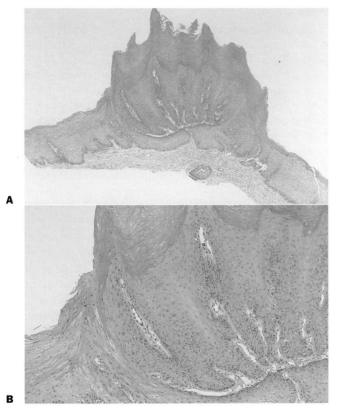

A

B

Figure 6-5 A and B, Oral wart.

> ### Box 6-2 Dysplastic Oral Warts
>
> HIV-positive patients only
> Multiple HPV subtypes, including 16, 18
> Oral mucosa only
> Histopathology—ranging from dysplasia to in situ carcinoma
> Invasive/metastatic potential unknown
>
> *HIV,* Human immunodeficiency virus; *HPV,* human papillomavirus.

olar ridge. A cause-and-effect relationship (e.g., lesion appearing under an ill-fitting denture) should be evident for inflammatory papillary hyperplasia. The condyloma would be larger than the papilloma, would have a broader base, and would appear pink to red as a result of less keratinization.

Treatment and Prognosis. Although many oral squamous papillomas appear to be virally induced, the infectivity of the HPV must be of a very low order. The route of transmission of the virus is unknown for oral lesions, although direct contact would be favored.

Surgical removal is the treatment of choice by either routine excision or laser ablation. Recurrence is uncommon, except for lesions in patients infected with human immunodeficiency virus (HIV). Patients who are HIV positive also often have multiple oral lesions.

Papillary Hyperplasia

Etiology. Papillary hyperplasia, or palatal papillomatosis, appears almost exclusively on the hard palate and

Differential Diagnosis. The differential diagnosis of oral squamous papilloma, when solitary, includes verruciform xanthoma, papillary hyperplasia, and condyloma acuminatum. Verruciform xanthoma may resemble squamous papilloma, although this lesion has a distinct predilection for the gingiva and the alve-

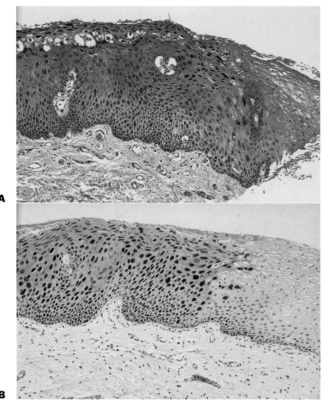

A

B

Figure 6-7   **Dysplastic oral wart. A,** Note normal epithelium at far right. **B,** Immunohistochemical stain for proliferation marker (PCNA) showing positive nuclear staining *(red)* in most keratinocytes.

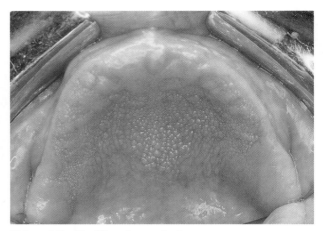

Figure 6-8   **Papillary hyperplasia.**

are tightly aggregated, producing an overall verrucous, granular, or cobblestone appearance. The projections may be slender and almost villous, although, in a majority of cases, each projection tends to be rounded and blunted, with narrow spaces on either side. Ulceration is rare, although intense erythema may at times provide an overall appearance of erosion. Focal telangiectatic sites may also be noted on occasion.

Histopathology. On perpendicular cross section, papillary hyperplasia appears as numerous small fronds or papillary projections covered with intact parakeratotic stratified squamous epithelium (Figure 6-9). The epithelium is supported by hyperplastic central cores of well-vascularized stromal tissue. The epithelium is hyperplastic and often demonstrates pseudoepitheliomatous features, occasionally severe enough to mimic squamous cell carcinoma. There is no evidence of dysplasia in association with this lesion and no increased risk of malignant transformation.

Differential Diagnosis. The range of possibilities in the differential diagnosis of papillary hyperplasia of the palate is rather narrow because this particular entity is seldom confused with other forms of pathology. The chief lesion to be separated from papillary hyperplasia is nicotine stomatitis involving the hard palate; however, nicotine stomatitis does not occur on the hard palate of those who wear complete maxillary removable appliances. Also, nicotine stomatitis tends to be more keratinized and usually demonstrates the presence of a small red dot or punctum in the center of each nodular excrescence, which represents the

almost always in association with a removable prosthesis. A definitive physical relationship with the mucosa covered by a removable denture base is seen; this may be noted in 1 in 10 people who wear appliances that cover the hard palatal mucosa.

The precise cause of papillary hyperplasia is not well understood, although it appears to be associated with ill-fitting or loose dentures that create a potential space between the denture base and tissue, predisposing to or potentiating growth of *Candida albicans* organisms. The tissue hyperplasia has been related to the presence of the fungal organism in the setting of low-grade chronic trauma.

Clinical Features. The area of mucosa over the palate that tends to be most commonly involved is the vault (Figure 6-8). Less commonly the alveolar ridge or the palatal incline is affected.

Presentation is characterized by multiple erythematous and edematous papillary projections that

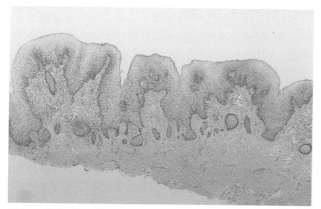

Figure 6-9 **Papillary hyperplasia.** Note pseudoepitheliomatous pattern.

orifice of the subjacent minor salivary gland duct. Rarely, in *Darier's disease,* the mucosa of the palate may demonstrate numerous papules. Numerous squamous papillomas may occur on the palate; however, these lesions tend to be more keratinized with more delicate projections. In the so-called malignant form of *acanthosis nigricans,* oral lesions are papillary in nature and may regress relative to the treatment response of the underlying distant malignancy. Finally, in the multiple hamartoma syndrome *(Cowden's syndrome)* the oral mucosa may exhibit numerous papillary mucosal nodules. These nodules, composed of benign fibroepithelial proliferations, may impart a cobblestone appearance, but usually to the tongue, buccal mucosa, and gingiva.

Treatment and Prognosis. Surgical removal is indicated before a denture is reconstructed for the patient. The actual surgical method is often a matter of individual preference and may include curettage, cryosurgery, electrosurgery, mucoabrasion, or laser ablation.

Removal of appliances at bedtime and soaking in a weak disinfecting or antifungal medium, as well as maintenance of good oral hygiene coupled with topical antifungal therapy, may significantly reduce the intensity of lesions. In mild cases the use of soft tissue conditioning agents and liners, with frequent changing of the lining material, can produce sufficient resolution to preclude surgery. Topical antifungal ointment, either alone or mixed with a corticosteroid ointment, may also help reduce the size and intensity of the lesions, although it will not effect a complete cure when used alone.

Condyloma Latum

Condyloma latum is one of the many and variable expressions of secondary syphilis. As with all forms of syphilis, cutaneous, mucosal, and systemic lesions that mimic other conditions or diseases can be seen. Characteristic of condyloma latum is the presence of exophytic, sometimes friable, papillary to polypoid lesions within the oral cavity. Condyloma latum contains abundant microorganisms *(Treponema pallidum)*, making it potentially infectious.

Condyloma latum usually appears on the skin, especially in the perianal and genital areas. Lesions may also be noted within the oral cavity. Here the tissue is formed into a soft, red, often mushroomlike mass with a generally smooth, lobulated surface.

Microscopically, the overlying epithelium demonstrates significant acanthosis, along with intracellular and intercellular edema and transmigration of neutrophils. A perivascular plasma cell infiltrate is common within the lamina propria in the absence of a true vasculitis.

Patients require systemic administration of antibiotics to eliminate the underlying bacteremia. The oral lesions generally regress as the systemic disease is brought under control.

Condyloma Acuminatum

Condyloma acuminatum is an infectious lesion that is characteristically located in the anogenital region but may also involve the oral mucosa. Common to these sites is a warm, moist squamous epithelial surface. An increasing frequency of this lesion has been noted in HIV-infected patients, reflecting an aspect of opportunistic infection.

Etiology and Pathogenesis. Condyloma acuminatum is a verrucous or papillary growth that has been etiologically related to HPV subtypes 6 and 11. The maturation of the various subtypes of HPV within oral and genital mucosal cells is essentially the same. The keratinized cells act as the hosts for the virus, with replication linked to the process of keratinization.

Clinical Features. Characteristic of early condyloma acuminatum formation is a group of numerous pink nodules that grow and ultimately coalesce (Figure 6-10). The result is a soft, broad-based, exophytic papillary growth that may be keratinized or nonkeratinized.

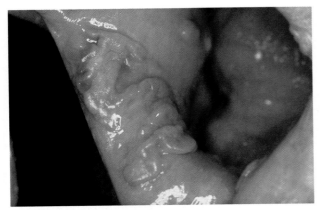

Figure 6-10   Condyloma acuminatum.

In 1 to 3 months after viral implantation, presumably as a result of orogenital contact with an infected partner, the disease becomes apparent. The lesions at times may be rather extensive, but they are generally self-limiting. The risk of autoinoculation is possible, thus offering a rationale for complete elimination of the lesions.

Histopathology. Papillary projections extending from the base of each lesion are covered by stratified squamous epithelium that is often parakeratotic but at times may be nonkeratinized. Koilocytosis of upper level epithelial cells is usually found. The epithelial layer itself is hyperplastic without evidence of dysplastic change. The underlying stroma is well vascularized and may contain a trace of chronic inflammatory cells.

Differential Diagnosis. Condyloma acuminatum may resemble focal epithelial hyperplasia in some cases. Multiple intraoral warts (verruca vulgaris) may be a consideration and indeed represent the same type of infection. Although condylomas tend to show more parakeratosis and acanthosis than verruca vulgaris, there are no universally accepted microscopic features that can be used to reliably separate the two. In situ DNA hybridization studies may be required to classify these lesions accurately.

Treatment and Prognosis. Treatment for these lesions is generally surgical excision, which may be cryosurgery, scalpel excision, electrodesiccation, or laser ablation. Recurrences are common and perhaps are related to surrounding normal-appearing tissue that may be harboring the infectious agent.

Focal Epithelial Hyperplasia

Focal epithelial hyperplasia (Heck's disease) was identified as a distinct entity in 1965. Early studies described lesions in Native Americans, in both the United States and Brazil, and in the Inuits of Greenland. More recent studies have also identified lesions in other populations and ethnic groups from South Africa, Mexico, and Central America, and clinical experience has demonstrated a wide ethnic incidence.

Etiology and Pathogenesis. Factors ranging from local low-grade irritation to vitamin deficiencies have been proposed as the cause of this condition. Convincing evidence, however, has been presented that HPV subtype 13 (and possibly 32) has an important etiologic role. Suggestions that genetic factors are involved have been made but not substantiated.

Clinical Features. This condition is characterized by the presence of numerous nodular soft tissue masses distributed over the mucosal surfaces, especially the buccal mucosa, labial mucosa, tongue, and gingiva (Figures 6-11 and 6-12). Lesions may appear as discrete or clustered papules, often similar in color to the surrounding mucosa. If found in areas of occlusal trauma, they may appear whitish because of keratosis. The lesions are asymptomatic and are often discovered incidentally. Initially described in children, this condition is now known to affect patients in a wide age range. An equal gender distribution has been noted.

Histopathology. Acanthosis and parakeratosis are consistent findings. Prominent clubbing and fusion of epithelial ridges is also seen. Enlarged ballooning cells with abnormal nuclear chromatin patterns are often seen within the spinous layer. More superficial elements demonstrate cytoplasmic granular changes and nuclear fragmentation. Cells immediately beneath the surface often show pyknotic nuclei with a surrounding clear zone.

Ultrastructurally, crystalline arrangements of viruslike particles may be noted. Such particles, which are located within the superficial spinous cells, measure approximately 50 nm in diameter. Viruses may be found within the nucleus, as well as the cytoplasm of spinous layer cells.

Differential Diagnosis. A differential diagnosis would include verruca vulgaris and multiple squamous papillomas. The oral mucosal lesions of *Cowden's (multiple hamartoma) syndrome* may present similarly and should

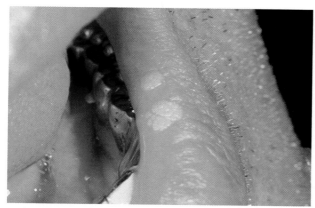

Figure 6-11 **Focal epithelial hyperplasia** of the lip.

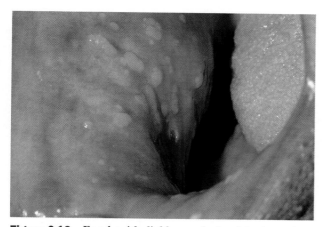

Figure 6-12 **Focal epithelial hyperplasia** of the buccal mucosa.

be ruled out. In addition, oral manifestations of Crohn's disease and pyostomatitis vegetans might be considered.

Treatment. No particular treatment is indicated, especially with widespread involvement. Surgical removal may be used if few lesions are present. Of significance is that spontaneous regression has been noted in many cases, perhaps as an expression of viral recognition and cell-mediated immunity.

NEOPLASMS

Keratoacanthoma

Etiology. Keratoacanthoma is a benign lesion of unknown cause that occurs chiefly on sun-exposed skin and, far less commonly, at the mucocutaneous junction. Very rarely has this lesion been reported to arise on mucous membranes. On the skin, keratoacanthomas originate within the pilosebaceous apparatus, which explains the predominance of this lesion there. It has been suggested that ectopic sebaceous glands may represent the site of origin intraorally. Viruslike intranuclear inclusions have been described in keratoacanthoma. However, attempts to produce such lesions in experimental animals by inoculation of tumor tissue have been unsuccessful. However, a rabbit skin model of keratoacanthoma was developed using topical carcinogens. In addition to sunlight and viruses, suspected etiologic agents include chemical carcinogens, trauma, and disordered cellular immunity.

Clinical Features. Keratoacanthomas may be solitary or multiple. The lesion usually begins as a small red macule that soon becomes a firm papule with a fine scale over its highest point. Rapid enlargement of the papule occurs over approximately 4 to 8 weeks, resulting ultimately in a hemispheric, firm, elevated, asymptomatic nodule. When fully developed, a keratoacanthoma contains a core of keratin surrounded by a concentric collar of raised skin or mucosa. A peripheral rim of erythema at the lesion's base may parallel the raised margin.

If the lesion is not removed, spontaneous regression occurs. The central keratin mass is exfoliated, leaving a saucer-shaped lesion that heals with superficial scar formation.

Histopathology. Keratoacanthoma is characterized by a central keratin plug with an overhanging lip or a marginal buttress of epithelium (Figure 6-13). Marked pseudoepitheliomatous hyperplasia is evident, along with an intense mixed inflammatory infiltrate.

Of great importance is the histologic similarity between a keratoacanthoma and a well-differentiated squamous cell carcinoma. Numerous histologic criteria, such as a high level of differentiation, the formation of keratin masses, smooth symmetric infiltration, abrupt epithelial changes at lateral margins, and transepidermal elimination of sun-damaged elastic fibers have been used to distinguish keratoacanthoma from carcinoma. Analysis of DNA indices and proliferative levels by flow cytometry of both well-differentiated squamous cell carcinomas and keratoacanthomas fails to separate the two lesions. Differences in various oncogene expression patterns and more recently the expression of angiotensin type

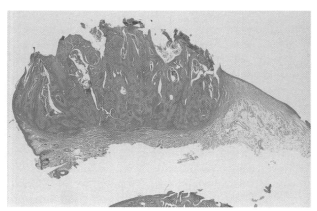

Figure 6-13 **Keratoacanthoma.** Note the "cup-shaped" symmetry and verruciform surface.

Box 6-3 Verrucous Carcinoma

ETIOLOGY

Tobacco and possibly HPV subtypes 16 and 18

CLINICAL FEATURES

Slow-growing verrucous patch
Locally destructive; rarely metastasizes
Buccal mucosa > gingiva > tongue > palate > other

MICROSCOPY

Well-differentiated carcinoma
Little or no dysplasia

TREATMENT

Excision; prognosis excellent

HPV, Human papillomavirus; >, more frequently affected than.

I receptors have either supported or refuted the theory that keratoacanthomas are a well-differentiated type of carcinoma.

Differential Diagnosis. The primary entity to be distinguished from a solitary keratoacanthoma is squamous cell carcinoma, from both a clinical and a microscopic perspective. Squamous cell carcinomas have a relatively slow growth rate, are of irregular shape, and generally begin later in life. For lesions on the lip, other conditions to be differentiated include molluscum contagiosum, solar keratosis, and verruca vulgaris. Most of these entities, however, can be easily excluded on the basis of histologic examination of the biopsy specimen.

Treatment and Prognosis. At the least, a very careful follow-up is required in all cases because of the difficulties in diagnosis and distinction from squamous cell carcinoma. Any dubious lesion should be treated because there are no absolutely reliable diagnostic, clinical, or histologic criteria to differentiate these two lesions. In addition, during the early phase of this lesion, prediction of its ultimate size may be impossible.

A solitary keratoacanthoma may be removed by surgical excision or by thorough curettage of the base; both methods are equally effective. No recurrence is expected. In cases in which no treatment is accomplished, spontaneous involution, often with scar formation, is seen.

Verrucous Carcinoma

Etiology. Verrucous carcinoma of oral mucous membranes (Box 6-3) is most closely associated with the use of tobacco in various forms, especially smokeless tobacco. A role for HPV in either a primary or an ancillary relationship is suspected. Identification of intratumor HPV DNA adds support for a possible role of this virus in tumor development.

Clinical Features. This form of carcinoma accounts for 5% of all intraoral squamous cell carcinomas (Figures 6-14 and 6-15). The buccal mucosa is the location for more than half of all cases, and the gingiva is the location for nearly one third of cases. The mandibular gingiva shows a slight predominance over the maxillary gingiva. There is a distinct male predominance, and most individuals are over 50 years of age.

Early lesions, which may initially be interpreted as verrucous hyperplasia, are relatively superficial and tend to appear white clinically. These lesions may arise in leukoplakia. In time, the lesion borders become irregular and indurated. As verrucous carcinoma develops, the lesion becomes exophytic with a whitish to gray shaggy surface. Although not highly infiltrative, the lesion pushes into surrounding tissues. When it involves the gingival tissues, it becomes fixed to the underlying periosteum. If it is untreated, gradual invasion of periosteum and destruction of bone occur.

Histopathology. At low magnification, surface papillary fronds are covered by a markedly acanthotic and highly keratinized epithelial surface. Bulbous, well-differentiated epithelial masses extend into the submucosa, with margins that are blunted and pushing

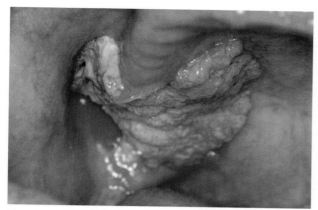

Figure 6-14 **Verrucous carcinoma** of the maxillary alveolar ridge.

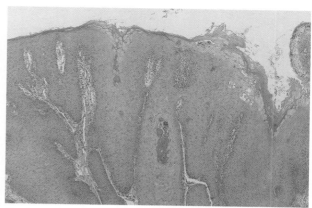

Figure 6-16 **Verrucous carcinoma** showing broad, "pushing," well-differentiated rete ridges.

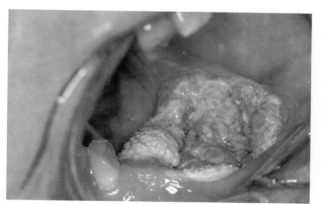

Figure 6-15 **Verrucous carcinoma** of the mandibular vestibule.

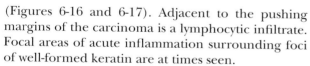

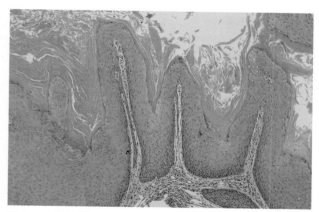

Figure 6-17 **Verrucous carcinoma** showing well-differentiated epithelium in a verruciform profile.

(Figures 6-16 and 6-17). Adjacent to the pushing margins of the carcinoma is a lymphocytic infiltrate. Focal areas of acute inflammation surrounding foci of well-formed keratin are at times seen.

Of importance is the deceptively benign microscopic pattern and the absence of significant cellular atypia. Diagnosis can be made only with a biopsy specimen of sufficient size to include the full thickness of the epithelial component, as well as the supporting connective tissue.

Papillary squamous cell carcinoma is a rarely seen malignancy of oral mucosa that has some resemblance to verrucous carcinoma. It exhibits a papillary profile and is moderately to well differentiated. Its prognosis is believed to be somewhat better than that for typical squamous cell carcinoma but worse than that for verrucous carcinoma.

Differential Diagnosis. In well-developed cases of verrucous carcinoma, the clinical pathologic diagnosis is relatively straightforward. However, in less than obvious situations, leukoplakia might be a clinical consideration. A differential diagnosis would also include papillary squamous carcinoma, which may be distinguished from verrucous carcinoma by its more infiltrative nature, its greater degree of cytologic atypia, and its more rapid growth. Verrucous carcinoma may develop from preexisting (and usually multiple) leukoplakia, representing part of the spectrum of *proliferative verrucous leukoplakia* (Box 6-4; Figures 6-18 to 6-23) (see also Chapter 3).

Treatment and Prognosis. Surgical methods are generally used as the primary form of therapy in most cases of verrucous carcinoma. This is chiefly because

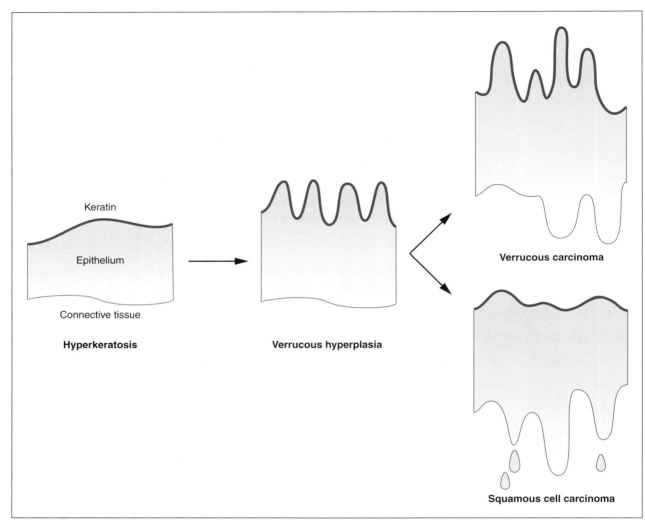

Figure 6-18   Proliferative verrucous leukoplakia.

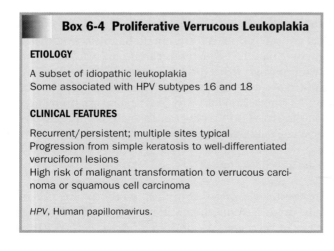

Box 6-4 Proliferative Verrucous Leukoplakia

ETIOLOGY

A subset of idiopathic leukoplakia
Some associated with HPV subtypes 16 and 18

CLINICAL FEATURES

Recurrent/persistent; multiple sites typical
Progression from simple keratosis to well-differentiated
verruciform lesions
High risk of malignant transformation to verrucous carcinoma or squamous cell carcinoma

HPV, Human papillomavirus.

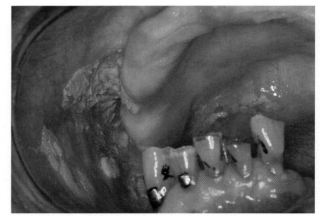

Figure 6-19   **Proliferative verrucous leukoplakia** of the
buccal mucosa and soft palate.

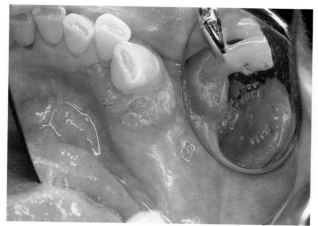

Figure 6-20 **Proliferative verrucous leukoplakia** of the gingiva.

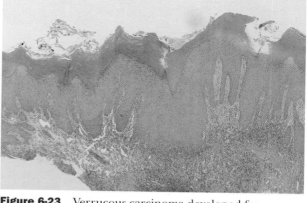

Figure 6-23 Verrucous carcinoma developed from persistent proliferative verrucous leukoplakia.

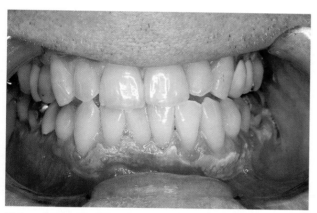

Figure 6-21 **Proliferative verrucous leukoplakia** of the gingiva. (Courtesy, Dr. Sol Silverman, Jr.)

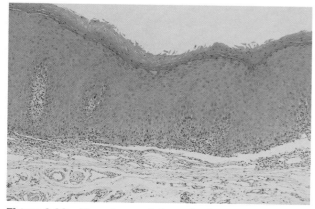

Figure 6-22 Hyperkeratosis in early phase of proliferative verrucous leukoplakia.

of early reports of dedifferentiation occurring in verrucous carcinoma after radiotherapy. The literature, however, now suggests that transformation to squamous cell carcinoma following radiotherapy occurs far less commonly than has been reported. Aggressive radiotherapy early or in combination with surgery may be a viable alternative treatment method.

Verrucous carcinoma rarely metastasizes, although it is locally destructive. In advanced cases in which the maxilla or the mandible exhibits significant destruction, resection may be necessary.

The prognosis for verrucous carcinoma is excellent, primarily because of its high level of differentiation and rarity of metastatic spread. Local recurrence, however, remains a distinct possibility if inadequate treatment is rendered.

IDIOPATHIC LESIONS

Pyostomatitis Vegetans

Originally described in 1949, pyostomatitis vegetans, a benign chronic and pustular form of mucocutaneous disease, is most often seen in association with inflammatory bowel disease. In two of the three original patients with oral disease, the lesions were confined to the oral mucosa. The cause of pyostomatitis vegetans is unknown, although it may be seen in association with ulcerative colitis, spastic colitis, chronic diarrhea, and Crohn's disease. More than 25% of cases are not associated with gastrointestinal disturbances.

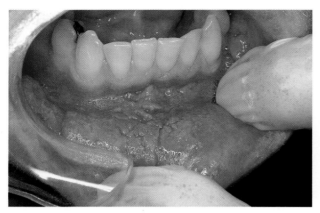

Figure 6-24   **Pyostomatitis vegetans.**

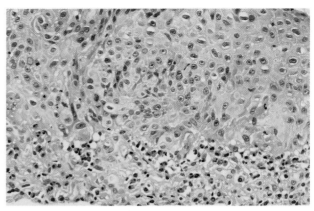

Figure 6-25   **Pyostomatitis vegetans** showing neutrophil and eosinophil infiltrate at epithelium–connective tissue junction.

Clinical Features. Early in the evolution of pyostomatitis vegetans, the oral mucosa (especially buccal mucosa) appears erythematous, edematous, nodular, and occasionally fissured (Figure 6-24). Numerous tiny yellow pustules, ranging from 2 to 3 mm in diameter, and small vegetating papillary projections may be seen over the surface of friable mucosa. Oral mucosal involvement may include the gingiva, hard and soft palate, buccal and labial mucosa, lateral and ventral aspects of the tongue, and floor of the mouth. Men are affected nearly twice as often as women, and the age range is generally between the third and sixth decades, with an average age of 34 years. Laboratory values are generally within normal limits, although in many patients peripheral eosinophilia or anemia may be noted.

Histopathology. The oral mucosa demonstrates hyperkeratosis and pronounced acanthosis, often with a papillary surface or with pseudoepitheliomatous hyperplasia (Figure 6-25). A pronounced inflammatory infiltrate composed of neutrophils and eosinophils is a constant finding. Superficial abscesses may be seen within the lamina propria, with extension into the parabasal regions of the overlying epithelium. Ulceration and superficial epithelial necrosis may also be noted.

Treatment and Prognosis. The management of this entity relates to controlling the associated bowel disease. Topical agents, such as corticosteroids, may be used intraorally. In addition, antibiotics, multivitamins, and

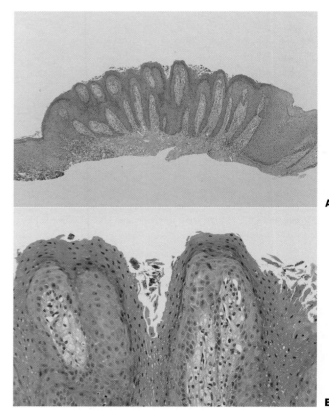

A

B

Figure 6-26   **Verruciform xanthoma. A** and **B,** Note xanthoma cells (foamy macrophages) in lamina propria.

nutritional supplements may be given; however, all are associated with variable results. Remission of oral lesions occurs when underlying bowel disease is medically controlled.

Verruciform Xanthoma

Verruciform xanthoma is an uncommon, benign oral mucosal lesion that occasionally may be found on the skin, typically on the genitalia. The cause is unknown.

Clinical Features. Clinically, verruciform xanthoma is well circumscribed, with a granular to papillary surface. The size of this lesion ranges from 2 mm to more than 2 cm. Either an exophytic or a depressed surface is present, and the lesion may occasionally be ulcerated. The level of keratinization of the surface influences the color, which ranges from white to red.

The majority of cases have been reported in whites; there is no gender predilection. The average age of patients is 45 years, with a few cases reported within the first and second decades. The lesions are usually discovered incidentally.

Histopathology. The architecture of the lesion is flat or slightly raised, with a papillomatous or verrucous surface composed of parakeratinized epithelial cells (Figure 6-26). Uniformly invaginated crypts alternate with papillary extensions. Elongated epithelial ridges extend into the lamina propria at a uniform depth. The epithelial component is normal, with no evidence of dysplasia or atypia.

Numerous foam or xanthoma cells are found within the lamina propria or connective tissue papillae. Characteristic of the foam cells is a granular to flocculent cytoplasm that may contain periodic acid–Schiff (PAS)–positive, diastase-resistant granules or lipid droplets, or both. Ultrastructurally, the foam cells are best characterized as macrophages.

Differential Diagnosis. A differential diagnosis for this entity would include squamous papilloma, papillary squamous carcinoma, and condyloma acuminatum.

Treatment. The treatment is conservative excision. No recurrences have been reported.

BIBLIOGRAPHY

SQUAMOUS PAPILLOMA/ORAL VERRUCA VULGARIS

Broich G, Saskai I: Electron microscopic demonstration of HPV in oral warts, *Microbiologica* 13:27-34, 1990.

Kellokoski J, Syrjanen S, Syrjanen K, et al: Oral mucosal changes in women with genital HPV infection, *J Oral Pathol Med* 19:142-148, 1990.

Regezi JA, Greenspan D, Greenspan JS, et al: HPV-associated epithelial atypia in oral warts in HIV+ patients, *J Cutan Pathol* 21:217-223, 1994.

Zeuss M, Miller C, White D: In situ hybridization analysis of human papilloma virus DNA in oral mucosal lesions, *Oral Surg Oral Med Oral Pathol* 71:714-720, 1991.

PAPILLARY HYPERPLASIA

Chang F, Syrjanen S, Kellokoski J, et al: Human papillomavirus (HPV) infections and their associations with oral disease, *J Oral Pathol* 20:305-307, 1991.

Kozlowski L, Nigra T: Esophageal acanthosis nigricans in association with adenocarcinoma from an unknown primary site, *J Am Acad Dermatol* 26:348-351, 1992.

Tyler MT, Ficarra G, Silverman S, et al: Malignant acanthosis nigricans with florid papillary oral lesions, *Oral Surg Oral Med Oral Pathol Oral Radiol Endod* 81:445-449, 1996.

Young S, Min K: In situ DNA hybridization analysis of oral papillomas, leukoplakias, and carcinomas for human papillomavirus, *Oral Surg Oral Med Oral Pathol* 71:726-729, 1991.

CONDYLOMA ACUMINATUM

Barone R, Ficarra G, Gaglioti D, et al: Prevalence of oral lesions among HIV-infected intravenous drug abusers and other risk groups, *Oral Surg Oral Med Oral Pathol* 69:169-173, 1990.

FOCAL EPITHELIAL HYPERPLASIA

Padayachee A, van Wyk C: Human papillomavirus (HPV) DNA in focal epithelial hyperplasia by in situ hybridization, *J Oral Pathol Med* 20:210-214, 1991.

KERATOACANTHOMA

Lawrence N, Reed RJ: Actinic keratoacanthoma speculations on the nature of the lesion and the role of cellular immunity in its evolution, *Am J Dermatopathol* 12:517-533, 1990.

Randall MB, Geisinger RR, Kute TE, et al: DNA content and proliferative index in cutaneous squamous cell carcinoma and keratoacanthoma, *Am J Clin Pathol* 93:159-262, 1990.

Street ML, White JW, Gibson LE: Multiple keratoacanthomas treated with oral retinoids, *J Am Acad Dermatol* 23:862-866, 1990.

Tsuji T: Keratoacanthoma and squamous cell carcinoma: study of PCNA and Le(Y) expression, *J Cutan Pathol* 7:409-415, 1997.

VERRUCOUS CARCINOMA

Greer RO Jr, Eversole LR, Crosby LK: Detection of human papillomavirus genome DNA in oral epithelial dysplasias, oral smokeless tobacco–associated leukoplakias and epithelial malignancies, *J Oral Maxillofac Surg* 48:1201-1209, 1990.

Mork J, Lie AK, Glattre E, et al: Human papillomavirus infection as a risk factor for squamous cell carcinoma of the head and neck, *N Engl J Med* 344:1125-1131, 2001.

Palefsky JM, Silverman S, Abdel-Salaam M, et al: Association between proliferative verrucous leukoplakia and infection with human papillomavirus type 16, *J Oral Pathol Med* 24:193-197, 1995.

Spiro RH: Verrucous carcinoma, then and now, *Am J Surg* 176(5):393-397, 1998.

Vidyasagar MS, Fernandes DJ, Kasturi P, et al: Radiotherapy and verrucous carcinoma of the oral cavity, *Acta Oncol* 31:43-47, 1992.

PYOSTOMATITIS VEGETANS

Healy CM, Farthing PM, Williams DM, et al: Pyostomatitis vegetans and associated systemic disease, *Oral Surg Oral Med Oral Pathol* 78:323-328, 1994.

Thornhill M, Zakrzawska J, Gilkes J: Pyostomatitis vegetans: report of 3 cases and review of the literature, *J Oral Pathol Med* 21:128-133, 1992.

VERRUCIFORM XANTHOMA

Olivera PT, Jaeger RG, Cabral LAG, et al: Verruciform xanthoma of the oral mucosa: report of four cases and a review of the literature, *Oral Oncol* 37:326-331, 2001.

CONNECTIVE TISSUE LESIONS

Connective tissue lesions comprise a large and diverse number of entities ranging from reactive lesions to neoplasms. Reactive conditions are derived from mesenchymal cells and are represented by fibrous hyperplasias or exuberant proliferations of granulation tissue. Tumors of connective tissue elements are heterogeneous and form a complex collection of diseases. Prediction of biologic behavior from histology alone is problematic and is reflected in the difficulties in grading individual tumors. Traditionally, tumors of connective tissues have been classified on the basis of a model based on presumed histogenetic lineage. Hence neoplasms are subdivided into tumors of fibrous, fibrohistiocytic, myofibroblastic, vascular, neural, muscular, adipose, and other types of tissue. Increasingly, it is becoming evident that many tumors do not arise from their mature, differentiated counterparts, since soft tissue tumors can arise in sites that are devoid of their mature tissue counterpart. For example, liposarcomas often arise at sites where there is no adipose tissue, and rhabdomyosarcomas often arise in sites that contain no striated muscle. It is likely that any soft tissue malignancy can develop along any differentiation pathway, which is dictated by the expression of specific differentiation genes. However, for the purposes of describing these entities, a histogenetic classification has been maintained here.

FIBROUS LESIONS

REACTIVE HYPERPLASIAS

Reactive hyperplasias comprise a group of fibrous connective tissue lesions that commonly occur in oral mucosa secondary to injury. They represent a chronic process in which overexuberant repair (granulation tissue and scar) follows injury. As a group, these lesions present as submucosal masses that may become secondarily ulcerated when traumatized during mastication. Their color ranges from lighter than the surrounding tissue (because of a relative increase in collagen) to red (because of an abundance of well-vascularized granulation tissue). Because nerve tissue does not proliferate with the reactive hyperplastic tissue, these lesions are painless. The reason for the overexuberant repair is unknown. Treatment is generally surgical excision and removal of the irritating factor(s).

Although these lesions are all pathogenically related, different names or subdivisions have been devised because of variations in the anatomic site, clinical appearance, or microscopic picture. Those lesions that present as prominent red masses are discussed in Chapter 4.

Peripheral Fibroma

Clinical Features. By definition, peripheral fibroma is a reactive hyperplastic mass that occurs on the gingiva and is believed to be derived from connective tissue of the submucosa or periodontal ligament (Figure 7-1). It may occur at any age, although it does have a predilection for young adults. Females develop these lesions more commonly than do males, and the gingiva anterior to the permanent molars is most often affected.

Peripheral fibroma presents clinically as either a pedunculated or a sessile mass that is similar in color to the surrounding connective tissue. Ulceration may

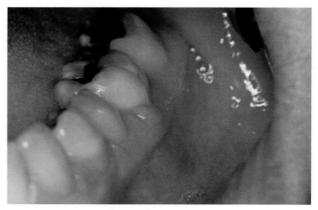

Figure 7-1   Peripheral fibroma.

be noted over the summit of the lesion. It rarely causes erosion of subjacent alveolar bone.

Histopathology. Peripheral fibroma is a focal fibrous hyperplasia that may also be called *hyperplastic scar.* It is highly collagenous and relatively avascular, and it may contain a mild to moderate chronic inflammatory cell infiltrate. This lesion is basically the gingival counterpart to traumatic fibroma occurring in other mucosal regions.

Microscopically, several subtypes of this lesion have been identified. These are essentially of academic interest, because biologic behavior and treatment of these microscopic variants are the same.

Peripheral ossifying fibroma is a gingival mass in which islands of woven (immature) bone and osteoid are seen. The bone is found within a lobular proliferation of plump, benign fibroblasts. Chronic inflammatory cells tend to be seen around the periphery of the lesion (Figure 7-2). The surface is typically ulcerated.

Peripheral odontogenic fibroma is a gingival mass composed of well-vascularized, nonencapsulated fibrous connective tissue. The distinguishing feature of this variant is the presence of strands of odontogenic epithelium, often abundant, throughout the connective tissue. Amorphous hard tissue resembling tertiary (reactive) dentin, so-called dentinoid, may also be present. The lesion is usually nonulcerated.

Giant cell fibroma is a focal fibrous hyperplasia in which connective tissue cells, many of which are multinucleated, assume a stellate shape. Immunohistochemical studies have shown that most of these stellate cells are fibroblasts (a few factor XIIIa–positive dendritic cells are also typically present) (Figure 7-3). These same peculiar stellate cells can also be found in focal

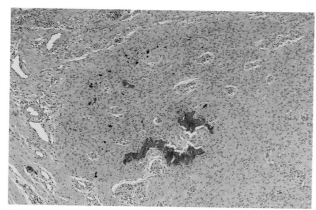

Figure 7-2   Peripheral ossifying fibroma. Note cellular fibroblastic proliferation with islands of new bone.

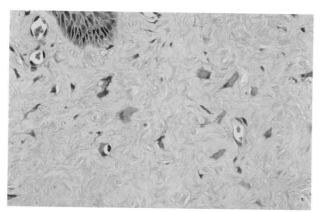

Figure 7-3   Peripheral fibroma with stellate-shaped fibroblasts.

fibrous hyperplastic lesions throughout the oral mucosa and occasionally on the skin (fibrous papule). One form of this lesion is known as *retrocuspid papilla* of the mandible.

Differential Diagnosis. Clinically, these lesions are usually not confused with anything else. There may, however, be some overlap with pyogenic granuloma and, rarely, peripheral giant cell granuloma, when these two lesions do not have a prominent vascular component.

Treatment. Peripheral fibroma should be treated by local excision that should include the periodontal ligament, if involved. Also, any identifiable etiologic agent, such as calculus or other foreign material, should be removed. Recurrence may occasionally be associated with the microscopic subtype, peripheral-ossifying fibroma. Reexcision to the periosteum or

---

Box 7-1 Gingival Hyperplasia: Causes/Modifiers

Local factors: plaque, calculus, bacteria
Hormonal imbalance: estrogen, testosterone
Drugs: phenytoin (Dilantin); cyclosporine; nifedipine and other calcium channel blockers
Leukemia (due to leukemic infiltrates and/or local factors)
Genetic factors/syndromes

---

periodontal ligament should prevent further recurrence.

Generalized Gingival Hyperplasia

Etiology. In generalized gingival hyperplasia, overgrowth of the gingiva may vary from mild enlargement of interdental papillae to such severe uniform enlargement that the crowns of the teeth may be covered by hyperplastic tissue (Box 7-1). Uniform or generalized gingival fibrous connective tissue hyperplasia may be due to one of several etiologic factors. Most cases are nonspecific and are a result of an unusual hyperplastic tissue response to chronic inflammation associated with local factors such as plaque, calculus, or bacteria. Why only some patients have a propensity for the development of connective tissue hyperplasia in response to local factors is unknown. Recent studies have stated a possible role for keratinocyte growth factor (a member of the fibroblast growth factor family) in this condition.

Other conditions such as hormonal changes and drugs can significantly potentiate or exaggerate the effects of local factors on gingival connective tissue. Hormonal changes occurring during pregnancy and puberty have long been known to be associated with generalized gingival hyperplasia. This hyper-responsiveness during pregnancy has led to the infrequently used and inappropriate term *pregnancy gingivitis*. Altered hormonal conditions act in concert with local irritants to produce the hyperplastic response. It is questionable whether significant gingival enlargement during periods of hormonal imbalance would occur in individuals with scrupulous oral hygiene.

Phenytoin (Dilantin), a drug used in the control of seizure disorders, is a well-known etiologic factor in generalized gingival enlargement. The extent or severity of so-called *dilantin hyperplasia* is dependent

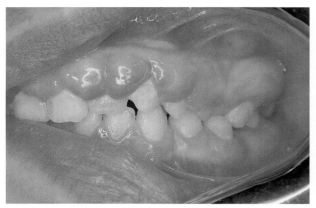

Figure 7-4 **Generalized gingival hyperplasia** associated with local factors and hormonal chenges.

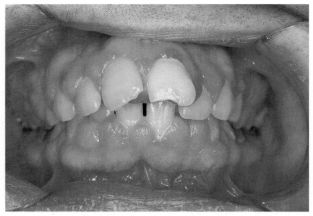

Figure 7-5 **Generalized gingival hyperplasia** associated with phenytoin therapy for seizures.

on the presence of local factors such as plaque and calculus. The effect of the time and dose of the drug on gingival tissue is not clear. The reported prevalence of this condition has ranged from 0% to 80%, depending on the investigator's clinical criteria and the number of patients observed. A 50% figure is generally accepted as the probable prevalence. In any event, the fact that not all patients taking phenytoin develop gingival hyperplasia indicates that some patients are predisposed to the development of this condition. It has only rarely been described in edentulous patients and in children before tooth eruption.

Cyclosporine, the immunosuppressant drug that is used to modulate T-lymphocyte function in transplant recipients and in patients with various autoimmune diseases, has also been linked to fibrous hyperplasia of the gingiva. Not all patients are affected (10% to 70%), and local factors have a synergistic role. Unlike phenytoin-related hyperplasia, cyclosporine-induced hyperplasia has been reported to be a reversible process following cessation of drug use.

Nifedipine and other calcium channel blockers used for treatment of angina, arrhythmias, and hypertension are also known to contribute to gingival hyperplasia. The process mimics phenytoin-related hyperplasia but, like cyclosporine-induced gingival hyperplasia, appears to be reversible.

Gingival enlargement is also known to occur in patients with leukemia, especially those with the chronic monocytic form. This is believed to be a result of infiltration of the gingival soft tissues by malignant white blood cells. It may also be modulated by

local factors such as plaque and calculus; because of the bleeding tendency associated with leukemia, patients may be unable or reluctant to practice correct oral hygiene, resulting in the accumulation of plaque and debris. This accumulation may provide the inflammatory stimulus for connective tissue hyperplasia.

Some rare types of gingival hyperplasia occurring in early childhood have a hereditary basis. The best recognized is hereditary gingival fibromatosis, which clinically can resemble dilantin-induced gingival hyperplasia. Patients with other rare syndromes such as Zimmerman-Laband, Cross', Rutherfurd's, Murray-Puretic-Drescher, and Cowden's syndromes can also develop varying degrees of fibrous gingival hyperplasia.

Clinical Features. The clinical feature common to the variously caused gingival hyperplasias is an increase in the bulk of the free and attached gingiva, especially the interdental papillae (Figures 7-4 to 7-6). Stippling is lost, and gingival margins become rolled and blunted. The consistency of the gingiva ranges from soft and spongy to firm and dense, depending directly on the degree of fibroplasia. A range of color from red-blue to lighter than the surrounding tissue is also seen; this depends on the severity of the inflammatory response as well. Generally, the hyperplasias associated with nonspecific local factors and hormonal changes appear more inflamed clinically than the drug-induced and idiopathic forms. The idiopathic type is particularly dense and fibrous, with relatively little inflammatory change.

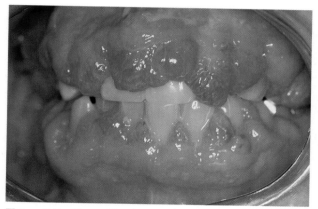

Figure 7-6 **Generalized gingival hyperplasia** associated with chronic monocytic leukemia.

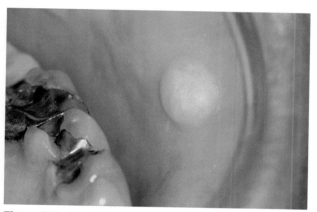

Figure 7-7 **Focal fibrous hyperplasia,** buccal mucosa.

Histopathology. There is an abundance of collagen. Fibroblasts are increased in number, and various degrees of chronic inflammation are seen. In some cases, especially those in which hormonal changes are important, capillaries may be increased and prominent. The overlying epithelium usually exhibits some hyperplasia. Occasionally, plasma cells dominate the histologic picture. In leukemic enlargements, atypical and immature white blood cells, representing a malignant infiltrate, may be found.

Treatment. In all forms of generalized gingival hyperplasia, attentive oral hygiene is necessary to minimize the effects of inflammation on fibrous proliferation and the effects of systemic factors. Gingivoplasty or gingivectomy may be required but should be done in combination with prophylaxis, oral hygiene instruction, and a comprehensive home care program.

Focal Fibrous Hyperplasia

Etiology. Focal fibrous hyperplasia is a reactive lesion usually caused by chronic trauma to oral mucous membranes. Overexuberant fibrous connective tissue repair results in a clinically evident submucosal mass. Although the terms *traumatic fibroma* and *oral fibroma* are often applied to these entities, they are misnomers, since these lesions are not benign tumors of fibroblasts, as the term *fibroma* implies (Box 7-2).

Clinical Features. There is no gender or racial predilection for the development of this intraoral lesion. It is a very common reactive hyperplasia that is typically found in frequently traumatized areas, such as the

> **Box 7-2 Oral Fibrous Hyperplasia: Synonyms**
>
> Traumatic fibroma
> Irritation fibroma
> Hyperplastic scar
> Inflammatory fibrous hyperplasia
> Peripheral fibroma of gingiva
> Fibrous epulis of gingiva
> Denture (induced fibrous) hyperplasia
> Epulis fissuratum (denture induced)

buccal mucosa, lateral border of the tongue, and lower lip (Figure 7-7). It is a painless, broad-based swelling that is more pale in color than the surrounding tissue because of its relative lack of vascular channels. The surface may occasionally be traumatically ulcerated, particularly in larger lesions. Lesions have limited growth potential and do not exceed 1 to 2 cm in diameter.

Multiple fibromas may be part of a rare autosomal-dominant syndrome known as *Cowden's syndrome* or *multiple hamartoma syndrome.* Many organ systems, such as the mucosa, skin, breast, thyroid, and colon, may be affected. Frequently encountered abnormalities include numerous oral fibromas and papillomas; cutaneous papules, keratoses, and trichilemmomas; benign and malignant neoplasms of the breast and thyroid; and colonic polyps. The underlying genetic problem appears to be related to germline mutations of the tumor suppressor gene *PTEN* found on chromosome 10q23.

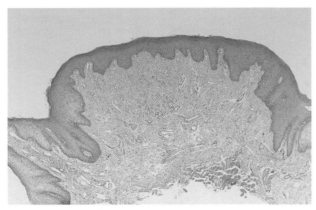

Figure 7-8   Focal fibrous hyperplasia.

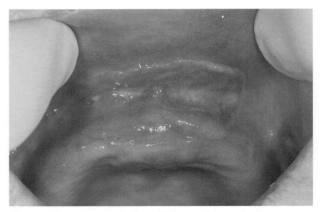

Figure 7-9   Denture-induced fibrous hyperplasia.

Histopathology. Collagen overproduction is the basic process that dominates the microscopy of this lesion. Fibroblasts are mature and widely scattered in a dense collagen matrix. Sparse chronic inflammatory cells may be seen, usually in a perivascular distribution (Figure 7-8). Overlying epithelium is often hyperkeratotic because of chronic low-grade friction.

Differential Diagnosis. This is a relatively trivial lesion that should be removed to rule out other pathologic processes. Depending on its location, several other entities might be included in a clinical differential diagnosis. Neurofibroma, neurilemmoma, and granular cell tumor would be possibilities for masses in the tongue. In the lower lip and buccal mucosa, lipoma, mucocele, and salivary gland tumors might be considered. Although rare, benign neoplasms of mesenchymal origin could present as submucosal masses not unlike focal fibrous hyperplasia.

Treatment. Simple surgical excision is usually effective. Infrequently, recurrences may be caused by continued trauma to the involved area. These lesions have no malignant potential.

Denture-induced Fibrous Hyperplasia

Etiology. Denture-induced fibrous hyperplasia of oral mucosa is related to the chronic trauma produced by an ill-fitting denture. The process is essentially the same as the one that leads to traumatic fibroma, except that a denture is specifically identified as the causative agent. This lesion has also been designated by the outdated synonyms *inflammatory hyperplasia, denture hyperplasia,* and *epulis fissuratum.*

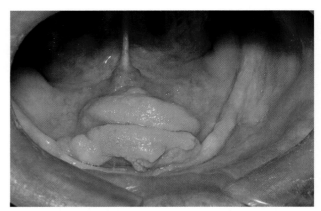

Figure 7-10   Denture-induced fibrous hyperplasia.

Clinical Features. Denture-induced fibrous hyperplasia is a common lesion that occurs in the vestibular mucosa and less commonly along the mandibular lingual sulcus where the denture flange contacts tissue (Figures 7-9 and 7-10). As the bony ridges of the mandible and the maxilla resorb with long-term denture use, the flanges gradually extend farther into the vestibule. There, chronic irritation and trauma may incite an overexuberant fibrous connective tissue reparative response. The result is the appearance of painless folds of fibrous tissue surrounding the overextended denture flange.

Treatment. Some reduction in size of the lesion may follow prolonged removal of the denture. However, because the hyperplastic scar is relatively permanent, surgical excision is usually required. Construction of a new denture or relining of the old one is also required to prevent recurrences.

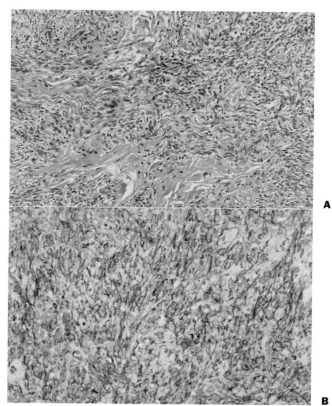

Figure 7-11 **Solitary fibrous tumor. A,** Haphazard spindle cell proliferation. **B,** Immunohistochemical stain for CD34 showing positive staining *(brown)* of tumor cells.

NEOPLASMS

Solitary Fibrous Tumor

Solitary fibrous tumor is a benign proliferation of spindle cells of disputed but probable fibroblastic origin (Box 7-3). This lesion was first described as a tumor of the pleura and has subsequently been described in many other sites. Oral lesions are seen in adults and present as submucosal masses predominantly in the buccal mucosa (Box 7-4).

Microscopically, lesions are circumscribed and are composed of a patternless proliferation of spindle cells (Figure 7-11). Some areas may suggest neurofibroma or neurilemmoma, whereas others may suggest pericytoma or leiomyoma. Tumor cells characteristically stain positive for CD34, CD99, and Bcl-2 by immunohistochemistry. Many factor XIIIa–positive cells may be found in solitary fibrous tumors.

Treatment is surgical excision, and recurrences are not seen. Malignant transformation has not been associated with oral tumors.

Myxoma

Clinical Features. Myxoma is a soft tissue neoplasm composed of gelatinous material that has a myxoid appearance histologically. The oral form of soft tissue myxoma is a rare lesion that presents as a slow-growing, asymptomatic submucosal mass, usually in the palate. There appears to be no gender predilection, and the lesion may occur at any age. Oral soft tissue myxomas have been reported in an autosomal dominantly inherited syndrome consisting of myxomas (including cardiac myxomas), mucocutaneous pigmentation, and endocrine abnormalities.

Histopathology. Oral myxomas are not encapsulated and may exhibit infiltration into surrounding soft tissue. Dispersed stellate and spindle-shaped fibroblasts are found in a loose myxoid stroma. Soft tissue myxomas may be confused with other myxoid lesions, such as nerve sheath myxoma and oral focal mucinosis (Table 7-1).

Nerve sheath myxoma arises from the endoneurium of a peripheral nerve. This lesion typically exhibits lobulated mucoid tissue containing stellate and spindle-shaped cells. Condensed connective tissue, representing perineurium, surrounds the lesion. With

TABLE 7-1 **Mucosal Myxoid Lesions: Microscopic Differentiation**

	Mast cells	Reticulin	Pattern	Periphery
Soft tissue myxoma	No	Yes	Diffuse, uniform	Blending, infiltration
Nerve sheath myxoma	Yes	Yes	Lobular	Condensed fibrous tissue
Focal mucinosis	No	No	Uniform	Circumscribed

special stains, a fine reticulin network is seen throughout. Mast cells are characteristically present in this lesion.

Oral focal mucinosis represents the mucosal counterpart of cutaneous focal mucinosis. The lesion appears as a well-circumscribed area of myxomatous connective tissue in the submucosa. It contains no mast cells and no reticulin network except that which surrounds supporting blood vessels.

Treatment. The treatment of choice for oral soft tissue myxoma, as well as other myxoid lesions, is surgical excision. Recurrence is not uncommon for myxomas but is unexpected for nerve sheath myxoma and focal mucinosis. All are benign processes and require conservative therapy only.

Nasopharyngeal Angiofibroma

Clinical Features. Nasopharyngeal angiofibroma is also known as *juvenile nasopharyngeal angiofibroma* because of its almost exclusive occurrence in the second decade of life. An uncommon to rare neoplasm that nearly always affects boys, this lesion characteristically produces a mass in the nasopharynx that arises along the posterolateral wall of the nasal roof. Over time it leads to obstruction or epistaxis that may, on occasion, be severe. Rarely this lesion may present intraorally, causing palatal expansion or inferior displacement of the soft palate, which appears blue because of the intense vascularity of the lesion. It can generally be described as benign and slow growing but unencapsulated and locally invasive. On occasion it may exhibit aggressive clinical behavior in which there is direct extension into the bones of the midface and the skull base. The symptom triad includes recurrent epistaxis, nasal obstruction, and mass effect within the nasopharynx.

Histopathology. Microscopically, nasopharyngeal angiofibroma has the appearance of a mature, well-collagenized lesion containing cleftlike vascular channels. The evenly spaced fibroblasts have a uniform, benign appearance with plump nuclei. The vascular channels vary in size and are lined by endothelium that may occasionally be rimmed by smooth muscle cells.

Treatment. Although numerous forms of treatment, such as radiation, exogenous hormone administration, sclerosant therapy, and embolization, have been used for nasopharyngeal angiofibroma, surgery remains the preferred form of therapy. Recurrences are common (up to 50% of cases) and are due to incomplete excision, the invasive nature of the lesion, and the surgically difficult anatomic location.

Giant Cell Angiofibroma

Clinical Features. Giant cell angiofibroma is a rare soft tissue tumor that was first described in the orbit. Since then, there have been several case reports describing this tumor in a number of extraorbital sites, including the submandibular region, parascapular area, and posterior mediastinum. The condition is also reported to occur in the oral cavity. The condition presents as a slowly growing nodule or mass with normal overlying mucosa. It behaves in a benign fashion with only rare local recurrences and no tendency to metastasize.

Histopathology. Microscopically, giant cell angiofibroma shows noninfiltrative growth of patternless round to spindle cells in a stroma that is composed of collagen fibers or occasionally myxoid material with irregular pseudovascular spaces. The giant cells are interspersed among the spindle cells and partially line the walls of the pseudovascular spaces. These cells are multinucleated floret-type giant cells with nuclei located at the periphery of the cell. Immunohistochemically, the spindle and giant cells are positive for both vimentin and CD34.

Treatment. The condition is benign, and local excision is curative.

Nodular Fasciitis

Clinical Features. Nodular fasciitis, also known as *pseudosarcomatous fasciitis,* is a well-recognized entity representing a fibrous connective tissue growth. A closely related lesion known as *proliferative myositis* occurs in muscle. The cause of this proliferation is unknown. Trauma is believed to be important in many cases because of the location of lesions over bony prominences, such as the angle of the mandible and the zygoma. Although traditionally considered a reactive condition, recent molecular evidence suggests that the cells in nodular fasciitis are clonal, thus supporting the concept that the lesion is a benign neoplasm. It typically presents as a firm mass in the dermis or the submucosa and exhibits such rapid growth clinically that malignancy may be suspected. Pain or tenderness often accompanies the process. There is no gender predilection, and young adults and adults are usually affected. The trunk and extremities are the areas most commonly involved, with about 10% of cases appearing in the head and neck, usually in the skin of the face and the parotid sheath. All of these lesions are benign and if left untreated ultimately regress on their own. Local recurrence occurs in only 2% of cases.

Histopathology. A nodular growth contains plump fibroblasts with vesicular nuclei in a haphazard to storiform arrangement (Figure 7-12). Myxoid areas are often found. Multinucleated giant cells are occasionally present and may originate from adjacent muscle or from fusion of macrophages. Mitotic figures may be frequent but are morphologically normal in appearance. Inflammatory cells and extravasated red blood cells are also microscopic features of nodular fasciitis.

Proliferative myositis, an analogous lesion occurring within muscle, is a reactive lesion that usually occurs in the trunk and rarely in the head and the neck (sternocleidomastoid muscle). It parallels the clinical course of nodular fasciitis, although it appears in an older age-group.

Differential Diagnosis. Diagnostic problems relative to nodular fasciitis occur because many of its microscopic features are shared by other fibrous proliferations, such as fibromatosis, fibrous histiocytoma, and fibrosarcoma (Table 7-2). Fibromatosis is more infiltrative than nodular fasciitis and may exhibit a fascicular growth pattern. It also produces more collagen, is generally less cellular, and has fewer mitotic figures. Fibrous histiocytoma is more cellular with a storiform pattern,

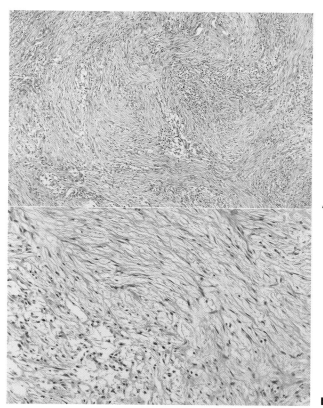

Figure 7-12 **Nodular fasciitis. A** and **B,** Lobular or nodular pattern with foci of lymphocytes.

TABLE 7-2 **Nodular Fasciitis, Fibrous Histiocytoma, Fibromatosis**

	Nodular Fasciitis	**Fibrous Histiocytoma**	**Fibromatosis**
Tumor type	Reactive	Benign	Benign, aggressive
Age	Young adults, adults	Adults	Children, young adults
Symptoms	Often	Infrequently	Infrequently
Sites	Trunk, extremities Head and neck 10%	Skin, mucosa	Shoulder, trunk Head and neck 10%
Growth rate	Rapid	Slow	Moderate
Periphery	Nodular	Circumscribed	Infiltrative
Recurrence	Rarely	Uncommon	Common
Treatment	Excision	Excision	Aggressive surgery

and it may not be as well circumscribed as nodular fasciitis. Fibrosarcoma is infiltrative and exhibits a herringbone pattern. Also, nuclei are pleomorphic and hyperchromatic, and mitoses are more abundant and atypical. By immunohistochemistry, the cells of nodular fasciitis express smooth muscle actin but not desmin. Some have described variable staining with the CD68 marker KP1.

Treatment. Conservative surgical excision is the treatment of choice for nodular fasciitis. Recurrences are rarely encountered.

Myofibroblastic Tumors

Clinical Features. Myofibromatosis and myofibromas represent proliferations of myofibroblasts. Myofibromatosis is multifocal and occurs in infants, and myofibroma is solitary and occurs over a wide age range. These lesions can appear in a variety of sites in the body but have a predilection for the head and neck—in particular, the oral cavity. They can occur in soft tissues or in bone and present as slowly growing, circumscribed masses.

Histopathology. Tumors show pushing, well-demarcated borders. Paucicellular lobules with hyalinized or collagenous stroma alternate with cellular zones, giving a hemangiopericytoma-like appearance The tumor cells are generally uniform, showing tapered nuclei, and express smooth muscle actin. They are negative for desmin, CD34, and S-100 but positive for smooth muscle actin (Figure 7-13). The lack of expression of desmin helps differentiate this tumor from leiomyoma and leiomyosarcoma, which are rare in the oral cavity.

Treatment. Myofibromas are benign, and local excision is generally curative. However, local recurrences are occasionally seen. Multiple lesions appearing in myofibromatosis likely do not represent recurrence or metastasis but multifocal disease.

Fibromatosis

Fibromatosis comprises a group of locally aggressive neoplasms that all show infiltrative, destructive, and recurrent growth but no tendency to metastasize. They are classified as superficial (palmar, plantar) or deep (desmoid). Superficial fibromatoses do not occur in the oral cavity. Deep fibromatoses are clinically diverse, deep-seated, fibrous proliferations. There are three

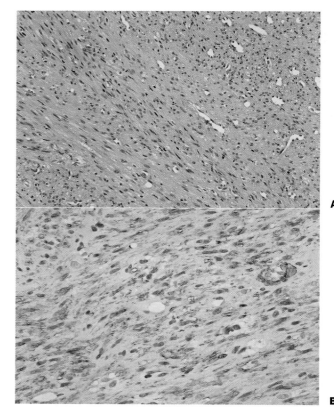

Figure 7-13   A, Myofibroma composed of fascicles of spindle cells. **B,** Positive *(brown)* immunohistochemical stain for smooth muscle actin; stain for desmin was negative.

types: sporadic, familial adenomatous polyposis (FAP) associated, and multicentric (familial). They can be further classified anatomically as extraabdominal (60% of cases), abdominal wall (25% of cases), or intraabdominal (15% of cases). Only extraabdominal desmoid fibromatoses occur in the head and neck. Although traditionally thought to be reactive lesions, cytogenetic and X-inactivation studies based on lyonization have shown clonality; thus fibromatoses are thought to be benign neoplasms.

Clinical Features. All extraabdominal desmoids are locally infiltrative lesions that have significant recurrence potential. Lesions typically present as firm asymptomatic masses. They are typically seen in children and young adults, with females affected twice as often as males. The most common site is the shoulder area and trunk, with about 10% of cases appearing in the soft tissues of the head and neck. The mandible and contiguous soft tissues are most often involved intraorally. The lesions are slower growing than those of nodular fasciitis and less likely to be symptomatic.

Histopathology. Fibromatosis is a nonencapsulated infiltrative lesion with a fascicular growth pattern (Figure 7-14). The lesion is composed of highly differentiated connective tissue containing uniform, compact fibroblasts, often surrounded by abundant collagen. Nuclei are not atypical, and mitotic figures are infrequent. When muscle invasion occurs, giant cells representing degenerate muscle cells may be seen. Slitlike vascular spaces are usually seen as well. Overall, the bland microscopic appearance of this lesion belies its locally aggressive behavior. By immunohistochemistry, actin, desmin, and S-100 are negative, although some cases may show patchy expression.

Treatment. Recurrence rates in the range of 20% to 60% have been reported for fibromatoses. Because of this and because of the locally destructive nature of fibromatosis, an aggressive surgical approach is recommended. There is no metastatic potential.

Fibrosarcoma

At one time, fibrosarcoma was the most common soft tissue sarcoma. With the introduction of electron microscopy and immunohistochemistry, it became evident that many previously diagnosed fibrosarcomas were other spindle cell malignancies. Today, fibrosarcoma is defined as a malignant spindle cell tumor showing a herringbone or interlacing fascicular pattern and no expression of other connective tissue cell markers.

Clinical Features. Fibrosarcoma is a rare soft tissue and bony malignancy of the head and neck. When it occurs in bone, the lesion may theoretically arise from periosteum, endosteum, or periodontal ligament (Figure 7-15).

A tumor results from proliferation of malignant mesenchymal cells at the site of origin. Secondary ulceration may be seen as the lesion enlarges. Young adults are most commonly affected. This is an infiltrative neoplasm that is more of a locally destructive problem than a metastatic problem.

Histopathology. Microscopically, fibrosarcoma exhibits malignant-appearing fibroblasts, typically in a herringbone or interlacing fascicular pattern (Figure 7-16). Collagen may be sparse, and mitotic figures frequent. The degree of cell differentiation from one tumor to another may be quite variable. The periphery of this lesion is ill defined because the neoplasm freely invades surrounding tissue. Fibrosarcoma is essentially a diagnosis of exclusion, and by definition there should be no expression of actin, S-100, epithelial membrane antigen, keratin, or desmin.

Treatment. Wide surgical excision is generally advocated for fibrosarcoma because of the difficulty in controlling local growth. Although recurrence is not uncommon, metastasis is infrequent. Bone lesions are more likely to metastasize via the bloodstream than are soft

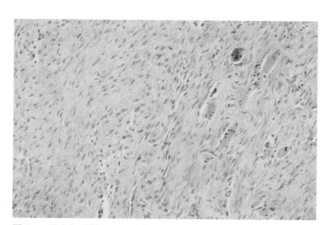

Figure 7-14 **Fibromatosis** appearing as deceptively bland fibroblastic proliferation. Note residual skeletal muscle (*right*) surrounded by invasive tumor.

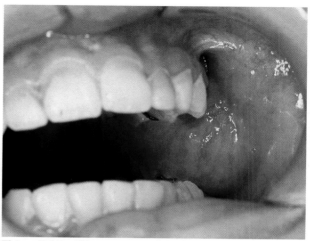

Figure 7-15 **Fibrosarcoma** of the buccal mucosa.

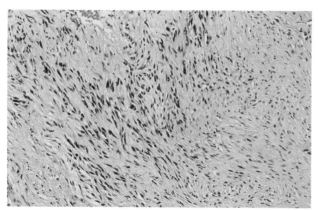

Figure 7-16 **Fibrosarcoma** composed of atypical spindle cells.

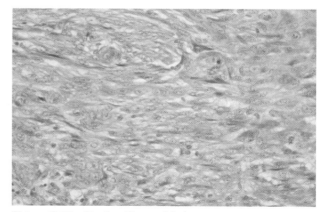

Figure 7-17 **Benign fibrous histiocytoma** composed of plump fibroblasts.

tissue lesions. The overall 5-year survival rate ranges between 30% and 50%. Generally, patients with soft tissue lesions fare better than patients with primary lesions of bone. Also, well-differentiated lesions have a better prognosis than do those with poorly differentiated features.

FIBROHISTIOCYTIC TUMORS

The original concept that some tumors show fibrohistiocytic differentiation was based on the notion that there exists a dual population of fibroblasts and histiocytes (macrophages) that in tissue culture show ameboid growth and phagocytic properties. It is now known that this concept is incorrect and that the tumors in this category show no histiocyte (macrophage) differentiation. Immunohistochemical evidence now favors a fibroblast cell of origin. However, the term *fibrous histiocytoma* has persisted to describe a group of likely unrelated benign and malignant tumors that share many histologic similarities.

Benign Fibrous Histiocytoma

Clinical Features. Benign fibrous histiocytomas are fibroblastic neoplasms that uncommonly or rarely occur in oral soft tissues, skin, or bone. They are lesions of adults, typically noted in the fifth decade, and present as painless masses that may be ulcerated. Intrabony lesions present as radiolucencies, often with ill-defined margins.

Histopathology. This tumor is fairly well demarcated and often circumscribed at the periphery. There is a

storiform (cartwheel or matlike) growth pattern of spindle cells (fibroblasts) with plump or vesicular nuclei admixed with some inflammatory cells (Figure 7-17). Tumor giant cells may be seen. There is no cellular atypia, and mitotic figures are infrequent and normal. Immunohistochemical stains are of little diagnostic value. Fibrous histiocytomas may show some positive staining for smooth muscle actin and/or CD34, but a consistent pattern has not been demonstrated.

Treatment. Surgical excision is the treatment of choice for benign fibrous histiocytoma. Lesions usually do not recur.

Malignant Fibrous Histiocytoma

Malignant fibrous histiocytoma is a controversial soft tissue malignancy whose pathogenesis continues to be redefined. It remains the most often used term for soft tissue sarcomas of late adult life. Five variants showing differing clinical and histologic features have been recognized: pleomorphic-storiform, myxoid (myxofibrosarcoma), giant cell, inflammatory, and angiomatoid. Recently it has been suggested that the prototypic form, pleomorphic-storiform MFH type, represents a heterogeneous group of malignancies. This would include pleomorphic variants of skeletal muscle (rhabdomyosarcoma), smooth muscle (leiomyosarcoma), and adipose (liposarcoma). Therefore MFH has become a diagnosis of exclusion. The angiomatoid type shows distinct clinical and histologic features and probably represents an entity that is distinct from other tumors in this category.

Clinical Features. MFH is an infrequently reported lesion in the head and neck, although it has been one of the most commonly made diagnoses of soft tissue sarcomas in the rest of the body—in par-ticular, the lower leg. It may also occur in bone, where it follows a more aggressive course than in soft tissue. Biologically, it has significant recurrence and metastatic potential that is dependent, in part, on clinical factors such as the anatomic site, depth of location, and size.

Overall, MFH occurs in late adult life and is rare in children. Men are affected more often than women. The extremities and retroperitoneum are favored sites. Intraoral soft tissue lesions appear to have no site predilection. Although only a small number have been reported, almost all regions have been affected. MFH has also been reported in the mandible and maxilla, resulting in radiolucencies with poorly defined margins.

Histopathology. Basic to all MFH is the proliferation of pleomorphic spindle cells showing fibroblastic morphology. Abnormal and frequent mitotic figures, necrosis, and extensive cellular atypia may be seen. In some lesions a storiform pattern may dominate the microscopic picture; in others, myxoid zones, giant cells, acute inflammatory cells, xanthoma cells, or blood vessels may be prominent. The recognition of these different microscopic features has led to the traditional subclassification into pleomorphic-storiform, myxoid (myxofibrosarcoma), giant cell, inflammatory, and angiomatoid types.

Treatment. Wide surgical excision is the usual treatment. Radiation or chemotherapy offers limited additional benefit. The 5-year survival rate ranges from 20% to 60%. Patients with oral lesions generally fare somewhat worse than others. Recurrence and metastatic rates are about 40%.

VASCULAR LESIONS

Reactive Lesions and Congenital Lesions

Lymphangioma

Etiology. Regarded as a congenital lesion, lymphangioma usually appears within the first 2 decades of life. Involution over time, in contrast to the situation with congenital hemangiomas, does not usually occur.

Clinical Features. Lymphangiomas present as painless, nodular, vesicle-like swellings when superficial or as a submucosal mass when located deeper. The color ranges from lighter than the surrounding tissue to red-blue when capillaries are part of the congenital malformation (Figures 7-18 and 7-19). On palpation the lesions may produce a crepitant sound as lymphatic fluid is pushed from one area to another.

The tongue is the most common intraoral site, and the lesions may be responsible for macroglossia when diffusely distributed throughout the submucosa (Box 7-5). Lymphangioma of the lip may cause a macrocheilia. Lymphangioma of the neck, known as *cystic hygroma, hygroma colli,* or *cavernous lymphangioma,* is a diffuse soft tissue swelling that may be life threatening because it involves vital structures of the neck. Respiratory distress, intralesional hemorrhage, and disfigurement are all potential sequelae to cystic hygroma.

Histopathology. Endothelium-lined lymphatic channels are diffusely distributed in the submucosa (Figure 7-

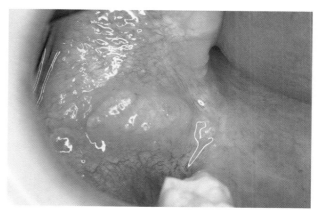

Figure 7-18 **Lymphangioma** of the buccal mucosa.

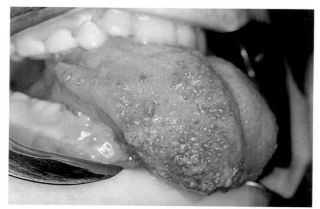

Figure 7-19 **Combined lymphangioma and hemangioma** of the tongue.

20). The channels contain eosinophilic lymph that occasionally includes red blood cells, especially in mixed lymphatic and capillary proliferations. There is no capsule. A characteristic feature is the location of lymphatic channels directly adjacent to overlying epithelium, without any apparent intervening connective tissue.

Treatment. Lymphangiomas are usually surgically removed, but because of their lack of encapsulation, recurrences are common. Large lymphangiomas, such as cystic hygromas, may require staged surgical procedures to gain control of the lesion.

NEOPLASMS

Hemangiopericytoma

Hemangiopericytoma is a rare neoplasm that was originally described as a vascular tumor derived from the pericyte. This cell is believed to be a modified smooth muscle cell and is normally found surrounding capillaries and venules, between the basement membrane and endothelium. The cell probably has a contractile property and serves as an endothelial reserve cell. Recent immunohistochemical evidence now suggests that conceptually this tumor is not derived from the pericyte because it does not express actin or myofibroblastic markers. It is likely that the neoplastic cell is an undifferentiated or fibroblastic cell. Recently it has been suggested that many tumors previously diagnosed histologically as hemangiopericytoma represent other soft tissue tumors that share similar features. For example, there is considerable histologic overlap between myofibroma, solitary fibrous tumor, synovial sarcoma, and mesenchymal chondrosarcoma, and it is conceivable that many hemangiopericytomas represent one of these entities. Increasingly, the diagnosis of hemangiopericytoma is a diagnosis of exclusion.

This neoplasm appears as a mass in any location of the body across a wide age spectrum. No distinguishing clinical signs would suggest a diagnosis of hemangiopericytoma.

Microscopically, the neoplasm is characterized by a proliferation of well-differentiated, oval to spindle-shaped mesenchymal cells separated by small, slitlike vascular channels. The vessels are thin walled and may exhibit "staghorn" profiles.

The biologic behavior of hemangiopericytoma is unpredictable, exhibiting on some occasions a benign course and on other occasions an aggressive, metastatic course. Unfortunately, there are no reliable histologic criteria that can be used to predict the clinical course, although necrosis, numerous mitotic figures, a high proliferation marker (Ki67 or proliferating cell nuclear antigen [PCNA]) labeling index, and hypercellularity may be suggestive of a more aggressive lesion. The treatment of choice is wide surgical excision. Recurrence and metastases are not uncommon.

Angiosarcoma

Angiosarcoma is a rare neoplasm of endothelial cell origin. A distinctive clinical pathologic variant of angiosarcoma is Kaposi's sarcoma.

The scalp is the usual location for angiosarcomas, although occasional lesions have been reported in the maxillary sinus and oral cavity. The lesion consists of an unencapsulated proliferation of anaplastic endothelial cells enclosing irregular luminal spaces.

Box 7-5   Macroglossia

Congenital hyperplasia/hypertrophy
Tumor: lymphangioma, vascular malformation, neurofibroma, granular cell tumors, salivary gland tumors
Endocrine abnormality: acromegaly, cretinism
Infections obstructing lymphatics
Beckwith-Wiedemann syndrome: macroglossia, exomphalos, gigantism
Amyloidosis
Angioedema

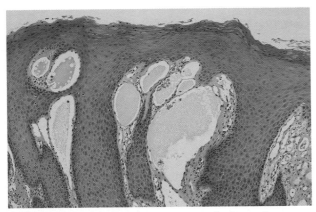

Figure 7-20   Lymphangioma composed of prominent lymphatic vessels. The vessels are characteristically apposed to the epithelium.

It has an aggressive clinical course and a poor prognosis.

NEURAL LESIONS

REACTIVE LESIONS

Traumatic Neuroma

Etiology. Traumatic neuromas are caused by injury to a peripheral nerve. In the oral cavity the injury may be in the form of trauma from a surgical procedure such as a tooth extraction, from a local anesthetic injection, or from an accident. Transection of a sensory nerve can result in inflammation and scarring in the area of injury. As the proximal nerve segment proliferates in an attempt to regenerate into the distal segment, it becomes entangled and trapped in the developing scar, resulting in a composite mass of fibrous tissue, Schwann cells, and axons.

Clinical Features. About half the patients with oral traumatic neuromas have associated pain. Pain ranges from occasional tenderness to constant, severe pain. Radiating facial pain may occasionally be caused by a traumatic neuroma (Figure 7-21). Injection of local anesthesia into the area of tumescence relieves the pain.

The lesions occur in a wide age range, although most are seen in adults. The mental foramen is the most common location, followed by extraction sites in the anterior maxilla and the posterior mandible. The lower lip, tongue, buccal mucosa, and palate are also relatively common soft tissue locations.

Histopathology. Microscopically, bundles of nerves in a haphazard or tortuous arrangement are found admixed with dense collagenous fibrous tissue (Figure 7-22). A chronic inflammatory cell infiltrate may be seen in a minority of cases, particularly those that are symptomatic.

Treatment. Even though surgical transection of a peripheral nerve may have caused the lesion, surgical excision is the treatment of choice. Recurrence is infrequent.

NEOPLASMS

Granular Cell Tumors

Etiology. *Granular cell tumor,* formerly known as *granular cell myoblastoma,* is an uncommon benign tumor of

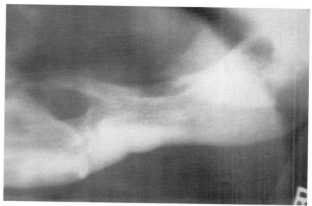

Figure 7-21   **Traumatic neuroma** presenting as a painful radiolucency at the mental foramen in an edentulous mandible (ramus to the right).

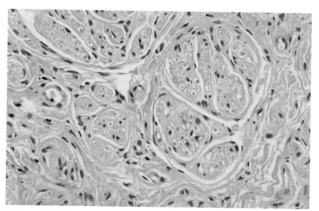

Figure 7-22   **Traumatic neuroma** composed of fibrous tissue and nerve bundles.

unknown cause. The unique granular cells that make up the lesion are believed to be of neural (Schwann cell) origin, predominantly on the basis of immunohistochemical studies. Origins from skeletal muscle, macrophages, undifferentiated mesenchymal cells, and pericytes have also been suggested but are unproven.

A related lesion known as *congenital gingival granular cell tumor* (congenital epulis) is composed of cells that are light microscopically identical to those of granular cell tumors. Slight differences have been noted by ultrastructural and immunohistochemical analysis and suggest that congenital gingival tumors have a different histogenesis from granular cell tumors.

Box 7-6 Oral Granular Cell Tumor

CLINICAL FEATURES

Benign tumor of neural sheath origin
Any age; females slightly more than males
Any site; usually tongue
Asymptomatic submucosal mass (1 to 2 cm)
 Same or lighter than mucosal color
 Intact overlying epithelium

HISTOPATHOLOGY

Large, uniform cells with granular cytoplasm
Overlying pseudoepitheliomatous hyperplasia
Cells positive for neural-associated proteins (e.g., S-100)
and negative for muscle proteins (actin)

TREATMENT

Excision; no recurrence

Box 7-7 Congenital Granular Cell Tumor

CLINICAL FEATURES

Benign tumor of disputed origin
Infants only
Gingiva only
Usually pedunculated, nonulcerated mass

HISTOPATHOLOGY

Large, uniform cells with granular cytoplasm
No overlying pseudoepitheliomatous hyperplasia
Cells negative for S-100 and actin

TREATMENT

Excision; no recurrence

Clinical Features. Granular cell tumors appear in a range of patients from children to the elderly, with the mean appearance usually in middle adult life. Some studies have shown a predilection for females; others have shown near-equal gender distribution (Box 7-6). In the head and neck, the tongue is by far the most common location for granular cell tumors (Figure 7-23). However, any oral location may be affected (Figure 7-24).

Presentation is typically as an uninflamed asymptomatic mass less than 2 cm in diameter. It often has a yellowish surface coloration. The overlying epithelium is intact. Multiple lesions have occasionally been described.

Congenital gingival granular cell tumors appear on the gingiva (usually anterior) of newborns (Box 7-7). This lesion presents as an uninflamed, pedunculated, or broad-based mass. The maxillary gingiva is more often involved than the mandibular gingiva, and girls are affected more often than boys. The lesion does not recur, and spontaneous regressions have been reported.

Histopathology. The clinical tumescence of granular cell tumors is due to the presence of unencapsulated sheets of large polygonal cells with pale granular or grainy cytoplasm (Figures 7-25 to 7-27). The nuclei are small, compact, and morphologically benign. Mitotic figures are rare. Pseudoepitheliomatous hyperplasia of the overlying oral epithelium is seen in about half the cases.

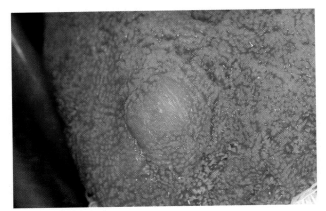

Figure 7-23 **Granular cell tumor** of the tongue.

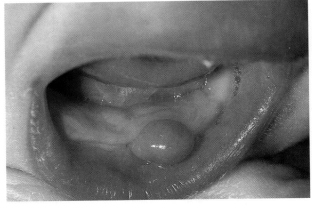

Figure 7-24 **Congenital gingival granular cell tumor.**

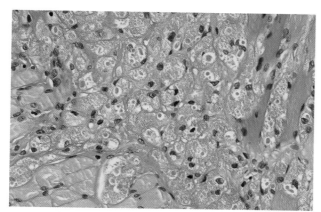

Figure 7-25 **Granular cell tumor.** Note uniform cells with granular cytoplasm found adjacent to skeletal muscle.

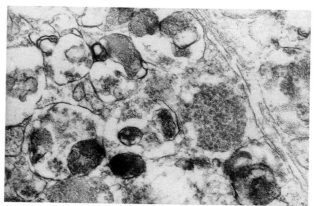

Figure 7-27 **Granular cell tumor.** Electron micrograph showing intracytoplasmic autophagic organelles.

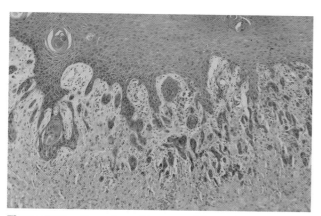

Figure 7-26 **Granular cell tumor** with overlying pseudoepitheliomatous hyperplasia.

This may be such a prominent feature that subjacent granular cells are overlooked, resulting in overdiagnosis of squamous cell carcinoma. The pseudoepitheliomatous hyperplasia overlying granular cell tumor is a completely benign process.

Ultrastructurally, granular cells of both the granular cell tumor and its congenital gingival counterpart contain autophagic vacuoles. One of the consistent differences noted has been the absence of angulate bodies in the gingival lesion. Also, in some gingival lesions, the presence of microfilaments with fusiform dense bodies, pinocytotic vesicles, and basement membrane has been noted.

Immunohistochemically, both lesions express carcinoembryonic antigens and human leukocyte antigens (HLA-DR). Granular cell tumors express neural-associated antigens, S-100 protein, CD57, and type IV collagen. Both lesions are negative for α_1-antichymotrypsin and muscle actin.

Differential Diagnosis. Clinically, granular cell tumors might be confused with other connective tissue lesions. Neurofibroma, schwannoma, and palisaded encapsulated neuroma would be prime considerations for tongue lesions. Salivary gland tumors, lipoma, and other benign mesenchymal neoplasms may present intraorally as asymptomatic lumps similar to granular cell tumor. Focal fibrous hyperplasia (traumatic fibroma) is a common reactive lesion that should be included in a differential diagnosis. A biopsy is the only way to achieve a definitive diagnosis.

Congenital gingival granular cell tumor is clinically distinctive because of the age of the patient and the location in which the mass is seen. Other submucosal masses that occur in the gingiva of infants, such as gingival cyst and neuroectodermal tumor of infancy, are more deeply seated and broad based. Rhabdomyosarcoma tends to grow more rapidly and is darker in color.

Treatment. Granular cell tumors are surgically excised and generally do not recur.

Schwannoma

Etiology. Schwannoma, or *neurilemmoma*, is a benign neoplasm that is derived from a proliferation of Schwann cells of the neurilemma, or nerve sheath. As the lesion

	Schwannoma	Neurofibroma	Mucosal Neuroma	PEN
Cell of origin	Schwann cell	Schwann cell and perineural fibroblast	Nerve tissue, hamartoma	Schwann cell
Age	Any	Any	Children, young adults	Adults
Site	Any, especially tongue	Any, especially tongue, buccal mucosa	Tongue, lip, buccal mucosa	Palate, lip
Number	Solitary	Solitary to multiple	Multiple	Solitary
Bone lesions	Occasionally	Frequently	No	No
Syndrome association	None	Neurofibromatosis	MEN III	None
Malignant potential	No	Yes, with syndrome	No	No

TABLE 7-3 **Neural Tumors: Comparative Features**

PEN, Palisaded encapsulated neuroma; *MEN III*, multiple endocrine neoplasia syndrome type III.

grows, the nerve is pushed aside and does not become enmeshed within the tumor.

Clinical Features. This lesion is an encapsulated submucosal mass that presents typically as an asymptomatic lump in patients of any age (Table 7-3). The tongue is the favored location, although lesions have been described throughout the mouth. Bony lesions produce a well-defined radiolucent pattern with a corticated periphery and may also cause pain or paresthesia. The lesion is usually slow growing but may undergo a sudden increase in size, which is thought in some cases to be due to intralesional hemorrhage. The fact that solitary schwannomas are usually not seen in neurofibromatosis is of clinical significance.

Histopathology. In this encapsulated tumor, spindle cells assume two different patterns (Figure 7-28). In one pattern, so-called Antoni A areas consist of spindle cells organized in palisaded whorls and waves. These cells often surround an acellular eosinophilic zone (Verocay body) representing reduplicated basement membrane. The other pattern is the so-called Antoni B tissue, consisting of spindle cells haphazardly distributed in a delicate fibrillar microcystic matrix. By immunohistochemistry this tumor strongly expresses S-100 protein. Stains for actin and desmin are negative.

A microscopic variant known as *ancient schwannoma* has been described to designate degenerative changes in a long-standing schwannoma. In this variant, fibrosis, inflammatory cells, and hemorrhage may be seen.

Treatment. Schwannomas are surgically excised, and recurrence is unlikely. The prognosis is excellent.

Neurofibroma

Etiology. Neurofibromas may appear as solitary lesions or as multiple lesions as part of the syndrome *neurofibromatosis (von Recklinghausen's disease of skin)*. The

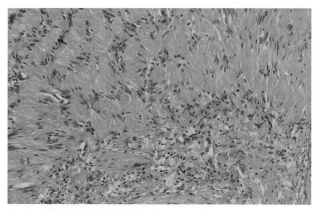

Figure 7-28 **Schwannoma** showing characteristic pattern of palisaded schwannoma cells around eosinophilic bodies.

cause of solitary neurofibroma is unknown. Neurofibromatosis, on the other hand, is inherited as an autosomal-dominant trait. It has variable expressivity and often (50% of cases) appears after spontaneous mutation. Two subsets have recently been defined: one associated with the NF1 gene and the other with the NF2 gene.

Clinical Features. Solitary neurofibroma presents at any age as an uninflamed asymptomatic, submucosal mass. The tongue, buccal mucosa, and vestibule are the oral regions most commonly affected (Figures 7-29 and 7-30).

Oral lesions are typically associated with neurofibromatosis 1. This condition includes multiple neurofibromas, cutaneous café-au-lait macules, bone abnormalities, central nervous system changes, and other stigmata. The neurofibromas range clinically from discrete, superficial nodules to deep, diffuse masses. Lesions may be so numerous and prominent that they become cosmetically significant. Intraoral

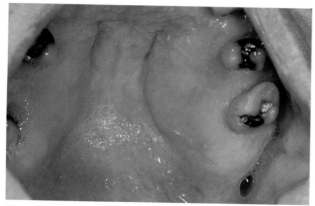

Figure 7-29 Neurofibroma of the left palate.

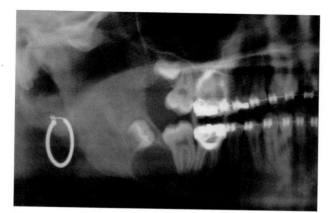

Figure 7-30 Intramandibular neurofibroma.

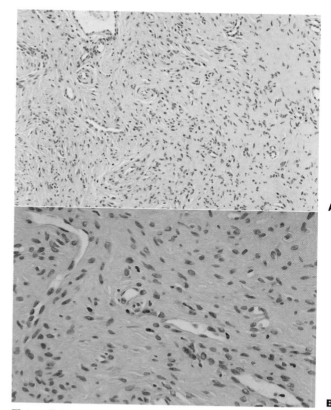

A

B

Figure 7-31 Neurofibroma. **A** and **B,** Haphazardly arranged spindle (Schwann) cells.

neurofibromas may be seen in as many as 25% of patients with neurofibromatosis. When other oral stigmata such as enlarged fungiform papillae and bone abnormalities are included, oral manifestations may be seen in as many as 70% of neurofibromatosis patients. Malignant degeneration of neurofibromas into neurogenic sarcoma is seen in 5% to 15% of patients with this syndrome.

The presence of six or more café-au-lait macules greater than 1.5 cm in diameter is generally regarded as being suggestive of neurofibromatosis. Other important diagnostic signs of the syndrome are axillary freckling (Crowe's sign) and iris freckling (Lisch spots).

Bone changes may be seen in half or more of patients with neurofibromatosis. The changes may be in the form of cortical erosion from adjacent soft tissue tumors or medullary resorption from intraosseous

lesions. In the mandible, lesions most commonly arise from the mandibular nerve and may result in pain or paresthesia. In such cases of mandibular involvement, an accompanying radiographic sign may be the formation of a flaring of the inferior alveolar foramen, the so-called blunderbuss foramen.

Histopathology. Solitary and multiple neurofibromas have the same microscopic features (Figure 7-31). They contain spindle-shaped cells, with fusiform or wavy nuclei found in a delicate connective tissue matrix; this matrix may be notably myxoid in character. These lesions may be well circumscribed or may blend into surrounding connective tissue. Mast cells are characteristically scattered throughout the lesion. A histologic subtype known as *plexiform neurofibroma* is regarded as being highly characteristic of neurofibromatosis. In this variety, extensive interlacing masses of nerve tissue are supported by a collagen matrix. Small axons may be seen among the proliferating Schwann cells and perineural cells. Demonstration of S-100 and neurofilament expression by immuno-

TABLE 7-4   Soft Tissue Tumors: Cytogenetic Abnormalities

Tumor Type	Cytogenetic Change	Gene Abnormality
Alveolar rhabdomyosarcoma	t(2;13), t(1;13)	PAX3-FKHR PAX7-FKHR
Synovial sarcoma	t(X;18)	SSX1-SYT SSX2-SYT
Lipoma	Translocations 12q13-15, rearranged 13q,6p	
Myxoid liposarcoma	t(12;16)	*CHOP* gene
Mucosal neuroma (MEN III)	Chromosome 10 mutation	*RET* gene

MEN III, Multiple endocrine neoplasia syndrome type III.

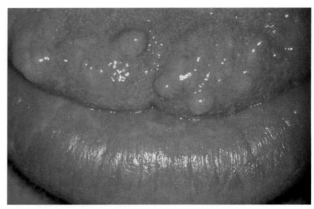

Figure 7-32   Mucosal neuromas of MEN III.

histochemistry are most useful in confirming the diagnosis.

Differential Diagnosis. A solitary nodular neurofibroma should be considered in a clinical differential diagnosis with other submucosal masses of connective tissue origin, such as traumatic fibroma, granular cell tumor, and lipoma. A diffuse neurofibroma resulting in macroglossia may require differentiation from lymphangioma and possibly amyloidosis.

Treatment. Solitary neurofibromas are treated by surgical excision and have little chance of recurrence. Multiple lesions of neurofibromatosis may be treated in the same way but may be so numerous that excision becomes impractical. The prognosis for a patient who has had neurosarcomatous change of a preexisting lesion is poor.

Mucosal Neuromas of Multiple Endocrine Neoplasia Syndrome Type III

Etiology. Multiple endocrine neoplasia syndrome type III (MEN III), of which mucosal neuromas are a prominent part, is inherited as an autosomal-dominant trait (Table 7-4). The clinical stigmata of this syndrome are related to a defect in neuroectodermal tissue. MEN III is caused by a mutation in the *RET* oncogene resulting in a single amino acid substitution that affects a critical region of the tyrosine kinase catalytic core. Although a mutation of the *RET* gene is also responsible for the MEN II syndrome, the mutations are different.

Clinical Features. MEN III consists of medullary carcinoma of the thyroid, pheochromocytoma of the adrenal, and mucosal neuromas (Figure 7-32).

Café-au-lait macules and neurofibromas of the skin may also be seen in this condition. MEN I and MEN II are related to MEN III in that patients with types I and II syndromes have neoplasms of various endocrine organs, but they do not have the oral manifestations of mucosal neuromas.

The mucosal neuromas of MEN III usually appear early in life as small, discrete nodules on the conjunctiva, labia, or larynx, or in the oral cavity. The oral lesions are seen on the tongue, lips, and buccal mucosa.

Histopathology. Mucosal neuromas are composed of serpiginous bands of nerve tissue surrounded by normal connective tissue (Figure 7-33). Axons have been found in the proliferating nerve tissue.

Treatment. Mucosal neuromas are surgically excised and are not expected to recur. The neuromas themselves are relatively trivial, but they are of considerable significance because they may be the first sign in this potentially fatal syndrome. The medullary carcinoma of the thyroid is a progressive malignancy that invades locally and has the ability to metastasize to local lymph nodes and distant organs. The 5-year survival rate of this malignancy is about 50%. Pheochromocytoma is a benign neoplasm that produces catecholamines that may cause significant hypertension and other cardiovascular abnormalities. Early detection of the mucosal neuromas is therefore of utmost importance in establishing the diagnosis or calling attention to other components of the syndrome.

Palisaded Encapsulated Neuroma

Palisaded encapsulated neuroma is another oral tumor of neural origin. It is not associated with neu-

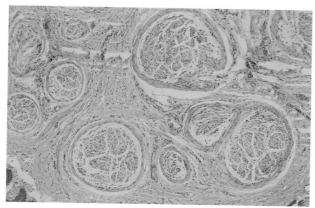

Figure 7-33 Mucosal neuroma of MEN III.

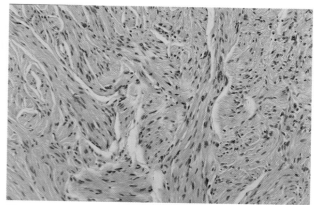

Figure 7-34 Palisaded and encapsulated neuroma showing a lobular pattern of spindle (Schwann) cells.

rofibromatosis or MEN III. It occurs typically in the palate and occasionally the lips. This dome-shaped nodule is encapsulated and exhibits a fascicular microscopic pattern with some suggestion of nuclear palisading (Figure 7-34). The tumor is composed of cells positive for S-100 protein (Schwann cells) and some axons. After surgical removal, recurrence is unexpected.

Malignant Peripheral Nerve Sheath Tumor

Malignant peripheral nerve sheath tumor (MPNST) is a rare malignancy that develops either from a preexisting neurofibroma or de novo. It can also complicate neurofibromatosis. The cell of origin is believed to be the Schwann cell and possibly other nerve sheath cells.

In soft tissues MPNST appears as an expansile mass that is usually asymptomatic. In bone, where it is believed to arise most often from the inferior alveolar nerve, it presents as a dilation of the mandibular canal or as a diffuse lucency. Pain or paresthesia may accompany the lesion in bone; this is also the case for other malignancies within the mandible or maxilla.

Microscopically, MPNST can be seen arising from a neurofibroma or from a nerve trunk. The lesion is composed of abundant spindle cells with variable numbers of abnormal mitotic figures. Streaming and palisading of nuclei are often seen, and nuclear pleomorphism may also be prominent. Microscopic separation of this lesion from fibrosarcoma and leiomyosarcoma may be difficult, making immunohistochemistry an important diagnostic adjunct.

The primary method of treatment is wide surgical excision. However, recurrence is common, and metas-

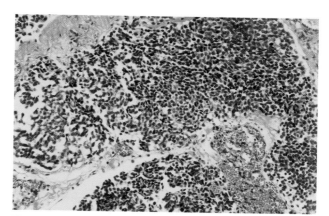

Figure 7-35 Olfactory neuroblastoma; "a round cell tumor."

tases are frequently seen. The prognosis varies from fair to good, depending on clinical circumstances.

Olfactory Neuroblastoma

Olfactory neuroblastoma, also known as *esthesioneuroblastoma*, is a rare malignant lesion that arises from olfactory tissue in the superior portion of the nasal cavity. This lesion, typically occurring in young adults, may result in epistaxis, rhinorrhea, or nasal obstruction, or it may present as polyps in the roof of the nasal cavity. It may also result in a nasopharyngeal mass or an invasive maxillary sinus lesion.

Microscopically, this lesion consists of small, undifferentiated, round cells with little visible cytoplasm (Figure 7-35). Compartmentalization and pseudorosette and rosette formations are often seen.

Immunohistochemistry study for chromogranin or synaptophysin can be used to confirm the light microscopic diagnosis. A microscopic differential diagnosis would include lymphoma, embryonal rhabdomyosarcoma, Ewing's sarcoma, and undifferentiated carcinoma.

Surgery or radiation is used to treat olfactory neuroblastoma. Recurrences are not uncommon, appearing in about half the patients. Metastasis, usually to local nodes or lung, occurs infrequently.

MUSCLE LESIONS

REACTIVE LESIONS

Myositis Ossificans

Myositis ossificans is an uncommon reactive lesion of skeletal muscle. It may appear in the muscles of the head and neck. As the name implies, the condition is an intramuscular inflammatory process in which ossification occurs. The reason for the appearance of bone within the muscle during the reparative process has not been fully explained.

Muscle ossification may be seen in either of two forms: as a progressive systemic disease (myositis ossificans progressiva) of unknown cause or as a focal single-muscle disorder (traumatic myositis ossificans). In the latter form, acute or chronic trauma may be responsible for the muscular change. The masseter and the sternocleidomastoid muscles are most commonly affected within the head and neck region. As the lesion matures, soft tissue radiographs show a delicate feathery opacification. The proliferating osteoblasts have occasionally been confused microscopically with the malignant cells of osteosarcoma. Maturation and organization of the osseous tissue peripheral to the central cellular zone is believed to be an important diagnostic feature of myositis ossificans. The lesion is treated with surgical excision and has little tendency to recur.

NEOPLASMS

Leiomyoma and Leiomyosarcoma

Smooth muscle neoplasms, in general, are relatively common and may arise anywhere in the body (Table 7-5). Leiomyomas most commonly arise in the muscularis layer of the gut and in the body of the uterus (Figure 7-36). Leiomyosarcomas most commonly arise

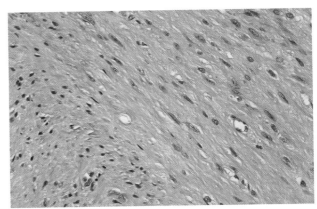

Figure 7-36   **Leiomyoma** composed of bland spindle cells.

	TABLE 7-5 Oral Spindle Cell Neoplasms: Differential Immunoprofile						
	S-100	Neurofilament	Muscle actin	Desmin	CD34	CD99	Factor VIII
Nerve sheath tumors (benign and malignant)	+	+	−	−	+/−	−	−
Myofibroma	−	−	+	−	−	−	−
Leiomyoma/sarcoma	−	−	+	+	−	−	−
Rhabdomyoma/sarcoma	−	−	−	+	−	−	−
Fibrous histiocytoma and MFH*	−	−	+/−	−	+/−	−	−
Solitary fibrous tumor	−	−	−	−	+	+	−
Kaposi's sarcoma	−	−	−	−	+	−	+

MFH, Malignant fibrous histiocytoma.
*Inconsistent staining. Angiomatoid MFH is positive for desmin and muscle actin.

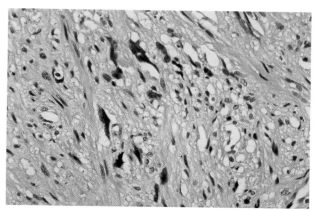

Figure 7-37 **Leiomyosarcoma** composed of spindle cells with atypical nuclei.

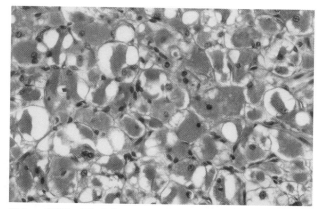

Figure 7-38 **Rhabdomyoma** mimicking adult skeletal muscle cells.

in the retroperitoneum, mesentery, omentum, or sub-cutaneous and deep tissues of the limbs (Figure 7-37).

Both leiomyoma and leiomyosarcoma are rare in the oral cavity. Oral *leiomyomas* present as slow-growing, asymptomatic submucosal masses, usually in the tongue, hard palate, or buccal mucosa. They may be seen at any age and are usually discovered when they are 1 to 2 cm in diameter.

Microscopic diagnosis may occasionally be difficult because the spindle cell proliferation shares many similarities with neurofibroma, schwannoma, fibromatosis, and myofibroma. Special stains that identify collagen may be helpful in distinguishing these lesions. Immunohistochemical demonstration of actin and desmin protein expression can confirm the diagnosis. A microscopic subtype known as *vascular leiomyoma* has numerous thick-walled vessels associated with well-differentiated smooth muscle cells. Leiomyomas are surgically excised, and recurrence is unexpected.

Oral *leiomyosarcomas* have been reported in all age-groups and most intraoral regions. Microscopic diagnosis is a considerable challenge because of similarities to other spindle cell sarcomas. As with the benign neoplasms, immunohistochemistry can be a valuable diagnostic tool to demonstrate the expression of desmin and actin proteins. This malignancy is usually treated with wide surgical excision. Metastasis to lymph nodes or lung is not uncommon.

Rhabdomyoma and Rhabdomyosarcoma

Rhabdomyomas are rare lesions, but they have a predilection for the soft tissues of the head and neck. The oral sites most frequently reported are the floor of the mouth, soft palate, tongue, and buccal mucosa. The mean age of patients is about 50 years, and the age range extends from children to older adults. Presentation is as an asymptomatic, well-defined submucosal mass.

Two microscopic variants are recognized. In the adult type, the neoplastic cells closely mimic their normal counterpart (Figure 7-38); in the fetal type, the neoplastic cells are elongated and less differentiated and exhibit fewer cross-striations. The latter type may be confused with rhabdomyo-sarcoma. Treatment is excision, and recurrence is unlikely.

Rhabdomyosarcomas are subdivided into three principal microscopic forms: embryonal, alveolar, and pleomorphic. The first two types occur in children, and the latter type occurs principally in adults. The embryonal type consists of primitive round cells in which striations are rarely found (Figure 7-39). Two subtypes are recognized: the spindle cell and botryoid types. Both confer an excellent prognosis. The alveolar variant is also composed of round cells but in a compartmentalized pattern. The pleomorphic type, the most well differentiated, contains strap or spindle cells that often exhibit cross-striations (Figure 7-40).

When it occurs in the head and neck, rhabdomyosarcoma is primarily found in children. When it occurs outside the head and neck, it is seen typically in adults. Rhabdomyosarcoma presents as a rapidly growing mass that may cause pain or paresthesia if there is jaw involvement. The most commonly affected oral sites are the tongue and soft palate. The embry-

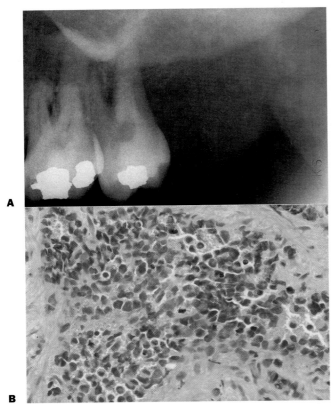

A

B

Figure 7-39 **Rhabdomyosarcoma** of the palate. **A,** Radiograph showing tumor destruction of tuberosity and alveolar bone around roots of second molar tooth. **B,** Biopsy specimen showing malignant round rhabdomyoblasts.

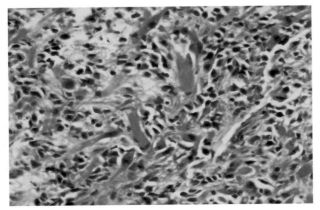

Figure 7-40 **Rhabdomyosarcoma,** pleomorphic type. Note straplike malignant cells.

onal type of rhabdomyosarcoma is the variety most commonly seen in the head and neck. Because of the relatively undifferentiated nature of this microscopic subtype, immunohistochemistry to demonstrate desmin, actin, and myogenin protein expression is typically used to support light microscopic interpretations. Two consistent and reproducible chromosome translocations are associated with alvelolar rhabdomyosarcoma. Most commonly there is t(12;13) (q35;q14), and less commonly there is t(1;13) (p36q14). This differs from the deletions on 11p that are seen in the embryonal forms.

The combination of surgery, radiation, and chemotherapy has been shown to produce far better clinical results than any one of these treatment methods alone. Survival rates have increased from less than 10% to better than 70% with this more aggressive treatment approach.

FAT LESIONS

Lipoma

Lipomas are uncommon neoplasms of the oral cavity that may occur in any region. The buccal mucosa, tongue, and floor of the mouth are among the more common locations (Figure 7-41). Clinical presentation is typically as an asymptomatic, yellowish submucosal mass. The overlying epithelium is intact, and superficial blood vessels are usually evident over the tumor. Other benign connective tissue lesions such as granular cell tumor, neurofibroma, traumatic fibroma, and salivary gland lesions (mucocele and mixed tumor) might be included in a differential diagnosis.

Numerous microscopic subtypes have been described, but they are primarily of academic interest. All types have adipocytes of various degrees of maturity. The usual simple lipoma consists of a well-circumscribed, lobulated mass of mature fat cells. The lesions are excised and are not expected to recur.

Liposarcoma

Liposarcoma is rarely encountered in soft tissues of the head and neck. It is a lesion of adulthood and may potentially occur in any site. It is generally slow growing and thus may be mistaken for a benign process. Considerable microscopic variation in these malignancies has led to subclassification into at least four

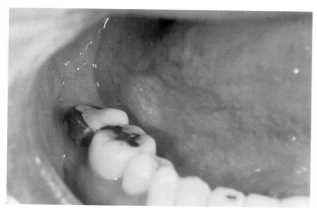

Figure 7-41 **Lipoma**, posterior floor of mouth.

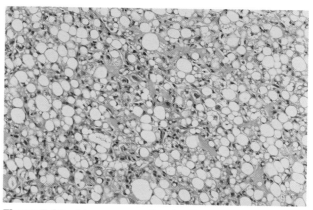

Figure 7-42 **Liposarcoma** showing irregular fat cells with atypical nuclei.

types: well differentiated, myxoid, round cell, and pleomorphic. Immunohistochemistry plays little role in the diagnosis of liposarcoma. The degree of tumor cell differentiation coupled with identification of the microscopic subtype is an important factor in predicting clinical behavior (Figure 7-42). These neoplasms may be treated with surgery or radiation, and the prognosis is fair to good.

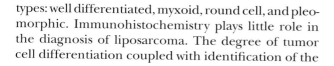

BIBLIOGRAPHY

FIBROUS CONNECTIVE TISSUE LESIONS

Alawi F, Stratton D, Freedman PD: Solitary fibrous tumor of the oral soft tissues: a clinicopathologic and immunohistochemical study of 16 cases, *Am J Surg Pathol* 25:900-910, 2001.

Brown R, Sein P, Corio R, et al: Nitrendipine-induced gingival hyperplasia, *Oral Surg Oral Med Oral Pathol* 70:593-596, 1990.

Das SJ, Olsen I: Keratinocyte growth factor is upregulated by the hyperplasia-inducing drug nifedipine, *Cytokine* 12(10):1566-1569, 2000.

Dent CD, DeBoom GW, Hamlin ML: Proliferative myositis of the head and neck, *Oral Surg Oral Med Oral Pathol* 78:354-358, 1994.

de Villiers-Slabbert H, Altini M: Peripheral odontogenic fibroma: a clinicopathologic study, *Oral Surg Oral Med Oral Pathol* 71:86-90, 1991.

Foss RD, Ellis G: Myxofibromas and myofibromatosis of the oral region: a clinicopathologic analysis of 79 cases, *Oral Surg Oral Med Oral Pathol Oral Radiol Endod* 89:57-65, 2000.

Fowler CB, Hartman KS, Brannon RB: Fibromatosis of the oral and paraoral region, *Oral Surg Oral Med Oral Pathol* 77:373-386, 1994.

Hajdu S: Fibrosarcoma: a historic commentary, *Cancer* 82:2081-2089, 1998.

Harel-Raviv M, Eckler M, Lalani K, et al: Nifedipine-induced gingival hyperplasia, *Oral Surg Oral Med Oral Pathol Oral Radiol Endod* 79:715-722, 1995.

Montgomery E, Speight PM, Fisher C: Myofibromas presenting in the oral cavity: a series of 9 cases, *Oral Surg Oral Med Oral Pathol Oral Radiol Endod* 89:343-348, 2000.

Odell E, Lock C, Lombardi T: Phenotypic characterization of stellate and giant cells in giant cell fibroma by immunocytochemistry, *J Oral Pathol Med* 23:284-287, 1994.

Perez-Ordonez B, Koutlas IG, Strich E, et al: Solitary fibrous tumor of the oral cavity, *Oral Surg Oral Med Oral Pathol Oral Radiol Endod* 87:589-593, 1999.

Rousseau A, Perez-Ordonez B, Jordan RCK: Giant cell angiofibroma of the oral cavity: report of a new location for a rare tumour, *Oral Surg Oral Med Oral Pathol Oral Radiol Endod* 88(5):581-585, 1999.

Vally I, Altini M: Fibromatosis of the oral and paraoral soft tissues and jaws, *Oral Surg Oral Med Oral Pathol* 69:191-198, 1990.

Vigneswaran N, Boyd D, Waldron C: Solitary infantile myofibromatosis of the mandible, *Oral Surg Oral Med Oral Pathol* 73:84-88, 1992.

NEURAL LESIONS

Chauvin P, Wysocki G, Daley T, et al: Palisaded encapsulated neuroma of oral mucosa, *Oral Surg Oral Med Oral Pathol* 73:71-74, 1992.

Chrysomali E, Papanicolaou S, Dekker NP, et al: Benign neural tumors of the oral cavity: a comparative immunohistochemical study, *Oral Surg Oral Med Oral Pathol Oral Radiol Endod* 84:381-390, 1997.

Gutmann DH, Aylsworth A, Carey JC, et al: The diagnostic evaluation and multidisciplinary management of neurofibromatosis 1 and neurofibromatosis 2, *JAMA* 278:51-57, 1997.

MUSCLE AND FAT LESIONS

Cessna MH, Zhou H, Perkins SL, et al: Are myogenin and MyoD1 expression specific for rhabdomyosarcoma? *Am J Surg Pathol* 25:1150-1157, 2001.

Parham DM: Pathologic classification of rhabdomyosarcomas and correlations with molecular studies, *Mod Pathol* 14:506-514, 2001.

SALIVARY GLAND DISEASES

REACTIVE LESIONS

Mucocele is a clinical term that includes mucus extravasation phenomenon and mucus retention cyst. Because each has a distinctive pathogenesis and microscopy, they are considered separately.

Ranula is a clinical term that also includes mucus extravasation phenomenon and mucus retention cyst, but it occurs specifically in the floor of the mouth. Ranula is associated with the sublingual or submandibular glands and presents as a fluctuant, unilateral, soft tissue mass. It often exhibits a bluish color that has been compared to a frog's belly; hence the term *ranula*. When it is significantly large, it can produce medial and superior deviation of the tongue. It may also cross the midline if the retained mucin dissects through the submucosa. A deep, so-called *plunging ranula* develops if mucus herniates through the mylohyoid muscle and along the fascial planes of the neck. On rare occasions it may progress into the mediastinum.

Mucus Extravasation Phenomenon

Etiology and Pathogenesis. The cause of mucus extravasation phenomenon is traumatic severance of a salivary gland excretory duct, resulting in mucus escape, or extravasation, into the surrounding connective tissue (Figure 8-1). An inflammatory reaction of neutrophils followed by macrophages ensues. Granulation tissue forms a wall around the mucin pool, and the contributing salivary gland undergoes inflammatory change. Ultimately, scarring occurs in and around the gland.

Clinical Features. The lower lip is the most common site of mucus extravasation phenomenon, but the buccal mucosa, anterior-ventral surface of the tongue (loca-

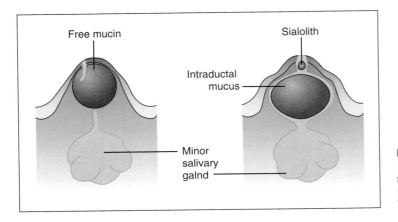

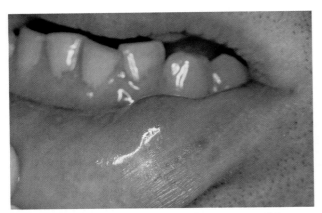

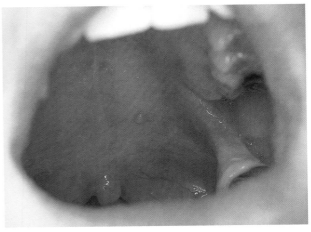

Figure 8-1   **Mucus extravasation phenomenon** (*left*) showing free mucin in submucosa and **mucus retention cyst** (*right*) showing mucin retained in the salivary excretory duct due to blockage by a sialolith.

Figure 8-2   **Mucus extravasation phenomenon** of the lower lip.

Figure 8-3   **Superficial mucocele** of the palate.

tion of Blandin-Nuhn glands), floor of the mouth, and retromolar region are often affected (Figures 8-2 and 8-3). Lesions are uncommonly found in other intraoral regions where salivary glands are located, probably because of a lower susceptibility to trauma.

Mucus extravasation phenomenon presents as a relatively painless smooth-surfaced mass ranging in size from a few millimeters to 2 cm in diameter. It has a bluish color when mucin is superficially located. Adolescents and children are more commonly affected than adults. Lesions may fluctuate in size because of mucosal rupture over the pooled mucin. Continued production of mucin leads to recurrence. The maximum size is usually reached within several days after injury, and a viscous material is found if aspiration is attempted.

Superficial mucocele is a variant of the extravasation-type mucocele. Rather than arising from traumatic duct rupture, this form of mucocele is believed to arise as a result of increased pressure in the outermost part of the excretory duct. These lesions are asymptomatic and numerous, occurring most commonly in the retromolar area, soft palate, and posterior buccal mucosa. Their clinical appearance suggests a vesiculobullous disease, but the lesions persist for an extended time. Other than being a diagnostic challenge, they are of little significance.

Histopathology. Extravasation of free mucin incites an inflammatory response that is followed by connective tissue repair. Neutrophils and macrophages are seen, and granulation tissue forms around the mucin pool (Figure 8-4). The adjacent salivary gland whose duct was transected shows ductal dilation, chronic inflammation, acinar degeneration, and interstitial fibrosis.

Differential Diagnosis. Although a history of a traumatic event followed by development of a bluish translucency

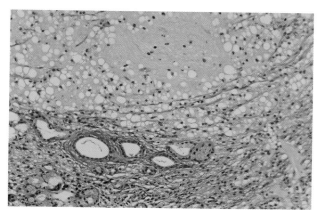

Figure 8-4   Mucus extravasation phenomenon showing free mucin *(top)* surrounded by inflamed connective tissue and salivary gland tissue.

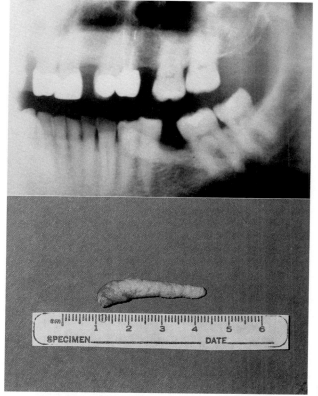

Figure 8-5   A, Sialolithiasis of the submandibular duct. **B,** Sialolith removed.

of the lower lip is characteristic of mucus extravasation phenomenon, other lesions might be considered when a typical history is absent. These include salivary gland neoplasm (especially mucoepidermoid carcinoma), vascular malformation, venous varix, and soft tissue neoplasm such as neurofibroma or lipoma. Rarely, a mucocele may appear in the alveolar gingival mucosa. When this is the case, an eruption cyst or gingival cyst should be included in the differential diagnosis.

Treatment and Prognosis.   The treatment of mucus extravasation phenomenon is surgical excision. Aspiration of the fluid content provides no lasting clinical benefit. Removal of the associated minor salivary glands along with the pooled mucus is necessary to prevent recurrence.

No treatment is required for superficial mucoceles, since they rupture spontaneously and are short-lived.

Mucus Retention Cyst

Etiology and Pathogenesis.   Mucus retention cysts result from obstruction of salivary flow because of a sialolith, periductal scar, or impinging tumor. The retained mucin is surrounded by ductal epithelium, giving the lesion a cystlike appearance microscopically.

Sialolithiasis.   Obstruction due to a salivary stone, or sialolith, is usually associated with the submandibular gland. The sialolith(s) may be found anywhere in the ductal system from the gland parenchyma to the excretory duct orifice. A *sialolith* represents the precipitation of calcium salts (predominantly calcium carbonate and calcium phosphate) around a central nidus of cellular debris or inspissated mucin.

Clinical Features.   Mucus retention cyst is less common than mucus extravasational phenomenon. It usually appears in an older age-group and is most commonly seen in the upper lip, palate, cheek, and floor of the mouth. Lesions present as asymptomatic swellings, usually without antecedent trauma (Figures 8-5 and 8-6). They vary in size from 3 to 10 mm and on palpation are mobile and nontender. The overlying mucosa is intact and of normal color. Mucin in floor-of-mouth lesions may penetrate musculature and escape into the soft tissues of the neck, causing a "plunging ranula."

Histopathology.   The cystlike cavity of a mucus retention cyst is lined by normal but compressed ductal epithelial cells (Figure 8-7). The type of lining formed by the epithelial cells ranges from pseudostratified to stratified squamous. The cyst lumen contains inspissated mucin or a calcified sialolith. The connective tissue

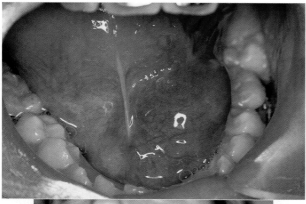

A

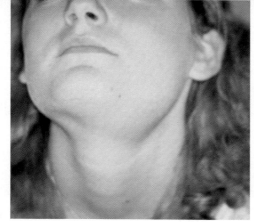

B

Figure 8-6   **A, Ranula** on the floor of the mouth. **B,** "Plunging ranula."

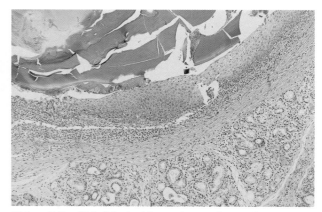

Figure 8-7   **Sialolith** *(top)* in a minor salivary gland *(bottom)* excretory duct of the upper lip.

around the lesion is minimally inflamed, although the associated gland shows obstructive change.

Differential Diagnosis. Salivary gland neoplasms, mucus extravasation phenomenon, and benign connective tissue neoplasms should be included in a clinical differential diagnosis. Dermoid cyst might also be included for lesions in the floor of the mouth.

Treatment and Prognosis. Treatment requires removal of the mucus retention cyst and the associated minor salivary gland to avoid postoperative mucus extravasation phenomenon. Lesions of the major salivary glands can be treated in a similar way or, on occasion, only by removal of the obstruction (sialolith) if it occurs in the distal part of the ductal system. The sialolith is either surgically removed or milked through the duct orifice. If a duct is surgically entered, special precautions are used to aid the healing process so that duct scarring is minimized. Constriction of the duct through excessive scar formation could result

in recurrence. Marsupialization by the placement of a silk suture in the roof of a large mucus retention cyst, particularly in one arising in the floor of the mouth, can be useful to reduce its size before surgical excision.

Maxillary Sinus Retention Cyst/Pseudocyst

Retention cysts and pseudocysts involving the lining of the maxillary antrum are common findings in panoramic radiographs. These lesions are discovered incidentally and are of little clinical significance.

Etiology and Pathogenesis. Retention cysts are thought to arise from blockage of an antral seromucous gland, resulting in a ductal epithelium-lined cystic structure filled with mucin. Pseudocysts are inflammatory in origin and result from fluid accumulation within the sinus membrane. They may be related to infection or allergy. Bacterial toxins, anoxia, or other factors presumably cause leakage of protein into surrounding soft tissue, thus raising the extravascular osmotic pressure with subsequent fluid increase.

Clinical Features. The great majority of these lesions are asymptomatic, although there may be some slight tenderness in the mucobuccal fold or, more rarely, palpable buccal expansion in this region. In panoramic and periapical radiographs, retention cysts and pseudocysts of the maxillary sinus are hemispheric, homogeneously opaque, and well delineated (Figure 8-8). They usually demonstrate an attachment to the floor of the antrum, with size being a function of the anatomic space rather than of duration. Uncommonly these lesions may appear bilaterally.

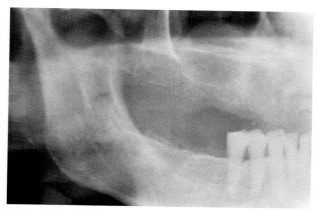

Figure 8-8 Maxillary sinus retention cyst.

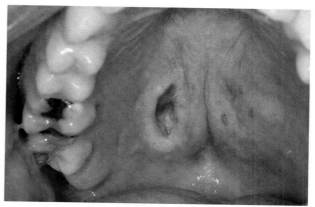

Figure 8-9 Necrotizing sialometaplasia of the hard palate.

Histopathology. The pathogenesis of the two forms of antral cysts is reflected in the histologic appearance. The retention cyst is lined by pseudostratified columnar epithelium with occasional mucous cells interspersed. The supportive elements are minimally inflamed. The pseudocyst shows no evidence of an epithelial lining but, rather, pools of mucoid material surrounded by slightly compressed connective tissue.

Differential Diagnosis. A clinical differential diagnosis of cysts and pseudocysts arising within the mucosa of the maxillary sinus would include polyps, hyperplasia of the sinus lining secondary to odontogenic infection, maxillary sinusitis, and neoplasms arising within the soft tissues of the antral lining.

Treatment. Antral retention cysts and pseudocysts are generally left untreated because they are limited in growth and are not destructive, and most spontaneously rupture. Therefore periodic observation is all that is required.

Necrotizing Sialometaplasia

Necrotizing sialometaplasia is a benign condition that typically affects the palate and rarely other sites containing salivary glands. Recognition of this entity is important because it mimics malignancy both clinically and microscopically. Unnecessary surgery has been performed because of an erroneous preoperative diagnosis of squamous cell carcinoma or mucoepidermoid carcinoma.

Etiology and Pathogenesis. The initiating event of necrotizing sialometaplasia is believed to be salivary gland ischemia precipitated by local trauma, surgical manipulation, or local anesthesia. Infarction of the gland follows, and squamous metaplasia of ductal remnants eventually appears.

This condition is believed to be due to local trauma or focal vascular compromise leading to discrete tissue necrosis in the area. Patients often have no history of a prior traumatic event.

Clinical Features. Intraorally, necrotizing sialometaplasia is characterized by a seemingly spontaneous appearance, most commonly at the junction of the hard and soft palates (Figure 8-9). Early in its evolution, the lesion may be noted as a tender swelling, often with a dusky erythema of the overlying mucosa. Subsequently the mucosa breaks down, with the formation of a sharply demarcated deep ulcer with a yellowish gray lobular base. In the palate the lesion may be unilateral or bilateral, with individual lesions ranging from 1 to 3 cm in diameter. Pain is generally disproportionately slight compared with the size of the lesion. Healing is generally protracted, taking from 6 to 10 weeks.

Histopathology. Submucosa adjacent to an ulcer shows necrosis of salivary glands and squamous metaplasia of salivary duct epithelium (Figure 8-10). Preservation of the lobular architecture of salivary glands serves to distinguish this process from neoplasia. The characteristic ductal squamous metaplasia shows no cytologic atypia, but the pattern may be misinterpreted as squamous cell carcinoma. When this metaplasia is seen in the presence of residual viable salivary gland, the lesion may be mistaken for mucoepidermoid carcinoma.

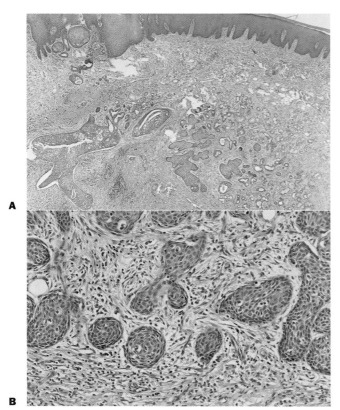

Figure 8-10 **Necrotizing sialometaplasia. A** and **B,** Squamous metaplasia of salivary ducts.

Differential Diagnosis. Clinically, squamous cell carcinoma and malignant minor salivary gland neoplasms must be ruled out, usually by a biopsy. Syphilitic gummas and deep fungal infections must likewise be ruled out, since they may present as punched-out lesions of the palate. Findings from serology, biopsy, and/or culture are usually needed to exclude these entities. In medically compromised patients, such as those with poorly controlled diabetes, opportunistic fungal infections such as mucormycosis may cause a similar clinical picture.

The entity *subacute necrotizing sialadenitis* has recently been described as a nonspecific, inflammatory condition of minor salivary glands of unknown etiology. It is characterized by an abrupt onset of pain and localized swelling, usually of the hard or soft palate, but unlike necrotizing sialometaplasia, is self-limiting without an ulcerative or metaplastic component.

Treatment and Prognosis. This condition is a benign, self-limiting process that does not require surgical inter-vention. However, an incisional biopsy should be performed to establish a definitive diagnosis. Healing takes place over several weeks by secondary intention. Patient reassurance, wound irrigation using a bland baking soda–and–water mouthrinse, and occasional use of analgesics are the only management steps necessary.

Adenomatoid Hyperplasia

Adenomatoid hyperplasia is a nonneoplastic enlargement of the minor salivary glands of the hard palate. The cause is unknown, although there is some evidence to suggest that trauma plays a role.

Clinical Features. The palate is the chief site of involvement of this salivary gland hyperplasia. There is a male predominance, and age ranges from 24 to 63 years. The clinical presentation is a unilateral swelling of the hard and/or soft palate. This lesion is asymptomatic, broad based, and covered with intact mucosa of normal color and quality.

Histopathology. Lobules of hyperplastic mucous glands extend beyond the submucosa and into the lamina propria. Individual acinar clusters are more numerous and larger than normal. Ducts exhibit a slight increase in relative prominence. The cytologic and morphologic features of acinar and ductal elements are within normal limits. There is generally no significant inflammatory cell infiltrate.

Differential Diagnosis. A clinical differential diagnosis would include salivary neoplasms, lymphoma, and extension of nasopharyngeal or sinonasal disease into the oral cavity. Periapical inflammatory disease should be excluded.

Treatment and Prognosis. Subsequent to identification by means of an incisional biopsy, no treatment is necessary, given the purely benign nature of this process. There is no neoplastic potential.

INFECTIOUS SIALADENITIS

Mumps

Mumps is an infectious, acute viral sialadenitis affecting primarily the parotid glands. Considered the most common of all salivary gland diseases before the advent of routine immunization, it has a year-round endemic pattern, although seasonal peaks are noted in the late winter and spring months.

Etiology and Pathogenesis. The causative agent of mumps is a paramyxovirus. A 2- to 3-week incubation period precedes clinical symptoms. Transmission is by direct contact with salivary droplets.

Clinical Features. Patients develop fever, malaise, headache, and chills in addition to preauricular pain. Salivary glands, usually the parotid, demonstrate a 70% incidence of bilateral infection. The parotid swelling tends to be asymmetric at the outset, reaching maximum proportions within 2 to 3 days. Severe local pain is often noted, especially on movement of the jaws in talking and chewing. Stensen's duct may become partially occluded as the gland swells, with sharp pain secondary to the stimulation of the secretory mechanism by food or drink. Perceptible diminution of swelling is noted approximately 10 days after the onset of symptoms. The disease affects males and females equally, especially young adults and children. Potentially serious complications (orchitis or oophoritis) can occur in adults. Mumps is a systemic infection, as evidenced by the widespread involvement of glandular and other tissues in the body, including the liver, pancreas, kidney, and nervous system.

Treatment and Prognosis. Treatment is symptomatic and includes bed rest. Analgesics are prescribed, and in severe cases corticosteroids may be used. Complete recovery is generally the rule, although fatalities have been associated with viral encephalitis, myocarditis, and nephritis. Nerve deafness and bilateral testicular atrophy have been noted but are uncommon.

Prevention of the disease is now possible using a live attenuated vaccine that induces a noncommunicable, subclinical infection. Antibody conversion occurs in approximately 90% of susceptible individuals, and immunity is lifelong.

Although mumps is the most common form of viral sialadenitis, it is important to note that parotitis may also be caused by other viral agents, including coxsackie A virus, echovirus, choriomeningitis virus, cytomegalovirus, and parainfluenza virus types 1 and 2.

Cytomegaloviral Sialadenitis

Cytomegalovirus infection of salivary glands, or so-called cytomegalic inclusion disease, is a rare condition that affects neonates as a result of transplacental infection. Systemic disease may cause debilitation, developmental retardation, and premature birth.

When encountered in adults who are immunosuppressed (e.g., human immunodeficiency virus [HIV] infection, organ transplants), infection may cause fever, salivary gland enlargement, hepatosplenomegaly, pneumonitis, and lymphocytosis. Retinitis can be a serious complication of this infection. Cytomegalovirus can be demonstrated in biopsy material, and with the use of in situ hybridization methods its presence can be easily confirmed in the tissue sections. Oral aphthouslike ulcers, particularly those arising in immunocompromised patients, may contain the virus, but the importance is undetermined. In severely infected immunocompromised patients, ganciclovir may be used to control cytomegalovirus infections.

Adults who are not immunosuppressed may also be infected with cytomegalovirus, as evidenced by demonstration of antibodies in serum. Symptomatology may be nonexistent, or there may be slight to debilitating fever and malaise. The significance of cytomegalovirus infections in this population is poorly understood.

Bacterial Sialadenitis

Etiology and Pathogenesis. Bacterial infections of salivary glands are generally due to microbial overgrowth in association with a reduction in salivary flow. Such reduction in flow may be noted subsequent to dehydration and debilitation. Traditionally, bacterial sialadenitis has been a common postoperative complication of surgery related to inadequate hydration. Numerous drugs associated with a decreased salivary flow rate likewise contribute to infections of the major salivary glands, especially the parotid. Other possible causes include trauma to the duct system and hematogenous spread of infection from other areas. The most commonly isolated organisms in parotitis are penicillin-resistant *Staphylococcus aureus, Streptococcus viridans,* and *Streptococcus pneumoniae.* It is of interest to note the marked reduction in the overall incidence of acute parotitis after the introduction of antibiotic preparations. As resistant strains of bacteria have appeared, the prevalence of acute parotitis has increased.

Clinical Features. Clinical features are chiefly characterized by the presence of a painful swelling, low-grade fever, malaise, and headache. Laboratory studies disclose an elevated erythrocyte sedimentation rate

(ESR) and leukocytosis, often with a characteristic shift to the left, indicating acute infection. The involved gland is extremely tender, with the patient often demonstrating guarding during examination. Trismus is often noted, and purulence at the duct orifice may be produced by gentle pressure on the involved gland or duct.

If the infection is not eliminated early, suppuration may extend beyond the limiting capsule of the parotid gland. Extension into surrounding tissues along fascial planes in the neck or extension posteriorly into the external auditory canal may follow.

Treatment and Prognosis. Management of bacterial sialadenitis is directed at elimination of the causative organism coupled with rehydration of the patient and drainage of purulence, if present. Culture and sensitivity testing of the exudate at the orifice of the duct is the first step in antibiotic management. After a culture is obtained, all patients should empirically be placed on a regimen of a penicillinase-resistant antibiotic such as semisynthetic penicillin. Along with rehydration and attempts at establishing and encouraging salivary flow, moist compresses, analgesics, and rest are in order. Medications containing parasympathomimetic agents, which reduce salivary flow, should be reduced or eliminated.

A biopsy and retrograde sialography should be avoided. The former may cause sinus tract formation, and the latter may allow infection to proceed beyond the boundaries of the gland into surrounding soft tissues. With prompt and effective treatment, recurrence is generally avoided. In cases of recurrent parotitis, considerable destructive glandular changes can be seen.

In the so-called *juvenile variant of parotitis,* intermittent unilateral or bilateral painful swelling is accompanied by fever and malaise. The initial attack usually occurs in individuals between ages 2 and 6 years, with numerous recurrences thereafter. Rarely a neonatal form of suppurative parotitis may develop, with *S. aureus* being the most common causative pathogen. Gross destruction of the parenchymal and ductal elements may be noted on sialographic examination. Absence of secretory acinar components and a damaged ductal system with numerous punctate globular spaces may be seen. Spontaneous regeneration of parotid salivary tissue has been reported in this condition. Finally, the rare example of childhood to adolescent–onset Sjögren's syndrome may be heralded by recurrent bilateral parotitis.

Sarcoidosis

Etiology. Sarcoidosis is a granulomatous disease of undetermined origin. Although no specific cause has been identified, it has been suggested that this disease represents an infection or a hypersensitivity response to atypical mycobacteria. As many as 90% of patients in some studies showed significant titers of serum antibodies to these organisms. In some patients with sarcoidosis, a transmissible agent from human sarcoid tissue has been identified. With the use of molecular biologic techniques, mycobacterial DNA and RNA have been identified in sarcoid tissues, raising the possibility of *Mycobacterium tuberculosis* or a related organism as a causative agent.

Susceptibility related to human leukocyte antigens (HLAs) has been studied. Patients with some histocompatibility antigens (HLA-B7, HLA-B5, HLA-A9) may have a greater incidence of sarcoidosis than do others. It has also been found that most patients with sarcoidosis are anergic, demonstrating decreased levels of cutaneous sensitization to dinitrochlorobenzene, as well as to tuberculin, mumps virus, *Candida* antigen, and pertussis antigen.

Clinical Features. The protean manifestations of this disease are well known. Clinical courses range from spontaneous resolution to chronic progression. The disease may affect individuals at any age, although most are affected in the second through fourth decades. Females show a higher incidence than do males, and African-Americans are more commonly affected than whites.

Sarcoidosis is usually a self-limiting, benign disease with an insidious onset and protracted course. Patients may complain of lethargy, chronic fatigue, and anorexia, with specific signs and symptoms related to the organ involved.

Pulmonary manifestations are the most characteristic of this disease. They are typified by bilateral, hilar, and less commonly, paratracheal lymphadenopathy. The disease may stabilize at this point, or it may advance to pulmonary fibrosis and a more ominous prognosis. The most serious complications of sarcoidosis are pulmonary hypertension, respiratory failure, and cor pulmonale.

The skin may be involved in approximately 25% of cases; most commonly, an erythema nodosum of acute onset and short duration is seen. Skin plaques characterized by nontender, dark purple, elevated areas on the limbs, abdomen, and buttocks may appear. Another form of cutaneous pathology includes lesions known as *lupus pernio*, a term used to describe symmetric, infiltrative, violaceous plaques on the nose, cheeks, ears, forehead, and hands.

Ocular involvement is variable, with inflammation of the anterior uveal tract most commonly seen. This may be associated with parotid gland swelling and fever, so-called *uveoparotid fever* or *Heerfordt's syndrome*.

Hepatic involvement is quite common, with approximately 60% of patients showing granulomatous lesions on liver biopsy specimens. However, clinical evidence of hepatic involvement appears in fewer than 50% of patients, as demonstrated in abnormal liver function test results.

Osseous lesions are uncommonly noted, with a 5% occurrence rate in most studies. When present, punched-out lesions involving the distal phalanges with erosions of cancellous bone and an intact cortex are seen. Destruction of alveolar bone with tooth mobility may be evident within the maxilla and mandible.

Oral soft tissue lesions of sarcoidosis are nodular and generally indistinguishable from those seen in Crohn's disease. Parotid swelling may occur either unilaterally or bilaterally with about equal frequency (Box 8-1). This is often associated with lassitude, fever, gastrointestinal upset, joint pains, and night sweats, which may precede glandular involvement by several days to weeks. Other salivary glands may also be involved in the granulomatous inflammatory process, leading to xerostomia.

The upper aerodigestive tract may be involved, with lesions developing in the nasal mucosa, especially in the inferior turbinate and septal regions. Granulomas may also occur in the nasal sinuses, pharynx, epiglottis, and larynx.

Serum chemistry, radiographic studies, and biopsy are useful laboratory tests. Serum chemistry studies should include calcium (for evidence of hypercalcemia) and angiotensin I–converting enzyme, lysozyme, and adenosine deaminase levels (for evidence of macrophage activity within granulomas). Gallium scintiscanning and routine chest radiographs and intraoral films may be used to demonstrate bone involvement.

Histopathology. Consistent microscopic findings of sarcoidosis are noncaseating granulomas (Figure 8-11). The granulomas may be well demarcated and discrete or confluent. Within the granulomas are epithelioid macrophages and multinucleated giant cells, which may contain stellate inclusions (asteroid bodies) and concentrically laminar calcifications (Schaumann bodies). A diffuse lymphocytic infiltrate may be seen around the periphery of the granulomas. Absent is the caseation-type necrosis that is typical of tuberculosis. Microorganisms are also absent.

A lip biopsy may occasionally provide evidence of sarcoid involvement of minor salivary glands in support of a clinical impression of pulmonary disease.

Diagnosis. The Kveim test has traditionally been used to establish the diagnosis of sarcoidosis; however, this test is no longer used. Of considerable value is a laboratory assay for angiotensin I–converting enzyme. Elevation of this enzyme in conjunction with a positive chest radiograph has a high diagnostic reliability.

The histologic differential diagnosis includes tuberculosis, Crohn's disease, leprosy, cat-scratch disease, fungal infections (blastomycosis, coccidioidomycosis,

---

Box 8-1 Salivary Gland Enlargement: Parotid Glands

Sjögren's syndrome
Neoplasms
  Adenomas and carcinomas
  Lymphoma
Infections
  Mumps
  Tuberculosis
  Sarcoidosis
  Other bacterial infections
Metabolic conditions
  Malnutrition, including anorexia and bulimia
  Diabetes mellitus
  Chronic alcoholism

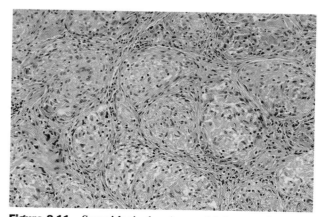

Figure 8-11 **Sarcoidosis** showing multiple granulomas.

and histoplasmosis), and parasitic diseases such as toxoplasmosis. Granulomas seen in association with beryllium and talc exposure must also be considered.

Treatment and Prognosis. Spontaneous resolution occurs in a significant number of patients. Corticosteroids are generally considered beneficial and remain the drugs of choice in treating symptomatic pulmonary sarcoidosis. Other agents may be used in addition to or instead of corticosteroids. Chloroquine has been found to be useful in the management of this disease, either alone or in combination with corticosteroids. Immunosuppressive drugs have been used with good results in individuals not responding to corticosteroid management. Immunomodulators such as levamisole may be useful in the management of arthritic symptoms caused by sarcoidosis.

In general, the prognosis for sarcoidosis is good, but patients must be monitored periodically with chest radiographs and serum angiotensin I–converting enzyme determinations. Clinical relapses are not usual in cases in which spontaneous resolution has occurred.

Metabolic Conditions

A generic term for a group of metabolic disorders that may cause salivary gland enlargement is *sialadenosis*, or *sialosis*. These conditions usually affect the parotid glands bilaterally, typically in the absence of inflammatory symptoms. Chronic alcoholism, dietary deficiency, obesity, diabetes mellitus, hypertension, and hyperlipidemia have been linked to this clinical salivary gland abnormality.

Alcoholic cirrhosis or chronic alcoholism and asymptomatic enlargement of the parotid glands occurs in 30% to 80% of patients. Salivary gland enlargement has been attributed to chronic protein deficiency. Comparable parotid gland enlargement in individuals with cirrhosis due to other causes apparently does not occur. Nutritional or protein deprivation may also lead to a similar salivary gland enlargement.

In diabetes mellitus, reduced flow rates have been reported in addition to bilateral parotid gland enlargement. The mechanism of acinar hypertrophy in this condition is unknown. Reduced flow rates from the parotid and other major salivary glands may lead to an increased risk of bacterial sialadenitis.

In cases of type I hyperlipoproteinemia a sicca-like syndrome has been described. This is characterized primarily by parotid enlargement with mild oral or ocular sicca symptoms; it is generally attributed to the presence of fatty replacement of functional salivary gland parenchyma.

Another endocrine-related salivary gland enlargement may be noted in acromegaly. This may merely be a reflection of a generalized organomegaly encountered in this endocrine-mediated disturbance. Apparent parotid enlargement (acinar hypertrophy) and increased levels of parotid flow have also been noted in patients having chronic relapsing pancreatitis.

Sjögren's Syndrome

Sjögren's syndrome is the expression of an autoimmune process that results principally in dry eyes (keratoconjunctivitis sicca) and dry mouth (xerostomia) owing to lymphocyte-mediated destruction of lacrimal and salivary gland parenchyma. Other autoimmune conditions, such as rheumatoid arthritis, may also be seen in this syndrome. The lacrimal and salivary gland involvement is often one expression of a generalized exocrinopathy that is lymphocyte mediated.

Etiology. Although the specific cause of this syndrome is unknown, numerous immunologic alterations indicate a disease of great complexity. The generalized alteration relates to a polyclonal B-cell hyperactivity that reflects a lack of regulation by T-cell subpopulations. As with the benign (salivary) lymphoepithelial lesion, the specific causes of this immunologic defect remain speculative.

This syndrome appears to be of autoimmune origin that may be limited to exocrine glands, or it may extend to include systemic connective tissue disorders. In instances of only exocrine involvement, the syndrome is known as *primary Sjögren's syndrome*. If, in addition to the xerostomia and keratoconjunctivitis sicca there is an associated connective tissue disorder, regardless of the specific type, it is known as *secondary Sjögren's syndrome*.

Viruses, particularly retroviruses and Epstein-Barr virus, have been implicated in the etiology of Sjögren's syndrome, but none are proven causes. Evidence suggesting a role for retroviruses has come from the demonstration of antibodies against HIV-associated proteins in a subset of patients with Sjögren's syndrome and from the clinical similarity of HIV-associated salivary gland disease to Sjögren's syndrome. The significance of anti-HIV antibodies in some patients with Sjögren's syndrome has not been determined. It has been suggested that these antibodies may be stimulated by another retrovirus that is related to HIV or that they may represent cross-reacting autoantibodies.

Epstein-Barr virus has been demonstrated in salivary gland tissue of patients with Sjögren's syndrome. However, the virus has also been found in the salivary glands of normal individuals, thus weakening the contention that Epstein-Barr virus has a primary role in the cause of this condition. If Epstein-Barr virus is involved, its role is likely secondary in nature.

Clinical Features. Sjögren's syndrome occurs in all ethnic and racial groups (Box 8-2). The peak age of onset is 50 years, and 90% of cases occur in women. Children and teenagers may be affected, but rarely. Distinguishing between primary and secondary forms of the syndrome, especially those associated with rheumatoid arthritis, is usually not difficult. This may be important because of an increased risk of lymphoreticular malignancy developing in the primary form—the relative risk is estimated to be approximately 44 times that in the general population. An interesting associated sign is a decrease in serum immunoglobulin levels accompanying or preceding the malignant change.

The chief oral complaint in Sjögren's syndrome is xerostomia, which may be the source of eating and speaking difficulties. These patients are also at greater risk for dental caries, periodontal disease, and oral candidiasis because of dry mouth. Parotid gland enlargement, which is often recurrent and symmetric, occurs in approximately 50% of patients (Figure 8-12). A significant percentage of these patients also present with complaints of arthralgia, myalgia, and fatigue.

The salivary component of Sjögren's syndrome may be assessed by sialochemical studies, nuclear imaging of the glands (scintigraphy), contrast sialography, flow rate analysis, and a minor salivary gland biopsy. The most commonly used and most reliable method of assessing salivary alteration in this syndrome currently is a labial salivary gland biopsy.

Nuclear medicine techniques using a technetium pertechnetate isotope and subsequent scintiscanning can yield functional information relative to the uptake of the isotope by salivary gland tissue. Contrast sialography aids in detecting filling defects within the gland being examined. A punctate sialectasia is characteristic in individuals with Sjögren's syndrome. This latter finding reflects significant ductal and acinar damage, with only the interlobular ducts remaining in cases of moderate to advanced disease. Over time, with further parenchymal and ductal damage, focal areas of nar-

---

Box 8-2 Sjögren's Syndrome: Potential Organopathy

SKIN

Dryness (reduced sweat production)
Scleroderma
Lupus erythematosus

SALIVARY AND LACRIMAL GLANDS

Enlargement
Xerostomia, dental caries, candidiasis
Keratoconjunctivitis sicca

GASTROINTESTINAL TRACT

Biliary cirrhosis
Hepatitis

RESPIRATORY TRACT

Rhinitis, pharyngitis
Obstructive pulmonary disease

CARDIOVASCULAR SYSTEM

Vasculitis

MUSCULOSKELETAL SYSTEM

Rheumatoid arthritis
Myositis

HEMATOPOIETIC SYSTEM

Lymphoma
Anemia, leukopenia

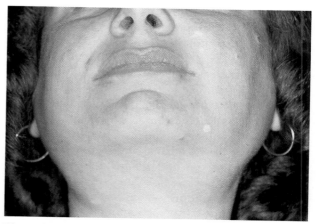

Figure 8-12 **Sjögren's syndrome** patient with bilateral parotid swelling.

rowing or stenosis of larger ducts take place and may be seen on a sialogram. Other forms of sialectasia may also be noted, including globular and cavitary types.

Other laboratory findings commonly found in primary and secondary Sjögren's syndrome include mild anemia, leukopenia, eosinophilia, an elevated ESR, and diffuse elevation of serum immunoglobulin levels. In addition, numerous autoantibodies may be found, including rheumatoid factor, antinuclear antibodies, and precipitating antinuclear antibodies such as anti–Sjögren's syndrome-A (SS-A) and anti–Sjögren's syndrome-B (SS-B). Antibodies SS-A and SS-B may be seen in association with both primary and secondary Sjögren's syndrome. Patients who have SS-B antibodies are more likely to develop extraglandular disease.

In the secondary form of Sjögren's syndrome, rheumatoid arthritis is the most common systemic autoimmune disease, although systemic lupus erythematosus is not infrequently encountered. Less commonly, diseases such as scleroderma, primary biliary cirrhosis, polymyositis, vasculitis, parotitis, and chronic active hepatitis may be associated with secondary Sjögren's syndrome.

Immunogenetic typing studies have indicated statistically significant expressions of various histocompatibility antigens in patients with primary and secondary forms of the syndrome. HLA-DR4 antigen is often identified in patients with secondary Sjögren's syndrome; antigens found in patients with the primary form are often HLA-B8 and HLA-DR3 types.

Histopathology. In individuals with Sjögren's syndrome, a benign lymphocytic infiltrate replaces major salivary gland parenchyma. The initial lesion is focal periductal aggregation of lymphocytes and occasionally plasma cells. As inflammatory foci enlarge, a corresponding level of acinar degeneration is seen (Figures 8-13 and 8-14). With increasing lymphocytic infiltration, confluence of inflammatory foci occurs. Epimyoepithelial islands are present in major glands in approximately 40% of cases and are only rarely seen in minor glands. There is a positive correlation in the pattern and extent of infiltration between labial salivary glands and submandibular and parotid glands in patients with Sjögren's syndrome.

An objective grading system has been developed for assessing the salivary component (lymphocytic sialadenitis) of Sjögren's syndrome in labial salivary gland biopsy specimens. A glandular area that con-

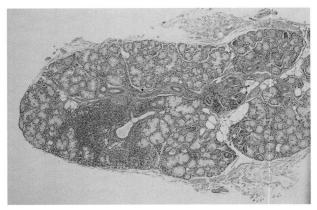

Figure 8-13 **Sjögren's syndrome,** minor salivary gland expression. Note lymphocytic focus adjacent to intact acini.

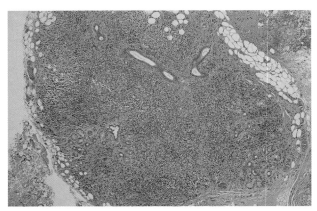

Figure 8-14 **Sjögren's syndrome,** minor salivary gland expression. Note confluent lymphocytic foci without evidence of scarring.

tains 50 or more lymphocytes is designated as a *focus.* More than one focus in 4 mm^2 is regarded as being consistent with the salivary component of Sjögren's syndrome. Interpretation of labial gland biopsy specimens should be done with the knowledge that infiltrates may be seen both in normal glands and in glands that are inflamed for other reasons, including myasthenia gravis, bone marrow transplantation, other connective tissue diseases, and obstructive phenomena.

Diagnosis. Diagnosis depends on the correlation between the patient history and laboratory data, clinical examination, and assessment of salivary function. An important consideration concerns the clinical manifestation of xerostomia. Although this is the main oral symptom and clinical sign in Sjögren's syndrome, other considerations of dry mouth must be evaluated. In addition, major salivary gland enlargement is a feature of Sjögren's syndrome but may be episodic in nature, and in some patients it may not be present at all. The sialographic and salivary scintigraphic findings are generally not specific and should be incorporated into other clinical and laboratory studies, including a minor salivary gland biopsy, as one considers the diagnosis of Sjögren's syndrome.

Treatment. Sjögren's syndrome and the complication of the sicca component are best managed symptomatically. Artificial saliva and artificial tears are available for this purpose. Preventive oral measures are extremely important relative to xerostomia. Scrupulous oral hygiene, dietary modification, topical fluoride therapy, and remineralizing solutions are important in maintaining oral and dental tissues. Use of sialagogues, such as pilocarpine and cevimeline, remains of limited value, especially in long-standing Sjögren's syndrome.

The prognosis of Sjögren's syndrome is complicated by an association with malignant transformation to lymphoma. This may occur in approximately 6% to 7% of cases; it is more common in those with only the sicca component of the syndrome. Less commonly observed is transformation of the epithelial component to undifferentiated carcinoma.

Generally, the course for Sjögren's syndrome is one of chronicity, requiring long-term symptomatic management. Careful follow-up and management by a dentist, ophthalmologist, and rheumatologist, among others, are critical.

Salivary Lymphoepithelial Lesion

An uncommon cause of major salivary gland enlargement is the so-called benign lymphoepithelial lesion (BLEL). The condition presents as a persistent, nonpainful, firm, unilateral or bilateral mass in a major salivary gland. Although this lesion most commonly occurs in the setting of Sjögren's syndrome, it has also been reported in the absence of the disease. The histopathology classically shows effacement of salivary tissue by a dense infiltrate of lymphocytes and plasma cells. This is associated with the proliferation of the ductal components to produce irregular islands of epithelium that are termed "epimyoepithelial islands" but that are principally composed of ductal cells with only occasional myoepithelial cells logic.

Although the term *benign lymphoepithelial lesion* has enjoyed common usage, other terms have been suggested, including *myoepithelial sialadenitis* and *immunosialadenitis*. Unfortunately, none of these appropriately reflect the biology of this lesion, since studies of the natural history, histopathology, immunology, and molecular biology now support the concept that many are not "benign" but, rather, represent occult lymphoma of the marginal zone type. Differentiation of benign lymphoid infiltrate in this setting from low-grade malignant lymphoma is difficult and rests on the identification of lymphocyte monotypia by molecular or immunohistochemical methods. More recently, the term *salivary lymphoepithelial lesion* has been proposed as a more accurate descriptor that better describes the basic pathologic lesion and its anatomic location without implicit reference to the underlying or potential biology of the disease.

BENIGN NEOPLASMS

At approximately 5 months of embryonic development, a characteristic lobular architecture of salivary glands becomes established. As branching morphogenesis continues, terminal tubular elements give rise to striated intralobular ducts, intercalated ducts, acini, and myoepithelial cells. Intralobular and interlobular ducts of the excretory system arise from the remaining progenitor stalk cells. A stem cell or reserve cell within the salivary duct system is believed by many to be the cell of origin of salivary gland neoplasms (Box 8-3). Because of their relatively undifferentiated ultrastructural appearance, intercalated duct cells are also thought to be capable of giving rise to these neoplasms. The importance of the myoepithelial cell in the composition and growth of numerous epithelial salivary tumors is considerable. Cells with a myoepithelial phenotype can be seen in all salivary gland tumors and are particularly abundant in mixed tumors, myoepitheliomas, adenoid cystic carcinomas, and epimyoepithelial carcinoma of intercalated duct origin.

The three major paired salivary glands—parotid, submandibular, and sublingual—plus the hundreds of small minor salivary glands located within the submucosa of the oral cavity and oropharynx are capable of giving rise to a wide range of neoplasms. The vast majority of salivary neoplasms are epithelial in origin; rarely, the interstitial connective tissue components of the major salivary glands give rise to primary neoplasms whose behavior is similar to that of their

Box 8-3 Benign Salivary Gland Tumors

Mixed tumor (pleomorphic adenoma)
Monomorphic adenomas
   Basal cell adenomas—solid, tubular, trabecular,
     membranous
   Canalicular adenoma
   Myoepithelioma
   Oncocytic tumors
     Oncocytoma
     Warthin's tumor and papillary cystadenoma
   Sebaceous adenoma
Ductal papillomas
   Inverted ductal papilloma
   Sialadenoma papilliferum
   Intraductal papilloma

Box 8-4 Mixed Tumor

CLINICAL FEATURES

Adults; men and women affected equally
Asymptomatic submucosal mass
Sites—palate > upper lip > buccal mucosa > other sites

HISTOPATHOLOGY

Encapsulated; variable glandular patterns; epithelial and
myoepithelial differentiation; no mitoses

TREATMENT

Excision; occasional recurrences in major glands

>, More frequently affected than.

TABLE 8-1   Salivary Gland Tumors

	Frequency (%)	% Malignant
Parotid glands	65	25
Submandibular glands	10	40
Sublingual glands	<1	90
Minor salivary glands	25	50

extraglandular counterparts. The ratio of benign to malignant salivary gland tumors is gland dependent (Table 8-1).

Mixed Tumor (Pleomorphic Adenoma)

The histogenesis of mixed tumor, or pleomorphic adenoma, relates to a dual proliferation of cells with ductal or myoepithelial features, separating it from monomorphic adenomas composed of only one cell type. The myoepithelial-differentiated cell assumes an important role in determining the overall composition and appearance of mixed tumors. A range of cell types and microscopic patterns are seen in mixed tumors—those composed almost completely of epithelial cells at one end of a spectrum and those composed almost completely of myoepithelial cells at the other end. Between these two extremes, less well developed cells with features of both myoepithelial and ductal elements may be seen. Alternatively, it has been theorized that rather than simultaneous proliferation of neoplastic epithelial and myoepithelial cells, a single cell with the potential to differentiate toward either

epithelial or myoepithelial cells may be responsible for these tumors.

Clinical Features. The mixed tumor, or pleomorphic adenoma, is the most common tumor of the major and minor salivary glands (Box 8-4). The parotid gland accounts for approximately 85% of these tumors, whereas the submandibular gland and the intraoral minor salivary glands account for 8% and 7%, respectively. Mixed tumors occur at any age, favor males slightly more than females, and are most prevalent in the fourth through sixth decades of life. They constitute approximately 50% of all intraoral minor salivary gland tumors. Generally, they are mobile except when they occur in the hard palate. They appear as firm, painless swellings and, in the vast majority of cases, do not cause ulceration of the overlying mucosa (Figure 8-15). The palate is the most common intraoral site, followed by the upper lip and buccal mucosa.

When they arise within the parotid gland, mixed tumors are generally painless and slow growing. They are usually located below the ear and posterior to the mandible. Some tumors may be grooved by the posterior extent of the mandibular ramus, with long-standing lesions capable of producing pressure atrophy on this bone. When they are situated within the inferior pole or tail of the parotid, the tumors may present below the angle of the mandible and anterior to the sternocleidomastoid muscle.

Mixed tumors range in size from a few millimeters to several centimeters in diameter and are capable of reaching giant proportions in the major salivary

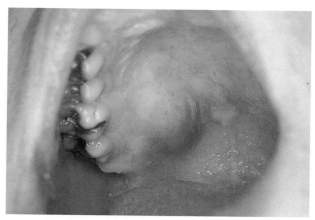

Figure 8-15   **Mixed tumor** of the palate.

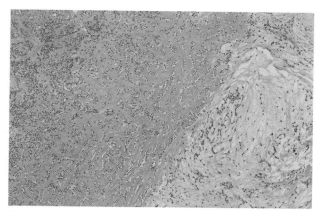

Figure 8-17   **Mixed tumor** with myxoid component *(right)* and fibrous/epithelial component *(left)*.

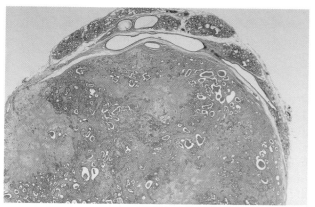

Figure 8-16   **Mixed tumor** showing encapsulation and heterogeneous pattern.

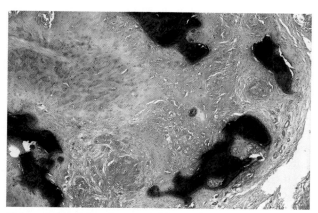

Figure 8-18   **Mixed tumor** with cartilage *(upper left)* and bone *(blue)* differentiation.

glands, especially the parotid. The tumor is typically lobulated and enclosed within a connective tissue pseudocapsule that varies in thickness. In areas where the capsule is deficient, neoplastic tissue may lie in direct contact with adjacent salivary tissue and may contribute to recurrences.

Histopathology. Microscopically, mixed tumors demonstrate a wide spectrum of histologic features (Figures 8-16 to 8-19). The pleomorphic patterns and the variable ratios of ductal to myoepithelial cells are responsible for the synonym *pleomorphic adenoma*. Approximately one third of mixed tumors show an almost equal ratio of epithelial and mesenchymal elements (believed to be derived from myoepithelial-

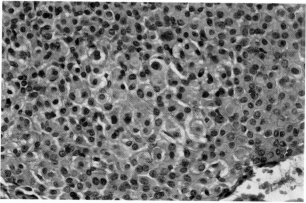

Figure 8-19   **Mixed tumor** showing plasmacytoid myoepithelial cells.

differentiated cells). The epithelial component may appear as ducts, tubules, ribbons, and solid sheets, and the mesenchymal component may appear as myxoid, hyalinized connective tissue. Infrequently, fat, cartilage, and/or bone may be seen. Myoepithelial cells may appear as plasmacytoid cells or spindled cells. The plasmacytoid cells, when seen, are highly characteristic of mixed tumors and are almost never found in other salivary gland tumors.

The pseudocapsule surrounding mixed tumors may demonstrate islands of tissue within it or extending through it. These islands represent outgrowths or pseudopods continuous with the main tumor mass and likely contribute to recurrences, particularly in the parotid.

Treatment and Prognosis. The treatment of choice is surgical excision. Enucleation of parotid mixed tumors is not advisable because of the risk of recurrence due to extension of tumor through capsular defects. Removal of mixed tumors arising within the parotid gland is complicated by the presence of the facial nerve. Any surgical approach, therefore, must include preservation of the uninvolved facial nerve. In most cases superficial parotidectomy (lateral lobectomy) with preservation of the facial nerve is the most appropriate management for those tumors arising within the parotid. Resection of the submandibular gland is the preferred treatment for mixed tumors in this location. Lesions of the palate or gingiva often involve or abut periosteum or bone, making complete removal difficult unless some bone is removed. Other oral benign mixed tumors can be more easily excised, preferably including tissue beyond the pseudocapsule.

Inadequate initial removal of mixed tumors in major glands may result in recurrence, often with multiple, discrete tumor foci. These recurrent lesions may be widely distributed within the area of previous surgery and may occur in association with the surgical scar. In most instances the recurrent tumor maintains the original pathology; however, with each recurrence there is an increased pos-sibility of malignant transformation (carcinoma ex-mixed tumor). The proportion of mixed tumors undergoing malignant transformation is not known with certainty, since almost all tumors are treated fairly early in their clinical course. However, if lesions are untreated for an extended length of time, typically years to decades, up to 25% may undergo malignant transformation. The probability of malignant change also increases if the area has previously been treated with surgery or radiotherapy.

Monomorphic Adenomas

Monomorphic adenomas are composed of an isomorphic epithelial cell population and lack the neoplastic connective elements that characterize mixed tumors. The classification scheme is based on the histologic pattern (see Box 8-3).

Basal Cell Adenomas. Basal cell adenomas constitute approximately 1% to 2% of all salivary gland adenomas. About 70% are found within the parotid. In minor salivary glands, most occur in the upper lip, followed in frequency by adenomas in the palate, buccal mucosa, and lower lip.

Clinical Features. Basal cell adenomas are generally slow growing and painless. The lesions tend to be clinically distinct on palpation, but they can be multifocal and multinodular. The age range of patients is between 35 and 80 years, with a mean age of approximately 60 years. A distinct male predilection is noted.

The *membranous adenoma (dermal analog tumor)* variant occurs in the parotid gland in more than 90% of cases, with no cases reported in the intraoral minor glands. These lesions vary from 1 to 5 cm in greatest dimension and generally present as an asymptomatic swelling. Several patients with this particular finding in the parotid gland have presented with synchronous or metachronous adnexal cutaneous tumors, including dermal cylindroma, trichoepithelioma, and eccrine spiradenoma.

Histopathology. In the *solid* variety of monomorphic adenoma, islands or sheets of basaloid cells often show peripheral palisading, with individual cells at the periphery appearing cuboidal to low columnar in profile (Figure 8-20). The *trabecular-tubular* form of basal cell adenoma exhibits trabecular cords of epithelial cells or tubular epithelial elements (Figures 8-21 and 8-22). *Membranous adenoma* grows in a nodular fashion with variable-sized islands of tumor tissue surrounded by a thick periodic-acid-Schiff (PAS)-positive hyaline membrane. Similar, if not identical, eosinophilic hyaline material is also noted in droplet form within the intercellular areas of the tumor islands, similar to those noted in so-called collagenous spherulosis of the breast and polycystic adenosis of salivary glands. Membranous adenomas may also contain foci of normal salivary gland, giving the erroneous impression of invasiveness and necessitating separation from adenoid cystic carcinoma.

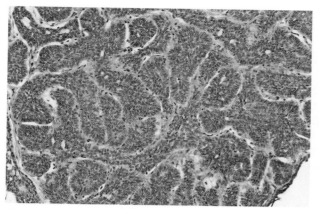

Figure 8-20   Basal cell adenoma, solid pattern.

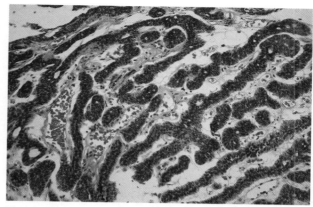

Figure 8-22   Basal cell adenoma, trabecular pattern.

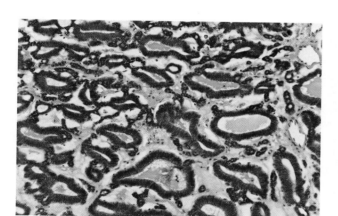

Figure 8-21   Basal cell adenoma, tubular pattern.

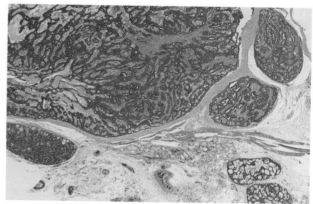

Figure 8-23   Canalicular adenoma with multiple foci.

Mitoses are rare in monomorphic adenomas. Nuclei are regular in shape and uniformly basophilic, and the amount of cytoplasm is generally slight.

Treatment and Prognosis. Except for membranous adenoma, monomorphic adenomas are benign and rarely recur. The membranous form of basal cell adenoma has a significant rate of recurrence because of its growth pattern and multifocal nature. Preferred management is conservative surgical excision including a margin of normal uninvolved tissue.

Canalicular Adenoma. *Canalicular adenoma* is generally separated from other monomorphic adenomas because it occurs almost exclusively within the oral cavity, commonly in the upper lip, and has distinctive histologic features. Its biologic behavior is, however, similar.

Clinical Features. A narrow age range is noted in patients with canalicular adenomas. Most patients tend to be older than 50 years of age, and most patients are women. The upper lip is by far the most common site for canalicular adenomas, with one series reporting 81% of lesions located in this region. The lesions tend to be freely movable and asymptomatic and range in size from a few millimeters to 2 to 3 cm.

Histopathology. Characteristically, canalicular adenomas show bilayered strands of basaloid cells that branch and anastomose within a delicate stroma that is highly vascular and contains few fibroblasts and little collagen (Figures 8-23 and 8-24). Individual cells are characteristically cuboidal to columnar, with moderate to abundant amounts of eosinophilic cytoplasm. Canalicular adenomas occasionally may not be totally encapsulated, and more than 20% of cases are also multifocal.

Treatment and Prognosis. The treatment of choice for canalicular adenoma is surgical excision with the inclu-

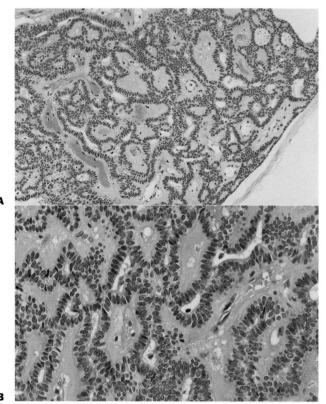

A

B

Figure 8-24   **A** and **B, Canalicular adenoma**. Note vascular stroma.

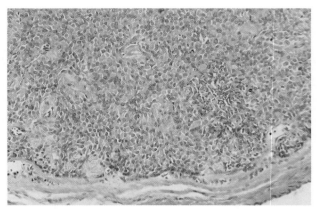

Figure 8-25   **Myoepithelioma** composed of plasmacytoid myoepithelial cells.

sion of a cuff of clinically normal tissue. The fact that more than 20% of lesions are multifocal may account for some recurrences.

Myoepithelioma. Benign salivary gland tumors composed entirely of myoepithelial cells are called *myoepitheliomas* (Figure 8-25). Although these tumors are of epithelial origin, the phenotypic expression of the tumor cells is more closely related to that of smooth muscle. Reflective of this is the immunohistochemical staining of myoepithelioma cells with antibodies to actins, cytokeratin, and S-100 protein.

Most myoepitheliomas arise within the parotid gland and, less commonly, the submandibular gland and intraoral minor salivary glands. Clinically, myoepitheliomas present as circumscribed painless masses. Lesions appear from the third through ninth decades (median age, 53 years) and in both genders equally.

Microscopically, sheets of either plasmacytoid or spindle cells make up these lesions. Approximately 70% of cases contain spindle cells, and approximately 20% are composed of plasmacytoid cells. Occasionally, both

cell forms may be seen in approximately equal quantity. Myoepithelial differentiation of tumor cells has been confirmed with immunohistochemical and electron microscopic studies. Rarely, clear cells may dominate the histologic presentation, leading to the designation of a "clear cell variant" of this entity.

Treatment of this benign lesion is identical to that of the benign mixed tumor. Conservative excision of lesions arising in minor salivary glands is advised, including a thin rim of surrounding normal tissue. When lesions are noted within the parotid gland, superficial parotidectomy is indicated. The overall prognosis is excellent, and recurrences are not expected.

Oncocytic Tumors

Oncocytoma. Oncocytoma, or oxyphilic adenoma, is a rare lesion seen predominantly in the parotid gland (Figures 8-26 to 8-28). This lesion is composed of *oncocytes*, large granular acidophilic cells filled with mitochondria. Such cells are normally found in salivary glands in the intralobular ducts, and they usually increase in number with age. The histogenetic origin of this lesion is believed to be from the salivary duct epithelium, in particular the striated duct.

Clinically, oncocytomas are solid, ovoid encapsulated lesions usually less than 5 cm in diameter when they are noted within the major salivary glands. In some instances bilateral occurrence may be noted. These lesions are rarely seen intraorally.

Within individual glands (most often the parotid) a nonneoplastic and multicentric cellular change known as *oncocytosis* may be seen. This metaplasia of salivary duct and acinar cells is seen in the context of

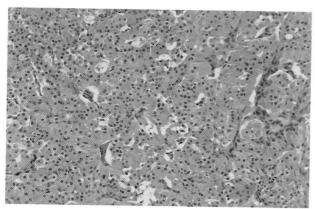

Figure 8-26 **Oncocytoma** composed of uniform cells with pink cytoplasm and centrally placed nuclei.

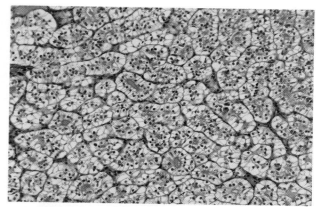

Figure 8-28 **Oncocytoma** with clear cell change.

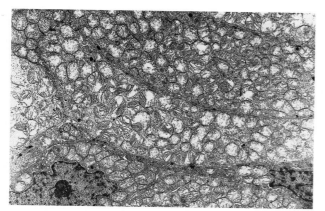

Figure 8-27 **Oncocytoma,** electron micrograph. Oncocytes filled with mitochondria; nuclei in lower left and right.

an otherwise normal gland. As oncocytic foci enlarge, confusion with oncocytoma may occur.

Microscopically, oncocytoma cells are polyhedral with granular eosinophilic cytoplasm. Nuclei are centrally placed and are typically vesicular. The histologic pattern is usually sheets of cells, although microcystic spaces and clear cell change may be seen. The histochemical stain phosphotungstic acid hematoxylin (PTAH), highlighting the intracytoplasmic mitochondria, is useful to confirm the diagnosis of oncocytoma. Antimitochondrial antibodies may also be used in an immunohistochemical approach to confirm diagnosis.

The growth rate is slow, and the course is benign. Treatment is conservative, with superficial parotidectomy as the treatment of choice for parotid lesions. In minor salivary glands, removal of the tumor with a margin of normal tissue is deemed to be adequate. Recurrence is rarely noted.

The malignant oncocytic tumor, or so-called malignant oncocytoma, is rare. The diagnosis is based on atypical nuclear changes in oncocytes in conjunction with an invasive pattern. Malignant change may arise de novo, or it may occur in a preexisting benign oncocytoma.

Papillary Cystadenoma Lymphomatosum (Warthin's Tumor). Papillary cystadenoma lymphomatosum, also known as Warthin's tumor, accounts for approximately 7% of epithelial neoplasms of salivary glands, with the vast majority occurring within the parotid gland (Figures 8-29 to 8-31). Intraorally, this lesion is rare. It is seen predominantly in men, typically between the fifth and eighth decades of life. Recent studies have shown a positive correlation between the development of Warthin's tumor and cigarette smoking.

Warthin's tumor is thought to arise within lymph nodes as a result of entrapment of salivary gland elements early in development. This theory is supported by the occasional case of multicentricity, as well as normal lymph node architecture surrounding many early or developing tumors. It is believed that some intraoral lesions may arise in an area of reactive lymphoid hyperplasia secondary to chronic inflammation.

When it occurs in the parotid, this tumor presents typically as a doughy to cystic mass in the inferior pole of the gland, adjacent and posterior to the angle of the mandible. In this situation the proximity of the submandibular gland may give the impression that the

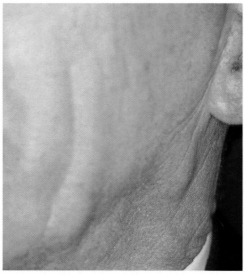

Figure 8-29 **Papillary cystadenoma lymphomatosum (Warthin's tumor)** in the tail of the parotid gland.

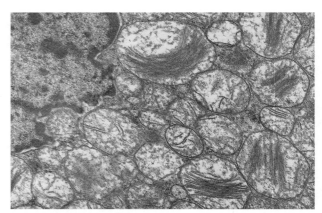

Figure 8-31 **Warthin's tumor.** Electron micrograph showing oncocytes in tumor cells. Note abundant mitochondria and nucleus *(upper left)*.

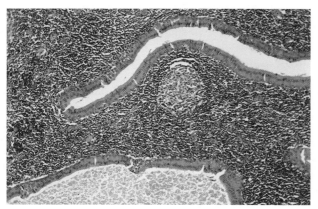

Figure 8-30 **Warthin's tumor** composed of pink oncocytes and lymphoid tissue.

lesion has developed within this gland rather than within the parotid.

This tumor is encapsulated and has a smooth to lobulated surface and a round outline. Microscopically, numerous cystic spaces of irregular outline contain papillary projections lined by columnar eosinophilic cells (oncocytes). The lining cells are supported by cuboidal cells that overlie lymphoid tissue with germinal centers.

Recurrences have been reported and documented but are believed to represent second primary lesions. Malignant transformation to carcinoma, especially as a complication of radiotherapy to the region, is rare.

Sebaceous Adenoma. The presence of sebaceous glands or evidence of sebaceous differentiation has been noted in submandibular and parotid salivary glands. This particular tissue, thought to originate in intralobular ducts, gives rise to sebaceous adenoma and to other sebaceous neoplasms designated as sebaceous lymphadenoma, sebaceous carcinoma, and sebaceous lymphadenocarcinoma. These rare lesions are composed predominantly of sebaceous gland–derived cells; they are well differentiated when benign, and moderately to poorly differentiated when malignant. In sebaceous lymphadenoma a benign lymphoid component is seen. The parotid gland is the site of chief involvement, although intraoral lesions have been reported. Parotidectomy is the treatment of choice when lesions arise in this gland. Surgical excision is used in cases of intraoral neoplasms.

Ductal Papillomas

Ductal papillomas comprise sialadenoma papilliferum, inverted ductal papilloma, and intraductal papilloma. These rare tumors are thought to arise within the interlobular and excretory duct portion of the salivary gland unit.

Sialadenoma papilliferum is an unusual benign salivary gland neoplasm that was first reported in 1969 as a distinct entity of minor and major salivary gland

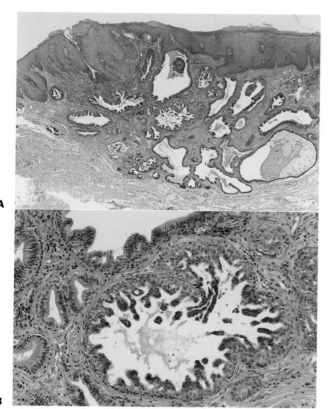

Figure 8-32   **Sialadenoma papilliferum. A and B,**
Papillary structures within cystlike spaces.

origin. The majority of cases reported subsequently have been found intraorally; the buccal mucosa and palate are the most common sites.

Sialadenoma papilliferum usually presents as a painless exophytic papillary lesion. Most cases have been reported in men between the fifth and eighth decades of life. The clinical impression before removal is that of a simple papilloma, owing to its frequent keratotic appearance and papillary surface configuration.

This tumor appears to originate from the superficial portion of the salivary gland excretory duct (Figure 8-32). Papillary processes develop, forming convoluted clefts and spaces. Each papillary projection is lined by a layer of epithelium approximately two to three cell layers thick and is supported by a core of fibrovascular connective tissue. The more superficial portions of the lesion demonstrate a squamous epithelial lining; deeper portions show more cuboidal to columnar cells, often oncocytic in appearance. As growth continues, the overlying mucous membrane becomes

papillary to verrucous in nature, much like a squamous papilloma. This lesion generally resembles syringocystadenoma papilliferum of the scalp, a lesion of eccrine sweat gland origin.

The behavior of this lesion is benign. Management is by conservative surgery; there is little chance of recurrence.

A related papillary lesion of salivary duct origin is *inverted ductal papilloma*. This is a rare entity that presents as a nodular submucosal mass resembling a fibroma or lipoma. It is seen in adults and has an equal gender distribution.

Microscopically, a marked proliferation of ductal epithelium is seen subjacent to intact mucosa (Figure 8-33). Crypts and cystlike spaces lined by columnar cells with polarized nuclei are interspersed with goblet cells and transitional forms of cuboidal to squamous cells.

The third form of ductal papilloma is *intraductal papilloma*. This rare lesion arises from a greater depth within the ductal system, often presenting as a salivary obstruction. Histologically, a single or double layer of cuboidal to columnar epithelium covers several papillary fronds that project into a duct, with no evidence of proliferation into the wall of the cyst (Figure 8-34). Treatment for this lesion, as well as inverted ductal papilloma, is simple excision. There is little risk of recurrence.

MALIGNANT NEOPLASMS

There are several ways to classify salivary gland malignancies. Box 8-5 lists them according to relative frequency, and Box 8-6 lists them according to biologic behavior. Box 8-7 is a summary of the general features that characterize malignancies of minor salivary glands. Table 8-2 compares features of benign and malignant salivary gland tumors.

Mucoepidermoid Carcinoma

Mucoepidermoid carcinomas exhibit biologic behaviors that range from low grade to high grade. All are capable of metastasis, but low-grade mucoepidermoid carcinomas typically pursue a locally invasive, relatively nonaggressive course. As the name implies, mucoepidermoid carcinomas are epithelial mucin-producing tumors. They are believed to arise from reserve cells in the interlobular and intralobular segments of the salivary duct system. The neoplastic mucous cells

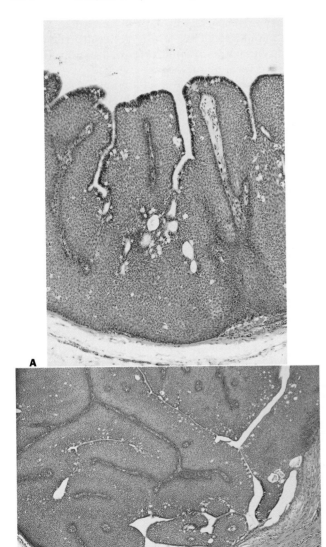

A

B

Figure 8-33 **Inverted ductal papilloma. A** and **B,** Circumscribed folds of bland ductal epithelial cells and occasional mucous cells.

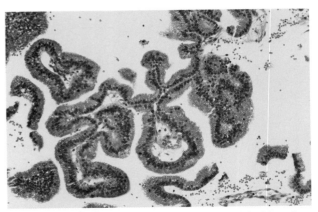

Figure 8-34 **Intraductal papilloma** composed of fronds of ductal cells. The duct from which this lesion is derived is not included in the photomicrograph.

Box 8-5 Malignant Salivary Gland Tumors

Mucoepidermoid carcinoma
Polymorphous low-grade adenocarcinoma
Adenoid cystic carcinoma
Clear cell carcinoma
Acinic cell carcinoma
Adenocarcinoma NOS
Rare, predominantly parotid tumors
   Carcinoma ex-mixed tumor/malignant mixed tumor
   Epimyoepithelial carcinoma
   Salivary duct carcinoma
   Basal cell adenocarcinoma
   Oncocytic adenocarcinoma
   Sebaceous adenocarcinoma
   Squamous cell carcinoma

NOS, Not otherwise specified.

contain neutral glycoproteins, acidic mucins, and sulfomucins; the epidermoid cells contain keratin intermediate filaments.

Clinical Features. The most common site of mucoepidermoid carcinomas is the parotid gland, where 60% to 90% of such lesions are encountered (Box 8-8). This lesion represents the most common malignant tumor of salivary glands and is also the most common salivary gland malignancy of childhood. Mucoepidermoid carcinomas account for approximately 34% of parotid malignancies, 20% of submandibular gland malignancies, and 30% of minor salivary gland malignancies. This lesion may also arise centrally within the mandible, presumably from embryonically entrapped salivary elements or from neoplastic transformation of mucous cells in odontogenic cysts.

The prevalence of mucoepidermoid carcinomas is noted to be highest in the third through fifth decades of life, and there is an equal gender representation. The clinical manifestations of this lesion depend greatly on the grade of malignancy (Figure 8-35). Tumors of low-grade malignancy present with a prolonged period of painless enlargement. Within the oral cavity mucoepidermoid carcinoma often resembles an

Box 8-6 Malignant Salivary Gland Tumors: Biologic Classification

LOW-GRADE MALIGNANCIES

Mucoepidermoid carcinoma (low grade)
Polymorphous low-grade adenocarcinoma
Acinic cell carcinoma (low to intermediate grade)
Clear cell carcinoma
Basal cell adenocarcinoma

INTERMEDIATE-GRADE MALIGNANCIES

Mucoepidermoid carcinoma (intermediate grade)
Epimyoepithelial carcinoma
Sebaceous adenocarcinoma

HIGH-GRADE MALIGNANCIES

Mucoepidermoid carcinoma (high grade)
Adenoid cystic carcinoma
Carcinoma ex-mixed tumor
Salivary duct carcinoma
Squamous cell carcinoma
Oncocytic adenocarcinoma

Box 8-7 Malignant Minor Salivary Tumors

CLINICAL FEATURES

Adults; men and women affected equally
Mass or ulcerated mass
Asymptomatic in early stages
Sites—palate > buccal mucosa > retromolar pad > upper lip > tongue
Low-grade mucoepidermoid carcinoma > polymorphous low-grade adenocarcinoma > adenoid cystic carcinoma

HISTOPATHOLOGY

Highly variable but characteristic patterns; infiltrative margins; rare mitoses; little pleomorphism

TREATMENT AND PROGNOSIS

Wide excision; radiation added for problematic cases
Ranges from low-grade to high-grade behavior (Adenoid cystic carcinoma has worst long-term prognosis.)

>, More frequently affected than/more common than.

TABLE 8-2   Comparison of Salivary Gland Tumors

	Benign	Malignant
Growth rate	Slow	Varied, usually rapid
Ulceration	No	Yes
Fixation	No	Yes
Facial nerve palsy	No	Yes
Encapsulated	Yes	No
Natural history	Slow growth	Slow to rapid growth
Metastasis	No	Yes
Treatment	Local excision	Surgery with or without radiation

Box 8-8 Mucoepidermoid Carcinoma

Most common malignancy of salivary glands
Adults
Most common salivary malignancy in children
Palate, most common intraoral site; rare primary intrabony (jaws) tumors
Low-, intermediate-, and high-grade lesions
    More ducts and mucous cells in low-grade lesions
    Most oral lesions are low grade
Low-grade lesions—excellent prognosis (~95%)
High-grade lesions—fair prognosis (~40%)

extravasation or retention-type mucocele that may at times be fluctuant as a result of mucous cyst formation. Tumors of high-grade malignancy, on the other hand, grow rapidly and are often accompanied by pain and mucosal ulceration. Within the major salivary glands, high-grade tumors may present with evidence of facial nerve involvement or obstructive signs. Mucoepidermoid carcinomas in the mandible or maxilla appear as radiolucent lesions within the molar and premolar area.

Histopathology. Mucoepidermoid carcinomas typically appear as a lobular infiltration of adjacent tissue, although they are often well circumscribed. Lesions are generally divided into low-grade, intermediate-grade, and high-grade types (Table 8-3). Low-grade mucoepidermoid carcinomas are composed of mucus-secreting cells arranged around microcystic structures, with an intermingling of epithelial, or "intermediate," cells (Figures 8-36 and 8-37). The mucin-containing cells are PAS and mucicarmine positive. Coalescence of small cysts into large cystic spaces is typical of low-grade malignancy. These cysts may distend the surrounding supportive tissue and rupture, allowing escape of mucus into the surrounding tissues, with a concomitant reactive inflammatory response. At the margin of low-grade tumors, the pattern is often one of broad, "pushing" fronts.

High-grade malignancies are characterized by neoplastic cell clusters composed chiefly of epidermoids

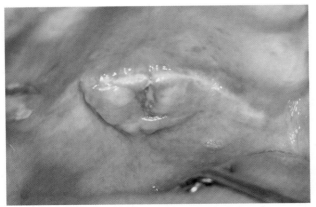

Figure 8-35 **Mucoepidermoid carcinoma** of the palate.

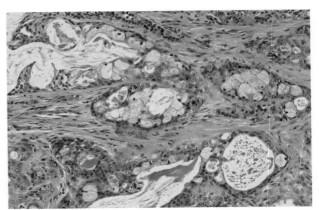

Figure 8-37 **Mucoepidermoid carcinoma**, low grade. Note cystic spaces and mucous tumor cells.

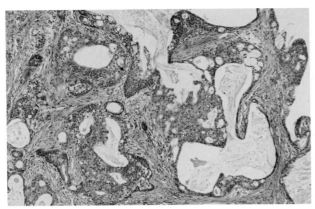

Figure 8-36 **Mucoepidermoid carcinoma**, low grade. Note cystic spaces and mucous tumor cells.

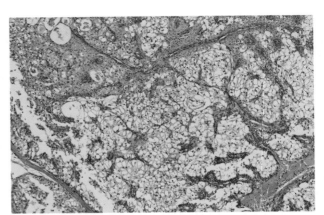

Figure 8-38 **Mucoepidermoid carcinoma** (intermediate grade) with a focus of clear cell change.

TABLE 8-3 **Mucoepidermoid Carcinoma: Histologic Grading**

	Low Grade (Good Prognosis)	High Grade (Fair Prognosis)
Cell type	Numerous mucous cells and intermediate cells Few epidermoid cells	Mainly epidermoid cells and few mucous cells; looks like squamous cell carcinoma
Microcystic spaces	Large and numerous cysts	Few cysts; mainly solid tumor
Cytologic atypia	None to little	Abundant

that are more solid with fewer cystic spaces and scattered mucous cells (Figures 8-38 and 8-39). Larger numbers of nonmucin-producing epithelial cells are seen at the expense of more-differentiated, mucous cells. Cellular pleomorphism, nuclear hyperchromatism, and mitotic figures may be noted within these tumors. In many high-grade mucoepidermoid carcinomas, much of the lesion may resemble squamous cell carcinoma, with only small numbers of mucous cells evident. In high-grade lesions, infiltration in the form of cords and strands of cells may be noted well beyond the obvious clinical focus of the tumor.

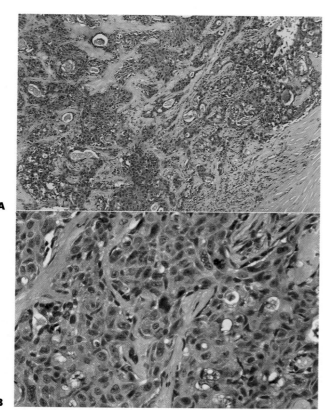

A

B

Figure 8-39 **A** and **B, Mucoepidermoid carcinoma,** high grade. Note that there are few tumor ducts and mucous cells.

Intermediate-grade lesions lie histologically and biologically between low- and high-grade lesions. Mucous cells and microcystic spaces are apparent, but not as numerous as in low-grade lesions. Cellular atypia is minimal.

Prognosis and Treatment. Prognostic significance may be ascribed to histologic grades of malignancy. Low-grade mucoepidermoid carcinomas characteristically follow a benign clinical course; however, in several instances low-grade lesions have metastasized widely. Clinical confirmation of the aggressiveness of high-grade carcinomas generally is evident within the first 5 years after the initial treatment, with local and distant metastases being evident in as many as 60% of cases. Incidences of metastases to cervical lymph nodes from mucoepidermoid carcinomas of the parotid gland (excluding low-grade lesions) have reached 44%. A 5-year survival rate of 95% or greater is associated with low-grade lesions. For high-grade lesions, however, sur-

vival rates are approximately 40%. In follow-up periods extended to 15 years, the cure rate for high-grade carcinomas drops to 25% or less.

Treatment of low-grade mucoepidermoid carcinomas is typically surgical. High-grade malignancies are usually managed with surgery plus postoperative radiotherapy to the primary site. Neck dissection is rarely performed in small lesions of low-grade malignancy; high-grade tumors usually require this form of management.

Central (intrabony) mucoepidermoid carcinomas are usually of low-grade histology and behavior. Most deaths occur because of uncontrolled local recurrence. When arising centrally in bone, these lesions have been associated with a 40% recurrence rate after simple curettage.

Polymorphous Low-Grade Adenocarcinoma

Polymorphous low-grade adenocarcinoma was first reported in 1983 by two different groups under the terms lobular carcinoma of salivary glands and terminal duct carcinoma. Today the term *polymorphous low-grade adenocarcinoma* is the accepted term for this entity. It has been segregated from other salivary tumors because of its distinctive clinical, histomorphologic, and behavioral aspects. This tumor is generally considered to be a low-grade malignancy with a relatively indolent course and low risk of recurrence and metastasis. The putative origin of the polymorphous low-grade adenocarcinoma is believed to be from reserve cells in the most proximal portion of the salivary duct. Myoepithelial-differentiated cells appear in this neoplasm, but only in slight to moderate numbers.

Clinical Features. This neoplasm occurs in the fifth through eighth decades of life, with a mean age of 59 years. There is no gender predilection. The lesion appears almost exclusively in minor salivary glands, with the palate being the most frequently reported site (Boxes 8-9 and 8-10). Polymorphous low-grade adenocarcinomas typically present as firm, elevated, nonulcerated nodular swellings that are usually nontender. A wide range in size has been noted, but most are between 1 and 4 cm in diameter. The slow growth rate is evidenced by the long duration—many months to years—before diagnosis and treatment. Neurologic symptoms are usually not reported in association with this tumor. Metastasis to local nodes is present at the time of diagnosis in approximately 10% of patients. Rare instances of lung metastasis have been reported.

Box 8-9 Polymorphous Low-Grade Adenocarcinoma

Malignancy of minor salivary gland; second in frequency to mucoepidermoid carcinoma
Presents as asymptomatic submucosal mass
Polymorphous microscopic pattern (Most cases show small nerve invasion, but no effect on prognosis.)
Low-grade malignancy; good prognosis
Treatment by wide excision; recurrence rate ~10%
Occasional metastasis
  Regional nodes ~10%
  Rare to lungs

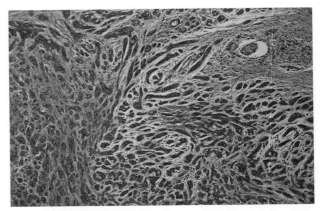

Figure 8-40   Polymorphous low-grade adenocarcinoma showing streaming pattern.

Box 8-10 Polymorphous Low-Grade Adenocarcinoma: Location

MINOR SALIVARY GLANDS

45% palate
20% lips
23% buccal mucosa
10% retromolar mucosa
1% floor of mouth
1% tongue

PAROTID GLAND

Few cases reported

SUBMANDIBULAR GLAND

Rare

NASAL/NASOPHARYNX

Few cases reported

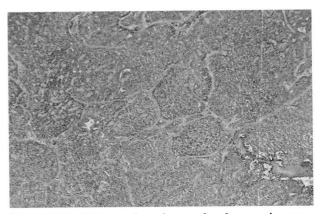

Figure 8-41   Polymorphous low-grade adenocarcinoma showing solid jigsaw pattern.

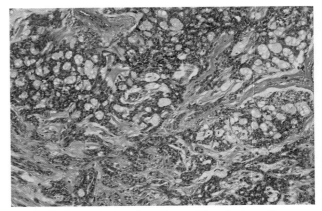

Figure 8-42   Polymorphous low-grade adenocarcinoma with a pseudocribriform pattern.

Histopathology. Absence of encapsulation together with infiltrating streams of cells and a general lobular morphology characterize this group of low-grade adenocarcinomas. Infiltration into the surrounding salivary gland and connective tissue is evident at low-power examination. In most areas the tumor is composed of a homogeneous population of cells with prominent, bland, often vesicular nuclei and minimal cytoplasm (Figures 8-40 to 8-45). These cells are arranged in lobules, as well as in solid nests. Tubules lined by a single layer of cells are also typical of this tumor. Cribriform structures bearing a resemblance to adenoid

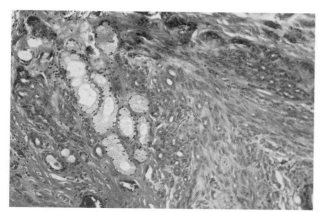

Figure 8-43 **Polymorphous low-grade adenocarcinoma** showing infiltrating tumor composed of single-layered ducts.

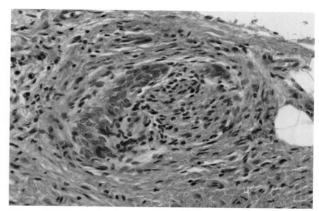

Figure 8-45 **Polymorphous low-grade adenocarcinoma** in perineural spaces.

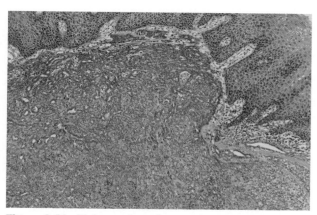

Figure 8-44 **Polymorphous low-grade adenocarcinoma** showing characteristic epithelial encroachment pattern.

cystic carcinoma may also be seen. Tumor cells, often spindled, are also arranged in trabeculae and narrow cords. Striking patterns in which concentric arrangements of individual cells appear around blood vessels and nerves may be noted. Perineural growth around small nerve twigs is evident in a majority of cases but appears to have no clinical relevance. Nuclear atypia, necrosis, and mitotic figures are absent.

Treatment and Prognosis. The indolent nature of this tumor mandates conservative surgical excision. With wide surgical excision the recurrence rate is approximately 10%. The role of radiation therapy in the primary treatment of polymorphous low-grade adenocarcinoma has yet to be fully assessed.

> **Box 8-11 Adenoid Cystic Carcinoma**
>
> High-grade salivary gland malignancy
> Adults; palatal mass/ulceration
> Cribriform microscopic pattern
> Spread through perineural spaces
> Local recurrence and metastasis; lung > nodes
> 5-year survival 70%; 15-year survival 10%
>
> >, More frequently than.

Adenoid Cystic Carcinoma

Adenoid cystic carcinoma is a high-grade malignancy that has a fair 5-year survival rate but a dismal 15-year survival rate. Typically showing little cellular atypia and only rare mitotic figures, it pursues an unrelenting course that defies most therapeutic measures.

Clinical Features. This lesion accounts for approximately 23% of all salivary gland carcinomas (Box 8-11). Approximately 50% to 70% of all reported cases of adenoid cystic carcinoma occur in minor salivary glands of the head and neck. In the major salivary glands the parotid gland is most often affected. Most patients with adenoid cystic carcinoma are in the fifth through seventh decades of life, and there is no gender predilection.

In the major salivary glands the clinical appearance is usually a unilobular mass that is firm on palpation, occasionally with some pain or tenderness. These lesions generally are characterized by a slow growth rate; they are often present for several years before

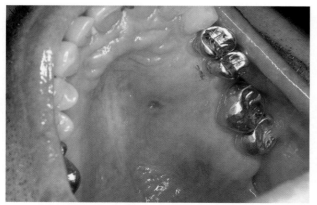

Figure 8-46 **Adenoid cystic carcinoma** of the palate.

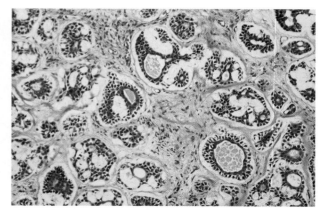

Figure 8-48 **Adenoid cystic carcinoma,** nests with retraction spaces.

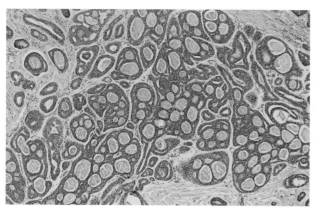

Figure 8-47 **Adenoid cystic carcinoma,** cribriform pattern.

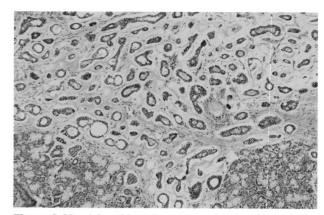

Figure 8-49 **Adenoid cystic carcinoma,** microinvasive pattern.

the patient seeks treatment. Facial nerve weakness or paralysis may occasionally be the initial presenting symptom, especially in late-stage lesions.

Bone invasion occurs often, initially without radiographic changes, because of infiltration through marrow spaces. Distant spread to the lungs is more common than metastasis to regional lymph nodes. It typically invades perineural spaces, leading to neoplasm well beyond the primary mass. A common feature of intraoral lesions, particularly those arising on the palate, is ulceration of the overlying mucosa, a point often used to help distinguish this lesion clinically from the more common benign mixed tumor (Figure 8-46).

Histopathology. There are three basic histomorphologic patterns: tubular, cribriform, and solid (Figures

8-47 to 8-53). The cribriform pattern is the best-recognized pattern and the prototypical one that typifies the tumor. The pseudocystic spaces contain sulfated mucopolysaccharides that are ultrastructurally characterized by multilayered or replicated basal lamina material. The tubular form is composed of smaller islands of cells with distinct ductlike structures centrally. The solid basaloid pattern shows little duct formation and is composed of larger islands of small-to medium-sized cells with small, dark nuclei. This type may also show more pleomorphism than the other forms and is associated with a poorer outcome. Areas of central necrosis within solid clusters of cells may indicate a more aggressive form of disease. Factors regarding prediction of behavior include the size of the histologic type, whether it is a primary lesion, the anatomic location, the presence or absence of metasta-

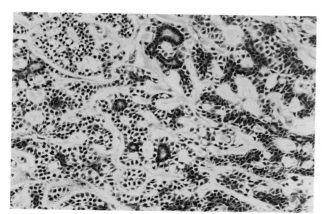

Figure 8-50 **Adenoid cystic carcinoma** with prominent clear cell layer surrounding inner ductal cells.

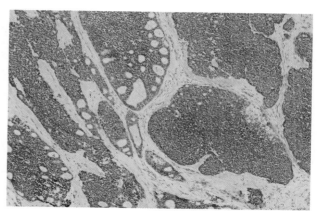

Figure 8-52 **Adenoid cystic carcinoma,** solid pattern.

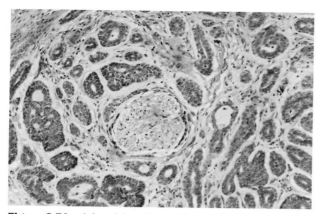

Figure 8-51 **Adenoid cystic carcinoma** showing perineural invasion.

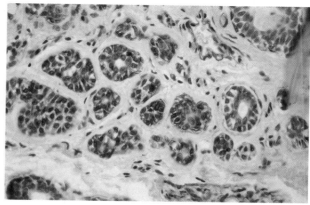

Figure 8-53 **Adenoid cystic carcinoma** stained for muscle-specific actin. Positive staining (*red*) is seen in outer layer of cells.

tic disease at the time of diagnosis, and facial nerve involvement.

Ductal structures are lined by cuboidal cells with uniform nuclei with condensed chromatin. An outer layer of cells with clear cytoplasm and angular nuclei characteristically surrounds the inner layer of cuboidal cells. The outer layer of cells exhibits myoepithelial differentiation and stains positive for actins. Nuclear atypia is absent or minimal, and mitotic figures are rare.

Treatment and Prognosis. Regardless of the site of the primary lesion, surgery is regarded as the treatment of choice for adenoid cystic carcinomas. When the parotid glands are involved, wide resection in the form of a superficial parotidectomy or superficial and deep

lobectomy is recommended. In the parotid region the debate is whether or not the facial nerve should be spared; most investigators recommend resection if the tumor surrounds or invades this nerve.

Intraorally, wide excision, often with removal of underlying bone, is the treatment of choice. Radical surgical excision may be justified to obtain surgical margins that are free of tumor.

Radiation therapy has shown promising results and has a role in the management of primary disease and recurrences, but to be effective, the radiation fields must be wide, reflecting the disseminated nature of the disease. Chemotherapy is generally regarded as ineffective, although multiple-agent chemotherapy has shown some promise in the management of widely metastatic disease. Immunohistochemical demon-

---

Box 8-12 Salivary Gland Clear Cell Tumors

CLEAR CELL TUMORS

Clear cell carcinoma
Epimyoepithelial carcinoma

CLEAR CELL CHANGE/ARTIFACT IN OTHER TUMORS

Adenoid cystic carcinoma
Oncocytoma
Acinic cell carcinoma
Mucoepidermoid carcinoma

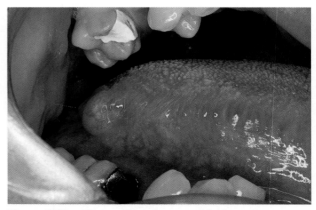

Figure 8-54   **Clear cell carcinoma** of the lateral tongue (Courtesy Dr. Francina Lozada-Nur).

stration of c-kit protein expression by this tumor may provide a basis for molecular therapeutic intervention.

The prognosis for patients with adenoid cystic carcinoma must be judged not in terms of 5-year survival rates but, rather, in terms of 15- to 20-year survival rates. Survival rates at 5 years approximate 70%; at 15 years the rate is only 10%. Factors that negatively influence the prognosis include the presence of tumor at the line of surgical excision, tumor size greater than 4 cm, and the presence of more than 30% of a solid pattern within the tumor. A long survival time has been positively correlated with a greater number of glandlike spaces per square millimeter within the tumor.

Clear Cell Carcinoma

There are four salivary gland tumors that, when poorly fixed, may have areas in which tumor cells exhibit clear cytoplasm, apparently as a result of autolysis of cytoplasmic organelles (Box 8-12). There are also two clear cell tumors—clear cell carcinoma and epimyoepithelial carcinoma (discussed later)—that exhibit clear cell changes that are due to cytoplasmic accumulation of glycogen and myofilaments, respectively. Clear cell carcinoma, formerly called hyalinizing clear cell carcinoma, is a low-grade tumor occurring predominantly in minor salivary glands (80% of cases). Most present as submucosal masses in the palate, although other sites may be affected (Figure 8-54). Microscopically, the neoplasm is composed of uniform bland cells, predominantly with clear cytoplasm (Figures 8-55 and 8-56). The pattern is typically trabecular, although nests and sheets of cells may be seen. The tumor cells stain positive for glycogen, but negative for mucin, S-100 protein, and muscle-specific actin. Treatment is by excision, and recurrences are very uncommon.

Acinic Cell Carcinoma

Acinic cell carcinoma occurs predominantly in the major salivary glands, especially the parotid. The putative origin of acinic cell carcinoma is from the intercalated duct reserve cell, although there is reason to believe that the acinic cell itself retains the potential for neoplastic transformation.

Clinical Features. Acinic cell carcinoma is found in all age-groups, including children, with the peak incidence noted within the fifth and sixth decades of life. There appears to be no gender predilection.

This lesion accounts for 14% of all parotid gland tumors and 9% of the total of salivary gland carcinomas of all sites. An unusual feature is the frequency of bilateral parotid gland involvement in approximately 3% of cases. Most cases develop within the superficial lobe and inferior pole of the parotid gland. Far fewer cases have been reported within the submandibular and intraoral minor salivary glands. Within the oral cavity most cases occur in the palate and buccal mucosa. Actinic cell carcinoma usually presents as a slow-growing lesion less than 3 cm in diameter. Although it is not indicative of the prognosis, pain is a common presenting symptom.

Histopathology. Acinic cell carcinoma typically grows in a solid pattern, although one third of lesions show a microcystic growth pattern (Figures 8-57 to 8-60). Papillary and follicular patterns may also be seen. Hemosiderin is often found, and there is little stromal tissue. Tumor cells are uniform and well differentiated. They often contain cytoplasmic PAS-positive, diastase. digestion-resistant granules similar to those found in normal acinic cells. Many acinic cell carcinomas

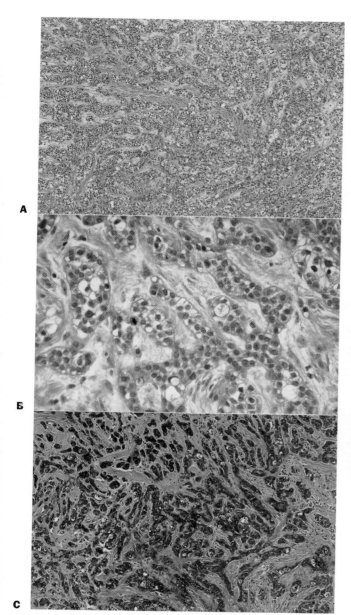

Figure 8-55 **A** and **B**, **Clear cell carcinoma,** trabecular arrangement of clear cells. **C,** Positive *(red)* PAS staining (glycogen) of tumor cells.

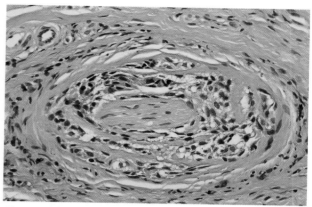

Figure 8-56 **Clear cell carcinoma** showing perineural invasion.

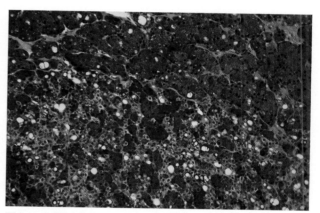

Figure 8-57 **Acinic cell carcinoma** with cells containing darkly staining zymogen granules.

demonstrate clear cell element zones, probably as a result of inadequate fixation.

Treatment and Prognosis. Surgery is the preferred treatment. In general, acinic cell carcinomas seldom metastasize, yet they have a tendency to recur. Determinant survival rates are 89% at 5 years and 56% at 20 years, indicating the overall malignant nature of these tumors. Metastases to regional lymph nodes

occur in approximately 10% of cases, whereas distant metastases occur in approximately 15% of cases. It has been found that neither the morphologic pattern nor the cell composition is a predictable prognostic feature. Unfavorable prognostic features include pain or fixation to surrounding tissue, gross tumor invasion into adjacent tissue, and microscopic features of desmoplasia, cellular atypia, and increased mitotic activity.

Adenocarcinoma Not Otherwise Specified

By definition, any malignancy arising from salivary duct epithelium or within salivary glands of epithelial origin is an adenocarcinoma. The term *adenocarcinoma not otherwise specified* is used as a diagnosis when lesions cannot be classified into existing categories. The "not

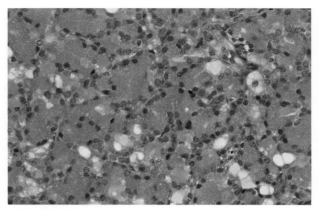

Figure 8-58 Acinic cell carcinoma.

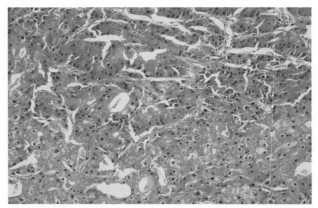

Figure 8-60 Acinic cell carcinoma with clear cell area (*bottom*).

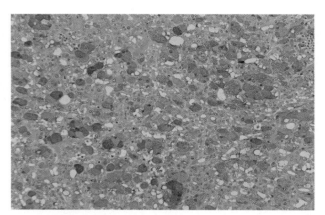

Figure 8-59 Acinic cell carcinoma.

otherwise specified (NOS)" label indicates that the microscopic appearance is nonspecific. Whether the lesion can be considered high grade depends on the presence of cellular atypia and an invasive growth pattern.

RARE TUMORS

Carcinoma Ex-Mixed Tumor/Malignant Mixed Tumor/Metastasizing Mixed Tumor

Carcinoma ex-mixed tumor represents an epithelial malignancy arising in a preexisting mixed tumor where such remnants may be identified. When metastatic disease occurs, only the malignant component metastasizes. This is more common than the so-called *malignant mixed tumor,* which has also been recognized. One type of the latter lesion is a malignancy in which both

the epithelial and the mesenchymal components are malignant; hence a carcinosarcoma designation could be used. In metastatic sites both elements are present. *Metastasizing mixed tumor* is characterized by a histologically benign mixed tumor that for some reason metastasizes while still retaining its bland, benign histologic appearance.

Carcinoma ex-mixed tumor usually arises from an untreated benign mixed tumor known to be present for several years or from a benign mixed tumor that has had many recurrences over many years (Figure 8-61). Malignancy occurring within a previously benign tumor is heralded by rapid growth after an extremely long period of minimally perceptible increase.

Approximately 68% of carcinoma ex-mixed tumors and malignant mixed tumors are found in the parotid gland, and 18% are found in the intraoral minor salivary glands. The average age when malignancy becomes evident is 60 years, approximately 20 years beyond the age noted for benign mixed tumors. Suspicious signs of malignancy include fixation of the mass to surrounding tissues, ulceration, and regional lymphadenopathy. Treatment is almost exclusively surgical, with radical neck dissection being part of the initial treatment in patients with evidence of cervical lymph node involvement.

Local recurrence is a problem in nearly half of patients with primary parotid neoplasms and in nearly three fourths of patients with submandibular and minor salivary gland tumors. Approximately 10% of cases present with uncontrollable lymphatic disease, with nearly one third of these showing metastasis to distant sites, usually lung and bone. Determinant cure

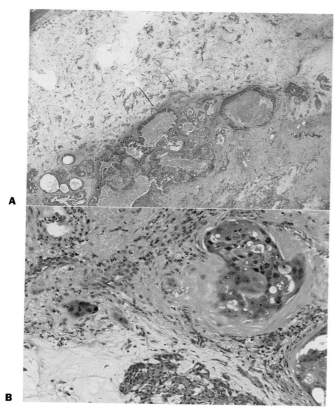

Figure 8-61 Carcinoma ex-mixed tumor. **A** and **B,** Note cellular atypia.

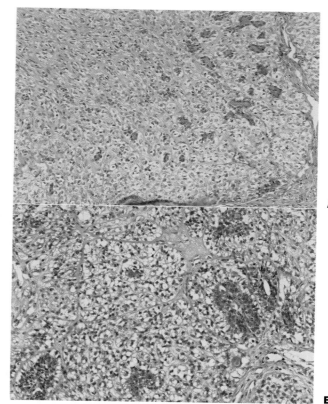

Figure 8-62 Epimyoepithelial carcinoma. **A** and **B,** Note clear cells surrounding darker-staining tumor ductal cells.

rates at 5, 10, and 15 years after treatment in one study were 40%, 24%, and 19%, respectively; in another study, 30% of those monitored for 10 years were free of disease.

Epimyoepithelial Carcinoma

Epimyoepithelial carcinoma is a clear cell containing malignancy of salivary gland (predominantly the major glands) origin. It is seen in the seventh and eighth decades of life, and there is a two-to-one female predilection.

A lobular growth is composed of two cell types: abundant clear cells with islands of cuboidal, darkly staining cells form a lumen. Glycogen, actins, and S-100 protein are present in these cells, supporting their myoepithelial origin (Figure 8-62).

Recurrences have most often been associated with lesions greater than 3 cm. The overall recurrence and metastasis rates suggest that this is a malignancy of intermediate grade.

Salivary Duct Carcinoma

Salivary duct carcinoma is a high-grade malignancy of the major salivary glands. It is characterized clinically by a distinctive predominance in the parotid gland (more than 80% of cases); the submandibular gland accounts for the remainder of cases. Nearly 80% of cases have been recorded in men, and the overall peak incidence is in the seventh decade. The lesion arises as a firm, painless mass. A striking microscopic resemblance to ductal carcinomas originating in the breast is noted, with architectural features that include papillary cribriform and solid growth patterns, along with a desmoplastic stroma and comedo necrosis. Nuclear atypia is noted, but few mitoses are seen. Most tumors have infiltrative margins, with neural invasion evident in approximately 50% of cases.

Surgical excision is the treatment of choice. Large series indicate that more than 50% of patients die of their disease within 5 months to 6 years after treatment. Pulmonary and osseous metastases are often noted.

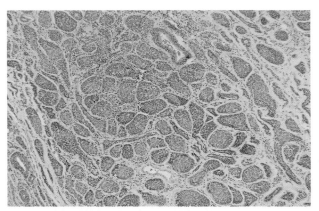

Figure 8-63   **Basal cell adenocarcinoma** in nested pattern.

Basal Cell Adenocarcinoma

Basal cell adenocarcinoma, a rare tumor of the major salivary glands, is believed to be the malignant counterpart of basal cell adenoma. It appears microscopically similar to basal cell adenoma, except that it exhibits an infiltrative growth pattern and has the ability to metastasize. These tumors are composed of nests, cords, and solid zones of basaloid cells (Figure 8-63). Two cytologic types of cells are often seen: small, compact cells and larger, polygonal cells. The former may often be seen surrounding the latter, often in a palisade fashion. The feature that separates this tumor from basal cell adenoma is the finding of small nests of neoplasm in adjacent normal structures. Infiltration of nerve is also seen. Local recurrence and distant metastasis seem to be distinct potentials for basal cell adenocarcinoma. Nonetheless, this tumor is generally regarded as a low-grade malignancy. With adequate surgical treatment, patients should have a favorable outcome.

Squamous Cell Carcinoma

Squamous cell carcinoma arising within the salivary glands is a relatively rare event and seems to be limited to the major salivary glands. The submandibular gland is most commonly involved, followed by the parotid. Obstructive sialadenitis (more common in the submandibular gland) has been thought to be a predisposing condition. Most patients are in the seventh decade of life or beyond.

Squamous cell carcinomas of the parotid and submandibular glands are generally well to moderately well differentiated with no evidence of mucin production. Metastatic squamous cell carcinoma and high-grade mucoepidermoid carcinoma are usually alternative diagnoses.

Local recurrence and regional lymph node metastasis are common events, and distant metastasis is unusual. Surgery is the treatment of choice. As with most other salivary gland malignancies, ultimate survival relates more to the clinical stage than to histologic differentiation.

BIBLIOGRAPHY

REACTIVE LESIONS (NONINFECTIOUS)

Brannon R, Fowler C, Hartman K: Necrotizing sialometaplasia: a clinico-pathologic study of sixty-nine cases and review of the literature, *Oral Surg Oral Med Oral Pathol* 72:317-325, 1991.

Bryant C, Manisali M, Barrett AW: Adenomatoid hyperplasia of palatal minor salivary glands, *J Laryngol Otol* 110(2):167-169, 1996.

Buchner A, Merrel PW, Carpenter WM, et al: Adenomatoid hyperplasia of minor salivary glands, *Oral Surg Oral Med Oral Pathol* 71:583-587, 1991.

Fowler CB, Brannon RB: Subacute necrotizing sialadenitis: report of 7 cases and a review of the literature, *Oral Surg Oral Med Oral Pathol Oral Radiol Endod* 89:600-609, 2000.

Jensen JL: Superficial mucoceles of the oral mucosa, *Am J Dermatopathol* 12:88-92, 1990.

McClatchey KD, Appelblatt NH, Zarbo RJ: Plunging ranula, *Oral Surg Oral Med Oral Pathol* 57:408-412, 1984.

Stephens LC, Schultheiss TE, Price RE, et al: Radiation apoptosis of serous acinar cells of salivary and lacrimal glands, *Cancer* 67:1539-1543, 1991.

Wolff A, Fox PC, Ship JA, et al: Oral mucosal status and major salivary gland function, *Oral Surg Oral Med Oral Pathol* 70:49-54, 1990.

INFECTIOUS CONDITIONS

Flaitz C: Parotitis as the initial sign of juvenile Sjögren's syndrome, *Pediatr Dent* 23:140-142, 2001.

Mitchell I, Turk J, Mitchell D: Detection of mycobacterial rRNA in sarcoidosis with liquid-phase hybridization, *Lancet* 339:1015-1017, 1992.

Saboor S, Johnson N, McFadden J: Detection of mycobacterial DNA in sarcoidosis and tuberculosis with polymerase chain reaction, *Lancet* 339:1012-1015, 1992.

Sabatino G, Verrotti A, de Martino M, et al: Neonatal suppurative parotitis: a study of five cases, *Eur J Pediatr* 158:312-314, 1999.

CONDITIONS ASSOCIATED WITH IMMUNE DEFECTS

Atkinson JC, Travis WD, Pillemer SR, et al: Major salivary function in primary Sjögren's syndrome and its relationship to clinical features, *J Rheumatol* 17:318-322, 1990.

Caselitz J, Osborn M, Wustrow J, et al: Immunohistochemical investigations on the epimyoepithelial islands in lymphoepithelial lesions, *Lab Invest* 55:427-432, 1986.

Daniels TE, Fox PC: Salivary and oral components of Sjögren's syndrome, *Rheum Dis Clin North Am* 18:571-589, 1992.

Daniels TE, Whitcher JP: Association of patterns of labial salivary gland inflammation with keratoconjunctivitis sicca, *Arthritis Rheum* 37:869-877, 1994.

Falzon M, Isaacson PG: The natural history of benign lymphoepithelial lesion of the salivary gland in which there is a monoclonal population of B-cells, *Am J Surg Pathol* 15:59-65, 1991.

Fox RI, Luppi M, Kang HI, et al: Reactivation of Epstein-Barr virus in Sjögren's syndrome, *Springer Semin Immunopathol* 13:217-231, 1991.

Garry RF, Fermin CD, Darrenn JH, et al: Detection of a human intracisternal A-type retroviral particle antigenically related to HIV, *Science* 250:1127-1129, 1990.

Jordan R, Diss TC, Lench NJ, et al: Immunoglobulin gene rearrangements in lymphoplasmacytic infiltrates of labial salivary glands in Sjögren's syndrome, *Oral Surg Oral Med Oral Pathol Oral Radiol Endod* 79:723-729, 1995.

Schiodt M: HIV-associated salivary gland disease: a review, *Oral Surg Oral Med Oral Pathol* 73:164-167, 1992.

Talal N: Immunologic and viral factors in Sjögren's syndrome, *Clin Exp Rheumatol* 8(suppl 5):23-26, 1990.

Talal N, Dauphinee MJ, Dang H, et al: Detection of serum antibodies to retroviral proteins in patients with primary Sjögren's syndrome (autoimmune exocrinopathy), *Arthritis Rheum* 33:774-781, 1990.

BENIGN NEOPLASMS

Batsakis JG, Luna MA, El-Naggar AK: Basaloid monomorphic adenomas, *Ann Otol Rhinol Laryngol* 100:687-690, 1991.

Brannon RB, Sciubba JJ, Giuliani M: Benign papillary intraoral minor salivary gland tumors: a report of 19 cases and a review of the literature, *Oral Surg Oral Med Oral Pathol Oral Radiol Endod* 92:68-77, 2001.

Chung YF, Khoo ML, Heng MK, et al: Epidemiology of Warthin's tumor of the parotid gland in an Asian population, *Br J Surg* 85:661-664, 1994.

Noguchi S, Aihara T, Yoshino K, et al: Demonstration of monoclonal origin of human parotid gland pleomorphic adenoma, *Cancer* 77:431-435, 1996.

Rousseau A, Mock D, Dover DG, et al: Multiple canalicular adenomas. A case report and review of the literature, *Oral Surg Oral Med Oral Pathol Oral Radiol Endod* 87:346-350, 1999.

Smith BC, Ellis GL, Slater L, et al: Sclerosing polycystic adenosis of major salivary glands: a clinicopathologic analysis of nine cases, *Am J Surg Pathol* 20:161-170, 1996.

MALIGNANT NEOPLASMS

Auclair PL, Goode RK, Ellis GL: Mucoepidermoid carcinoma of minor salivary glands, *Cancer* 69:2021-2030, 1992.

Batsakis JG, El-Naggar AK: Terminal duct adenocarcinomas of salivary tissues, *Ann Otol Rhinol Laryngol* 100:251-253, 1991.

Brandwein MS, Jagirdar J, Patil J, et al: Salivary duct carcinoma (cribriform salivary carcinoma of excretory ducts), *Cancer* 65:2307-2314, 1990.

Brookstone MS, Huvos AS: Central salivary gland tumors of the maxilla and mandible: a clinicopathologic study of 11 cases with an analysis of the literature, *J Oral Maxillofac Surg* 50:229-236, 1992.

Callendar DL, Frankenthaler RA, Luna MA, et al: Salivary gland neoplasms in children, *Arch Otolaryngol Head Neck Surg* 118:472-476, 1992.

Castle JT, Thompson LDR, Frommelt RA, et al: Polymorphous low grade adenocarcinoma: a clinicopathologic study of 164 cases, *Cancer* 86:207-219, 1999.

Dardick I, Gliniecki MR, Heathcote J, et al: Comparative histogenesis and morphogenesis of mucoepidermoid carcinoma and pleomorphic adenoma, *Virchows Arch A Pathol Anat Histopathol* 417:405-417, 1990.

Goode RK, Auclair PL, Ellis GL: Mucoepidermoid carcinoma of the major salivary glands, *Cancer* 82:1217-1224, 1998.

Hamper K, Lazar F, Dietel M, et al: Prognostic factors for adenoid cystic carcinoma of the head and neck, *J Oral Pathol Med* 19:101-107, 1990.

Holst VA, Marshall CE, Moskaluk CA, et al: KIT protein expression and analysis of c-kit gene mutation in adenoid cystic carcinoma. *Mod Pathol* 12:956-960, 1999.

Jeng YM, Lin CY, Hsu HC: Expression of the c-kit protein is associated with certain subtypes of salivary glnad carcinomas. *Cancer Lett* 154:107-111, 2000.

Lewis JE, Olsen KD, Sebo TJ: Carcinoma ex pleomorphic adenoma: pathologic analysis of 73 cases, *Hum Pathol* 32:596-604, 2001.

Lewis JE, Olsen KD, Weiland LH: Acinic cell carcinoma: clinicopathologic review, *Cancer* 67:172-179, 1991.

Milchgrub S, Gnepp DR, Vuitch F, et al: Hyalinizing clear cell carcinoma of salivary gland, *Am J Surg Pathol* 18:74-82, 1994.

Norberg LE, Burford-Mason AP, Dardick I: Cellular differentiation and morphologic heterogeneity in polymorphous low-grade adenocarcinoma, *J Oral Pathol Med* 20:373-379, 1991.

Ogawa Y, Hong SS, Toyosawa S, et al: Expression of major histocompatibility complex class II antigens and interleukin-1 by epithelial cells of Warthin's tumor, *Cancer* 66:2111-2117, 1990.

Seifert G, Brocheriou C, Cardesa A, et al: WHO International Classification of Tumors: tentative histological classification of salivary gland tumors, *Pathol Res Pract* 186:555-581, 1990.

Simpson RHW, Clarke TJ, Sarsfield PTL, et al: Epithelial-myoepithelial carcinoma of salivary glands, *J Clin Pathol* 44:419-423, 1991.

Simpson R, Sarsfield P, Clarke T, et al: Clear cell carcinoma of minor salivary glands, *Histopathology* 17:433-438, 1990.

van der Waal JE, Snow GB, van der Waal I: Intraoral adenoid cystic carcinoma: the presence of perineural spread in relation to site, size, local extension and metastatic spread in 22 cases, *Cancer* 66:2031-2033, 1990.

Vincent SD, Hammond HL, Finkelstein MW: Clinical and therapeutic features of polymorphous low-grade adenocarcinoma, *Oral Surg Oral Med Oral Pathol* 77:41-47, 1994.

Waldron CA, Koh ML: Central mucoepidermoid carcinoma of the jaws: report of four cases with analysis of the literature and discussion of the relationship to mucoepidermoid, sialodontogenic and glandular odontogenic cysts, *J Oral Maxillofac Surg* 48:871-877, 1990.

Yoo J, Robinson RA: H-ras gene mutations in salivary gland mucoepidermoid carcinomas, *Cancer* 88:518-523, 2000.

LYMPHOID LESIONS

REACTIVE LESIONS

In this chapter three primary groupings of lesions—reactive, developmental, and neoplastic—are considered. An important point in the discussion of lymphoid lesions involving the oral cavity and adjacent areas is that many lesions, especially those arising in lymph nodes, are capable of simulating malignancy.

Lymphoid Hyperplasia

It is sometimes difficult to distinguish reactive from neoplastic lymphoid proliferations, especially when they occur in unusual sites such as the peritonsillar area, palate, buccal mucosa, lymph nodes, and salivary glands. There is also an increasing incidence of benign cystic lymphoepithelial lesions within the parotid and submandibular glands in patients with acquired immunodeficiency syndrome (AIDS).

One of the normal sites of lymphoid tissue is the posterolateral portion of the tongue. The aggregations of lymphoid tissue within this area are part of the *foliate papillae,* or lingual tonsil. They may be distinguished from other lymphoid tissues by deep crypts lined by stratified squamous epithelium. These papillae occasionally become inflamed or irritated, with associated enlargement and tenderness. In such instances patients may become symptomatic. On examination these areas are enlarged and somewhat lobular in outline, with an intact overlying mucosa and prominent superficial vessels. In instances in which such lesions are removed for diagnostic purposes, the chief finding is reactive lymphoid hyperplasia. Within the enlarged germinal centers, mitoses and macrophages containing cellular debris may be seen. In addition to the foliate papillae, other zones where lymphoid tissue is found include the anterior floor of the mouth on either side of the lingual frenum, the anterior tonsillar pillar, and the posterior portion of the soft palate (Figures 9-1 and 9-2). Because lymphoid tissues are not always found in these areas, they are usually regarded as ectopic. The term *oral tonsil* also refers to this tissue.

Reactive lymphoid hyperplasia (oral tonsil) has male predominance and is noted within the second and third decades of life. In one study, a mean of 23 years was found. The lesions range from 1 to 15 mm in diameter and may persist for years.

The *buccal* or *facial lymph node* is often the site of a reactive hyperplastic process. This is characterized as a freely movable submucosal nodule in the buccal mucosa that is usually adjacent to the second premolar and first molar teeth and can often be palpated extraorally. The cause of the process is unknown, but it may be a reaction to irritation or localized trauma. Gingivitis or periapical pathology may occasionally stimulate or initiate enlargement of this particular lymph node.

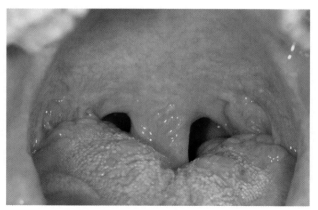

Figure 9-1 **Hyperplastic lymphoid tissue** in uvula and tonsillar areas.

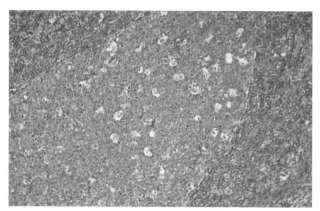

Figure 9-2 **Hyperplastic lymphoid follicle** with prominent macrophages (light-staining cells).

Management should be directed toward elimination of the cause of the problem if it can be identified, followed by simple observation.

Follicular lymphoid hyperplasia may be seen in the palate. This reactive polyclonal proliferation of lymphocytes is often difficult to separate from *lymphoproliferative disease of the palate*, a condition that may signify lymphoma. Histologically, follicular lymphoid hyperplasia of the palate is characterized by irregularly sized, well-demarcated germinal centers with a crisply defined rim or mantle of small, mature lymphocytes. Within the germinal centers, macrophages contain phagocytosed nuclear debris. Using immunohistochemical techniques, a mixture of kappa and lambda light chains (B-lymphocytes) is seen, indicating polyclonality. In addition, the mantle zones are composed of both mature and immature B cells, whereas the extramantle zones contain both B and T lymphocytes, plasma cells, macrophages, and eosinophils. Indefinite follow-up is prudent because of possible progression to lymphoma.

Angiolymphoid Hyperplasia With Eosinophilia

Angiolymphoid hyperplasia with eosinophilia (ALHE), also known as *epithelioid hemangioma,* was first described in 1948 as a nodular subcutaneous benign disease in young men. Later, however, cases with the same clinical and histologic features were reported in the oral cavity. In addition to nodular aggregates of lymphocytes and eosinophils, regional lymphadenopathy and blood (peripheral) eosinophilia were noted. Similar findings were also noted under the headings of *Kimura's disease,* eosinophilic granuloma of soft tissue, and eosinophilic lymphofolliculosis. Because Kimura's disease was originally described as having a distinct male predilection without the associated regional lymphadenopathy, some clinicians believe that the two conditions represent different entities. Histologically, some differences have also been described, adding to the tendency to split ALHE and Kimura's disease into two separate but related entities.

Etiology. Because of vascular proliferation and an intensive inflammatory infiltrate, a reactive etiology has been suggested. Increased serum immunoglobulin E (IgE) levels and deposition of IgE within the lymphoid follicles further suggest a reactive immune cause. Also demonstrated has been the presence of anti–*Candida albicans* antibody within the lesions and improvement after hyposensitization to this allergen.

Clinical Features. ALHE is found predominantly in the head and neck area, accounting for approximately 85% of all cases. However, oral mucous membrane involvement is rare. The labial mucosa is the oral site most commonly affected. There is a wide age range from 7 to 79 years and a mean age of 35 years. Lesions generally are solitary, with a mean size of 1.7 cm reported. Peripheral eosinophilia greater than 4% has been noted in 60% of the cases in which peripheral blood counts have been studied. The clinical course is characterized by the presence of a painless, mobile, submucosal nodule that enlarges gradually. Multiple lesions have been reported in more than 40% of cases.

Histopathology. Lesions are circumscribed and usually are grossly separable from surrounding tissue. A nodular mass of hyperplastic lymphoid tissue with well-developed lymphoid follicles containing germinal centers may be seen. Proliferating capillaries with plump endothelial cells are found in a dense, patchy infiltrate of lymphocytes, with eosinophils and fewer numbers of macrophages noted. Toward the periphery, this infiltrate may extend into surrounding soft tissue. Arterial intimal proliferation and disruption of the internal elastic lamina may be seen. Early lesions or those in an active growth phase may be dominated by a vascular element; older or quiescent lesions may contain a larger percentage of inflammatory cells.

Differential Diagnosis. When it involves the labial mucosa, ALHE's characteristic nodule may be indistinguishable from a minor salivary gland neoplasm or a mucus retention cyst or mucocele. Other benign soft tissue neoplasms, such as lipoma and schwannoma, might be included in the differential diagnosis.

Because of the presence of eosinophils within tissue, a microscopic differential diagnosis should include Langerhans cell disease (eosinophilic granuloma), traumatic (eosinophilic) granuloma, and possibly a drug reaction or parasitic infection.

Treatment. Excision is the treatment of choice. Intralesional steroid injections have also been used with variable results. Recurrences are occasionally noted. The presence of blood or peripheral eosinophilia has generally been reported with numerous or recurrent lesions.

DEVELOPMENTAL LESIONS

Lymphoepithelial Cyst

Lymphoepithelial cyst is an uncommon lesion of the mouth, major salivary glands, or neck that is thought to arise from an entrapment of epithelium within lymph nodes or lymphoid tissue during development. Subsequent epithelial proliferation results in a clinically evident mass.

Oral lymphoepithelial cysts (see also the discussion on ectopic lymphoid tissue in Chapter 3) present as asymptomatic mucosal elevations that are well defined and yellowish pink (Figure 9-3). The site most commonly affected is the floor of the mouth, where approximately 50% of cases are found. The ventral and posterolateral portions of the tongue constitute an additional 40% of cases; the balance is shared among the soft palate, mucobuccal fold, and anterior facial pillars. A wide age range is noted, from adolescence to the seventh decade of life. The gender distribution is essentially equal. Except for the small central cystic

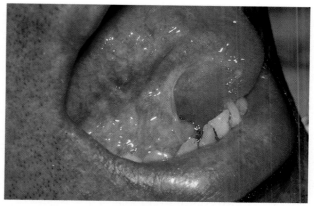

Figure 9-3   **Lymphoepithelial cyst** in lingual frenum.

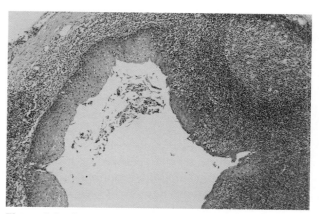

Figure 9-4   **Lymphoepithelial cyst.** Squamous epithelial lining and lymphoid tissue in surrounding tissue.

space, these lesions are identical to ectopic lymphoid aggregates.

A marked increase in the incidence of lymphoepithelial cysts of the major salivary glands has been noticed recently, particularly in those testing positive for the human immunodeficiency virus (HIV). The mechanism of cyst formation is unclear.

Histopathology. The lymphoepithelial cyst is lined by stratified squamous epithelium that is often parakeratotic. There may be focal areas of pseudostratified columnar cells or mucous cells. The epithelial lining is surrounded by a discrete, well-circumscribed lymphoid component, often with germinal center formation and a sharply defined zone of mantle lymphocytes. In addition, the cyst wall may contain variable proportions of lymphocytes, macrophages, plasma cells, and occasional multinucleated giant T cells (Figure 9-4). Continuity of the cyst lining with the surface oral epithelium may occasionally be noted.

Differential Diagnosis. In the anterior floor of the mouth, a sialolith may be similar in appearance to a lymphoepithelial cyst. However, a history of pain and swelling of the associated salivary gland would be expected with a salivary duct stone. Developmental anomalies such as teratomas or dermoid cysts, benign mesenchymal neoplasms, and salivary gland tumors might also be considered in a differential diagnosis for a floor-of-mouth soft tissue mass. When it involves the parotid gland, a lymphoepithelial cyst must be distinguished from salivary lymphoma, Warthin's tumor, and cystic neoplasms of salivary origin.

Treatment. Conservative excisional biopsy is generally used for definitive diagnosis, as well as for treatment. Recurrence is not expected.

NEOPLASMS

Lymphoma

Lymphomas are malignant neoplasms of component cells of lymphoid tissues. A broad division of the group into Hodgkin's disease and non-Hodgkin's lymphoma is widely accepted. Hodgkin's disease is primarily a disease of lymph nodes characterized by the presence of Reed-Sternberg cells and a lymphoid stroma composed of large numbers of nonneoplastic cells. These are very rare in the oral cavity.

Non-Hodgkin's Lymphoma

Non-Hodgkin's lymphomas (NHLs) are a relatively common group of neoplasms (more than 50,000 cases per year) that often occur in extranodal head and neck sites, especially in HIV-infected (AIDS) patients. NHLs comprise a heterogeneous group of lymphoid neoplasms with a spectrum of behavior. Some are indolent but ultimately fatal; others are aggressive and if left untreated kill the patient rapidly. NHL can arise in lymph nodes (nodal) and extranodal sites. Up to 40% of all NHLs arise at extranodal sites, with the most common site being the gastrointestinal tract. In the West they most commonly occur in the stomach, but in the Middle East the intestine is the most common location. The head and neck is the second most common site for extranodal NHL, with the majority of cases arising in Waldeyer's ring.

　　Similar to lymphomas arising in lymph nodes, B-cell lymphomas are the most common phenotype in extranodal sites. A wide histologic and biologic spectrum of B-cell lymphomas occurs in the head and neck. Although most are diffuse large B-cell lymphomas, other types are seen in specific sites and populations of patients. These include Burkitt's lymphoma occurring in the facial bones of young patients and T-cell and natural killer cell lymphomas in the nasofacial region, producing the clinical condition termed *midline granuloma*. A large proportion of lymphomas arise within lymph nodes embedded in the salivary tissues. Lymphomas may also arise within salivary gland parenchyma and resemble those arising in mucosa-associated lymphoid tissue (MALT). This group of tumors, now known as extranodal marginal zone lymphomas, is genotypically and phenotypically unique and is characterized by a relatively long natural history.

Classification. The microscopic classification of NHL continues to be a source of controversy. At least eight classifications have been proposed over the past 30 years, but none have gained universal acceptance. The current and most widely adopted system is known as the *Revised European American Lymphoma (REAL)* scheme, proposed by the International Lymphoma Study group (Table 9-1). This scheme divides lymphomas into T- and B-cell groups and includes a number of entities that arise at extranodal sites. This system focuses on distinct biologic entities defined by a combination of clinical, morphologic, immunophenotypic, and genotypic features. It has been shown to be highly reproducible and clinically relevant. Moreover, since it is a list of entities, new lymphomas can be added when they are identified and characterized. However, the REAL classification has been criticized for its heavy reliance on immuno-histochemical phenotyping and its problematic application when there is missing or limited clinical information. Moreover, since it is a list of entities without biologic groupings, learning the system is difficult. The most recent World Health Organization (WHO) lymphoma classification is essentially based on the REAL system with some minor modifications.

Etiology. Little is known of the etiology of NHL. Variations in the incidence in different ethnic groups suggest that there is a strong genetic predisposition. Immunodeficiency, whether acquired or congenital, is an important risk factor for the development of some lymphomas and may be related to a defective immune response to the Epstein-Barr virus (EBV), permitting clonal expansion of infected cells. Some lymphomas are also clearly associated with specific chromosome

TABLE 9-1 Revised European-American Lymphoma (REAL) Classification of Lymphoid Neoplasms

	B-Cell Neoplasms	T-Cell and Postulated NK-Cell Neoplasms
Precursor cell neoplasms	Precursor B-lymphoblastic lymphoma/leukemia	Precursor T-lymphoblastic lymphoma/leukemia
Peripheral (mature) cell neoplasms	B-cell chronic lymphocytic leukemia/small lymphocytic lymphoma (B-CLL/SLL) Lymphoplasmacytoid lymphoma Mantle cell lymphoma Marginal zone B-cell lymphoma (extranodal or nodal) Splenic marginal zone B-cell lymphoma Hairy cell leukemia Plasmacytoma Diffuse large B-cell lymphoma Burkitt's lymphoma	T-cell chronic lymphocytic leukemia Large granular lymphocytic leukemia (T-cell or NK-cell type) Mycosis fungoides Peripheral T-cell lymphoma, unspecified Angioimmunoblastic lymphoma Intestinal T-cell lymphoma Adult T-cell lymphoma/leukemia Anaplastic large cell lymphoma

NK, Natural killer; *B-CLL/SLL*, B-cell chronic lymphocytic leukemia/small lymphocytic lymphoma.

TABLE 9-2 Characteristic Cytogenetic Findings in Selected, Specific Lymphomas

Lymphoma Type	Translocation	Oncogene or Tumor Suppressor Genes	Mechanism
Follicular lymphoma	t(14;18)	*Bcl-2*	Juxtaposition of *Bcl-2* with IgH promoter results in overexpressed antiapoptotic protein Bcl-2
Extranodal marginal zone lymphoma	t(11;18) t(1;14)	*API2, MLT* *Bcl-10*	Chimeric protein that inhibits apoptosis Juxtaposition of *Bcl-10* with IgH promoter results in overexpressed Bcl-10 protein
Mantle cell lymphoma	t(11;14)	*Bcl-1 (Cyclin D-1)*	Juxtaposition of *Bcl-1* with IgH promoter results in overexpressed cyclin D1 protein
Burkitt's lymphoma	t(8;14) t(8;22) t(2;8)	*c-Myc*	Overexpression of *myc* is due to juxtaposition of the *c-Myc* gene with IgH, Igκ, or Igλ
Anaplastic large cell lymphoma	t(2;5)	*NPM, ALK*	Production of chimeric NPM-ALK protein, which has tyrosine kinase activity

Ig, Immunoglobulin.

translocations such as t(8;14), t(8;22), and t(2;8) in Burkitt's lymphoma and t(11;14) in mantle cell lymphoma (Table 9-2). These specific chromosome translocations result in the dysregulation of oncogenes or tumor suppressor genes, producing unregulated cell proliferation. Why specific translocations occur is not known.

Staging. The importance of proper staging (determining the clinical extent of disease) for patients with lymphoma in the oral region cannot be overempha-

sized. Staging serves a number of important purposes, including the determination of the type and intensity of therapy, the overall prognosis for the patient, and the potential complications associated with the disease. The Ann Arbor method, although initially designed to stage Hodgkin's disease, is now widely used for NHL (Box 9-1). Generally, patients are assigned a stage between I and IV, depending on the site and extent of their tumor. In addition, patients are classified as being "A" (no symptoms) or "B'"(constitutional symptoms).

The staging procedure often differs for the type and site of lymphoma. Gastrointestinal assessment is performed for lymphomas of Waldeyer's ring, since these tumors are often accompanied by gastrointestinal involvement. Extranodal marginal zone lymphoma tends to remain localized for prolonged periods and has a relatively indolent clinical course; hence less extensive investigation is often required. Assessment of the central nervous system (CNS) is performed for lymphomas of the nose and paranasal sinuses, and for lymphoblastic lymphoma and undifferentiated types. Bone marrow biopsy is generally performed for all extranodal lymphomas of the head and neck, but staging laparotomy is rarely done, since visceral organ involvement is unlikely.

Clinical Features. Clinically, three broad groups of NHL can be discerned on the basis of biologic behavior (Table 9-3). These may be indolent, aggressive, or highly aggressive lymphomas. The indolent lymphomas are characterized by slow growth, wide dissemination at presentation, a long natural history, and relative incurability. By contrast, the aggressive and highly aggressive groups are characterized by rapid growth, frequent localized presentation, a short natural history, and frequent responsiveness to chemotherapeutic agents. It is a paradox that the most aggressive lymphomas are the ones most likely to be cured and that the indolent lymphomas are the ones least likely to be cured. Most lymphomas in adults are diffuse B-cell lymphoma or follicular lymphoma, which together make up more than 50% of all types. Follicular lymphoma is predominantly a tumor of lymph nodes and rarely occurs in the oral cavity. By contrast, T-cell lymphomas are considerably less common at all sites, including the oral cavity. In children, aggressive and highly aggressive lymphomas are the most common, with Burkitt's lymphoma accounting for more than 40% of types.

Box 9-1 Ann Arbor Staging System for Non-Hodgkin's Lymphoma

STAGE	DEFINITION
I	Involvement of a single lymph node region or of a single extranodal organ or site (I_E)
II	Involvement of two or more lymph node regions on the same side of the diaphragm, or localized involvement of an extranodal site or organ (II_E) and one or more lymph node regions on the same side of the diaphragm
III	Involvement of lymph node regions on both sides of the diaphragm, which may also be accompanied by localized involvement of an extranodal organ or site (III_E) or spleen (III_S), or both (III_{SE})
IV	Diffuse or disseminated involvement of one or more distant extranodal organs with or without associated lymph node involvement

SUBCLASSIFICATION

A. Without systemic symptoms
B. Systemic symptoms: unexplained fever > 38°C; unexplained weight loss > 10% of body weight in past 6 months; night sweats

---

TABLE 9-3   Comparison of Features of Indolent, Aggressive, and Highly Aggressive Lymphomas

	Indolent	Aggressive	Highly Aggressive
Examples of types	Follicular lymphoma B-CLL/SLL Mantle cell lymphoma	Diffuse B-cell lymphoma Peripheral T-cell lymphoma	Burkitt's lymphoma
Age	Adults	Any	Children, young adults
Stage at presentation	High (>80% stages III and IV)	Any	High
Tumor growth rate	Slow; proliferative fraction is low	Fast	Very fast; proliferative fraction >95%
Bone marrow involvement	Yes	Uncommon	Common
Natural history if untreated	Indolent; usually takes years to kill patient	Kills patient in 1 to 2 years	Kills patient in weeks to months
Response to treatment	Poor	Responsive	Very responsive

Modified from Chan JKC: Chapter 21. In Fletcher CDM: Diagnostic histopathology of tumors, ed 2. London, 2000, Churchill Livingstone.
B-CLL/SLL, B-Cell chronic lymphocytic leukemia/small lymphocytic lymphoma.

The clinical presentation of lymphomas of the oral region varies with their site of origin and tumor type, but most present as a mass or an ulcerated mass and resemble squamous cell carcinoma or salivary neoplasm. Other lymphoid malignancies, such as plasmacytoma and Burkitt's lymphoma, show a striking predilection for primary involvement of bone. The microscopic characterization of specific lymphoma types is important because staging procedures and therapy may differ for each type. The only reliable method of distinguishing and characterizing these lesions is a biopsy coupled with tissue-based immunologic studies. Lymphomas arising within the oral cavity account for fewer than 5% of oral malignancies. In the head and neck, lymphomas may be seen within regional lymph nodes and within extranodal lymphoid sites in areas known as gut associated or MALT (extending from the oral cavity to the anal region) (Figure 9-5). Within the oral cavity, lymphoid tissue is chiefly represented in Waldeyer's ring; elsewhere within the oral cavity it appears as unencapsulated lymphoid tissue within the base of the tongue and soft palate, as well as within the major and minor salivary glands. The tonsils are the most common oropharyngeal site, followed by the palate (Figures 9-6 to 9-8). If bone is the primary site, alveolar bone loss and tooth mobility are often presenting signs (Figure 9-9). Swelling, pain, numbness of the lip, and pathologic fracture may also be associated with bone lesions.

Treatment and Prognosis. The treatment of NHL depends on a number of factors, including the histologic type and grade of the tumor; the stage of the disease; the patient's age, health, and immune status; and the patient's wishes. Two modes of treatment are available: radiation therapy and chemotherapy. Radiation therapy is used if there is tumor in a specific localized field, and chemotherapy is used for nonlocalized disease. Radiation is typically delivered to the level of 40 to 50 Gy. Chemotherapy is given as a single- or multiple-drug regimen. The goal of chemotherapy is to maximize tumor toxicity but minimize damage to normal tissues, particularly the hematopoietic tissues. Disease relapse during the course of treatment is a poor prognostic sign and is likely related to the evolution of drug-resistant clones. If there is a relapse years after the discontinuation of therapy, the tumor is likely still susceptible to the original chemotherapeutic agent. For some patients with indolent lymphomas no treatment may be needed initially. Later both radiation and chemotherapy can be used if necessary. In general,

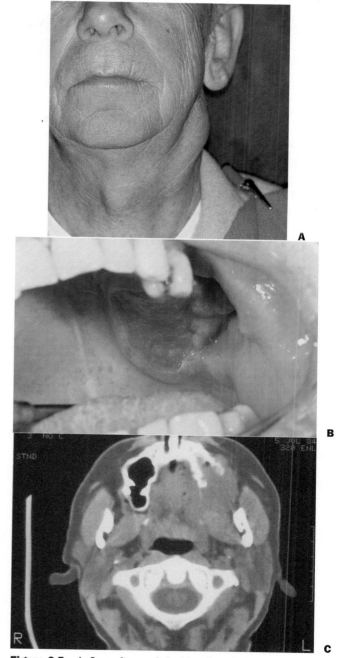

Figure 9-5 **A, Lymphoma,** left side of neck. **B,** Lesion also in the maxillary alveolar ridge. **C,** CT scan showing mass in left maxilla.

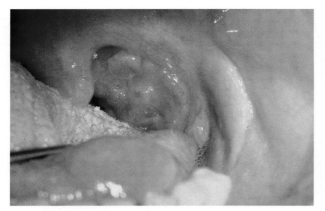

Figure 9-6　**Lymphoma** of the left tonsil.

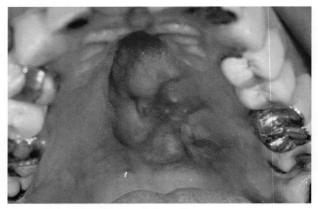

Figure 9-8　**Lymphoma** of the palate.

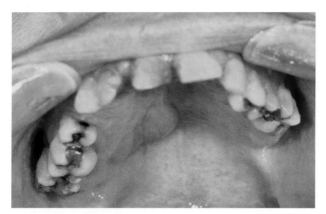

Figure 9-7　**Lymphoma** of the palate.

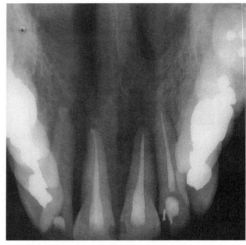

Figure 9-9　**Lymphoma** presenting as lucencies around apices of anterior maxillary teeth.

the prognosis of indolent lymphomas is poor. Although survival is long with a mean time of 8 years, this group is considered incurable. For aggressive lymphomas, more than 90% of patients receive chemotherapy. Multiple-agent chemotherapy will induce remission in about 40% of patients. The goal of treatment is to extend the dose to the limits of tolerance by the patient. For patients who respond, the outlook is good, with cures expected. For patients who do not respond, the outlook is poor. Similarly, highly aggressive lymphomas respond well to chemotherapy, with many patients having resolution of the disease after only one course of treatment. For nonresponders, however, the disease is usually fatal within weeks.

Specific Lymphomas.　In general, two basic histomorphologic groups of lymphomas are recognized: follicular (nodular) and diffuse forms; the former group shows a more favorable prognosis. Follicular lymphomas show malignant cells arranged in a pattern characterized by uniformly sized nodules distributed throughout a lymph node or extranodal site. In lymphomas showing a diffuse pattern, abnormal cells are distributed uniformly throughout the involved tissue. In either case the normal architecture of the lymphoid tissue is destroyed. Cytology, or the predominant cell type within the lesion, is of great significance. Not all classified forms of lymphoma are discussed here—only entities of relevance to the head and neck. Specific antibodies used in the diagnosis of each type of lymphoma are detailed in Table 9-4. The cytogenetics and immunophenotyping of specific lymphomas are shown in Tables 9-2 and Table 9-5, respectively.

TABLE 9-4   Antibodies to CD Markers Useful in the Diagnosis of Lymphoma

CD Marker	Expression in Normal Tissues	Expression in Malignancy
CD1a	Langerhans cells	Langerhans cell disease
CD3	T cells NK cells	T-cell neoplasms NK neoplasms
CD4	Helper/inducer T cells Monocytes Histiocytes Langerhans cells	Some T-cell neoplasms Langerhans cell disease
CD8	Suppressor/cytotoxic T cells NK cells	Some T-cell neoplasms Some NK-cell neoplasms
CD10 (CALLA)	Follicular center B cells Granulocytes	Follicular center cell lymphomas Burkitt's lymphoma
CD15 (LeuM1)	Granulocytes Monocytes	Classic Hodgkin's disease
CD20	B cells but not pre–B cells or plasma cells	B-cell neoplasms Weak in B-CLL/SLL Nodular lymphocyte predominant Hodgkin's disease
CD22	B cells but not plasma cells	B-cell neoplasms
CD23	B cells Follicular dendritic cells	B-CLL/SLL Some follicular center cell lymphomas
CD30	Activated T and B cells	Classic Hodgkin's disease ALCL
CD43	T cells Histiocytes	T-cell neoplasms Some B-cell neoplasms
CD45RB	All leukocytes Not plasma cells	Lymphomas and leukemias
CD45RO (UCHL-1)	T cells Histiocytes Myeloid cells	T-cell neoplasms
CD56	NK cells	NK-cell neoplasms Some peripheral T-cell lymphomas
CD79a	B cells, including plasma cells	B-cell neoplasms including plasma cell tumors Nodular lymphocyte predominant Hodgkin's disease

NK, Natural killer; *B-CLL/SLL*, B-Cell chronic lymphocytic leukemia/small lymphocytic lymphoma.

TABLE 9-5   Antibody Panel for Immunophenotyping of Lymphomas

Lymphoma Type	CD5	CD20	CD23	CD10	CD30	Cyclin D1	Bcl-2	CD3
B-CLL/SLL	+	−	+	−	−	−	−	−
Mantle cell	+	+	−	−	−	+	−	−
Marginal zone	−	+	−	−	−	−	−	−
Diffuse B-cell	−	+	−	−	−	−	+/−	−
Follicular	−	+	−	+	−	−	+	−
ALCL	−	−	−	−	+	−	+/−	+*

B-CLL/SLL, B-Cell chronic lymphocytic leukemia/small lymphocytic lymphoma; *ALCL*, anaplastic large cell lymphoma.
*Positive in only about 25% of ALCL and negative in NK-cell type. Other positive T-cell markers, such as CD4 and CD2, are usually needed to confirm ALCL.

Diffuse B-Cell Lymphoma. Diffuse B-cell lymphoma is an aggressive, rapidly growing neoplasm of large lymphoid cells. Diffuse B-cell lymphomas usually arise de novo but may also represent transformation of a lower-grade lymphoma. They occur over a wide age range with a slight male predilection. Diffuse B-cell lymphomas may present as lymphadenopathy or in extranodal sites (Figure 9-10). Within bone the tumor produces extensive destruction. Approximately 50% of all tumors present in stages I or II, and with treatment 50% to 60% of these patients can achieve prolonged disease-free survival.

Histologically, the tumor is composed of sheets of large lymphoid cells showing abundant cytoplasm and nuclei comparable in size or larger than reactive histiocytes. Within lymph nodes, normal lymphoid architecture is effaced and necrosis is common.

Follicular B-Cell Lymphoma. Follicular B-cell lymphomas are tumors composed of follicular center B lymphocytes showing follicular organization. This category of tumor accounts for 22% to 40% of all NHLs in whites, but only 5% to 10% of NHLs in Asians. It is typically a disease of older adults, presenting as a slowly growing, painless enlargement of one or several lymph nodes. It is rare in the oral cavity. The tumor is characterized by a protracted course highlighted by numerous recurrences over several years. This tumor is essentially incurable, with a median survival of 5 to 10 years. Histologically, there is complete effacement of normal lymph node architecture by neoplastic follicles composed of a range of follicular center–like cells, including small and large cleaved cells and, occasionally, large noncleaved cells.

Extranodal Marginal Zone Lymphoma. Extranodal marginal zone lymphoma was previously known as lymphoma of MALT. This lesion is an indolent lymphoma occurring in mucosal sites and in extranodal tissues, including the gastrointestinal tract, salivary glands, lung, thyroid gland, and skin. Any age-group or gender can be affected, although in some settings, such as those associated with Sjögren's syndrome, there is a striking female predominance. There are a number of predisposing factors for extranodal marginal zone lymphoma, including Hashimoto's thyroiditis, Sjögren's syndrome, *Helicobacter pylori* gastritis, and *Borrelia burgdorferi* skin infections (Lyme disease). These lymphomas tend to localize to an involved organ for a protracted time before dissemination. Most cases are treated with local-regional therapy, and the prognosis is excellent, with 5-year survival on the order of 75%.

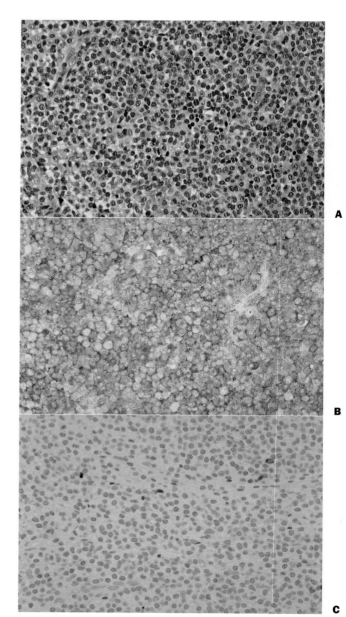

Figure 9-10 **A, Diffuse B-cell lymphoma. B** and **C,** Immunohistochemical stains for kappa **(B)** and lambda **(C)** light chains demonstrating monoclonality of infiltrate.

Histologically, there is unifocal or multifocal involvement of extranodal tissues. All extranodal marginal zone lymphomas share a number of histopathologic features regardless of site. The tumor is composed predominantly of centrocyte-like (CCL) cells morphologically resembling a range from lymphocytes to monocytoid cells. In some tumors the proportion of CCL cells showing plasmacytoid differentiation can be so extensive as to resemble a plasmacytoma. Clusters of CCL cells typically invade and destroy the epithelium to form lymphoepithelial lesions, which can be few or extensive. The tumor cells begin proliferation in the marginal zone and gradually expand around reactive lymphoid follicles. With time the neoplastic CCL cells infiltrate the reactive follicles in one of three patterns termed *follicular colonization*. Occasionally this can give the tumors a vague nodularity, which can lead to the misdiagnosis of a follicular lymphoma.

Mantle Cell Lymphoma. Mantle cell lymphoma is an indolent B-cell lymphoma derived from mantle zone cells or primary lymphoid follicles. The hallmark of this disease is the inappropriate overexpression of cyclin D1 protein. Mantle zone lymphoma occurs in middle-aged or older adults and has a striking male predominance. The condition typically presents as lymphadenopathy, but extranodal disease, including that in the spleen and gastrointestinal tract, is common. The clinical course is progressive, with an almost uniformly poor outcome. Most patients relapse within 24 months, with a 5-year survival rate of 30%. Histology shows a diffuse, vaguely nodular or nodular pattern of lymphocytes around residual reactive germinal centers. Cells are monotonous and small with indented or angulate nuclei but a spherical shape.

B-Cell Chronic Lymphocytic Leukemia/Small Lymphocytic Lymphoma. B-cell chronic lymphocytic leukemia/small lymphocytic lymphoma (B-CLL/SLL) is an indolent lymphoma composed of a neoplastic proliferation of small, well-differentiated lymphocytes (Figure 9-11). Most cases have a leukemic presentation and are rarely localized. The condition affects older patients and is typically an incidental finding in the peripheral blood. Bone marrow involvement at presentation is common, and about 40% of patients have symptoms (B-type). Many have infectious complications, and some develop autoimmune hemolytic anemia. Since the condition is indolent and slowly progressive, many asymptomatic patients are not treated. B-CLL/SLL responds to single-agent chemotherapy, but cures are almost never achieved. The course of the disease is characterized by frequent relapses and death after many years. The median survival is 5 to 8 years. Histologically, there is effacement of lymph nodes by small lymphocytes with small, rounded nuclei; condensed chromatin; inconspicuous nucleoli; and little cytoplasm.

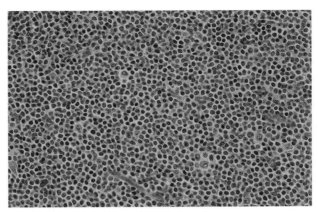

Figure 9-11 Small lymphocytic lymphoma.

Burkitt's Lymphoma. Burkitt's lymphoma (BL) is a highly aggressive B-cell lymphoma that primarily afflicts children and adolescents. Three forms of the disease are recognized: an endemic type in Africa, a sporadic form occurring in North America and Europe, and a form associated with immunodeficiency.

Endemic BL is a disease of children occurring in equatorial Africa, where endemic malaria may serve as a pathogenetic co-factor. Approximately 95% of this form is associated with EBV infection. Jaw involvement is characteristic of endemic BL, with up to 50% of those afflicted having lesions of the maxilla or mandible. Other organs are also commonly involved, including the kidneys, liver, retroperitoneum, and gonads. Sporadic BL occurs in non-African countries, primarily affecting young adults. This variety of BL often presents as an abdominal mass, and bone marrow involvement is more common than in the endemic form. Jaw lesions in sporadic BL are considerably less common than in endemic BL, occurring in approximately 10% of cases. BL can also complicate HIV infection. Most patients are adults with marked immunosuppression. There is tumor presentation both in lymph nodes and at extranodal sites, particularly the CNS, bone marrow, and the gastrointestinal tract. Although EBV has been identified in a large proportion of endemic BL, only 10% of cases of sporadic BL are associated with EBV infection. The outcome for endemic and sporadic BL depends on the stage at presentation. With aggressive chemotherapy protocols the 5-year survival rate is more than 75% for stages I to III, but only 25% for stage IV disease. For AIDS-associated BL, the prognosis is poor.

Histologically, all forms of BL show similar findings consisting of monomorphic sheets of densely packed, medium-sized neoplastic lymphocytes. The cytoplasm of the cells is deeply basophilic and often forms acute angles with neighboring cells in well-fixed sections. The tumor has a very high mitotic rate, with more than 10 mitoses per high-power field, and Ki-67 staining demonstrates that almost 100% of the tumor cells are dividing. Numerous macrophages containing cellular debris give the classic starry sky appearance to the tumor (Figure 9-12).

Lymphomas Associated With Human Immunodeficiency Virus Infection. The development of NHL has long been recognized as a rare complication of many congenital immunodeficiency states. The increase in organ transplantation coupled with immunosuppression techniques has also witnessed a marked increase in the development of many lymphoproliferative disorders. The development of lymphoma in the setting of HIV infection is now seen as an important complication of AIDS (Figure 9-13). It is a relatively late complication of HIV infection, with some lymphomas, particularly immunoblastic lymphoproliferations, occurring primarily when there is a marked depression of CD4+ T cells.

In contrast to lymphomas complicating other immunodeficiency states, up to 75% of those arising in HIV infection are extranodal, and almost one fifth occur in the CNS. Sites of involvement are relatively distinct in AIDS-related lymphomas and include the CNS, anorectal region, and oral cavity. NHLs account for 3% of all malignant tumors within the oral cavity in patients with HIV infection. The most commonly affected sites include the fauces or gingiva, typically exhibiting a rapidly growing mass and/or tooth mobility. Characteristically, these lymphomas present as widespread disease with systemic symptoms. Also, a large proportion of patients will develop spread to the CNS and bone marrow during the course of their disease. The prognosis for lymphomas arising in HIV infection is generally very poor. The advanced stage at presentation, the aggressive behavior of both low- and high-grade forms, and the profound immunosuppression contribute to a generally poor prognosis. The median survival for all patients with AIDS-associated lymphoma is 6.5 months.

In AIDS, B-cell lymphomas predominate, although T-cell lymphomas are also seen. Most of the B-cell lymphomas are immunoblastic or Burkitt's-like lym-

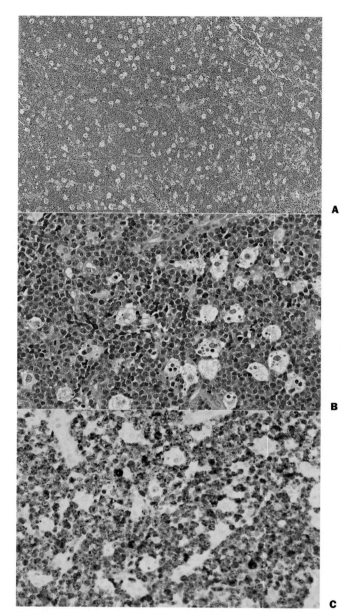

Figure 9-12 **A** and **B, Burkitt's lymphoma.** Note starry sky effect due to scattered light-staining tingible body macrophages. **C,** Immunohistochemical stain for Ki-67 proliferation marker showing positive reaction in nearly all tumor cells.

phoma. Both tumors resemble their counterparts, arising in the nonimmunosuppressed, although there are some histologic differences.

Anaplastic Large Cell Lymphoma. Anaplastic large cell lymphoma (ALCL) is an aggressive lymphoma of T-cell or NK-cell lineage that characteristically expresses

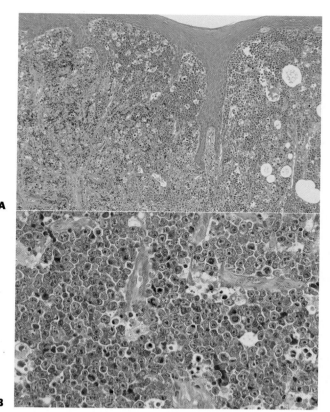

Figure 9-13 **A** and **B, High-grade lymphoma** from a palatal mass in an AIDS patient.

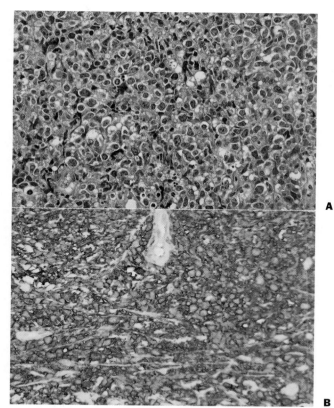

Figure 9-14 **A, Anaplastic large cell lymphoma. B,** Immunohistochemical stain for CD20 confirming B-cell lineage of tumor.

the CD30 (Ki-1 or Ber-H2) antigen (Figure 9-14). Although expression of this antigen was thought to be specific for ALCL, it is now recognized that CD30 is an activation marker that can be expressed by other B-cell and T-cell lymphomas. It has been determined recently that the cytogenetic abnormality t(2;5) involving the *NPM* and *ALK* genes is an important characteristic of ALCL. That up to 80% of ALCLs express the ALK protein in nuclei and cytoplasm of tumor cells makes this an important diagnostic feature.

ALCL has a characteristic bimodal age distribution, affecting both adolescents and older adults. Males are affected more often than females. The lymphoma has a variable clinical presentation with both lymph node and extranodal presentations, including skin, the gastrointestinal tract, and bone. Bone marrow involvement at presentation is variable, ranging from 10% to 40%, depending on whether morphologic or immunohistochemical methods are used for detection. Bone marrow involvement at presentation is a poor prognostic sign. Although the tumor is aggres-

sive, it responds well to single- or multiple-agent chemotherapy, with a 5-year median survival rate of 77%. Histologically, there are many different patterns. The prototypic form consists of large or very large cells with rounded or horseshoe-shaped single or multiple nuclei. Occasionally the nuclei are arranged in a wreathlike pattern. The cytoplasm is amphophilic, and abundant. ALCL may be difficult to differentiate from other large cell neoplasms such as undifferentiated carcinoma and malignant melanoma, hence the need for immunophenotyping to diagnose the condition.

Nasofacial Natural Killer/T-Cell Lymphoma. Progressive, ulcerative destruction of the palate, nose, and paranasal structures has long been recognized as a striking and potentially fatal condition. The term *midline lethal granuloma* was originally used to describe this condition, but a number of other terms have been suggested, including *polymorphous reticulosis, lymphomatoid granulomatosis, idiopathic destructive disease,* and *midline malig-*

nant reticulosis. Evidence now shows that a variety of diseases, including Wegener's granulomatosis, infectious agents, and lymphoma, were diagnosed as midline (lethal) granuloma. After exclusion of Wegener's granulomatosis and infection, the remainder of cases appear to be T-cell or natural killer (NK)–cell (NK/T-cell) lymphomas. At this site it is often difficult to histologically separate T-cell lymphoma from NK-cell lymphoma; hence the term *nasofacial NK/T-cell lymphoma* is now preferred.

Nasofacial NK/T-cell lymphoma is an aggressive lymphoma of adults, with a median age at presentation of 53 years. Men are affected more often than women. Nasal symptoms are often the most common presenting feature, with epistaxis occasionally present. Some patients may present early on with swelling of the soft or hard palate. With time this evolves to frank ulceration and destruction of the palatal and nasal tissues, often leading to an oronasal fistula. Without treatment the relentless destruction of midface structures by the lymphomatous infiltrate can lead to death from hemorrhage or secondary infection. Typically, the condition is treated with chemotherapy, radiation therapy, or a combination of both. Reports of long-term survival vary, in part because of the confusion regarding the diagnosis of the condition. Overall survival from the time of diagnosis has been reported as ranging from 3 months to 14 years. More aggressive management has improved the prognosis to a 5-year disease-free survival of 78% for patients with early-stage lesions and 19% for those with more widely disseminated disease.

The histologic appearance of nasofacial NK/T-cell lymphoma is characterized by the presence of varying amounts of granulation tissue and necrosis. An inflammatory infiltrate consists of a mixture of acute and chronic inflammatory cells intermingled with atypical lymphocytes that can range from a few in number to a predominant proportion of the infiltrate. These cells are medium sized or large with a clear cytoplasm and an irregular nuclear outline. Some have prominent nucleoli and may resemble immunoblasts. Angiocentricity and epitheliotropism are also common histopathologic features of nasofacial NK/T-cell lymphomas. A minority of cases of midface destructive disease are caused by other types of lymphoma, including various B-cell lymphomas.

Hodgkin's Lymphoma

Hodgkin's lymphoma rarely involves the oral cavity, although there are cases in which this disease has appeared in the soft tissues, as well as in the mandible and maxilla. On occasion the oral manifestations may represent the primary site of involvement; in other cases, associated cervical lymphadenopathy or more widespread disease may be noted concurrently.

Clinical Features. Generally, Hodgkin's lymphoma occurs over a wide age spectrum, with clustering of patients between 15 and 35 years of age and beyond 55 years of age. There is a slight male predilection. Clinically, Hodgkin's disease is characterized by painless enlargement of lymph nodes or extranodal lymphoid tissue. Within the oral cavity, tonsillar enlargement, usually unilateral, may be seen in the early phases. When extranodal sites are involved, submucosal swellings may be seen, sometimes with mucosal ulceration or erosion of underlying bone. Subsequent to microscopic diagnosis, clinical staging must be undertaken. This may consist of physical examination, radiographic imaging, lymphangiography, and laparotomy. After the staging procedure a definitive treatment plan is established. Box 9-1 provides details of the Ann Arbor system of clinical staging.

Histopathology. Of greatest significance is the identification of the Reed-Sternberg cell, which must be present for the diagnosis of Hodgkin's lymphoma to be established. This cell of lymphocytic origin is characterized by its large size and bilobed nucleus; each lobe contains a large amphophilic or eosinophilic nucleolus. The nuclear chromatin pattern is vesicular and condensed at the periphery. Other Reed-Sternberg cells may be characterized by two nuclei with a prominent nucleolus or by multiple nuclei. Cells similar to Reed-Sternberg cells may be seen in certain viral diseases, such as infectious mononucleosis and BL, as well as in patients with treated lymphocytic lymphoma, chronic lymphocytic leukemia, or some benign immunoblastic proliferations.

The REAL/WHO system for classifying Hodgkin's lymphoma is the most current and widely used system and is based on two earlier systems: the Lukes-Butler and Rye schemes. Classic Hodgkin's lymphoma comprises four entities: (1) lymphocyte-rich, classic; (2) nodular sclerosis; (3) mixed cellularity; and (4) lymphocyte depletion types. The REAL/WHO system has added lymphocyte predominant, nodular, which is not a classic type. The lymphocyte-rich, classic type has the most favorable prognosis, and the lymphocyte depletion type has the least favorable prognosis. In the lymphocyte-rich, classic form, a small, mature lymphocyte is the most prevalent cell, but it is mixed with scattered macrophages. Few Reed-Sternberg cells are seen in this form of the disease.

The most common form of Hodgkin's lymphoma is the nodular-sclerosing type, accounting for more than 50% of cases. It is characterized by bands of collagen that originate from the periphery and penetrate into the lymph node, subdividing it into islands of tumor that contain Reed-Sternberg cells.

The mixed cellularity type of Hodgkin's lymphoma contains a combination of lymphocytes, eosinophils, neutrophils, plasma cells, macrophages, and many Reed-Sternberg cells. The mixed cellularity type of Hodgkin's lymphoma carries a prognosis that is intermediate between the nodular-sclerosing type and the lymphocyte depletion form.

In the lymphocyte depletion form of Hodgkin's disease, the chief microscopic characteristic is abundant pleomorphic Reed-Sternberg cells and relatively few lymphocytes.

Differential Diagnosis. Cervical lymphadenopathy would suggest conditions ranging from inflammatory to neoplastic. Specified entities that can produce lymph node enlargement include chronic lymphadenitis, infectious diseases, and lymphoma. In young patients infectious mononucleosis should be considered. Nonlymphoid lateral neck lesions that could be included in a clinical differential diagnosis include salivary gland tumors, cervical lymphoepithelial cyst, carotid body tumor, and metastatic cancer.

Treatment and Prognosis. The clinical staging and histologic classification of Hodgkin's disease are critical in determining management and prognosis. The lymphocyte-rich, classic form of disease carries with it the most favorable prognosis, and the lymphocyte depletion form has the worst prognosis. Stage I disease has the best prognosis, and stage IV (disseminated disease) the worst. Generally, the clinical stage has a greater influence on the overall prognosis than does the histologic subtype. Management of Hodgkin's disease consists of external radiation therapy and multiple-agent chemotherapy. What was once a fatal illness with poor survival statistics has become a curable disease. Most patients with Hodgkin's disease are cured because of treatment with intensive radiotherapy and/or chemotherapy.

Multiple Myeloma/Plasmacytoma

Plasma cell neoplasms include multiple myeloma, solitary plasmacytoma of bone, and extramedullary

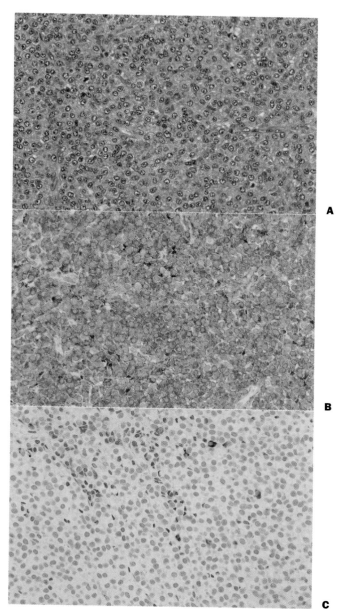

Figure 9-15 **A, Multiple myeloma** composed of neoplastic plasma cells. **B** and **C,** Immunohistochemical stains for kappa (**B**) and lambda (**C**) light chains demonstrating monoclonality of the plasma cells.

plasmacytoma and are characterized by an expansion of a clone of immunoglobulin-secreting cells (Figure 9-15) (see also Chapter 14). The biologic behavior of these conditions varies, although histologically, all contain monotonous sheets of neoplastic cells resembling plasma cells. The cell population may vary from small, well-differentiated cells

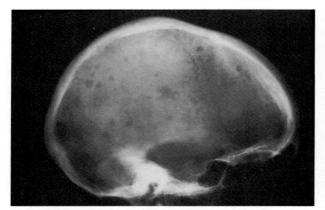

Figure 9-16 **Multiple myeloma** showing multiple punched-out lesions of the skull.

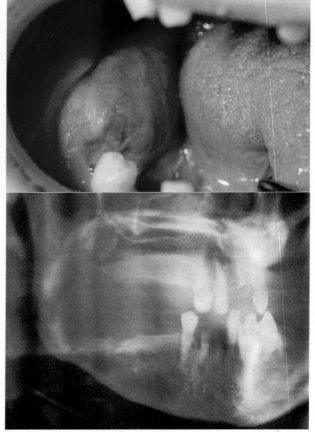

Figure 9-17 **Multiple myeloma. A** and **B,** Right mandibular mass.

with an eccentric nucleus and basophilic cytoplasm to less well differentiated, atypical cells resembling immunoblasts.

The most common and important plasma cell dyscrasia is multiple myeloma characterized by multiple osteolytic bone lesions, serum or urinary M proteins, and bone marrow biopsy findings showing greater than a 10% plasma cell composition (Figure 9-16). Symptoms are related to infiltration of organs by neoplastic plasma cells and by the excessive production of immunoglobulins having abnormal biochemical properties. Pathologic fractures occur in 20% of patients. Advanced disease is associated with hypercalcemia and renal failure. Bone marrow infiltration leads to anemia, thrombocytopenia, and leukocytopenia, with the latter resulting in an increased susceptibility to infection. Jaw lesions can be identified in 30% of cases of multiple myeloma and radiographically appear as noncorticated, well-defined radiolucencies that are more common in the mandible than in the maxilla (Figures 9-17 to 9-19). The posterior portions of the jaw are more commonly affected, since the marrow spaces are larger. The formation of amyloid from the aggregation of immunoglobulin light-chain proteins is a common sequela of multiple myeloma and when deposited in the tongue can produce macroglossia. Treatment of multiple myeloma is directed at reducing the tumor burden and reversing complications of the disease, such as those related to renal failure. Single–alkylating agent chemotherapy is the treatment of choice for multiple myeloma.

A solitary focus of lytic bone destruction showing a plasma cell tumor without bone marrow involvement

is termed *solitary plasmacytoma of bone.* This lesion constitutes 3% of all plasma cell neoplasms and is believed to represent a localized myeloma. Involvement of the facial bones is rare and, when present, typically represents disseminated disease. Progression to myeloma occurs in 30% to 75% of cases, although long-term survival is also common. Solitary lesions are typically treated with radiation therapy supplemented by chemotherapy. When the disease is disseminated, it is treated as myeloma.

Isolated plasma cell tumors within soft tissues are termed *extramedullary plasmacytoma.* This definition excludes tumors that have arisen in bone and involved soft tissues secondarily, following perforation of the bone cortex. More than 80% of all extramedullary plasmacytomas arise in the upper respiratory tract and oral cavity, forming 4% of all nonepithelial neoplasms of the nose, nasopharynx, and paranasal sinuses. The clin-

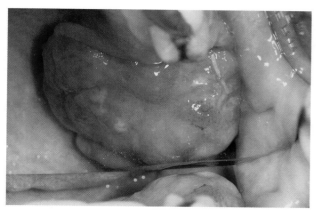

Figure 9-18 **Multiple myeloma** involving the left maxillary tuberosity.

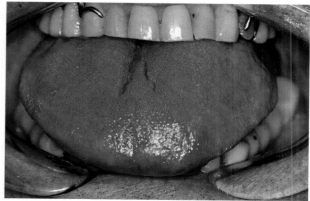

Figure 9-20 **Amyloidosis** of the tongue resulting in macroglossia.

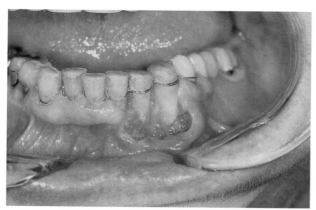

Figure 9-19 **Multiple myeloma** presenting orally as an ulcerated gingival mass.

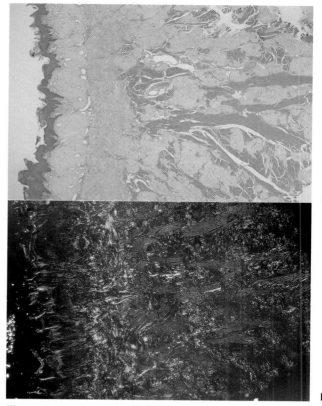

A

B

Figure 9-21 **A, Amyloidosis** of the tongue exhibiting pale eosinophilic deposits between skeletal muscle bundles *(right)*. **B,** Congo red stain in polarized light showing characteristic apple green birefringence of amyloid deposits. (Note: Mucosa is to the left in **A** and **B**.)

ical appearance is of a dark red, fleshy mass that rarely ulcerates. Multiple lesions at other sites in the head and neck are seen in 20% of patients, and up to 40% may have regional lymph nodes involved. Unlike multiple myeloma and solitary plasmacytoma of bone, wide dissemination is rare and typically shows no preference for active hematopoietic sites. In contrast to the behavior of solitary plasmacytoma of bone, many reports have shown that the progression of extramedullary plasmacytoma to myeloma is distinctly uncommon. Extramedullary plasmacytomas are radiosensitive, and regional control rates of 80% can be achieved.

A complication not infrequently associated with multiple myeloma is *amyloidosis* (Figures 9-20 and 9-21). Amyloid is the deposition of complex proteins in tissues that, when stained with the dye Congo red, shows apple green birefringence under polarized light. There are several forms of amyloid occurring in a number of differing clinical conditions, including multiple myeloma, some chronic inflammatory diseases, and a number of hereditary conditions. The constituent proteins of each condition differ, but common to all is a unique protein folding pattern known as a "β-pleated sheet." By electron microscopy all amyloid has a fibrillar appearance. The most common proteins making up amyloid are immunoglobulin light chains (Table 9-6). Other proteins that can aggregate into amyloid include liver-derived amyloid-associated nonimmunoglobulin protein, transthyretin, α_2-microglobulin, and some keratins. In multiple myeloma, excess immunoglobulin light chains are produced, which combine to form amyloid. These are deposited in organs such as the kidney, replacing normal tissues and resulting in organ dysfunction. Also in multiple myeloma, nodular or diffuse deposits of amyloid can occur in the tongue, producing macroglossia.

Leukemias

Leukemias encompass a group of disorders characterized by neoplastic proliferation of bone marrow lymphocyte or myeloid precursors that replace the marrow and can be identified in the peripheral blood. Neoplastic cells can also infiltrate other organs such as the liver, spleen, lymph nodes, and other tissues. A number of different causes have been attributed to the development of specific forms of leukemia, including genetic factors such as specific chromosome translocations (t[9;22] in chronic myeloid leukemia), environmental agents such as benzene, ionizing radiation, and viruses such as human T-cell lymphotrophic virus type 1 (HTLV1) in adult T-cell leukemia.

Leukemias are classified on the basis of the type of progenitor cell (myeloid or lymphoid lineage) and the clinical presentation (acute or chronic). Acute leukemias are characterized by the presence of immature cells and a fulminant clinical course. Chronic leukemias are characterized by the presence of better-differentiated, mature cells and a more indolent clinical course.

Acute Leukemias. Acute myeloid leukemia (AML) is a disease of adults, and acute lymphocytic leukemia (ALL) is predominantly a disease of children. Patients with AML or ALL present with bleeding (due to thrombocytopenia), fatigue (due to anemia), and infection (due to agranulocytosis). Diagnosis is established by examination of the peripheral blood differential and count and is confirmed by bone marrow biopsy findings showing greater than 5% blast cells. Between 50% and 80% of patients with AML achieve complete remission with aggressive chemotherapy, but for those who relapse, cure is rare without bone marrow transplantation. Between 60% and 90% of patients with ALL achieve remission.

Chronic Leukemias. Both chronic myeloid leukemia (CML) and chronic lymphocytic leukemia (CLL) are diseases of adults. The incidence of CML is highest in the fourth and fifth decades of life and rare in children. CLL occurs more commonly than other types of leukemia and has a median age at diagnosis in the seventh decade of life. Most patients with CML are asymptomatic. Some may have fatigue, weight loss, fever, and night sweats. Symptoms related to splenomegaly may also occur. CLL is also most commonly asymptomatic at diagnosis, although as the disease progresses, there may be lymphadenopathy, splenomegaly, and hepatomegaly. The diagnosis of chronic leukemias is made by examination of the peripheral blood and by bone marrow biopsy. A

TABLE 9-6   Amyloidosis Classification According to Fibril-Forming Protein

Disease	Amyloid Subtype and protein	Precursor Protein
Primary amyloidosis (myeloma associated)	AL	Igκ, Igλ
Secondary amyloidosis (chronic inflammatory disease associated)	AA	Serum amyloid A (apoSAA)
Chronic renal failure	$A\beta_2M$	β_2-Microglobulin
Alzheimer's disease	Aβ	Amyloid β-precursor protein
Medullary carcinoma of thyroid	ACa	Calcitonin

common complication of CML, particularly the myelomonocytic and monocytic forms, is generalized gingival hypertrophy (Figure 9-22). The gingiva is red, boggy, and edematous, and it bleeds easily. Sometimes this may be the initial presenting feature of CML. The

gingival appearance is due to infiltration by neoplastic myeloid cells. Both CML and CLL are difficult to cure. CML is managed by chemotherapy, typically with hydroxyurea or busulfan. More recently, interferon-alpha and a tyrosine kinase inhibitor have been used with clinical efficacy. CLL is often not treated if the patient is elderly or asymptomatic. Symptomatic CLL patients or those with extensive disease will receive alkylating chemotherapy, although cure is unlikely.

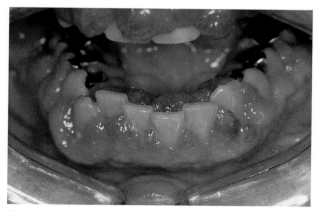

Figure 9-22   **Chronic monocytic leukemia** of the gingiva.

Granulocytic Sarcoma

Granulocytic sarcoma, also known as extramedullary myeloid tumor, is a localized infiltrate of immature granulocytes in an extramedullary site that superficially resembles sarcoma clinically. Oral granulocytic sarcoma presents as a localized soft tissue mass, although less frequently intraosseous presentation has been reported. Clinically, granulocytic sarcoma may occur in three settings: in a patient previously known to have AML; as a sign of blast transformation in a

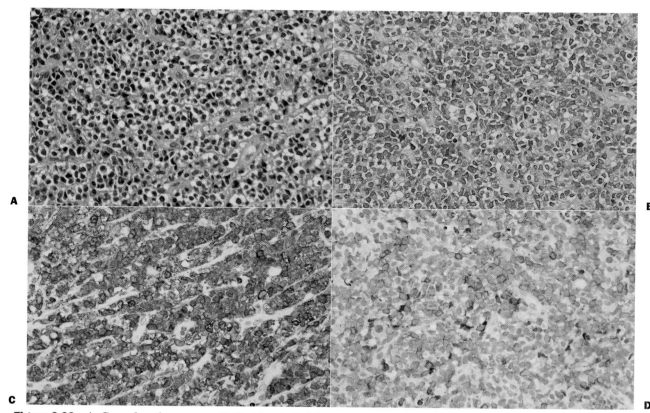

Figure 9-23   **A,** Granulocytic sarcoma. **B,** Positive *(red)* chloroacetate esterase stain of tumor cells. **C** and **D,** Positive *(brown)* immunohistochemical stains for CD43 and myeloperoxidase. Stains shown confirm the granulocyte lineage of the tumor infiltrate.

patient with CML or other chronic myeloproliferative disorders; or in a patient who was previously well.

Granulocytic sarcoma may be difficult to differentiate histologically from other malignancies such as large cell lymphoma, poorly differentiated carcinoma, or even plasmacytoma (Figure 9-23). Crystalline, rodlike, intracytoplasmic acidophilic bodies (Auer rods) can establish the diagnosis of both granulocytic sarcoma and AML; however, they may be present in less than 10% of cases. Diagnostic confirmation usually requires histochemical stains to demonstrate the presence of myeloperoxidase. Naphthol ASD chloroacetate esterase and β-naphthol acetate esterase demonstrate the presence of granulocytic esterases. Specific markers of cluster differentiation (CD) typical of myeloid (granulocytic) lineage, including CD15, can also be demonstrated using immunohistochemistry.

The prognosis for granulocytic sarcoma is poor. In patients with no history of leukemia, the frequent association with AML has prompted some clinicians to recommend chemotherapy regimens for patients with granulocytic sarcoma that are typical for the management of acute leukemia. Although few long-term survivors have been described, these individuals have generally received chemotherapy shortly after diagnosis.

BIBLIOGRAPHY

REACTIVE LESIONS

d'Agay MF, de Roquancourt A, Peuchamaur M, et al: Cystic benign lymphoepithelial lesion of the salivary glands in HIV-positive patients, *Virchows Arch A Pathol Anat Histopathol* 417:353-356, 1990.

Finfer MD, Gallo L, Perchick A, et al: Fine needle aspiration of cystic benign lymphoepithelial lesion of the parotid gland in patients at risk for the acquired immune deficiency syndrome, *Acta Cytol* 34:821-826, 1990.

Napier SS, Newlands C: Benign lymphoid hyperplasia of the palate: report of two cases and immunohistochemical profile, *J Oral Pathol Med* 19:221-225, 1990.

DEVELOPMENTAL LESIONS

Elliott JN, Oertel YC: Lymphoepithelial cysts of the salivary glands: histologic and cytologic features, *Am J Clin Pathol* 93:39-43, 1990.

Hong SS, Ogawa Y, Yagi T, et al: Benign lymphoepithelial lesion with large cysts, *Oral Surg Oral Med Oral Pathol* 19:266-270, 1990.

NEOPLASMS

Carbone A, Vaccher E, Barzan L, et al: Head and neck lymphomas associated with human immunodeficiency virus infection, *Arch Otolaryngol Head Neck Surg* 121:210-218, 1995.

Chan JKC: Advances in immunohistochemical techniques: toward making things simpler, cheaper, more sensitive, and more reproducible, *Adv Anat Pathol* 5:314-325, 1998.

Chan JKC: Tumors of the lymphoreticular system, including spleen and thymus. In Fletcher CDM, editor: *Diagnostic histopathology of tumors,* ed 2, London, 2001, Churchill Livingstone.

Chu PG, Chang KL, Arber DA, et al: Practical applications of immuno-histochemistry in hematolymphoid neoplasms, *Ann Diagn Pathol* 3:104-133, 1999.

Dardick I, Moher D, Cavell S, et al: An ultrastructural morphometric study of follicular center lymphocytes. III. The control of lymphocyte nuclear size in reactive hyperplasia and non-Hodgkin's lymphoma, *Mod Pathol* 3:176-185, 1990.

Druker BJ, Talpaz M, Resta DJ, et al: Efficacy and safety of a specific inhibitor of the BCR-ABL tyrosine kinase in chronic myeloid leukemia. *N Engl J Med* 344:1031-1037, 2001.

Economopoulos T, Asprou N, Stathakis N, et al: Primary extranodal non-Hodgkin's lymphoma in adults: clinicopathological and survival characteristics, *Leuk Lymphoma* 21:131-136, 1996.

Fukuda Y, Ishida T, Fujimoto M, et al: Malignant lymphoma of the oral cavity: clinicopathologic analysis of 20 cases, *J Oral Pathol* 16:8-12, 1987.

Green JD, Neel HB, Witzig TE: Lymphoproliferative disorders of the head and neck, *Am J Otolaryngol* 12:26-32, 1991.

Grogan TM, Miller TP, Fisher RI: A southwest oncology group perspective on the revised European-American Lymphoma Classification, *Hematol/Oncol Clin North Am* 11:819-842, 1997.

Hamilton-Dutoit SJ, Pallesen G, et al: AIDS-related lymphoma, *Am J Pathol* 138:149-163, 1991.

Harris NL, Jaffe ES, Stein H, et al: A revised European-American classification of lymphoid neoplasms: a proposal from the International Lymphoma Study Group, *Blood* 84:1361-1392, 1994.

Ioachim HL, Dorsett B, Cronin W, et al: Acquired immunodeficiency syndrome-associated lymphomas: clinical, pathologic, immunologic, and viral characteristics of 111 cases, *Hum Pathol* 22:659-673, 1991.

Jaffe ES, Chan JK, Su IJ, et al: Report of the Workshop on Nasal and Related Extranodal Angiocentric T/Natural Killer Cell Lymphomas: definitions, differential diagnosis, and epidemiology, *Am J Surg Pathol* 20:103-111, 1996.

Jordan RCK, Speight PM: Extranodal non-Hodgkin's lymphomas of the oral cavity, *Curr Top Pathol* 90:125-146, 1996.

Jordan RCK, Chong L, Dipierdomenico S, et al: Oral lymphoma in human immunodeficiency virus infection: a report of six cases and review of the literature, *Otolaryngol Head Neck Surg* 119:672-677, 1998.

Jordan RCK, Speight PM: Extra-nodal Non-Hodgkin's lymphomas of the oral cavity. In Seifert G et al, editors: *Current topics in pathology,* Berlin, 1996, Springer-Verlag.

Kantarjian HM, Smith TL, O'Brien S, et al: Prolonged survival in chronic myelogenous leukemia after cytogenetic response to interferon-alpha therapy. The leukemia service. *Ann Intern Med* 122:254-261, 1995.

Leong IT, Fernandes BJ, Mock D: Epstein-Barr virus detection in non-Hodgkin's lymphoma of the oral cavity: an immunocyto-chemical and in situ hybridization study, *Oral Surg Oral Med Oral Pathol Oral Radiol Endod* 92:184-193, 2001.

Lozada-Nur F, de Sanz S, Silverman S, et al: Intraoral non-Hodgkin's lymphoma in seven patients with acquired immunodeficiency syndrome, *Oral Surg Oral Med Oral Pathol Oral Radiol Endod* 82: 173-178, 1996.

Morra E: The biological markers of non-Hodgkin's lymphomas: their role in diagnosis, prognostic assessment and therapeutic strategy, *Int J Biol Markers* 14:149-153, 1999.

Parker SL, Tong T, Bolden S, et al: Cancer statistics, 1997, *CA Cancer J Clin* 47:5-27, 1997.

Raphael M, Gentilhomme O, Tuillez M, et al: Histopathologic features of high-grade non-Hodgkin's lymphomas in acquired immunodeficiency syndrome, *Arch Pathol Lab Med* 115:15-20, 1991.

Razquin S, Mayayo E, Citores MA, et al: Angiolymphoid hyperplasia with eosinophilia of the tongue: report of a case and review of the literature, *Hum Pathol* 22:837-839, 1991.

Regezi JA, Zarbo RJ, Stewart JCB: Extranodal oral lymphomas: histologic subtypes and immunophenotypes (in routinely processed tissue), *Oral Surg Oral Med Oral Pathol* 72:702-708, 1991.

Serraino D, Pezzotti P, Dorrucci M, et al: Cancer incidence in a cohort of human immunodeficiency virus seroconverters, *Cancer* 79:1004-1008, 1997.

Soderholm AL, Lindqvist C, Heikinheimo K, et al: Non-Hodgkin's lymphomas presenting through oral symptoms, *Int J Oral Maxillofac Surg* 19:131-134, 1990.

CYSTS OF THE JAWS AND NECK

A cyst is defined as an epithelium-lined pathologic cavity. Cysts of the maxilla, mandible, and perioral regions vary markedly in histogenesis, incidence, behavior, and treatment. Cysts are divided into odontogenic cysts, nonodontogenic cysts, pseudocysts, and neck cysts. Pseudocysts differ from true cysts in that they lack an epithelial lining.

ODONTOGENIC CYSTS

Periapical (Radicular) Cyst

Periapical (radicular or apical periodontal) cysts are by far the most common cysts of the jaws. These inflammatory cysts derive their epithelial lining from the proliferation of small odontogenic epithelial residues (rests of Malassez) within the periodontal ligament.

Etiology and Pathogenesis. A periapical cyst develops from a preexisting *periapical granuloma*, which is a focus of chronically inflamed granulation tissue in bone located at the apex of a nonvital tooth (Figures 10-1 and 10-2). Periapical granulomas are initiated and maintained by the degradation products of necrotic pulp tissue. Stimulation of the resident epithelial rests of Malassez occurs in response to the products of inflammation (Table 10-1). Cyst formation occurs as a result of epithelial proliferation, which helps to separate the inflammatory stimulus (necrotic pulp) from the surrounding bone (Figure 10-3).

Breakdown of cellular debris within the cyst lumen raises the protein concentration, producing an increase in osmotic pressure. The result is fluid transport across the epithelial lining into the lumen from the connective tissue side. Fluid ingress assists in outward growth of the cyst. With osteoclastic bone resorption, the cyst expands. Other bone-resorbing factors, such as prostaglandins, interleukins, and proteinases, from inflammatory cells and cells in the peripheral portion of the lesion permit additional cyst enlargement.

Clinical Features. Periapical cysts constitute approximately one half to three fourths of all cysts in the jaws. The age distribution peaks in the third through sixth

TABLE 10-1   **Cysts of the Jaws: Epithelial Origin**

Type	Source	Origin of Rests	Cyst Examples
Odontogenic rests	Rests of Malassez	Epithelial root sheath	Periapical (radicular) cyst
	Reduced enamel epithelium	Enamel organ	Dentigerous cyst
	Rests of dental lamina (rests of Serres)	Epithelial connection between mucosa and enamel organ	Odontogenic keratocyst Lateral periodontal cyst Gingival cyst of adult Gingival cyst of newborn Glandular odontogenic cyst
Nonodontogenic rests	Remnants of nasopalatine duct	Paired nasopalatine ducts (vestigial)	Nasopalatine canal cyst

decades. Of note is the relative rarity of periapical cysts in the first decade, even though caries and nonvital teeth are rather common in this age-group. Most cysts are located in the maxilla, especially the anterior region, followed by the maxillary posterior region, the mandibular posterior region, and finally the mandibular anterior region.

Periapical cysts are usually asymptomatic and are often discovered incidentally during routine dental radiographic examination (Figures 10-4 and 10-5). They cause bone resorption but generally do not produce bone expansion. By definition, a nonvital tooth is necessary for the diagnosis of a periapical cyst.

Radiographically, a periapical cyst cannot be differentiated from a periapical granuloma. The radiolucency associated with a periapical cyst is generally round to ovoid, with a narrow, opaque margin that is contiguous with the lamina dura of the involved tooth. This peripheral radiopaque component may not be apparent if the cyst is rapidly enlarging. Cysts range from a few millimeters to several centimeters in diameter, although the majority tend to be less than 1.5 cm. In long-standing cysts, root resorption of the offending tooth and occasionally of adjacent teeth may be seen.

Histopathology. The periapical cyst is lined by nonkeratinized stratified squamous epithelium of variable thickness (Figures 10-6 and 10-7). Transmigration of inflammatory cells through the epithelium is common, with large numbers of polymorphonuclear leukocytes (PMNs) and fewer numbers of lymphocytes involved. The underlying supportive connective tissue may be focally or diffusely infiltrated with a mixed inflammatory cell population. Plasma cell infiltrates and

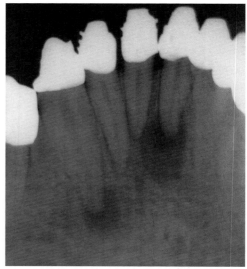

Figure 10-1   **Periapical granulomas** associated with nonvital teeth.

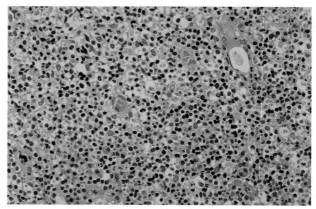

Figure 10-2   **Periapical granuloma** composed of a mixed inflammatory cell infiltrate in a connective tissue stroma.

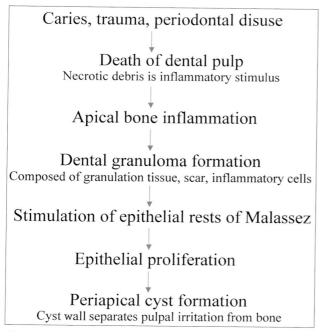

Caries, trauma, periodontal disuse

↓

Death of dental pulp
Necrotic debris is inflammatory stimulus

↓

Apical bone inflammation

↓

Dental granuloma formation
Composed of granulation tissue, scar, inflammatory cells

↓

Stimulation of epithelial rests of Malassez

↓

Epithelial proliferation

↓

Periapical cyst formation
Cyst wall separates pulpal irritation from bone

Figure 10-3   **Periapical (radicular) cyst** developmental sequence.

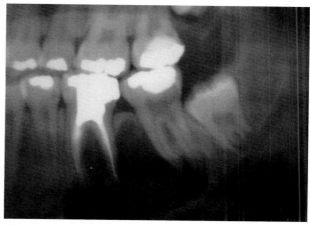

Figure 10-5   **Periapical cyst** associated with a mandibular first molar.

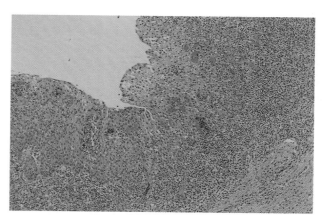

Figure 10-6   **Periapical cyst** with a chronic inflammatory cell infiltrate and nonkeratinized epithelial lining.

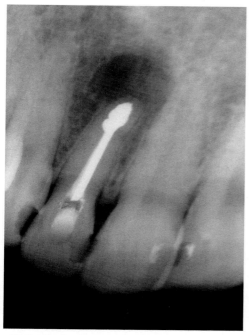

Figure 10-4   **Periapical cyst** associated with a nonvital lateral incisor.

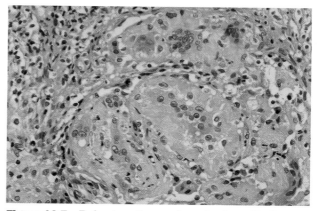

Figure 10-7   **Pulse (seed) granuloma** in the wall of a periapical cyst.

associated refractile and spherical intracellular *Russell bodies*, representing accumulated gamma globulin, are often found and sometimes dominate the microscopic picture. Foci of dystrophic calcification, cholesterol clefts, and multinucleated foreign body–type giant cells may be seen subsequent to hemorrhage in the cyst wall. Pulse or seed granulomas are also occasionally found in periapical cyst walls, indicating apical communication with the oral cavity through the root canal and carious lesion.

In a small percentage of periapical cysts (and dentigerous cysts), hyaline bodies, so-called *Rushton bodies,* may be found. Such bodies within the epithelial lining are characterized by a hairpin or slightly curved shape, concentric lamination, and occasional basophilic mineralization. The origin of these bodies is believed to be related to previous hemorrhage. They are of no clinical significance.

Differential Diagnosis. Radiographically, a differential diagnosis of the periapical cyst must include periapical granuloma. In areas of previously treated apical pathology, a surgical defect or periapical scar might also be considered. In the anterior mandible a periapical radiolucency should be distinguished from the earliest developmental phase of periapical cemento-osseous dysplasia. In the posterior quadrants apical radiolucencies must be distinguished from a traumatic bone cyst. Occasionally, odontogenic tumors, giant cell lesions, metastatic disease, and primary osseous tumors may mimic a periapical cyst radiographically. In all the above considerations, the associated teeth are vital.

Treatment and Prognosis. A periapical lesion (cyst/granuloma) may be successfully managed by extraction of the associated nonvital tooth and curettage of the apical zone. Alternatively, a root canal filling may be performed in association with an apicoectomy (direct curettage of the lesion). The third, and most often used, option involves performing a root canal filling only, since most periapical lesions are granulomas and resolve after removal of the inflammatory stimulus (necrotic pulp). Surgery (apicoectomy and curettage) is done for lesions that are persistent, indicating the presence of a cyst or inadequate root canal treatment.

When the necrotic tooth is extracted but the cyst lining is incompletely removed, a *residual cyst* may develop from months to years after the initial extirpation (Figure 10-8). If either a residual cyst or the

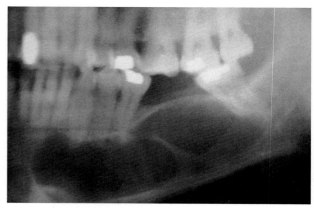

Figure 10-8 Residual cyst.

original periapical cyst remains untreated, continued growth can cause significant bone resorption and weakening of the mandible or maxilla. Complete bone repair is usually seen in adequately treated periapical and residual cysts.

Lateral Periodontal Cyst

A lateral periodontal cyst is a nonkeratinized developmental cyst occurring adjacent or lateral to the root of a tooth. *Gingival cysts of the adult* are histogenetically and pathologically similar and are also discussed here.

Etiology and Pathogenesis. The origin of this cyst is believed to be related to proliferation of rests of dental lamina. The lateral periodontal cyst has been pathogenetically linked to the gingival cyst of the adult; the former is believed to arise from dental lamina remnants within bone, and the latter from dental lamina remnants in soft tissue between the oral epithelium and the periosteum (rests of Serres). The close relationship between the two entities is further supported by their similar distribution in sites containing a higher concentration of dental lamina rests, and their identical histology. By contrast, periapical cysts are most common at the apices of teeth, where rests of Malassez are more plentiful.

Clinical Features. The majority of lateral periodontal cysts and gingival cysts of the adult occur in the mandibular premolar and cuspid region and occasionally in the incisor area (Figure 10-9). In the maxilla, lesions are noted primarily in the lateral incisor region. A distinct male predilection is noted for lateral periodon-

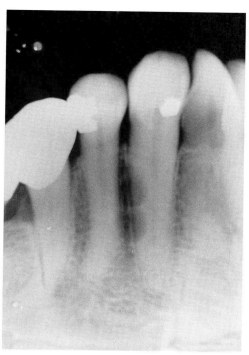

Figure 10-9 **Lateral periodontal cyst,** loculated.

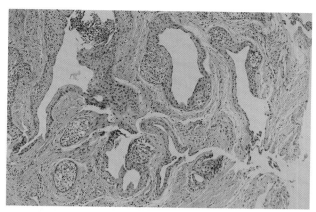

Figure 10-11 **Lateral periodontal cyst.** Note loculations lined by thick and thin epithelium.

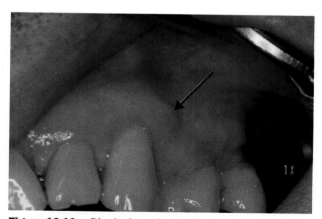

Figure 10-10 **Gingival cyst** located between canine and premolar.

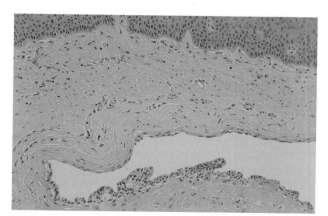

Figure 10-12 **Gingival cyst** of the adult lined by thin, nonkeratinized epithelium.

tal cysts, with a greater than 2-to-1 distribution. Gingival cysts show a nearly equal gender predilection. The median age for both types of cysts is between the fifth and sixth decades of life, with a range of 20 to 85 years for lateral periodontal cysts and 40 to 75 years for gingival cysts of the adult.

Clinically, a gingival cyst appears as a small soft tissue swelling within or slightly inferior to the interdental papilla (Figure 10-10). It may assume a slightly bluish discoloration when it is relatively large. Most cysts are less than 1 cm in diameter. There are no radiographic findings.

A lateral periodontal cyst presents as an asymptomatic, well-delineated, round or teardrop-shaped unilocular (and occasionally multilocular) radiolucency with an opaque margin along the lateral surface of a vital tooth root. Root divergence is rarely seen. The term *botryoid odontogenic cyst* is sometimes used when the lesion is multilocular.

Histopathology. Both the lateral periodontal cyst (Figure 10-11) and the gingival cyst of the adult (Figure 10-12) are lined by a thin, nonkeratinized epithelium. Clusters of glycogen-rich, clear epithelial cells may be noted in nodular thickenings of the cyst lining.

Differential Diagnosis. The lateral periodontal cyst must be distinguished from a cyst resulting from an inflammatory stimulus through a lateral root canal of a nonvital tooth (a lateral radicular cyst), an odontogenic keratocyst along the lateral root surface, and radiolucent odontogenic tumors. A differential diagnosis for the gingival cyst would include gingival mucocele, Fordyce's granules, parulis, and possibly a peripheral odontogenic tumor.

Treatment and Prognosis. Local excision of both gingival and lateral periodontal cysts is generally curative. The multilocular variant *botryoid odontogenic cyst* seems to have increased recurrence potential. Follow-up, therefore, is suggested for treated multilocular odontogenic cysts.

Gingival Cyst of the Newborn

Gingival cysts of the newborn are also known as dental lamina cysts of the newborn or Bohn's nodules. These cysts appear typically as multiple nodules along the alveolar ridge in neonates. It is believed that fragments of the dental lamina that remain within the alveolar ridge mucosa after tooth formation proliferate to form these small, keratinized cysts. In the vast majority of cases these cysts degenerate and involute or rupture into the oral cavity.

Histologically, this cyst is lined by a bland stratified squamous epithelium (Figure 10-13). Treatment is not necessary, because nearly all involute spontaneously or rupture before the patient is 3 months of age.

Similar epithelial inclusional cysts may occur along the midline of the palate (*palatine cysts of the newborn, or Epstein's pearls*). These are of developmental origin and are derived from epithelium that is included in the fusion line between the palatal shelves and the nasal processes. No treatment is necessary, because they fuse with the overlying oral epithelium and resolve spontaneously.

Dentigerous Cyst

Dentigerous or follicular cysts are the second most common type of odontogenic cyst, and the most common developmental cysts of the jaws. By definition, a dentigerous cyst is attached to the tooth cervix (enamel-cementum junction) and encloses the crown of the unerupted tooth.

Etiology and Pathogenesis. A dentigerous cyst develops from proliferation of the enamel organ remnant or reduced enamel epithelium.

As with other cysts, expansion of the dentigerous cyst is related to epithelial proliferation, release of bone-resorbing factors, and an increase in cyst fluid osmolality.

Clinical Features. Dentigerous cysts are most commonly seen in association with third molars and maxillary canines, which are the most commonly impacted teeth (Box 10-1; Figures 10-14 and 10-15). The highest incidence of dentigerous cysts occurs during the second and third decades. There is a greater incidence in males, with a ratio of 1.6 to 1 reported.

Symptoms are generally absent, with delayed eruption being the most common indication of dentigerous cyst formation. This cyst is capable of achieving significant size, occasionally with associated cortical bone expansion but rarely to a size that predisposes the patient to a pathologic fracture.

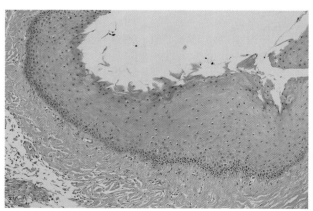

Figure 10-13 **Gingival cyst** of the newborn lined by stratified squamous epithelium.

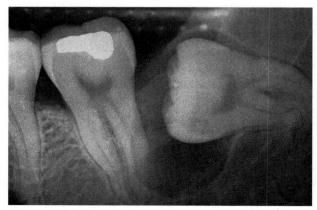

Figure 10-14 **Dentigerous cyst** surrounding the crown of an impacted molar.

Radiographically, a dentigerous cyst presents as a well-defined, unilocular or occasionally multilocular radiolucency with corticated margins in association with the crown of an unerupted tooth. The unerupted tooth is often displaced. In the mandible the associated radiolucency may extend superiorly from the third molar site into the ramus or anteriorly and inferiorly along the body of the mandible. In maxillary dentigerous cysts involving the canine region, extension into the maxillary sinus or to the orbital floor may be noted.

Resorption of roots of adjacent erupted teeth may occasionally be seen.

A variant of the dentigerous cyst arising at the bifurcation of molar teeth is the *paradental cyst or buccal bifurcation cyst* (Figure 10-16). Originally this cyst was described along the buccal root surface of partially erupted mandibular third molar teeth, but later involvement of other mandibular molar teeth was recognized. Often in these latter circumstances the molar teeth are fully erupted. Radiographically, paradental cysts are characterized as well-circumscribed radiolucencies in the buccal bifurcation region. Often there is buccal tipping of the crown that can be demonstrated by occlusal radiography. Histologically, they are identical to the wall of a dentigerous cyst with or without secondary inflammation.

Histopathology. The supporting fibrous connective tissue wall of the cyst is lined by stratified squamous epithelium (Figures 10-17 to 10-19). In an uninflamed dentigerous cyst the epithelial lining is nonkeratinized and tends to be approximately four to six cell layers thick. On occasion, numerous mucous cells, ciliated cells, and rarely, sebaceous cells may be found in the lining of the epithelium. The epithelium–connective tissue junction is generally flat, although in cases in which there is secondary inflammation, epithelial hyperplasia may be noted.

Differential Diagnosis. A differential diagnosis of pericoronal radiolucency should include odontogenic keratocyst, ameloblastoma, and other odontogenic tumors. Ameloblastic transformation of a dentigerous cyst lining should also be part of the differential

---

Box 10-1 Dentigerous Cyst

Second most common odontogenic cyst after periapical cyst

RADIOGRAPHIC FEATURES

Lucency associated with crown of impacted tooth
Third molars and canine teeth most commonly affected

HISTOPATHOLOGY

Lined by nonkeratinized stratified squamous epithelium
Proliferation of reduced enamel epithelium—stimulus unknown

POSSIBLE COMPLICATIONS

Extensive bone destruction with growth
Resorption of adjacent tooth roots
Displacement of teeth
Neoplastic transformation of lining (rare)—ameloblastoma formation; carcinoma very rarely

---

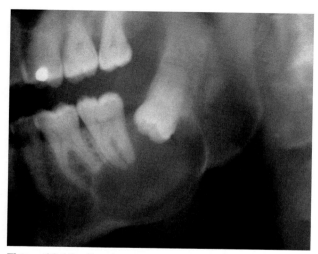

Figure 10-15 **Dentigerous cyst** exhibiting cortical expansion.

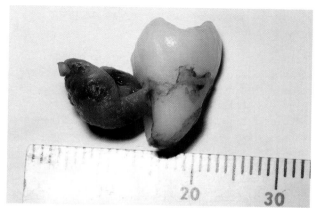

Figure 10-16 **Paradental cyst** associated with a mandibular molar, gross specimen.

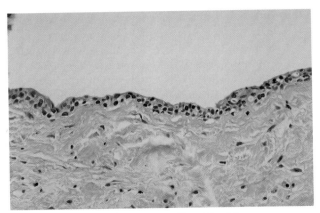

Figure 10-17 **Dentigerous cyst** lined by thin, nonkeratinized epithelium.

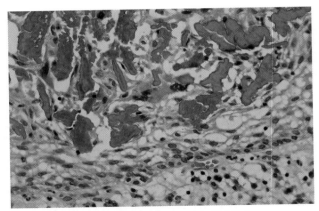

Figure 10-19 **Dentigerous cyst** epithelial lining containing Rushton bodies; an incidental finding of no significance.

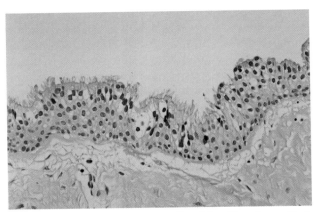

Figure 10-18 **Dentigerous cyst** lined by ciliated stratified squamous epithelium.

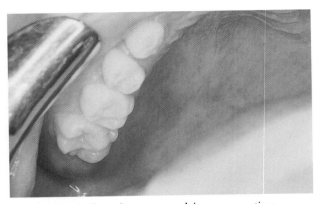

Figure 10-20 **Eruption cyst** overlying an erupting maxillary molar.

diagnosis. Adenomatoid odontogenic tumor would be a further consideration with anterior pericoronal radiolucencies, and ameloblastic fibroma would be a possibility for lesions occurring in the posterior jaws of young patients.

Treatment. Removal of the associated tooth and enucleation of the soft tissue component is definitive therapy in most instances. In cases in which cysts affect significant portions of the mandible, an acceptable early treatment approach involves exteriorization or marsupialization of the cyst to allow for decompression and subsequent shrinkage of the lesion, thereby reducing the extent of surgery to be done at a later date.

Potential complications of untreated dentigerous cysts include transformation of the epithelial lining into an ameloblastoma and, rarely, carcinomatous transformation of the epithelial lining. In cases in which mucous cells are present, the potential for development of the rarely seen intraosseous mucoepidermoid carcinoma is believed to exist.

Eruption Cyst

An eruption cyst results from fluid accumulation within the follicular space of an erupting tooth (Figure 10-20). The epithelium lining this space is simply reduced enamel epithelium. With trauma, blood may appear within the tissue space, forming a so-called *eruption hematoma*. No treatment is needed, because the tooth erupts through the lesion. Subsequent to eruption, the cyst disappears spontaneously without complication.

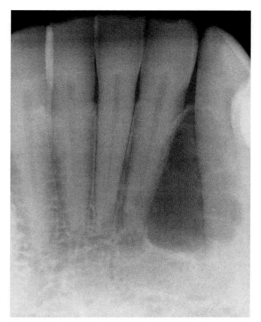

Figure 10-21 Glandular odontogenic cyst.

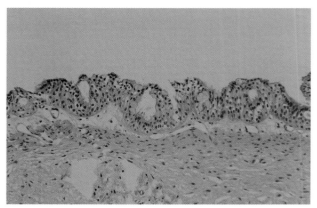

Figure 10-22 Glandular odontogenic cyst lined by epithelium showing ductlike features and mucous cells.

Glandular Odontogenic Cyst

The rare glandular odontogenic cyst, or *sialoodontogenic cyst*, was first described in 1987 and has some histologic features that suggest a mucus-producing salivary gland tumor.

Clinical Features. A strong predilection is seen for the mandible (80%), especially the anterior mandible (Box 10-2; Figure 10-21). Maxillary lesions tend to be localized to the anterior segment. Jaw expansion is not uncommon, particularly in association with mandibular lesions. The gender ratio is approximately 1 to 1. The mean age is 50 years, with a wide age range from the second through ninth decades.

Radiographic Features. Most cases are radiographically multiloculated. In cases in which a unilocular radiolucency has been noted initially, recurrent lesions have tended to be multiloculated. Lesions that have been reported have exhibited a wide variation in size, from less than 1 cm to those involving most of the mandible bilaterally. Radiographic margins may be well defined and sclerotic. More aggressive lesions have shown an ill-defined peripheral border.

Histopathology. Histologically, this multilocular cyst is lined by nonkeratinized epithelium with focal thick-

---

> **Box 10-2 Glandular Odontogenic Cyst (Sialoodontogenic Cyst)**
>
> Rare developmental cyst
>
> **CLINICAL FEATURES**
>
> Adults
> Either jaw (anterior > posterior)
>
> **HISTOPATHOLOGY**
>
> Focal mucous cells, pseudoducts
> Resembles low-grade mucoepidermoid carcinoma
>
> **BEHAVIOR**
>
> Locally aggressive; recurrence potential
>
> >, More frequently affected than.

---

enings in which the epithelial cells assume a swirled appearance. The epithelial lining consists of cuboidal cells, often with cilia at the luminal surface. Mucous cells are clustered in the cyst lining along with mucin pools. The overall histomorphology is reminiscent of a cystic low-grade mucoepidermoid carcinoma (Figures 10-22 and 10-23).

Treatment and Prognosis. This lesion can be considered locally aggressive; therefore surgical management should be dictated by the clinical and radiographic extent of the disease. Where adequate healthy bone remains beyond the extent of the cystic lesion,

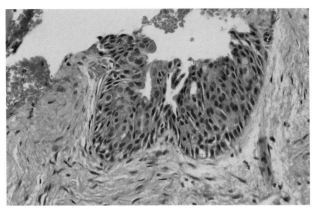

Figure 10-23   Glandular odontogenic cyst lined by epithelium showing a few ductlike changes.

peripheral curettage or marginal excision is appropriate. Long-term follow-up is essential given the local aggressiveness and recurrence rate (approximately 25%) of this lesion.

Odontogenic Keratocyst

Odontogenic keratocysts (OKCs) may exhibit aggressive clinical behavior, a significant recurrence rate, and an association with *nevoid basal cell carcinoma syndrome (NBCCS)*. They are found anywhere in the jaws and can radiographically mimic other types of cysts. Microscopically, however, they have a consistent and unique appearance.

Etiology and Pathogenesis. There is general agreement that OKCs develop from dental lamina remnants in the mandible and maxilla. However, an origin of this cyst from extension of basal cells of the overlying oral epithelium has also been suggested.

Pathogenetic mechanisms that favor growth and expansion of OKCs include a high proliferation rate, overexpression of antiapoptotic protein Bcl-2, and expression of matrix metalloproteinases (MMPs 2 and 9) (Box 10-3).

The defective gene associated with NBCCS was first identified on chromosome 9p22.3 and found to be homologous to the *Drosophila* (fruit fly) patched *(PTCH)* gene. The protein product of the *PTCH* gene (a tumor suppressor gene) is a component of the hedgehog signaling pathway and is essential for development during embryogenesis and cell signaling in the adult. The *PTCH* gene product normally represses the activity of the so-called sonic hedgehog protein and other signaling proteins, such as smoothened proteins. If the *PTCH* gene is nonfunctional, then there is overexpression of sonic hedgehog and/or smoothened proteins, leading to increased cell proliferation.

Mutations of the *PTCH* gene are involved in the development of human syndromic basal cell carcinomas and are also present in a proportion of sporadic basal cell carcinomas (as well as medulloblastomas), providing further evidence of the crucial role of *PTCH* as a tumor suppressor in human keratinocytes. *PTCH* mutations are also found in OKCs in NBCCS patients and probably in some OKCs that occur sporadically. Recently mutation of the *SUFU* gene that encodes a component of the sonic hedgehog pathway has been identified as a second genetic alteration that may occur in NBCCS and medulloblastoma.

Clinical Features. OKCs are relatively common jaw cysts (Box 10-4; Figures 10-24 and 10-25). They occur at any age and have a peak incidence within the second and third decades. Lesions found in children are often reflective of multiple OKCs as a component of NBCCS. OKCs represent 5% to 15% of all odontogenic cysts. Approximately 5% of patients with OKCs have multiple cysts (Figure 10-26), and another 5% have NBCCS (Figure 10-27).

OKCs are found in the mandible in approximately a 2-to-1 ratio. In the mandible the posterior portion of the body and the ramus region are most commonly affected, and in the maxilla the third molar area is most commonly affected (Figures 10-28 and 10-29).

Radiographically, an OKC characteristically presents as a well-circumscribed radiolucency with smooth

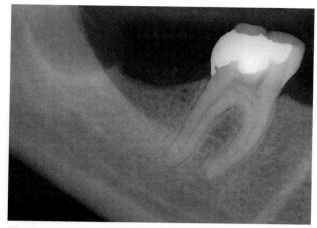

Figure 10-24   Odontogenic keratocyst.

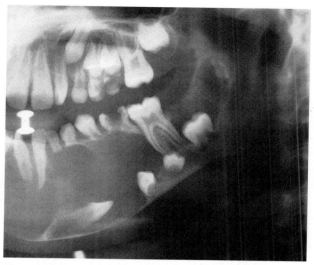

Figure 10-26   **Multiple odontogenic keratocysts** in patient with nevoid basal cell carcinoma syndrome.

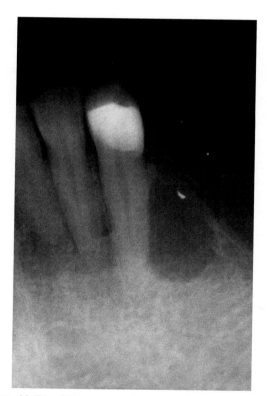

Figure 10-25   **Odontogenic keratocyst** in a lateral root position.

Box 10-4 Odontogenic Keratocyst: Clinical Features

Aggressive; recurrence risk; association with nevoid basal cell carcinoma syndrome

Solitary cysts—common (5% to 15% of odontogenic cysts); recurrence rate 10% to 30%

Multiple cysts—5% of OKC patients; recurrence greater than with solitary cysts

Syndrome-associated, multiple cysts—5% of OKC patients; recurrence greater than with multiple cysts

OKC, Odontogenic keratocyst.

radiopaque margins. Multilocularity is often present and tends to be seen more commonly in larger lesions. Most lesions, however, are unilocular, with as many as 40% noted adjacent to the crown of an unerupted tooth (dentigerous cyst presentation). Approximately 30% of maxillary and 50% of mandibular lesions produce buccal expansion. Mandibular lingual enlargement is occasionally seen.

Histopathology. The epithelial lining is uniformly thin, generally ranging from 8 to 10 cell layers thick. The basal layer exhibits a characteristic palisaded pattern with polarized and intensely stained nuclei of uniform diameter. The luminal epithelial cells are parakeratinized and produce an uneven or corrugated profile. Focal zones of orthokeratin are rarely seen. Additional histologic features that may occasionally be encountered include budding of the basal cells into the connective tissue wall and microcyst formation. The fibrous connective tissue component of the cyst wall is often

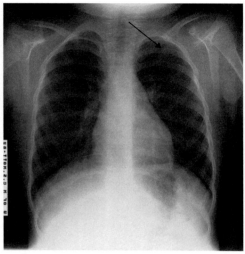

Figure 10-27   Nevoid basal cell carcinoma syndrome patient. Note bifid *(arrow)*.

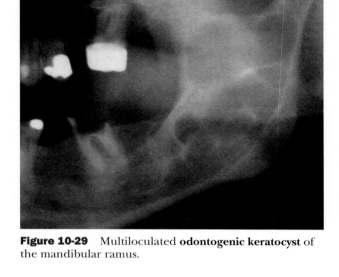

Figure 10-29   Multiloculated **odontogenic keratocyst** of the mandibular ramus.

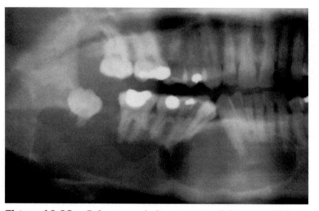

Figure 10-28   **Odontogenic keratocyst** of the mandible.

Box 10-5 Odontogenic Keratocyst: Diagnosis

Thin epithelium (6 to 10 cell layers)
Refractile, *parakeratotic* lining
Epithelial budding and "daughter cysts"
Characteristic features lost with inflammation
Orthokeratinized odontogenic cyst
  Less common
  Not syndrome associated
  Lower recurrence rate

free of an inflammatory cell infiltrate and is relatively thin. The epithelium–connective tissue interface is characteristically flattened, with no epithelial ridge formation. All so-called primordial cysts (cyst in place of a tooth), when examined microscopically, are OKCs (Box 10-5; Figures 10-30 to 10-34).

An *orthokeratinized odontogenic cyst* has been described and is about one twentieth as common as the OKC (Figure 10-35). Histologic distinction between parakeratinized and orthokeratinized cysts is made because the latter type of cyst is less aggressive, has a lower rate of recurrence, and is generally not syndrome associated. In the orthokeratotic odontogenic cyst a prominent granular layer is found immediately below a flat, noncorrugated surface. The basal cell layer is less prominent, with a more flattened or squamoid appearance in comparison with the parakeratotic type.

Differential Diagnosis. When cysts are associated with teeth, several entities might be considered, such as dentigerous cyst, ameloblastoma, odontogenic myxoma, adenomatoid odontogenic tumor, and ameloblastic fibroma. Lucent, nonodontogenic tumors, such as central giant cell granuloma, traumatic bone cyst, and aneurysmal bone cyst, might be included in a differential diagnosis of this entity in young patients.

Treatment and Prognosis. Surgical excision with peripheral osseous curettage or ostectomy is the preferred method of management. This more aggressive approach for a cystic lesion is justified because of the

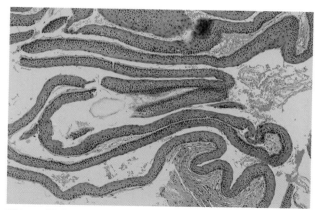

Figure 10-30 **Odontogenic keratocyst** epithelium exhibiting characteristic loss of adhesion to underlying connective tissue.

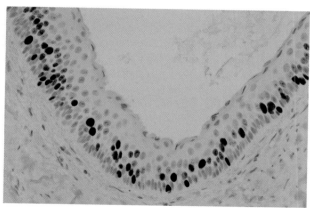

Figure 10-33 **Odontogenic keratocyst.** Note numerous positive staining nuclei *(brown)* in immunohistochemical stain for proliferation protein Ki-67.

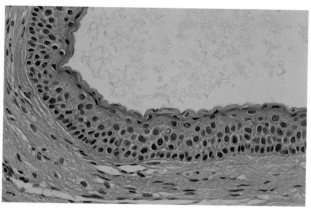

Figure 10-31 **Odontogenic keratocyst** showing characteristic parakeratinized lining with basal cell polarization.

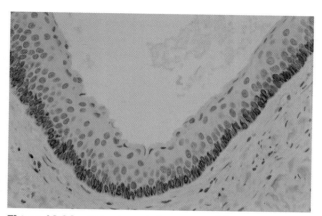

Figure 10-34 **Odontogenic keratocyst.** Note numerous positive staining cells *(brown)* in immunohistochemical stain for antiapoptosis protein Bcl-2.

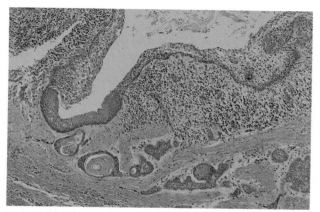

Figure 10-32 **Odontogenic keratocyst** showing loss of characteristic features in areas of inflammation, as well as mural daughter cysts/rests.

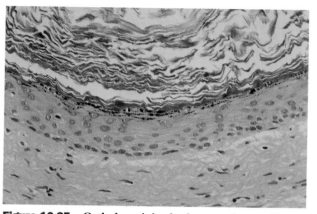

Figure 10-35 **Orthokeratinized odontogenic cyst.** Note granular layer subjacent to keratin and lack of basal cell organization.

high recurrence rate associated with OKCs. Some have also advocated the use of chemical cauterization of the cyst using Carnoy's solution (biologic fixative). In selected cases of large OKCs, marsupialization to permit cyst shrinkage, followed by enucleation, may be an attractive alternative.

The recurrence rate of 10% to 30% appears to be associated with several physical factors. The friable, thin connective tissue wall of the cyst may lead to incomplete removal. Small dental lamina remnants or satellite cysts in the bone adjacent to the primary lesion may contribute to recurrence. Also, cystic proliferation of the overlying oral epithelial basal cell layer, if not excised during cyst removal, is thought by some to be significant. The actual biologic qualities of the cyst epithelium, such as an increased mitotic index and production of bone-resorbing factors, may be associated with recurrences.

Follow-up examinations are important for patients with this lesion. Patients should be evaluated for completeness of excision, new keratocysts, and NBCCS. Most recurrences become clinically evident within 5 years of treatment. Aside from the recurrence potential, ameloblastic transformation is a rare complication. Patients with multiple keratocysts have a significantly higher rate of recurrence than do those with single keratocysts: 30% and 10%, respectively.

Clinical manifestations of NBCCS include multiple OKCs, bone defects, and multiple basal cell carcinomas. The other cutaneous abnormalities include palmar and plantar keratotic pitting, multiple milia, and dermal calcinosis. Common bone defects include bifid ribs, as well as vertebral and metacarpal abnormalities. Mild mandibular prognathism has been recorded in a small percentage of cases. Facial dysmorphogenesis, including a broad nasal bridge with corresponding ocular hypertelorism and laterally displaced inner ocular canthi (dystopia canthorum), may be seen. Neurologic abnormalities, including medulloblastoma, dysgenesis or agenesis of the corpus callosum, calcification of the falx cerebri, and less often, calcification of the falx cerebelli, have also been documented.

Calcifying Odontogenic Cyst

Calcifying odontogenic cysts (COCs) are developmental odontogenic lesions that occasionally exhibit recurrence (Box 10-6). A solid variant known as *odontogenic ghost cell tumor* is believed to potentially exhibit more aggressive clinical behavior.

Box 10-6 Calcifying Odontogenic Cyst

CLINICAL FEATURES

No distinctive age, gender, or location
Lucent to mixed radiographic patterns

HISTOPATHOLOGY

Basal palisading
Ghost cells and dystrophic calcification
Similar to pilomatrixoma of skin

BEHAVIOR

Unpredictable

VARIANTS

Odontogenic ghost cell tumor—solid
Odontogenic ghost cell carcinoma—cytologic atypia

Etiology and Pathogenesis. COCs are believed to be derived from odontogenic epithelial remnants within the gingiva or within the mandible or maxilla. "Ghost cell keratinization," the characteristic microscopic feature of this cyst, is also a defining feature of the cutaneous lesion known as *calcifying epithelioma of Malherbe* or *pilomatrixoma*. In the jaws, ghost cells may also be seen in other odontogenic tumors, including odontomas, ameloblastomas, adenomatoid odontogenic tumors, ameloblastic fibroodontomas, and ameloblastic fibromas.

Clinical Features. There is a wide age range for this cyst, with a peak incidence in the second decade. It usually appears in individuals younger than 40 years of age and has a decided predilection for females. More than 70% of COCs are seen in the maxilla (Figures 10-36 and 10-37). Rarely COCs may present as localized extraosseous masses involving the gingiva. Those presenting in an extraosseous or peripheral location are usually noted in individuals older than 50 years of age and are found anterior to the first molar region.

Radiographically, COCs may present as unilocular or multilocular radiolucencies with discrete, well-demarcated margins. Within the radiolucency there may be scattered, irregularly sized calcifications. Such opacities may produce a salt-and-pepper type of pattern, with an equal and diffuse distribution. In some cases mineralization may develop to such an extent that the radiographic margins of the lesion are difficult to determine.

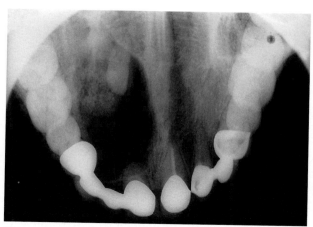

Figure 10-36 **Calcifying odontogenic cyst** of the maxilla seen in association with an impacted tooth.

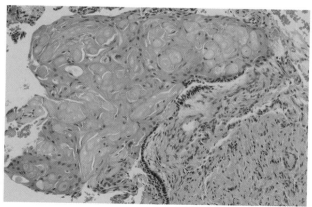

Figure 10-38 **Calcifying odontogenic cyst** showing keratinized epithelial cells (ghost cells) filling the lumen *(left)*.

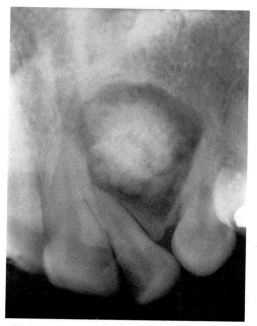

Figure 10-37 **Calcifying odontogenic cyst.**

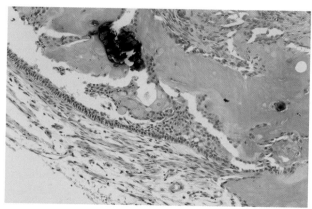

Figure 10-39 **Calcifying odontogenic cyst** showing calcification of ghost cells *(upper left)*.

Histopathology. Most COCs present as well-delineated cystic proliferations with a fibrous connective tissue wall lined by odontogenic epithelium. Intraluminal epithelial proliferation occasionally obscures the cyst lumen, thereby producing the impression of a solid tumor. The epithelial lining is of variable thickness. The basal epithelium may focally be quite prominent, with hyperchromatic nuclei and a cuboidal to columnar pattern. Above the basal layer are more loosely arranged epithelial cells, sometimes resembling the stellate reticulum of the enamel organ. The most prominent and unique microscopic feature is the presence of so-called ghost cell keratinization. The ghost cells are anucleate and retain the outline of the cell membrane. These cells undergo dystrophic mineralization characterized by fine basophilic granularity, which may eventually result in large sheets of calcified material (Figures 10-38 and 10-39). On occasion, ghost cells may become displaced in the connective tissue wall, eliciting a foreign-body giant cell response.

Differential Diagnosis. In the early stages of formation, COCs may have little or no mineralization and therefore may present as radiolucencies. The differential diagnosis in these instances includes dentigerous cyst,

OKC, and ameloblastoma. In later stages when a mixed radiolucent-radiopaque appearance is present, a differential diagnosis would include adenomatoid odontogenic tumor, a partially mineralized odontoma, calcifying epithelial odontogenic tumor, and ameloblastic fibroodontoma.

Treatment and Prognosis. Because of the unpredictable biologic behavior of this lesion, treatment is usually more aggressive than simple curettage. Patients should be monitored following treatment because recurrences are not uncommon. Management of the extraosseous or peripheral variant is conservative because recurrence is not characteristic.

NONODONTOGENIC CYSTS

Globulomaxillary Cyst/Lesion

Globulomaxillary cysts were once considered fissural cysts, located between the globular and maxillary processes. The former theory of origin related to epithelial entrapment within a line of embryologic closure with subsequent cystic change. Embryologic evidence now shows that the premaxilla and maxillary processes do not fuse in this manner, and thus there can be no fusion-related mechanism to account for a distinct globulomaxillary cyst in this location. Radiolucencies in this location, when reviewed microscopically, have been shown to represent radicular cysts, periapical granulomas, lateral periodontal cysts, OKCs, central giant cell granulomas, calcifying odontogenic cysts, and odontogenic myxomas. Thus today the term *globulomaxillary* can be justified only in an anatomic sense, with definitive diagnosis of lesions located in this area made by combined clinical and microscopic examination (Box 10-7).

Radiologically, a globulomaxillary lesion appears as a well-defined radiolucency, often producing divergence of the roots of the maxillary lateral incisor and canine teeth. Radicular cyst and periapical granuloma can be ruled out with pulp vitality testing.

Because of the array of potential diagnoses, the histology varies considerably from case to case. Specific histologic features of the entities included in the differential diagnosis are found in the discussions of those entities.

Treatment and prognosis are determined by the definitive microscopic diagnosis.

Nasolabial Cyst

Nasolabial cysts are soft tissue cysts of the upper lip. The pathogenesis of the nasolabial cyst is unclear, although it has been suggested that this lesion represents cystic change of the solid cord remnants of cells that form the nasolacrimal duct.

The nasolabial cyst is a rare lesion with a peak incidence noted in the fourth and fifth decades. There is a distinct female predilection of nearly 4 to 1. The chief clinical sign is a soft tissue swelling that may present in the soft tissue over the canine region or the mucobuccal fold.

The epithelial lining of this cyst is characteristically a pseudostratified columnar type with numerous goblet cells. Stratified squamous epithelium may be present in addition to cuboidal epithelium in some cases. The cyst is treated by curettage with few recurrences expected.

Median Mandibular Cyst

Median mandibular cysts, like globulomaxillary cysts, were once considered fissural cysts. Justification for a fissural origin was based on the no-longer-tenable theory of epithelial entrapment in the midline of the mandible during the "fusion" of each half of the mandibular arch. There is now embryologic evidence of an isthmus of mesenchyme between the mandibular processes that is gradually eliminated as growth continues, and therefore no evidence of epithelial fusion. Cases diagnosed clinically as median mandibular cysts represent a microscopic spectrum of odontogenic cysts and tumors.

Nasopalatine Canal Cyst

Nasopalatine canal cysts, also known as *incisive canal cysts*, are located within the nasopalatine canal or within the palatal soft tissues at the point of the opening of

---

Box 10-7 Globulomaxillary Lesions

Nonspecific designation for any lesion in the globulomaxillary area (between maxillary lateral incisor and canine)
Inverted pear-shaped radiolucency
Asymptomatic; teeth vital; divergence of roots
May represent odontogenic cyst or neoplasm, or nonodontogenic tumor
Biopsy necessary to establish definitive diagnosis

the canal, where the lesions are called *cysts of the palatine papilla*. The so-called *median palatine cyst* is believed to represent a more posterior presentation of a nasopalatine canal cyst rather than cystic degeneration of epithelial rests in the line of fusion of the palatine shelves.

Etiology and Pathogenesis. A nasopalatine canal cyst develops from the proliferation of epithelial remnants of paired embryonic nasopalatine ducts within the incisive canal. The canal itself forms secondary to the fusion of the premaxilla with the right and left palatal processes. The anatomic exit of the canal is slightly posterior to the incisive papilla.

The stimulus for cyst formation from the epithelial remnants of the nasopalatine canals is uncertain, although bacterial infection and/or trauma is thought to have a role. Alternatively, it has been suggested that the mucous glands within the lining may cause cyst formation as a result of mucin secretion.

Clinical Features. This is a relatively common cyst that may present as a symmetric swelling in the anterior region of the palatal midline or as a midline radiolucency (Figure 10-40). The majority of cases occur between the fourth and sixth decades of life. Men are affected more often than women—differences range as high as 3 to 1.

Most cases are asymptomatic, with the clinical sign of swelling usually calling attention to the lesion. Symptoms may follow secondary infection. Sinus formation and drainage occur occasionally at the most prominent portion of the palatine papilla.

Radiographically, a nasopalatine canal cyst is purely radiolucent, with sharply defined margins. The lesion may produce divergence of the roots of the maxillary incisor teeth and, less commonly, induce external root resorption. The anterior nasal spine is often centrally superimposed on the lucent defect, producing a heart shape. The radiolucency may occasionally be unilateral, with the midline forming the most medial aspect of the radiolucency.

Histopathology. The epithelial lining of this cyst ranges from stratified squamous to pseudostratified columnar (when located near the nasal cavity). In many instances a mixture of two or more types of lining cells is seen. The connective tissue wall contains small arteries and nerves, representing the nasopalatine neurovascular bundle (Figure 10-41).

Differential Diagnosis. The entities periapical granuloma and periapical (radicular) cyst must be separated from the nasopalatine canal cyst. This can be done simply by determining tooth vitality. A normal but widened canal might also be considered.

Treatment and Prognosis. This cyst requires surgical enucleation. In cases of large cysts, marsupialization may be considered before definitive enucleation. The recurrence rate is very low.

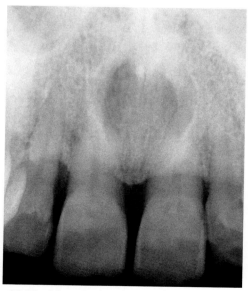

Figure 10-40 **Nasopalatine canal cyst** in the midline of the maxilla.

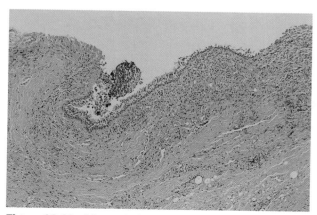

Figure 10-41 **Nasopalatine canal cyst** exhibiting respiratory-type epithelium and mural inflammation.

PSEUDOCYSTS

Aneurysmal Bone Cyst

Aneurysmal bone cysts are pseudocysts because they appear radiographically as cystlike lesions but microscopically exhibit no epithelial lining (Box 10-8). This lesion represents a benign lesion of bone that may arise in the mandible, maxilla, or other bones. Within the craniofacial complex, approximately 40% of these lesions are located in the mandible and 25% are located in the maxilla.

Etiology and Pathogenesis. Although the pathogenesis of the aneurysmal bone cyst is obscure, the process is generally regarded as reactive. An unrelated antecedent primary lesion of bone, such as fibrous dysplasia, central giant cell granuloma, nonossifying fibroma, chondroblastoma, and other primary bone lesions, is believed to initiate a vascular malformation, resulting in a secondary lesion or aneurysmal bone cyst.

Clinical Features. Aneurysmal bone cysts typically occur in persons younger than 30 years of age. The peak incidence occurs within the second decade of life. There is a slight female predilection.

When the mandible and maxilla are involved, the more posterior regions are affected, chiefly the molar areas (Figure 10-42). Pain is described in approximately half the cases, and a firm, nonpulsatile swelling is a common clinical sign. On auscultation, a bruit is not heard, indicating that the blood is not located within an arterial space, and on firm palpation, crepitus may be noted.

Radiographic features include the presence of a destructive or osteolytic process with slightly irregular margins. A multilocular pattern is noted in some instances. When the alveolar segment of the mandible and maxilla is involved, teeth may be displaced with or without concomitant external root resorption.

Histopathology. A fibrous connective tissue stroma contains variable numbers of multinucleated giant cells (Figure 10-43). Sinusoidal blood spaces are lined by fibroblasts and macrophages. With the exception of the sinusoids, the aneurysmal bone cyst is similar to

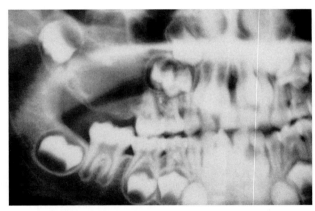

Figure 10-42 **Aneurysmal bone cyst** of the right maxilla.

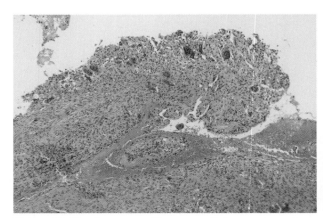

Figure 10-43 **Aneurysmal bone cyst** lining composed of connective tissue and scattered multinucleated giant cells.

Box 10-8 Aneurysmal Bone Cyst

ETIOLOGY

Unknown; may be related to altered hemodynamics or abnormal healing of bone hemorrhage

CLINICAL FEATURES

Teenagers and young adults affected
Multilocular lucency
No associated thrill or bruit on auscultation

HISTOPATHOLOGY

Blood-filled spaces lined by connective tissue and multinucleated giant cells
Differential diagnosis includes central giant cell granuloma, hyperparathyroidism, cherubism

TREATMENT

Excision
No bleeding hazard

central giant cell granuloma. Reactive new bone formation is also commonly noted.

Differential Diagnosis. Odontogenic keratocyst, central giant cell granuloma, and ameloblastic fibroma should be included in a differential diagnosis. Ameloblastoma and odontogenic myxoma could be included, although these lesions more typically appear in older patients.

Treatment and Prognosis. A relatively high recurrence rate has been associated with simple curettage. Excision or curettage with supplemental cryotherapy is the treatment of choice.

Traumatic (Simple) Bone Cyst

A traumatic bone cyst is an empty intrabony cavity that lacks an epithelial lining. The designation of pseudocyst relates to the cystic radiographic appearance and gross surgical presentation of this lesion (Box 10-9). It is seen mostly in the mandible.

Pathogenesis. The pathogenesis is not known, although some cases seem to be associated with antecedent trauma. Assuming this to be the case, it has been hypothesized that a traumatically induced hematoma forms within the intramedullary portion of bone. Rather than organizing, the clot breaks down, leaving an empty bony cavity. Alternative developmental pathways include cystic degeneration of primary tumors of bone, such as central giant cell granuloma, disorders of calcium metabolism, and ischemic necrosis of bone marrow.

Clinical Features. Teenagers are most commonly affected, although traumatic bone cysts have been reported over a wide age range. An equal gender distribution has been noted.

By far, the most common site of occurrence is the mandible (Figure 10-44). The lesion may be seen in either anterior or posterior regions. Rare bilateral cases have been described. Swelling is occasionally seen, and pain is infrequently noted.

Radiographically, a well-delineated area of radiolucency with an irregular but defined edge is noted. Interradicular scalloping of varying degrees is characteristic, and occasionally slight root resorption may be noted.

Traumatic bone cysts have often been seen in association with florid osseous dysplasia. The relationship between these two entities is not understood.

Histopathology. Grossly, only minimal amounts of fibrous tissue from the bony wall are seen. The lesion may occasionally contain blood or serosanguineous fluid. Microscopically, delicate, well-vascularized, fibrous connective tissue without evidence of an epithelial component is identified (Figure 10-45).

Treatment and Prognosis. Once entry into the cavity is accomplished, the clinician need merely establish bleeding into the lesion before closure. Organization of the bony clot results in complete bony repair without recurrence.

Static Bone Cyst (Stafne's Bone Defect)

A static bone cyst is an anatomic indentation of the posterior lingual mandible that appears to resemble a cyst on radiographic examination (Box 10-10; Figure 10-46). This depression of the mandible is believed to

---

Box 10-9 Traumatic Bone Cyst

ETIOLOGY

Unknown; trauma sometimes suggested
May be related to bleeding in the jaw with clot resorption

CLINICAL FEATURES

Lucency discovered on routine examination
Empty "dead" space in medullary bone, especially mandible
Teenagers most commonly affected

TREATMENT

Surgical entry to initiate bleeding and stimulate healing
Some may heal spontaneously

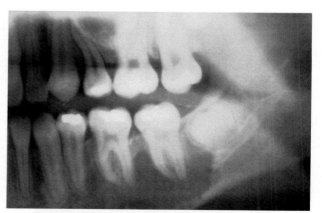

Figure 10-44 **Traumatic bone cyst** of the body of the mandible.

be developmental, although almost all cases appear in adults, particularly men. The cause is unknown, but some have suggested that the lesion is due to entrapment of salivary gland or other soft tissue during the development of the mandible. Others have suggested that the cause is lingual mandibular cortical erosion from hyperplastic salivary gland tissue. Both demo-

graphic and anatomic findings are more consistent with the latter hypothesis. These defects may occasionally be noted bilaterally and, rarely, anterior to the first molar region of the mandible.

This lesion is entirely asymptomatic and is often observed as an incidental finding in panoramic radiographic films. It appears as a sharply circumscribed oval radiolucency beneath the level of the inferior alveolar canal, with encroachment on the inferior border of the mandible. The presence of salivary tissue within the defect may be confirmed by sialography. The appearance of a static bone cyst is usually pathognomonic, and no treatment is required. Other depressions of the cortical surface of the mandible have been reported, albeit rarely, within the parotid gland along the lateral or facial aspect of the mandibular ramus.

Box 10-10 Static (Stafne's) Bone Cyst

Developmental defect
Located below mandibular canal in molar region
Salivary gland or adipose tissue in defect
Discrete corticated margin
Diagnostic on panoramic film
No symptoms
No biopsy or treatment

Focal Osteoporotic Bone Marrow Defect

Focal osteoporotic bone marrow defects (*hematopoietic bone marrow defects*) are uncommon lesions that typically present as asymptomatic, focal radiolucencies in areas where hematopoiesis is normally seen (angle of the mandible and maxillary tuberosity). Approximately 70% of these lesions occur in the posterior mandible; 70% occur in females.

The pathogenesis of the osteoporotic marrow defect is unknown, although three theories have been proposed. One theory states that abnormal healing following tooth extraction may be responsible (Figure 10-47). Another theory states that residual remnants

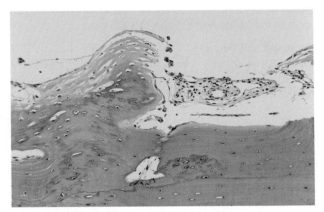

Figure 10-45 **Traumatic bone cyst** consisting of connective tissue fragments lining surrounding bone *(bottom).*

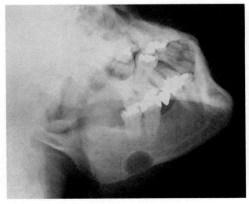

Figure 10-46 **Static bone cyst.**

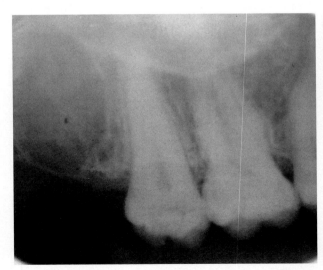

Figure 10-47 **Focal osteoporotic bone marrow defect** in a maxillary molar extraction site.

of fetal marrow may persist into adulthood, thus presenting as a focal lucency. Finally, this tissue may merely represent a focus of extramedullary hematopoesis that becomes hyperplastic in adult life.

Microscopic findings show a predominance of hematopoietic cells with relatively fewer fat cells. Within the cellular marrow, small lymphoid aggregates may be found, as well as megakaryocytes (Figure 10-48).

Because of nonspecific radiographic findings, diagnosis by an incisional biopsy is generally desirable. Subsequent to the establishment of this diagnosis, no further treatment is necessary.

SOFT TISSUE CYSTS OF THE NECK

Branchial Cyst/Cervical Lymphoepithelial Cyst

Branchial (cleft) cysts, or cervical lymphoepithelial cysts, are located in the lateral portion of the neck, usually anterior to the sternomastoid muscle (Figure 10-49). These lesions may also appear in the sub-

mandibular area, adjacent to the parotid gland, or around the sternomastoid muscle. There is an intra-oral *lymphoepithelial cyst* counterpart (Figure 10-50). The floor of the mouth is the most common site for these lesions, followed by the posterior lateral tongue.

At one time the branchial cyst was thought to occur because of incomplete obliteration of the branchial clefts with epithelial remnants ultimately undergoing cystic change. Current theory of origin proposes that epithelium is entrapped in cervical lymph nodes during embryogenesis (Box 10-11). This epithelium, thought to be of salivary origin, would undergo cystic change at a later date.

Clinical Features. These asymptomatic cysts usually become clinically apparent in late childhood or young adulthood as a result of enlargement. Drainage may

---

Box 10-11 Branchial Cyst

Developmental cyst—arises from epithelium entrapped in lymph node
Lateral neck mass—along anterior border of sternocleido-mastoid muscle
Fluctuant texture
Young adults
Lymphoid tissue surrounds a squamous or pseudostratified epithelial lining

---

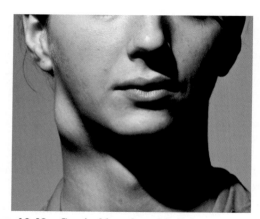

Figure 10-49 Cervical lymphoepithelial cyst.

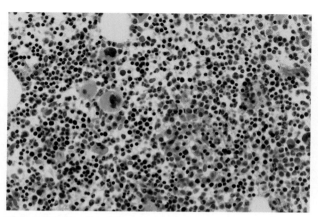

Figure 10-48 Focal osteoporotic bone marrow defect composed of maturing blood cells and megakaryocytes.

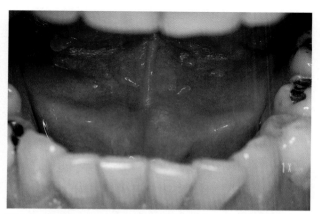

Figure 10-50 Lymphoepithelial cyst located at the left submandibular caruncle.

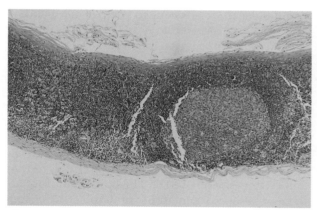

Figure 10-51 **Lymphoepithelial cyst** lined by squamous epithelium *(top)* and supported by lymphoid tissue.

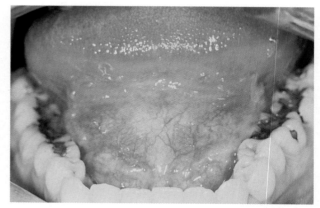

Figure 10-52 **Dermoid cyst** presenting intraorally as a midline swelling in the floor of the mouth.

> ### Box 10-12 Dermoid Cyst
>
> Mass in midline of neck or floor of mouth (location depends on relationship to mylohyoid and geniohyoid muscles)
> Young adults
> Doughy by palpation because of sebum in lumen
> Lined by epithelium and secondary skin structures (sebaceous glands, hair)
> Designated as teratoma if all three germ layers are represented

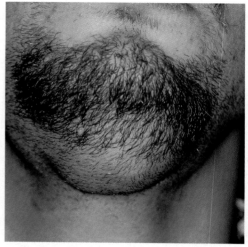

Figure 10-53 **Dermoid cyst** presenting as a midline swelling in the neck.

occur along the anterior margin of the sternomastoid muscle.

Histopathology. The branchial cyst is lined with stratified squamous epithelium, pseudostratified columnar epithelium, or both (Figure 10-51). The epithelium is supported by connective tissue containing lymphoid aggregates.

Differential Diagnosis. Preoperative diagnoses may include cervical lymphadenitis, skin inclusion cyst, lymphangioma, and tumor of the tail of the parotid. Laterally displaced thyroglossal tract cyst and dermoid cyst might also be considered.

Treatment. Treatment is surgical excision.

Dermoid Cyst

Dermoid cysts are developmental lesions that may occur in many areas of the body (Box 10-12). When found in the oral cavity, the lesion is usually in the anterior portion of the floor of the mouth in the midline. The cause of the lesion in this area is believed to be developmental entrapment of multipotential cells or possibly implantation of epithelium.

Clinical Features. Clinically, these cysts, when located above the mylohyoid muscle, displace the tongue superiorly and posteriorly (Figure 10-52). When they are located below the mylohyoid muscle, a midline swelling of the neck occurs (Figure 10-53). These cysts are painless and slow growing; there is no gender predilection. Lesions are generally less than 2 cm in diameter; however, extreme examples may range up to 8 to 12 cm. On palpation, the cysts are soft

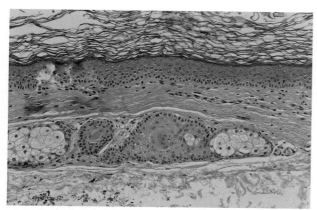

Figure 10-54 **Dermoid cyst** lined by keratinized epithelium with sebaceous glands and rudimentary hair in the supporting connective tissue.

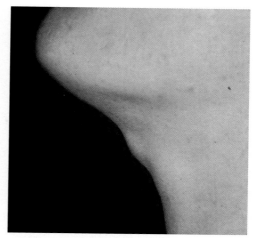

Figure 10-55 **Thyroglossal tract cyst** in the midline of the neck.

Box 10-13 Thyroglossal Tract Cyst

Arises from epithelial remnants of thyroid gland development
Occurs in midline of neck—anywhere between thyroid embryonic origin (foramen caecum of tongue) and thyroid gland
Lingual thyroid
   Mass in tongue base due to failed descent of thyroid tissue
   May be only functional thyroid tissue in patient
Treatment by excision; may recur because of tortuous configuration

---

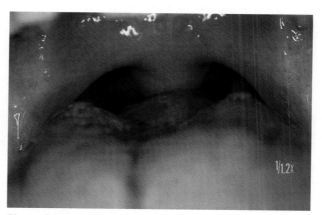

Figure 10-56 **Lingual thyroid** posterior to circumvallate papillae in the midline of the tongue.

and doughy because of keratin and sebum in the lumen.

Histopathology. Microscopically, the dermoid cyst is lined by stratified squamous epithelium supported by a fibrous connective tissue wall (Figure 10-54). Numerous secondary skin structures, including hair follicles, sebaceous glands, and sweat glands (and occasionally teeth), may be found.

Treatment. Treatment is surgical excision. Most lesions can be removed through the mouth with little risk of recurrence.

Thyroglossal Tract Cyst

Thyroglossal tract cysts are the most common developmental cysts of the neck, accounting for nearly three fourths of such lesions (Box 10-13). The basis of this cystic pathology relates to thyroid gland development. The thyroid tissue becomes evident in the fourth week of gestation, when derivatives of first and second branchial arches form the posterior portion of the tongue in the region of the foramen caecum. The thyroid anlage grows downward from the foramen caecum area to its permanent location in the neck. Residual epithelial elements along this pathway that do not completely atrophy may give rise to cysts in later life from the posterior portion of the tongue (*lingual thyroid*) to the midline of the neck (Figures 10-55 and 10-56).

Clinical Features. Approximately 30% of cases are found in patients older than 30 years of age, with a similar percentage in patients younger than 10 years of age. Most cysts occur in the midline, with 60% occurring in the thyrohyoid membrane and only 2% occurring within the tongue itself. The overriding majority (70%

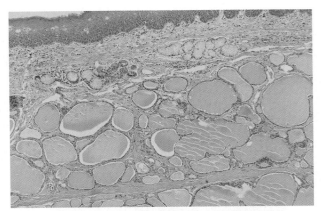

Figure 10-57   **Lingual thyroid** showing thyroid acini in submucosa.

to 80%) occur below the level of the hyoid bone. These cysts are generally asymptomatic. When attached to the hyoid bone and tongue, they may retract on swallowing or extension of the tongue. If infected, drainage through a sinus tract may occur. Rarely, malignant transformation has been described in these lesions.

Histopathology. Microscopic findings vary depending on the location of the cyst (Figure 10-57). Lesions occurring above the level of the hyoid bone demonstrate a lining chiefly of stratified squamous epithelium. A ciliated or columnar type of epithelium is usually found in cysts occurring below the hyoid bone. However, wide variation may be seen within a single cyst. Thyroid tissue may be seen within the connective tissue wall. Rare malignancies arising within the thyroglossal tract are usually papillary thyroid adenocarcinomas.

Differential Diagnosis. A differential diagnosis of the thyroglossal tract cyst should include dermoid cyst, thyroid neoplasm, branchial cyst, and sebaceous cyst.

Treatment. Treatment is surgical excision. It is important to establish before surgery whether the thyroglossal duct cyst represents the only functioning thyroid tissue in the patient. Because the lesion may be rather tortuous in configuration, recurrence may be seen. It is often recommended that the central portion of the hyoid bone be removed in an effort to eliminate any residual thyroglossal tract epithelium from this site.

BIBLIOGRAPHY

ODONTOGENIC CYSTS

Androulakis M, Johnson JT, Wagner RL: Thyroglossal duct and second branchial cleft anomalies in adults, *Ear Nose Throat J* 69:318-322, 1990.

Aszterbaum M, Rothman A, Johnson RL, et al: Identification of mutations in the human PATCHED gene in sporadic basal cell carcinomas and in patients with basal cell nevus syndrome, *J Invest Dermatol* 110:885-888, 1998.

Buchner A: The central (intraosseous) calcifying odontogenic cyst: an analysis of 215 cases, *J Oral Maxillofac Surg* 49:330-339, 1991.

Crowley TE, Kaugars GE, Gunsolley JC: Odontogenic keratocysts: a clinical and histologic comparison of the parakeratin and orthokeratin variants, *J Oral Maxillofac Surg* 50:22-26, 1992.

Fantasia JE: Lateral periodontal cysts, botryoid odontogenic cysts and glandular odontogenic cysts, *Oral Maxillofac Surg Clin North Am* 3:127-136, 1991.

Kenealy JF, Torsiglieri AJ Jr, Tom LW: Branchial cleft anomalies: a five year retrospective review, *Trans Pa Acad Ophthalmol Otolaryngol* 42:1022-1025, 1990.

Lench NJ, High AS, Markham AF, et al: Investigation of chromosome 9q22.3-q31 DNA marker loss in odontogenic keratocysts, *Oral Oncol* 32B:202-206, 1996.

Lo Muzio L, Staibano S, Pannone G, et al: Expression of cell cycle and apoptosis-related proteins in sporadic odontogenic keratocysts and odontogenic keratocysts associated with the nevoid basal cell carcinoma syndrome, *J Dent Res* 78:1345-1353, 1999.

Pavelic B, Levanat S, Crnic I, et al: *PTCH* gene altered in dentigerous cysts, *J Oral Pathol Med* 30:569-576, 2001.

Ramer M, Montazem A, Lane SL, et al: Glandular odontogenic cyst, *Oral Surg Oral Med Oral Pathol Oral Radiol Endod* 84:54-57, 1997.

Redman RS, Whitestone BW, Winne CE, et al: Botryoid odontogenic cyst: report of a case with histologic evidence of multicentric origin, *Int J Oral Maxillofac Surg* 19:144-146, 1990.

Renard TH, Choucair RJ, Stevenson WD, et al: Carcinoma of the thyroglossal duct, *Surg Gynecol Obstet* 171:305-308, 1990.

Sadeghi EM, Weldon LL, Kwon PH, et al: Mucoepidermoid odontogenic cyst, *Int J Oral Maxillofac Surg* 29:142-143, 1991.

Sciubba JJ, Fantasia JE, Kahn LB: *Tumors and cysts of the jaws*, Washington, DC, 2001, Armed Forces Institute of Pathology.

Spatafore CM, Griffin JA Jr, Keyes GG, et al: Periapical biopsy report: an analysis over a ten year period, *J Endod* 16:239-241, 1990.

Taylor MD, Liu L, Raffel C, et al: Mutations in SUFU predispose to medulloblastoma. *Nat Genet* Jun 17 (e-pub ahead of print), 2002.

Teronen O, Konttinen YT, Rifkin B, et al: Identification and characterization of gelatinase/type IV collagenases in jaw cysts, *J Oral Pathol Med* 24:78-84, 1995.

vanHeerden WFP, Raubenheimer EJ, Turner M: Glandular odontogenic cyst, *Head Neck* 14:316-320, 1992.

Waldron CA, Koh ML: Central mucoepidermoid carcinoma of the jaws: report of four cases with analysis of the literature and discussion of the relationship to mucoepidermoid, sialo-odontogenic and glandular odontogenic cysts, *J Oral Maxillofac Surg* 48:871-877, 1990.

Wolf J, Hietanen J: The mandibular infected buccal cyst (paradental cyst): a radiographic and histologic study, *Br J Oral Maxillofac Surg* 28:322-325, 1990.

Yaskima M, Ogura M, Abiko Y: Studies on cholesterol accumulation in radicular cyst fluid—origin of heat-stable cholesterol-binding protein, *Int J Biochem* 22:165-169, 1990.

Zedan W, Robinson PA, Markham AF, et al: Expression of the Sonic Hedgehog receptor "PATCHED" in basal cell carcinomas and odontogenic keratocysts, *J Pathol* 194:473-477, 2001.

Nonodontogenic Cysts

Revel MP, Vanel D, Sigal R, et al: Aneurysmal bone cysts of the jaws: CT and MR findings, *J Comput Assist Tomogr* 16:84-86, 1992.

Soft Tissue Cysts of the Neck

Fernandez JF, Ordonez NG, Schultz PN, et al: Thyroglossal duct carcinoma, *Surgery* 6:928-934, 1991.

ODONTOGENIC TUMORS

Epithelial Tumors

  Ameloblastoma

  Calcifying Epithelial Odontogenic Tumor

  Adenomatoid Odontogenic Tumor

  Squamous Odontogenic Tumor

  Clear Cell Odontogenic Tumor (Carcinoma)

Mesenchymal Tumors

  Odontogenic Myxoma

  Central Odontogenic Fibroma

  Cementifying Fibroma

  Cementoblastoma

  Periapical Cementoosseous Dysplasia

Mixed (Epithelial and Mesenchymal) Tumors

  Ameloblastic Fibroma and Ameloblastic Fibroodontoma

  Odontoma

Odontogenic tumors are lesions derived from the epithelial and/or mesenchymal remnants of the tooth-forming apparatus. They are therefore found exclusively in the mandible and maxilla (and occasionally gingiva) and must be considered in differential diagnoses of lesions involving these sites.

The etiology and pathogenesis of this group of lesions are unknown. Clinically, odontogenic tumors are typically asymptomatic, although they may cause jaw expansion, movement of teeth, root resorption, and bone loss. Knowledge of typical basic features such as age, location, and radiographic appearance of the various odontogenic tumors can be extremely valuable in developing a clinical differential diagnosis.

Like neoplasms elsewhere in the body, odontogenic tumors tend to mimic microscopically the cell or tissue of origin. Histologically, they may resemble soft tissues

of the enamel organ or dental pulp, or they may contain hard tissue elements of enamel, dentin, and/or cementum.

Lesions in this group range from hamartomatous proliferations to malignant neoplasms with metastatic capabilities. An understanding of the biologic behavior of the various odontogenic tumors is of fundamental importance to the overall treatment of patients.

Several histologic classification schemes have been devised for this complex group of lesions. Common to all is the division of tumors into those that are composed of odontogenic epithelial elements, those that are composed of odontogenic mesenchyme, and those that are proliferations of both epithelium and mesenchyme. Classified according to biologic behavior, they range from clinically trivial (i.e., benign, no recurrence potential) to malignant (Box 11-1).

EPITHELIAL TUMORS

Ameloblastoma

Historically, ameloblastoma has been recognized for over a century and a half. Its frequency, persistent local growth, and ability to produce marked deformity before leading to serious debilitation probably account for its early recognition. Recurrence, especially after conservative treatment, has also contributed to the awareness of this lesion.

Pathogenesis. This neoplasm originates within the mandible or maxilla from epithelium that is involved in the formation of teeth. Potential epithelial sources include the enamel organ, odontogenic rests (rests of Malassez, rests of Serres), reduced enamel epithelium, and the epithelial lining of odontogenic cysts, especially dentigerous cysts. The trigger or stimulus for neo-

Box 11-1 Biologic Classification of Odontogenic Tumors

BENIGN, NO RECURRENCE POTENTIAL

Adenomatoid odontogenic tumor
Squamous odontogenic tumor
Cementoblastoma
Periapical cementoosseous dysplasia
Odontoma

BENIGN, SOME RECURRENCE POTENTIAL

Cystic ameloblastoma
Calcifying epithelial odontogenic tumor
Central odontogenic fibroma
Florid cementoosseous dysplasia
Ameloblastic fibroma and fibroodontoma

BENIGN AGGRESSIVE

Ameloblastoma
Clear cell odontogenic tumor
Odontogenic ghost cell tumor
Odontogenic myxoma
Odontoameloblastoma

MALIGNANT

Malignant ameloblastoma
Ameloblastic carcinoma
Primary intraosseous carcinoma
Odontogenic ghost cell carcinoma
Ameloblastic fibrosarcoma

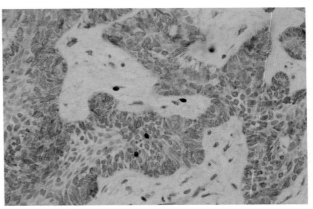

Figure 11-1   **Ameloblastoma** exhibiting overexpression (brown cytoplasmic stain) of antiapoptotic protein Bcl-2.

Box 11-2 Ameloblastoma: Pathogenetic Mechanisms

CELL CYCLE–RELATED FACTORS

Low proliferation rate; few cells in cell cycle based on low Ki-67 expression
Antiapoptotic proteins expressed; overexpression of Bcl-2 and Bcl-x_L
Some positive p53 staining; probably wild-type protein inactivated by MDM2 binding

INTERFACE FACTORS

Invasive properties enhanced
    Altered laminin 5 at interface
    Expression of FGF and interleukins (1 and 6)
    Overexpression of proteinases (MMPs 9 and 20; EMSP1)

MDM2, Murine double minute; *FGF*, fibroblast growth factor; *MMPs*, matrix metalloproteinases; *EMSP1*, enamel matrix serine proteinase.

plastic transformation of these epithelial residues is totally unknown.

Mechanisms by which ameloblastomas gain a growth and invasion advantage include overexpression of anti-apoptotic proteins (Bcl-2, Bcl-x_L) and interface proteins (fibroblast growth factor [FGF], matrix metalloproteinases [MMPs]) (Figure 11-1 and Box 11-2). Ameloblastomas, however, have a low proliferation rate, as shown by staining for the cell cycle–related protein, Ki-67. Mutations of the p53 gene do not appear to play a role in the development or growth of ameloblastoma.

Clinical Features. Ameloblastoma is chiefly a lesion of adults. It occurs predominantly in the fourth and fifth decades of life, and the age range is very broad, extending from childhood to late adulthood (mean age, approximately 40 years). The rare lesions occurring in children are usually cystic and appear clinically as odontogenic cysts. There appears to be no gender predilection for this tumor.

Ameloblastomas may occur anywhere in the mandible or maxilla, although the mandibular molar-ramus area is the most favored site. In the maxilla the molar area is more commonly affected than the premolar and anterior regions. Lesions are usually asymptomatic and are discovered either during routine radiographic examination or because of asymptomatic jaw expansion (Figures 11-2 and 11-3). Occasionally, tooth movement or malocclusion may be the initial presenting sign.

Radiographically, ameloblastomas are osteolytic, typically found in the tooth-bearing areas of the jaws, and may be either unilocular or multilocular (Figures

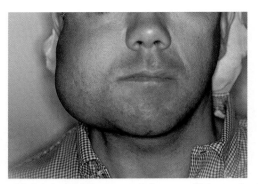

Figure 11-2 **Ameloblastoma** of the mandible producing marked cortical expansion.

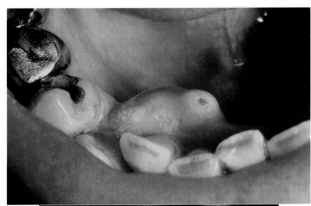

A

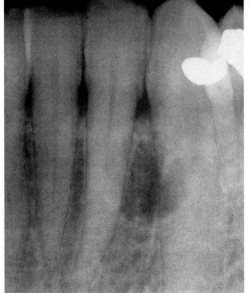

B

Figure 11-3 **A** and **B, Ameloblastoma** of the mandible with oral expression.

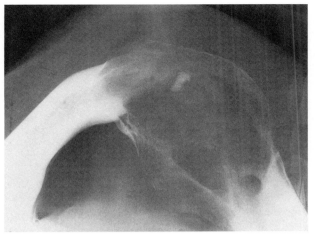

Figure 11-4 **Ameloblastoma** in an edentulous anterior mandible. Occlusal view shows a destructive multilocular lesion.

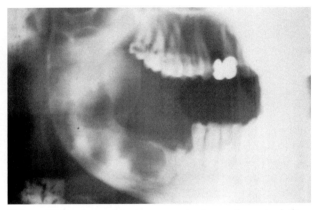

Figure 11-5 **Ameloblastoma** producing a characteristic multilocular lesion of the molar-ramus area of the mandible.

11-4 and 11-5). Because ameloblastomas are slow growing, the radiographic margins are usually well defined and sclerotic. In cases in which connective tissue desmoplasia occurs in conjunction with tumor proliferation, ill-defined radiographic margins are typically seen. This variety, known as *desmoplastic ameloblastoma,* also has a predilection for the anterior jaws and radiographically resembles a fibroosseous lesion. The generally slow tumor growth rate may also be responsible for the movement of tooth roots. Root resorption occasionally occurs in association with ameloblastoma growth.

Biologic Subtypes. *Peripheral or extraosseous ameloblastomas* may occur in the gingiva and very rarely in the buccal

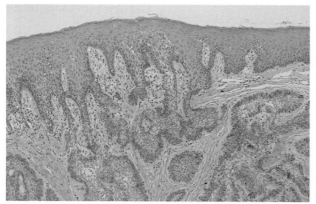

Figure 11-6 **Peripheral ameloblastoma** showing communication with overlying epithelium.

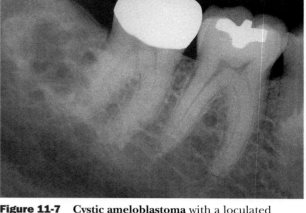

Figure 11-7 **Cystic ameloblastoma** with a loculated appearance in retromolar mandibular bone.

Box 11-3 Ameloblastoma: Biologic Subtypes

Solid ameloblastoma
Cystic ameloblastoma
Peripheral ameloblastoma
Malignant ameloblastoma
Ameloblastic carcinoma

Box 11-4 Cystic Ameloblastoma*

CLINICAL FEATURES

Multilocularity and cortical perforation (25% of cases)

HISTOPATHOLOGY

Thin, nonkeratinized epithelium
Basal palisading
Spongiosis
Epithelial invaginations
Subepithelial hyalinization

MICROSCOPIC PATTERNS

Simple cystic
Intraluminal
Mural invasion

TREATMENT

Excision
Curettage; recurrence rate of as high as 40% (seen as late as 9 years after surgery)

*Also known as unicystic ameloblastoma.

---

mucosa (Box 11-3 and Figure 11-6). These lesions are seen in older adults, usually between 40 and 60 years of age. They may arise from overlying epithelium or rests of Serres. They exhibit a benign, nonaggressive course and generally do not invade underlying bone. Following local excision, recurrence is rare.

Cystic ameloblastoma was formerly referred to as *unicystic ameloblastoma*. We prefer the term *cystic ameloblastoma* because these entities are often multilocular, show cortical perforation in 25% of cases, and have a recurrence rate as high as 40% (treated with curettage) (seen as late as 9 years following surgery) (Box 11-4 and Figures 11-7 and 11-8). They are seen in a younger age-group (mean age approximately 35 years) than solid tumors. The microscopy is deceptive because the lesions are nearly completely cystic and can be confused with a simple odontogenic cyst (Figures 11-9 and 11-10).

Malignant variants of ameloblastomas may rarely be encountered. These lesions occur in a relatively young age-group (thirties) and appear in the mandible more commonly than in the maxilla. By definition, these are lesions that metastasize to local lymph nodes or distant organs. Direct extension into contiguous areas does not qualify for a malignant classification.

Malignant lesions have been divided into two subtypes: *malignant ameloblastoma* (Figure 11-11), in which the primary and metastatic lesions are microscopically well differentiated with the characteristic histologic features of ameloblastoma, and *ameloblastic carcinoma* (Figure 11-12), in which the lesions (primary and/or metastatic) exhibit less microscopic differentiation, showing cytologic atypia and mitotic figures. Malignant vari-

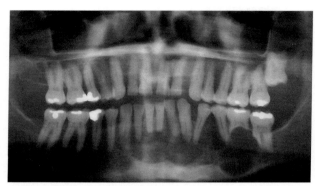

Figure 11-8 **Cystic ameloblastoma** occupying the body of the mandible. The lesion recurred twice following curettage.

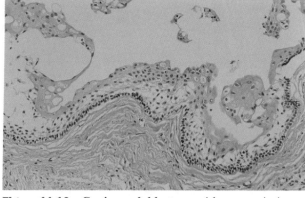

Figure 11-10 **Cystic ameloblastoma** with a spongiotic epithelial lining.

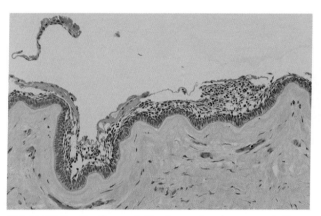

Figure 11-9 **Cystic ameloblastoma** showing spongiotic epithelium and basal palisading.

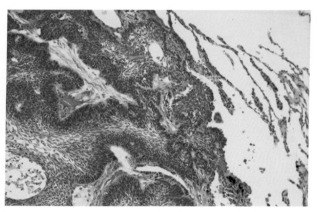

Figure 11-11 **Malignant ameloblastoma** in the lung (lung septa at *right*).

ants of ameloblastomas are difficult to control locally. Metastases may appear usually in the lung, presumably because of aspiration of tumor cells. Regional lymph nodes are the second most common metastatic site, followed by the skull, liver, spleen, kidney, and skin.

An epithelial odontogenic malignancy of the mandible and maxilla that is believed to arise from odontogenic rests has been designated as *primary intraosseous carcinoma*. This lesion does not have histologic features of ameloblastoma and is regarded as a primary jaw carcinoma. It does not have its origin from a preexisting odontogenic cyst. This rare lesion of adults affects men more than women, and it is seen in the mandible more than the maxilla. Microscopically, about half of these lesions exhibit keratin formation and about half show peripheral palisading of

epithelial cell nests. This lesion must be differentiated microscopically from acanthomatous ameloblastoma and squamous odontogenic tumor. The prognosis is poor, with a 2-year survival rate reported at 40%.

Another ameloblastoma that might be considered a subtype has been designated as *sinonasal ameloblastoma*. A mean age of 61 years and male dominance have been noted. Signs of nasal obstruction, epistaxis, and opacification are seen. The "totipotential" sinonasal lining cells are the putative cells of origin. A plexiform microscopic pattern is most commonly seen.

Histopathology. Numerous histologic patterns of no clinical relevance may be seen in solid ameloblastomas (Box 11-5). Some may exhibit a single histologic subtype; others may display several histologic patterns

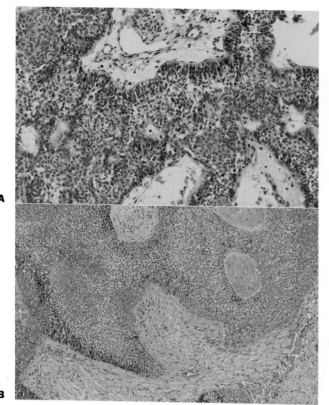

A

B

Figure 11-12   A, Ameloblastic carcinoma exhibiting cellular atypia and mitotic figures. **B,** Second recurrence of the lesion in **A.**

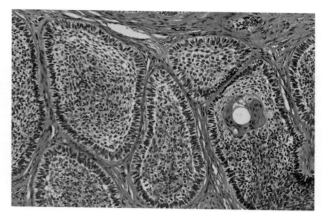

Figure 11-13   Ameloblastoma, follicular pattern.

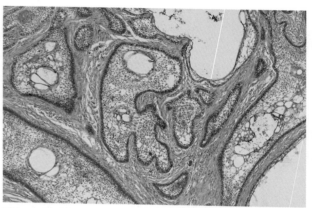

Figure 11-14   Ameloblastoma, follicular pattern with microcystic change.

> **Box 11-5 Ameloblastoma: Histologic Subtypes/Patterns**
>
> All subtypes mimic enamel organ
>   Peripheral palisades and budding
>   No hard tissue formation
> No clinical significance to subtypes
> Microscopic—desmoplastic, follicular, plexiform, granular cell, basaloid

within the same lesion. Common to all subtypes is the palisading of columnar cells around epithelial nests in a pattern similar to that of ameloblasts of the enamel organ. Central to these cells are loosely arranged cells that mimic the stellate reticulum of the enamel organ. Another typical feature is the budding of tumor cells from neoplastic foci in a pattern reminiscent of tooth development.

The microscopic subtype most commonly seen in solid ameloblastoma is the *follicular* type (Figure 11-

13). It is composed of islands of tumor cells that mimic the normal dental follicle. Central cystic degeneration of the follicular islands leads to a microcystic pattern (Figure 11-14). The neoplastic cells occasionally develop into a network of epithelium, prompting the term *plexiform ameloblastoma* (Figure 11-15). When the stroma is desmoplastic and the tumor islands become squamoid or elongated, the term *desmoplastic ameloblastoma* is used (Figure 11-16). Some tumors are microscopically similar to basal cell carcinoma and are called *basal cell* or *basaloid ameloblastomas*. A type of solid ameloblastoma in which the central neoplastic cells exhibit prominent cytoplasmic granularity (and swelling) is known as *granular cell ameloblastoma* (Figure 11-17). Clear tumor cells and cells expressing ghost cell–type keratinization have also been seen in ameloblastomas. Separation of ameloblastomas into the various microscopic groups described is essentially

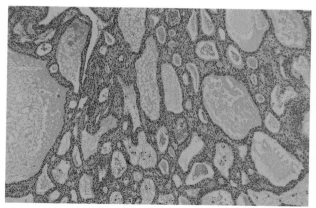

Figure 11-15 **Ameloblastoma,** plexiform pattern.

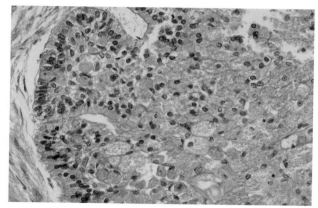

Figure 11-17 **Ameloblastoma** with granular cell change.

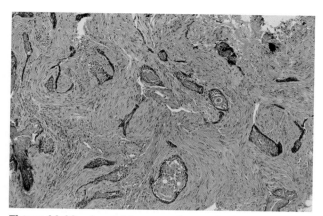

Figure 11-16 **Ameloblastoma,** desmoplastic type.

an academic exercise, because there appears to be no correlation between clinical behavior and these microscopic patterns.

Cystic ameloblastoma is a type of ameloblastoma that has a major cystic space or spaces lined by thin epithelium showing basal palisading. There is often epithelial invagination into supporting connective tissue, and occasionally, mural islands may be seen. There is also a characteristic spongiotic change in the epithelial lining, and occasionally subepithelial hyalinization. Some lesions have an intraluminal component, usually in a plexiform pattern. Diagnosis is often retrospective after enucleation for what was thought to be an odontogenic cyst.

Differential Diagnosis. When age, location, and radiographic features are considered together, the clinical differential diagnosis can generally be limited to several entities in the three categories of jaw disease— odontogenic tumors, cysts, and benign nonodontogenic lesions. Among the odontogenic tumors the radiolucent form of the calcifying epithelial odontogenic tumor and odontogenic myxomas are prime considerations. The dentigerous cyst and the odontogenic keratocyst can also be included. In relatively young individuals, lesions that are radiographically similar to ameloblastoma include nonodontogenic lesions such as central giant cell granuloma, ossifying fibroma, central hemangioma, and possibly idiopathic histiocytosis.

Treatment and Prognosis. No single standard type of therapy can be advocated for patients with ameloblastoma. Rather, each case should be judged on its own merits. Of prime considerations are whether the lesion is solid, cystic, extraosseous, or malignant, and location. The solid lesions require at least surgical excision, because recurrence follows curettage in 50% to 90% of cases. Block excision or resection is generally reserved for larger lesions. Cystic ameloblastomas may be treated less aggressively, but with the knowledge that recurrences are often associated with simple curettage. Peripheral ameloblastomas should be treated in a conservative fashion. Malignant lesions should be managed as carcinomas. Patients with all forms of central ameloblastoma should be followed indefinitely, since recurrences may be seen as long as 10 to 20 years after primary therapy. Ameloblastomas of the maxilla are generally more difficult to manage than those of the mandible due to anatomic relationships and due to the high content of cancellous bone in the maxilla. Thus intraosseous maxillary ameloblastomas are often excised with a wider normal margin than mandibular tumors.

Radiotherapy has rarely been used in the treatment of ameloblastomas, because it is generally believed that these tumors are radioresistant. Until more is known about tumor responsiveness, radiation should be reserved for exceptional cases that are difficult or impossible to control surgically.

Calcifying Epithelial Odontogenic Tumor

Calcifying epithelial odontogenic tumor (CEOT), also known as *Pindborg tumor* after the oral pathologist who first described the entity, shares many clinical features with ameloblastoma (Box 11-6). Microscopically, however, there is no resemblance to ameloblastoma, and radiographically distinct differences will often be noted. CEOTs are of odontogenic origin. The cells from which these tumors are derived are unknown, although the dental lamina remnants and the stratum intermedium of the enamel organ have been suggested.

Clinical Features. CEOTs are seen in patients ranging in age from the second to the tenth decade, with a mean age of about 40 years. There is no gender predilection. The mandible is affected twice as often as the maxilla, and there is a predilection for the molar-ramus region, although any site may be affected (Figure 11-18). Peripheral lesions, usually in the anterior gingiva, are rarely seen.

Jaw expansion or incidental observation on a routine radiographic survey is the usual way in which these lesions are discovered. Radiographically, the lesions are often associated with impacted teeth. The lesions may be unilocular or multilocular. Small loculations in some lesions have prompted the use of the term *honeycomb* to describe this lucent pattern. A CEOT may be completely radiolucent, or it may contain opaque foci—a reflection of the calcified amyloid seen microscopically. The lesions are usually well circumscribed radiographically, although sclerotic margins may not always be evident.

Histopathology. The CEOT has a unique and sometimes bizarre microscopic pattern. Large polygonal epithelial cells, seen in sheets or islands, contain nuclei that show considerable variation in size and shape (Figure 11-19). Mitotic figures are rare. The cytoplasm is abundant and eosinophilic. Focal zones of clear cells can occasionally be seen in a so-called clear cell variant. Extracellular amyloid of epithelial origin is also typical of these tumors (Figures 11-20 and 11-21). This homogeneous, pale-staining eosinophilic material can be stained with Congo red or thioflavine T (Figure 11-22). Immunohistochemical staining for cytokeratins is also positive, suggesting that keratin proteins form an important component of the amyloid in this tumor. Concentric calcific deposits (Liesegang rings), seen in the amyloid material, are responsible for radiopacities when sufficiently dense.

Box 11-6 Calcifying Epithelial Odontogenic Tumor (Pindborg Tumor)

HISTOGENESIS

Unknown; may be dental lamina or stratum intermedium

CLINICAL FEATURES

Adults between 30 and 50 years of age
Posterior mandible favored

HISTOPATHOLOGY

Epithelioid strands/nests/sheets
Amyloid and calcification
Rare clear cell variant

BEHAVIOR

Benign; recurrence potential (<20%)

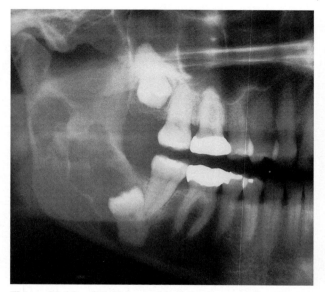

Figure 11-18   **Calcifying epithelial odontogenic tumor.** The multiloculated lesion extends from the third molar to the condyle. (Courtesy Dr. Bruce A. Shapton.)

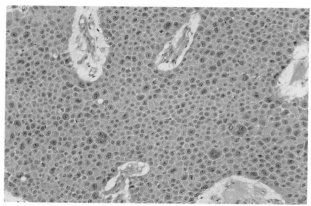

Figure 11-19 **Calcifying epithelial odontogenic tumor** composed of a sheet of atypical and multinucleated tumor epithelial cells.

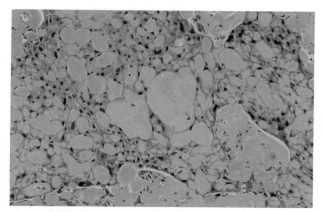

Figure 11-20 **Calcifying epithelial odontogenic tumor** showing amyloid deposits.

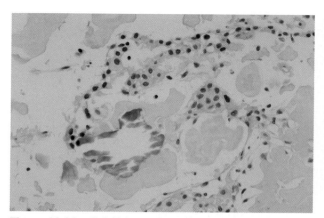

Figure 11-21 **Calcifying epithelial odontogenic tumor** showing nuclear atypia, amyloid, and calcification.

Differential Diagnosis. When this lesion is radiolucent, it must be separated clinically from dentigerous cyst, odontogenic keratocyst, ameloblastoma, and odontogenic myxoma. Some benign nonodontogenic jaw tumors might also be considered, but these would be less likely, on the basis of age and location.

When a mixed radiolucent-radiopaque pattern is encountered, calcified odontogenic cyst should be considered in a clinical differential diagnosis. Other, less likely possibilities include adenomatoid odontogenic tumor, ameloblastic fibroodontoma, ossifying fibroma, and osteoblastoma.

Treatment. This tumor has invasive potential but apparently not to the extent of ameloblastoma. It is slow growing and compromises the patient through direct extension. Metastases have not been reported. Various forms of surgery, ranging from enucleation to resection, have been used to treat CEOTs. The overall recurrence rate has been less than 20%,

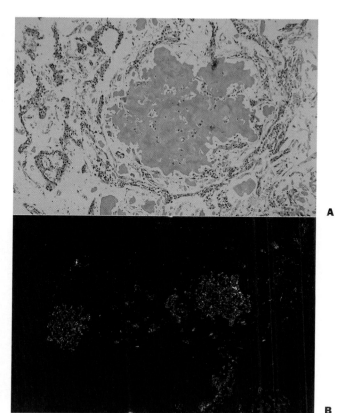

Figure 11-22 **Calcifying epithelial odontogenic tumor.** **A,** Congo red stain. **B,** Congo red stain viewed through polarized light. Amyloid is apple green.

indicating that aggressive surgery is not indicated for the management of most of these benign neoplasms.

Adenomatoid Odontogenic Tumor

Although adenomatoid odontogenic tumor (AOT) is an odontogenic lesion that contains ductlike or gland-like structures, until its distinctive characteristics were fully appreciated, it was thought to be a subtype of ameloblastoma and was known by the name *adenoameloblastoma*. Clinically, microscopically, and behaviorally, it is clearly different from ameloblastoma, behaving more like a hamartoma than a neoplasm (Box 11-7).

Clinical Features. AOTs are seen in a rather narrow age range, between 5 and 30 years, with most cases appearing in the second decade. Females are more commonly affected than males. Most lesions appear in the anterior portion of the jaws and more often in the anterior maxilla, generally in association with the crowns of impacted teeth (Figure 11-23). Rarely, this lesion is seen in a peripheral gingival location.

Radiographically, the AOT is a well-circumscribed unilocular lesion usually around the crown of an impacted tooth. Lesions are typically radiolucent but may have small opaque foci distributed throughout, reflecting the presence of calcifications in the tumor tissue (Figure 11-24). When they are located between anterior teeth, divergence of roots may be seen.

Histopathology. An intracystic epithelial proliferation is composed of polyhedral to spindle cells. The pattern is typically lobular, although some areas may show a syncytial arrangement of cells. Rosettes and ductlike structures of columnar epithelial cells give the lesion its characteristic microscopic features (Figures 11-25 and 11-26). Foci of PAS-positive material are scattered

throughout the lesion. The number, size, and degree of calcification of these foci determine how the lesion presents radiographically.

Differential Diagnosis. Other lesions that might be included in a differential diagnosis of AOT are

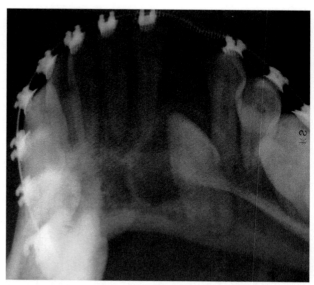

Figure 11-23 **Adenomatoid odontogenic tumor** surrounding the crown of an impacted tooth.

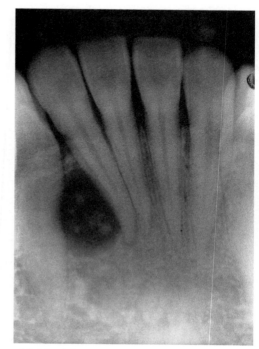

Figure 11-24 **Adenomatoid odontogenic tumor** with opaque islands.

Box 11-7 Adenomatoid Odontogenic Tumor

Epithelial odontogenic hamartoma containing pseudoducts and enameloid
Tumor of two thirds—maxilla, females, anterior jaws, crown of impacted tooth
Teenagers most commonly affected; rarely seen over the age of 30 years
Lucent and lucent-opaque patterns
Treatment by enucleation; no recurrences

dentigerous cyst (because of frequent association with impacted teeth) and lateral root cyst (because of its occasional location adjacent to roots of anterior teeth). If opacities are evident, calcifying odontogenic cyst and CEOT should receive consideration.

Treatment. Conservative treatment (enucleation) is all that is required. AOTs are benign, encapsulated lesions that do not recur.

Squamous Odontogenic Tumor

Because squamous odontogenic tumor involves the alveolar process, the lesion is believed to be derived from neoplastic transformation of the rests of Malassez. It occurs in the mandible and maxilla with equal frequency, favoring the anterior region of the maxilla and the posterior region of the mandible. Multiple lesions have been described in about 20% of affected patients, as have multicentric familial lesions.

The age range for this tumor extends from the second through the seventh decades, with a mean age of 40 years. There is no gender predilection. Patients usually experience no symptoms, although tenderness and tooth mobility have been reported. Radiographically, this lesion is typically a well-circumscribed, often semilunar lesion associated with the cervical region of roots of teeth. Microscopically, it has some similarity to ameloblastoma, although it lacks the columnar peripherally palisaded layer of epithelial cells (Figure 11-27). Although proliferation is robust, there is also some similarity to proliferating odontogenic rests.

Squamous odontogenic tumors have some invasive capacity and infrequently recur after conservative therapy. Curettage or excision is the treatment of choice.

Clear Cell Odontogenic Tumor (Carcinoma)

Clear cell odontogenic tumor (carcinoma) is a rare neoplasm of the mandible and maxilla (Box 11-8). The etiology is unknown, but the location and histologic appearance of this lesion suggest an odontogenic source. Usually found in women older than 60 years of age, it is a locally aggressive, poorly circumscribed neoplasm composed of sheets of cells with relatively clear cytoplasm (Figure 11-28). Metastases to lung and regional lymph nodes have been reported. The microscopic differential diagnosis includes other jaw tumors that may have a clear cell component, such as CEOT, central mucoepidermoid carcinoma, metastatic acinic cell carcinoma, metastatic renal cell carcinoma, and ameloblastoma. Stains often need to be performed to rule out other local clear cell carcinomas that produce mucin or glycogen, and a metastatic survey needs to

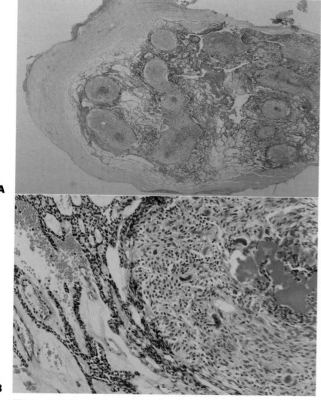

Figure 11-25 **Adenomatoid odontogenic tumor.**
A and **B,** Characteristic thick capsule and intraluminal nodular proliferation. Note calcified material in **B** *(right).*

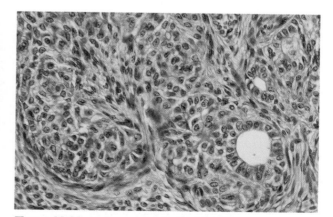

Figure 11-26 **Adenomatoid odontogenic tumor** exhibiting pseudoducts and rosettes.

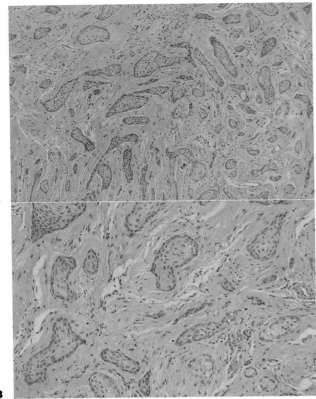

A

B

Figure 11-27 **Squamous odontogenic tumor. A** and **B,** Bland proliferation of squamous islands.

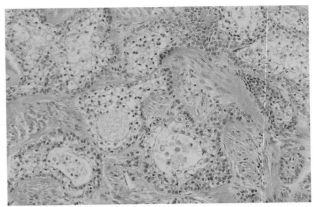

Figure 11-28 **Clear cell odontogenic tumor** as nests of odontogenic epithelium with relatively clear cytoplasm.

Box 11-8 Clear Cell Odontogenic Tumor

HISTOGENESIS

Unknown; probably odontogenic

CLINICAL FEATURES

Age over 60 years; women affected more often than men
Either jaw
Occasionally painful

HISTOPATHOLOGY

Nests/cords of clear cells, some palisades
Some glycogen; mucin negative

MICROSCOPIC DIFFERENTIAL DIAGNOSIS

Calcifying epithelial odontogenic tumor
Mucoepidermoid carcinoma
Renal cell carcinoma

BEHAVIOR

Recurrence and metastasis (neck nodes/lung)

---

be done to exclude clear cell malignancies from other sites in the body.

MESENCHYMAL TUMORS

Odontogenic Myxoma

Odontogenic myxoma is a mesenchymal lesion that mimics microscopically the dental pulp or follicular connective tissue. When relatively large amounts of collagen are evident, the term *fibromyxoma* may be used. This is a benign neoplasm that may be infiltrative and aggressive and that may recur (Box 11-9).

Clinical Features. The age range in which this lesion appears extends from 10 to 50 years, with a mean of about 30 years. There is no gender predilection, and the lesions are seen anywhere in the mandible and maxilla with about equal frequency (Figure 11-29).

Radiographically, this lesion is always lucent, although the pattern may be quite variable. It may appear as a well-circumscribed or a diffuse lesion. It is often multilocular and often has a honeycomb pattern (Figure 11-30). Cortical expansion or perforation and root displacement or resorption may be seen.

Histopathology. This tumor is composed of bland, relatively acellular myxomatous connective tissue (Figure 11-31). Benign fibroblasts and myofibroblasts with variable amounts of collagen are found in a mucopolysaccharide matrix. Bony islands, representing residual trabeculae, and capillaries are found scattered throughout the lesion (Figure 11-32). Odontogenic rests are

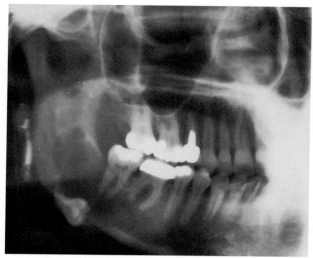

Figure 11-29 **Odontogenic myxoma** of the right mandible. Note malpositioned third molar.

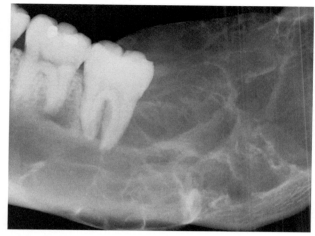

Figure 11-30 **Odontogenic myxoma** showing characteristic multilocularity.

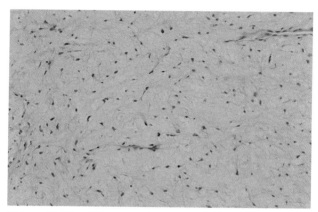

Figure 11-31 **Odontogenic myxoma** exhibiting typical bland myxoid appearance.

Box 11-9 Odontogenic Myxoma (Fibromyxoma)

HISTOGENESIS

Periodontal ligament or dental pulp

CLINICAL FEATURES

Adults (median of about 30 years of age)
Either jaw

HISTOPATHOLOGY

Bland myxoid
No epithelial rests
Variable amounts of collagen

MICROSCOPIC DIFFERENTIAL DIAGNOSIS

Hyperplastic follicular sac and dental pulp
Odontogenic fibroma
Desmoplastic fibroma

BEHAVIOR

Recurrences
No capsule and loose tumor consistency

---

typically absent in these tumors and are not required for the diagnosis. Odontogenic myxomas have a very low proliferation rate. However, they express some anti-apoptotic proteins that, in part, may explain their persistence. Myxomatous follicular sacs with odontogenic rests should not be confused with this neoplasm (Figure 11-33).

Differential Diagnosis. The clinical differential diagnosis is essentially the same as that described for ameloblastoma. In addition, central hemangioma is a serious consideration for a lesion with a honeycomb radiographic appearance. An important note is that the microscopic differential diagnosis should include developing dental pulp and hyperplastic follicular connective tissue surrounding a developing or mature impacted tooth. Nerve sheath myxoma might also be considered, although this entity is rare in the jaws. Clinical pathologic correlation is important in the definitive diagnosis of odontogenic myxoma.

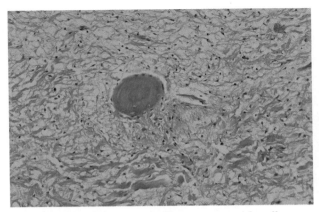

Figure 11-32 **Odontogenic fibromyxoma** with collagen bundles and residual bony trabecula *(center)* evident.

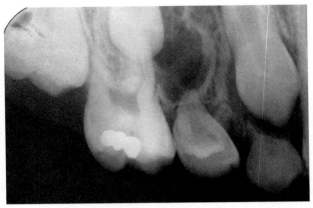

Figure 11-34 **Central odontogenic fibroma** of the right maxilla.

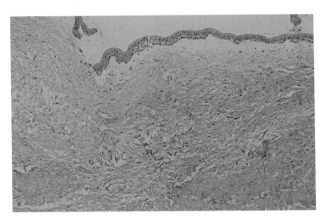

Figure 11-33 **Follicular sac** with myxomatous change. Note residual reduced enamel epithelium at top.

Box 11-10 Central Odontogenic Fibroma

HISTOGENESIS

Origin unknown; may be from periodontal ligament or dental pulp

CLINICAL FEATURES

Adults
Well-defined lucency

HISTOPATHOLOGY

Collagenous with epithelial strands

MICROSCOPIC DIFFERENTIAL DIAGNOSIS

Desmoplastic fibroma
Fibromyxoma
Hyperplastic follicular sac

BEHAVIOR

Few recurrences

Treatment. Surgical excision is the treatment of choice. Because of an often loose, gelatinous consistency, curettage may result in incomplete removal of the neoplasm. The absence of encapsulation may also contribute to recurrence if the lesion is treated too conservatively. Although these lesions exhibit some aggressiveness and have a moderate recurrence rate, the prognosis is very good. Repeated surgical procedures do not appear to stimulate growth or metastasis.

Central Odontogenic Fibroma

Central odontogenic fibroma is a rare lesion that is regarded as the central counterpart to peripheral odontogenic fibroma (Box 11-10). It has been seen in all age-groups, and it is found in both the mandible and the maxilla (Figure 11-34). It results in a radiolucent lesion that is usually multilocular, often causing cortical expansion. The clinical differential diagnosis is similar to that described for ameloblastoma.

Microscopically, two patterns are generally ascribed to central odontogenic fibroma (Figure 11-35). In the simple type, the lesion is composed of a mass of mature fibrous tissue containing few epithelial rests. In the World Health Organization type, mature connective tissue contains abundant rests and calcific deposits of what is regarded as dentin or cementum. This microscopic differentiation may be academic, since there appears to be no difference in clinical behavior

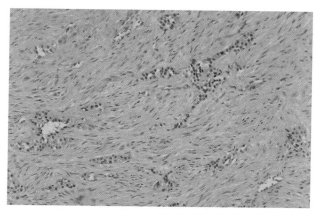

Figure 11-35 **Central odontogenic fibroma** containing strands of odontogenic epithelium.

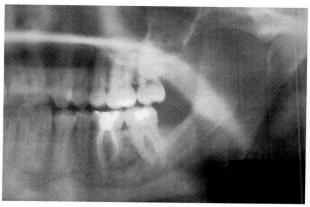

Figure 11-36 **Cementoblastoma** around the roots of a mandibular first molar.

between the two subtypes. A microscopic differential diagnosis would include *desmoplastic fibroma* (the bony counterpart of fibromatosis). This purely fibrous connective tissue lesion may be difficult to separate from central odontogenic fibroma because of overlapping microscopy. Clinical correlation should help, since desmoplastic fibroma would exhibit a more aggressive and recurrent behavior. Treatment of odontogenic fibroma is enucleation or excision, and recurrence is very uncommon.

Cementifying Fibroma

See discussion of ossifying fibroma in Chapter 12.

Cementoblastoma

Clinical Features. Cementoblastoma, also known as *true cementoma*, is a rare benign neoplasm of cementoblast origin (Box 11-11). It occurs predominantly in the second and third decades of life, typically before 25 years of age. There is no gender predilection. It is more often seen in the mandible than in the maxilla and more often in posterior than in anterior regions. It is intimately associated with the root of a tooth, and the tooth remains vital. Cementoblastoma may cause cortical expansion and, occasionally, low-grade intermittent pain.

Radiographically, this neoplasm is an opaque lesion that replaces the root of the tooth (Figure 11-36). It is usually surrounded by a radiolucent ring representing the periodontal ligament space and the advancing front of the tumor.

Box 11-11 Cementoblastoma

Benign fibroosseous/cementum jaw lesion
Young adults, mandible > maxilla
Attached to and replaces tooth root
Periodontal ligament space surrounds lesion
Opaque mass; may rarely cause cortical expansion
Histologic features of osteoblastoma
Attached to tooth; tooth removed with lesion
No recurrence

>, More frequently affected than.

Histopathology. This lesion appears microscopically as a dense mass of mineralized cementum-like material with numerous reversal lines (Figure 11-37). Intervening well-vascularized soft tissue contains cementoblasts—often numerous, large, and hyperchromatic. Occasional cementoclasts are also evident. This lesion has histologic features similar to those of osteoblastoma but is attached to a tooth root.

Differential Diagnosis. The characteristic radiographic appearance of this lesion is usually diagnostic. Other opaque lesions that share some features include odontoma, osteoblastoma, focal sclerosing osteomyelitis, and hypercementosis.

Treatment. Because of the intimate association of this neoplasm with the tooth root, it cannot be removed without sacrificing the tooth. Bone relief is typically required to remove this well-circumscribed mass. Recurrence is not seen.

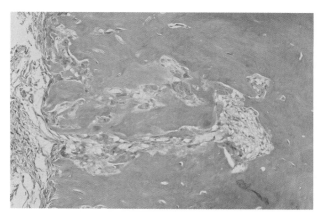

Figure 11-37 **Cementoblastoma** with a periphery showing numerous pale cementoblasts *(left)* against a dense network of cementum.

Periapical Cementoosseous Dysplasia

As the name implies, periapical cementoosseous dysplasia (formerly known as *cementoma*) represents a reactive or dysplastic process rather than a neoplastic one. This lesion appears to be an unusual response of periapical bone and cementum to some undetermined local factor (Box 11-12). When not associated with a tooth apex the term *focal cementoosseous dysplasia* is used.

Clinical Features. This is a relatively common phenomenon that occurs at the apex of vital teeth. A biopsy is unnecessary because the condition is usually diagnostic by clinical and radiographic features. Women, especially black women, are affected more than men. Periapical cementoosseous dysplasia appears in middle age (around 40 years) and rarely before the age of 20. The mandible, especially the anterior periapical region, is far more commonly affected than other areas. More often, the apices of two or more teeth are affected.

This condition is typically discovered on routine radiographic examination, because patients are asymptomatic. It appears first as a periapical lucency that is continuous with the periodontal ligament space. Although this initial pattern simulates radiographically a periapical granuloma or cyst, the teeth are always vital. As the condition progresses or matures, the lucent lesion develops into a mixed or mottled pattern because of bone repair. The final stage appears as a solid, opaque mass that is often surrounded by a thin, lucent ring. This process takes months to years to reach the final stages of development and, obviously, may be discovered at any stage (Figures 11-38 to 11-40).

A less common condition known as *florid cementoosseous dysplasia (FCOD)* appears to be an exuberant

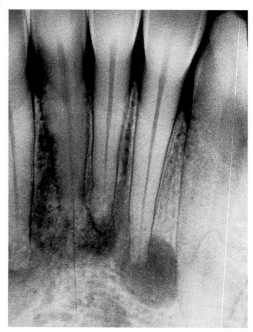

Figure 11-38 **Periapical cementoosseous dysplasia,** radiolucent phase.

Box 11-12 Periapical Cementoosseous Dysplasia

CLINICAL FEATURES

Reactive, unknown stimulus, teeth vital
Common in anterior mandible of adults
No symptoms
Progresses from lucent to opaque lesion
Exuberant variant—florid cementoosseous dysplasia

HISTOPATHOLOGY

Fibroosseous lesion
Mature and immature bone
Heterogeneous pattern
Few inflammatory cells

OTHER

No treatment
Clinical radiographic correlation is diagnostic

---

form of periapical cemental dysplasia (Box 11-13 and Figure 11-41). FCOD represents the severe end of the spectrum of this unusual process. There is no apparent cause, and patients are asymptomatic except when the complication of osteomyelitis occurs. Women,

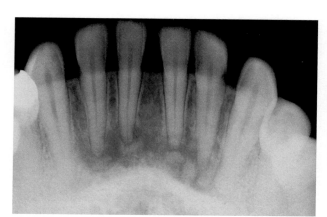

Figure 11-39 Periapical cementoosseous dysplasia, radiopaque phase.

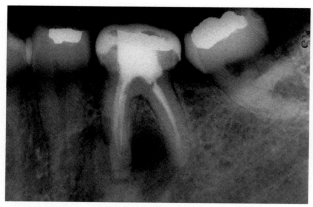

Figure 11-40 Periapical cementoosseous dysplasia associated with a molar tooth.

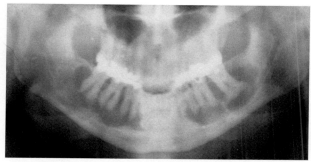

Figure 11-41 Florid cementoosseous dysplasia of the mandible.

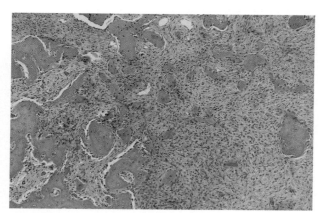

Figure 11-42 Periapical cementoosseous dysplasia. This lesion has a heterogeneous benign fibroosseous appearance.

especially black women, are predominantly affected, usually between 25 and 60 years of age. The condition is typically bilateral and may affect all four quadrants. A curious finding has been the concomitant appearance of traumatic (simple) bone cysts in affected tissue. Radiographically, FCOD appears as diffuse radiopaque masses throughout the alveolar segment of the jaws. A ground-glass or cystlike appearance may also be seen.

Histopathology. Periapical cementoosseous dysplasia is a mixture of benign fibrous tissue, bone, and cementum (Figure 11-42). The calcified tissue is arranged in trabeculae, spicules, or larger irregular masses. Reversal lines are eventually seen, and osteoblasts or cementoblasts, or both, line the islands of hard tissue. Chronic inflammatory cells may also be seen. Microscopically, periapical cementoosseous dysplasia may

---

Box 11-13 Florid Cementoosseous Dysplasia

Exuberant variant of periapical cementoosseous dysplasia
Large lucency with opaque zones
Predominantly mandible in adults
Confused clinically with diffuse sclerosing osteomyelitis
Asymptomatic unless secondarily infected
Teeth are vital
Diagnosis from clinical radiographic correlation
No treatment unless secondarily infected

---

appear very similar to chronic osteomyelitis and ossifying fibroma.

Microscopically, FCOD is a heterogeneous lesion consisting of a benign fibrous stroma containing irregular trabeculae of mature and immature bone and cementum-like material (Figure 11-43). Because FCOD is an asymptomatic, self-limited process, no treatment is required. In cases in which secondary

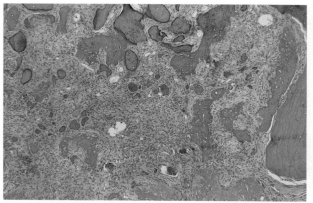

Figure 11-43   **Florid cementoosseous dysplasia.** This lesion has a heterogeneous benign fibroosseous appearance.

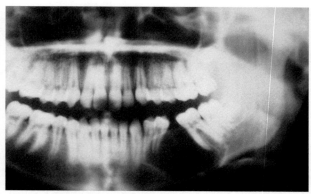

Figure 11-44   **Ameloblastic fibroma** of the left mandible. The lesion is a well-circumscribed lucency.

infection occurs, antibiotics and sequestrectomy may be necessary.

Differential Diagnosis. Age, gender, location, radiographic appearance, and tooth vitality considered together are diagnostic of this condition. When one or more of these factors are atypical, other diagnostic considerations include chronic osteomyelitis, ossifying fibroma, and periapical granuloma or cyst. In the opaque stage, odontoma, osteoblastoma, and focal sclerosing osteomyelitis are diagnostic possibilities.

The clinical differential diagnosis of FCOD includes diffuse sclerosing osteomyelitis, Paget's disease, and familial gigantiform cementoma. Paget's disease can be ruled out with a biopsy and determination of serum alkaline phosphatase (elevated in Paget's disease, normal in FCOD). Chronic diffuse sclerosing osteomyelitis would be symptomatic, and it would have a different radiographic appearance. Also, inflammatory cells would appear in biopsy tissue.

Treatment. No treatment is required for either periapical cementoosseous dysplasia or FCOD. Once the opaque stage is reached, the lesion stabilizes and causes no complications. Because teeth remain vital throughout the entire process, they should not be extracted, and endodontic procedures should not be done.

MIXED (EPITHELIAL AND MESENCHYMAL) TUMORS

Ameloblastic Fibroma and Ameloblastic Fibroodontoma

Ameloblastic fibroma and ameloblastic fibroodontoma are considered together because they appear to be

> **Box 11-14 Ameloblastic Fibroma/Fibroodontoma**
>
> Occurs in children and teenagers
> Often associated with an impacted tooth
> Composed of neoplastic epithelium and neoplastic myxomatous connective tissue
> Treatment by curettage or excision
> Excellent prognosis; rarely recurs
> Malignant counterpart is rare

slight variations of the same process (Box 11-14). Except for the presence of an odontoma, people affected with either of these two lesions share similar features of age, gender, and location. The biologic behaviors of these lesions are also similar. Both are benign mixed odontogenic tumors composed of neoplastic epithelium and mesenchyme with microscopically identical soft tissue components.

Clinical Features. These neoplasms occur predominantly in children and young adults. The mean age is about 12 years, and the upper age limit seems to be 40 years. The mandibular molar-ramus area is the favored location for these lesions, although any region may be affected (Figures 11-44 and 11-45). There is no gender predilection.

Radiographically, these lesions are well circumscribed and are usually surrounded by a sclerotic margin. They may be either unilocular or multilocular and may be associated with the crown of an impacted tooth. An opaque focus that appears within the ameloblastic fibroodontoma is due to the presence of

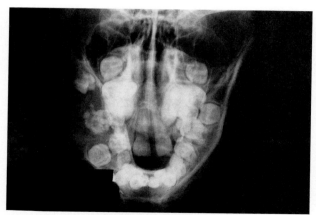

Figure 11-45 **Ameloblastic fibroodontoma** as represented in the right molar-ramus area of this skull radiograph. Note odontoma between impacted teeth.

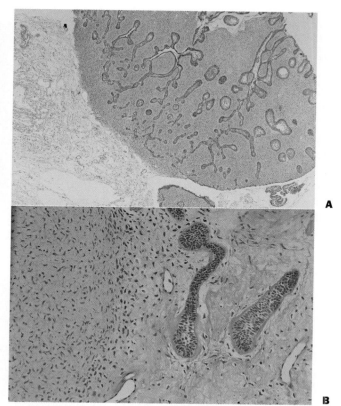

Figure 11-47 **Ameloblastic fibroma. A,** Lobular circumscribed pattern. **B,** Myxoid stroma and odontogenic strands.

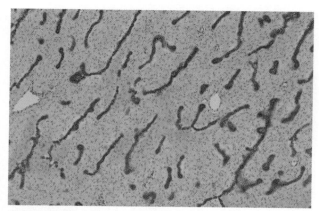

Figure 11-46 **Ameloblastic fibroma** composed of pale myxoid stroma with numerous strands of odontogenic epithelium.

an odontoma. This lesion therefore presents as a combined lucent-opaque lesion; the ameloblastic fibroma is completely lucent radiographically.

Histopathology. These lesions are lobulated in general configuration and are usually surrounded by a fibrous capsule. The tumor mass is composed predominantly of a primitive-appearing myxoid connective tissue (Figures 11-46 and 11-47). The general absence of collagen gives this component a resemblance to dental pulp. Evenly distributed throughout the tumor mesenchyme are ribbons or strands of odontogenic epithelium that are typically two cells wide. Rarely the epithelium may be more follicular in appearance, resembling ameloblastoma. The epithelial component has been compared microscopically to the dental lamina that proliferates from oral epithelium in the early stages of tooth development.

In ameloblastic fibroodontoma, one or more foci contain enamel and dentin. This may be in the form of a compound or complex odontoma, the presence of which does not alter the treatment or prognosis (Figure 11-48).

Differential Diagnosis. When ameloblastic fibroma (fibroodontoma) presents with the clinical features (age, location) and radiographic pattern that are typical for these lesions, the diagnosis is usually apparent. When clinical features are outside the usual boundaries, a differential diagnosis for ameloblastic fibroma should include ameloblastoma, odontogenic myxoma, dentigerous cyst, odontogenic keratocyst, central giant cell granuloma, and histiocytosis. The differential diagnosis for ameloblastic fibroodontoma includes lesions with mixed radiographic patterns such as calcifying epithelial odontogenic tumor, calcifying odontogenic cyst, developing odontoma, and possibly adenomatoid

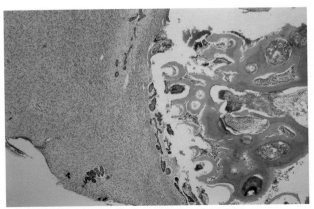

Figure 11-48   Ameloblastic fibroodontoma. Note odontoma at right.

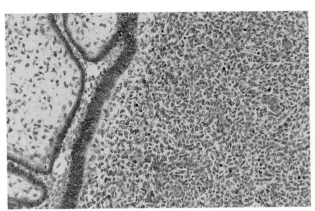

Figure 11-49   Ameloblastic fibrosarcoma with a malignant mesenchymal component.

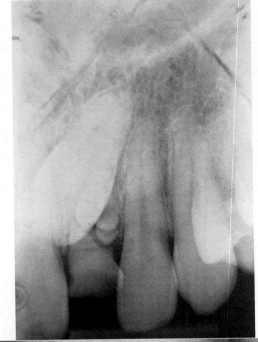

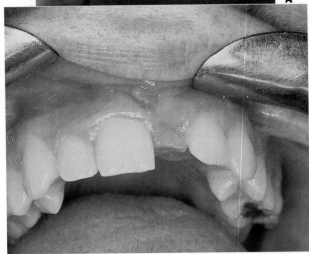

Figure 11-50   A, Compound odontoma blocking the eruption of a permanent tooth. **B,** Retained deciduous tooth overlying compound odontoma.

odontogenic tumor. Microscopically, this lesion must be differentiated from the hyperplastic follicular sacs, in which there is proliferation of odontogenic rests.

Treatment. Because of tumor encapsulation and the general lack of invasive capacity, this lesion is treated with a conservative surgical procedure such as curettage or excision. Recurrences have been documented, but they are uncommon.

A rare malignant counterpart known as *ameloblastic fibrosarcoma* has been documented as arising in the jaws either de novo or from preexisting or recurrent ameloblastic fibroma (Figure 11-49). In this lesion the mesenchymal component has the appearance of a fibrosarcoma and the epithelial component appears as it does in the benign lesion. Clinically, ameloblastic fibrosarcoma occurs at an age of about 30 years and more often in the mandible than in the maxilla. Symp-

toms of pain and paresthesia may be present. This is a locally aggressive lesion that has metastatic potential. Resection is therefore the treatment of choice.

Odontoma

Odontomas are *mixed odontogenic tumors*, since they are composed of both epithelial and mesenchymal dental

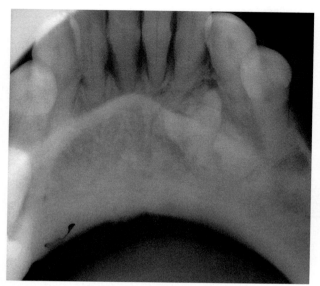

Figure 11-51 **Complex odontoma** in the anterior mandible.

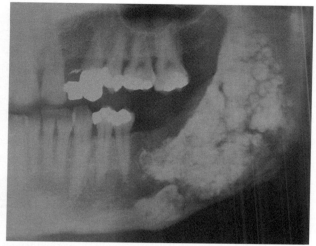

Figure 11-52 **Complex odontoma** occupying most of the mandibular ramus.

hard tissues. These fully differentiated tissues are a composite of enamel and dentin. Biologically, odontomas can be regarded as hamartomas rather than neoplasms.

These calcified lesions take one of two general configurations. They may appear as numerous miniature or rudimentary teeth, in which case they are known as *compound odontomas*, or they may appear as amorphous conglomerations of hard tissue, in which case they are known as *complex odontomas*. They are the most common odontogenic tumors.

Clinical Features. Odontomas are lesions of children and young adults; most are discovered in the second decade of life. The range does, however, extend into later adulthood. The maxilla is affected slightly more often than the mandible. There is also a tendency for compound odontomas to occur in the anterior jaws and for complex odontomas to occur in the posterior jaws. There does not appear to be a significant gender predilection. Clinical signs suggestive of an odontoma include a retained deciduous tooth, an impacted tooth, and alveolar swelling (Figure 11-50). These lesions generally produce no symptoms.

Radiographically, compound odontomas typically appear as numerous tiny teeth in a single focus. This focus is typically in a tooth-bearing area, between roots or over the crown of an impacted tooth. Complex odontomas appear in the same regions but as amorphous, opaque masses (Figures 11-51 and 11-52). Lesions dis-

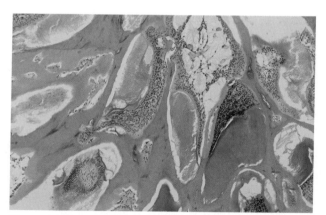

Figure 11-53 **Complex odontoma** (decalcified) showing a network of pink dentin and islands of bluish enamel matrix.

covered during early stages of tumor development are primarily radiolucent, with focal areas of opacity representing early calcification of dentin and enamel.

Histopathology. Normal-appearing enamel, dentin, cementum, and pulp may be seen in these lesions. Prominent enamel matrix and the associated enamel organ are often seen before final maturation of hard tissues (Figure 11-53). So-called ghost cell keratinization is occasionally seen in the enamel-forming cells of some odontomas. This microscopic feature has no significance other than to indicate the potential of these epithelial cells to keratinize.

Differential Diagnosis. Compound odontomas are diagnostic on radiographic examination. Complex odontomas usually present a typical radiographic appearance because of their solid opacification in relationship to teeth. However, a differential diagnosis might include other opaque jaw lesions such as focal sclerosing osteitis, osteoma, periapical cemental dysplasia, ossifying fibroma, and cementoblastoma.

Treatment. Odontomas have very limited growth potential, although an occasional complex odontoma may achieve a considerable mass. Enucleation is curative, and recurrence is not a problem.

A rare variant known as *odontoameloblastoma* has been described. This is essentially an ameloblastoma in which there is focal differentiation into an odontoma. Until more is known of the behavior of this rare lesion, it should be treated as an ameloblastoma.

BIBLIOGRAPHY

ODONTOGENIC TUMORS

Aviel-Ronen S, Liokumovich P, Rahima D, et al: The amyloid deposit in calcifying epithelial odontogenic tumor is immunoreactive for cytokeratins, *Arch Pathol Lab Med* 124:872-876, 2000.

Daley TD, Wysocki GP: Relative incidence of odontogenic tumors and oral and jaw cysts in a Canadian population, *Oral Surg Oral Med Oral Pathol* 77:276-228, 1994.

Handlers J, Abrams A, Melrose R, et al: Central odontogenic fibroma, *J Oral Maxillofac Surg* 49:46-54, 1991.

Kumamoto H, Ooya K: Immunohistochemical analysis of Bcl-2 family proteins in benign and malignant ameloblastomas, *J Oral Pathol Med* 28:343-349, 1999.

Li TJ, Browne RM, Matthews JB: Expression of proliferating cell nuclear antigen (PCNA) and Ki-67 in unicystic ameloblastoma, *Histopathology* 26:219-228, 1995.

Lu Y, Mock D, Takata T, et al: Odontogenic ghost cell tumor: report of four new cases and review of the literature, *J Oral Pathol Med* 28:323-329, 1999.

Nakamura N, Mitsuyasu T, Higuchi Y, et al: Growth characteristics of ameloblastoma involving the inferior alveolar nerve: a clinical and histopathologic study, *Oral Surg Oral Med Oral Pathol Oral Radiol Endod* 91:557-562, 2001.

Philipsen HP, Reichert PA: Unicystic ameloblastoma: a review of 193 cases from the literature, *Oral Oncol* 34:317-325, 1998.

Philipsen HP, Reichert PA, Nikai H, et al: Peripheral ameloblastoma: biological profile based on 160 cases from the literature, *Oral Oncol* 37:17-27, 2001.

Philipsen HP, Reichart PA, Zhang K, et al: Adenomatoid odontogenic tumor: biologic profile based on 499 cases, *J Oral Pathol Med* 20:149-158, 1991.

Rosenstein T, Pogrel MA, Smith RA, et al: Cystic ameloblastoma: behavior and treatment of 21 cases, *J Oral Maxillofac Surg* 59:1311-1316, 2001.

Sciubba JJ, Fantasia JE, Kahn LB: *Tumors and cysts of the jaws*, Washington, DC, 2001, Armed Forces Institute of Pathology.

Slootweg PJ: p53 protein and Ki-67 reactivity in epithelial odontogenic lesions: an immunohistochemical study, *J Oral Pathol Med* 24:393-397, 1995.

Thomas G, Pandey M, Mathew A, et al: Primary intraosseous carcinoma of the jaw: pooled analysis of the world literature and report of two cases, *Int J Oral Maxillofac Surg* 30:349-355, 2001.

Thompson IO, van Rensberg LJ, Phillips VM: Desmoplastic ameloblastoma: correlative histopathology, radiology, and CT-MR imaging, *J Oral Pathol Med* 25:405-410, 1996.

BENIGN NONODONTOGENIC TUMORS

Jeffery C.B. Stewart, DDS, MS

Ossifying Fibroma

Fibrous Dysplasia

Cementoosseous Dysplasia

Osteoblastoma/Osteoid Osteoma

Osteoma

Desmoplastic Fibroma

Chondroma

Central Giant Cell Granuloma

Giant Cell Tumor

Hemangioma of Bone

Langerhans Cell Disease

Tori and Exostoses

   Torus Palatinus

   Torus Mandibularis

   Exostoses

Coronoid Hyperplasia

OSSIFYING FIBROMA

Ossifying fibroma is a benign neoplasm of bone that has the potential for excessive growth, bone destruction, and recurrence. It is clinically and microscopically similar, if not identical, to cementifying fibroma. Composed of a fibrous connective tissue stroma in which new bone is formed, it is classified as one of the benign fibroosseous lesions of the jaws (Boxes 12-1 and 12-2).

Etiology and Pathogenesis. Ossifying fibroma is of undetermined cause (Box 12-3). Although chromosome translocations have been identified in a few cases of ossifying fibroma, genetic studies have been insufficient to determine the molecular mechanisms that underlie the development of this tumor.

Clinical Features. Ossifying fibroma is an uncommon lesion that tends to occur during the third and fourth decades of life, and in women more than men. It is a slow-growing, asymptomatic, and expansile lesion. In the head and neck, ossifying fibroma may be seen in the jaws and craniofacial bones. Lesions of the jaws characteristically arise in the tooth-bearing regions, most often in the mandibular premolar-molar area (Figure 12-1). The slow but persistent growth of the tumor may ultimately produce expansion and thinning of the buccal and lingual cortical plates, although perforation and mucosal ulceration are rare (Figure 12-2). Most of these lesions are solitary, although instances of multiple synchronous lesions have been reported; there is rarely a familial background for synchronous lesions.

The most important radiographic feature of this lesion is the well-circumscribed, sharply defined border. Ossifying fibromas otherwise present a variable appearance, depending on the density of calcifications present. Lesions may be relatively radiolucent because of evenly dispersed, calcified new bone. Lesions may also appear as unilocular or multilocular radiolucencies that bear a resemblance to odontogenic lesions. A mixed radiolucent-radiopaque image is seen when islands of tumor bone are densely calcified. The roots of teeth may be displaced and, less commonly, tooth resorption is seen.

A variant of ossifying fibroma, *juvenile (aggressive) ossifying fibroma*, has been described in children and young adults (Box 12-4). Most affected individuals are younger than 15 years of age. This lesion most commonly involves the paranasal sinuses and periorbital

Box 12-1 Fibroosseous Lesions of the Jaws

Generic microscopic term
Benign fibrous stroma with immature bone
Includes reactive, dysplastic, neoplastic lesions
Histologic overlap
Diagnosis based on clinical pathologic correlation

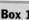

Box 12-2 Fibroosseous Lesions of the Jaws: Entities Most Commonly Included

Ossifying fibroma
Fibrous dysplasia
Cementoosseous dysplasia
  Periapical/focal
  Florid
Chronic osteomyelitis

Box 12-3 Ossifying Fibroma

CLINICAL FEATURES

Third and fourth decades
Mandible > maxilla
Well circumscribed
Lucent or lucent/opaque pattern
Continuous growth

HISTOPATHOLOGY

Cellular fibrous matrix
Islands/trabeculae of new bone
Osteoblasts; no osteoclasts
Relatively homogeneous pattern
No inflammatory cells

TREATMENT

Curettage/excision

>, More frequently affected than.

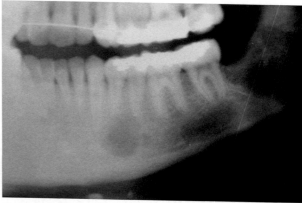

Figure 12-1 **Ossifying fibroma** of the left mandible. The lesion is relatively radiolucent at apices of premolars.

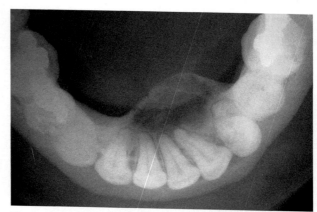

Figure 12-2 **Ossifying fibroma** in the anterior mandible showing cortical expansion.

Cementifying fibroma, cementoossifying fibroma, and *psammomatoid ossifying fibroma* are terms occasionally used when the bony islands in these lesions have a round or spheroidal shape. These tumors occur in similar age-groups and locations, exhibit comparable clinical characteristics, and have the same biologic behavior. They are, for all practical purposes, the same lesion as ossifying fibroma.

Histopathology. Ossifying fibroma is composed of fibrous connective tissue with well-differentiated spindled fibroblasts. Cellularity is uniform but may vary from one lesion to the next. Collagen fibers are arranged haphazardly, although a whorled, storiform pattern may be evident. Bony spheroids, trabeculae, or islands are evenly distributed throughout the fibrous stroma (Figures 12-3 to 12-5). Bone is immature and often

bones, where it may cause exophthalmos, proptosis, sinusitis, and nasal symptoms. This rare tumor behaves in a more aggressive fashion than does ossifying fibroma, and it may require more extensive surgery when encountered. Microscopically, juvenile ossifying fibroma is highly cellular and contains trabeculae or spheroids of new bone.

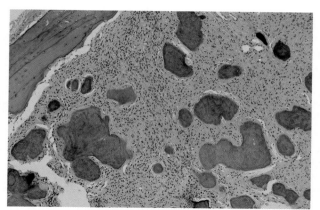

Figure 12-3 **Ossifying fibroma** exhibiting islands of new bone in fibroblastic matrix. Note cortex at upper left.

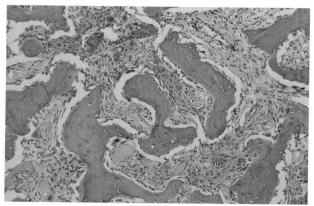

Figure 12-5 **Ossifying fibroma** composed of bony trabeculae in benign fibroblast matrix.

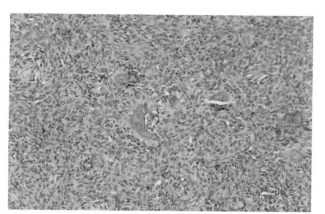

Figure 12-4 **Ossifying fibroma** with cellular stroma and small bony islands.

Box 12-4 Ossifying Fibroma Variants

JUVENILE OSSIFYING FIBROMA

Younger patients
Aggressive clinical course
Cellular (benign) stroma
Trabecular or spherical bone

CEMENTO/PSAMMATOID OSSIFYING FIBROMA

Biologically same as ossifying fibroma
Spherical islands of bone (cementum)
Bone and cementum microscopically identical

surrounded by osteoblasts. Osteoclasts are infrequently seen.

Differential Diagnosis. Distinguishing between ossifying fibroma and fibrous dysplasia is the primary diagnostic challenge. Both lesions may exhibit similar clinical, radiographic, and microscopic features. The most helpful feature in distinguishing the two is the well-circumscribed radiographic appearance of ossifying fibroma and the ease with which it can be separated from normal bone. In most cases the well-defined appearance of ossifying fibroma is evident radiographically. Historically, differentiating the two lesions was based primarily on histologic criteria. Fibrous dysplasia was reported to contain only woven bone, without evidence of osteoblastic rim-

ming of bone. The presence of more mature lamellar bone was believed to be characteristic of ossifying fibroma. Most authorities now acknowledge that these criteria are unreliable, because both types of bone and cellular features may be found in either lesion.

Other differential considerations are osteoblastoma, focal cementoosseous dysplasia, and focal osteomyelitis. Osteoblastoma is evident in a slightly younger age-group and is often characterized by pain. In addition, osseous trabeculae in these lesions are rimmed by abundant plump osteoblasts, and a central nidus may be evident. Periapical cementoosseous dysplasia in posterior teeth may appear radiographically similar and require a biopsy to separate it from ossifying fibroma. Focal osteomyelitis is associated with a source of inflammation and is possibly accompanied by pain and swelling.

Treatment and Prognosis. Treatment of ossifying fibroma is most often accomplished by surgical removal using curettage or enucleation. The lesion can typically be separated easily from the surrounding normal bone. Recurrence is described only rarely after removal.

FIBROUS DYSPLASIA

Fibrous dysplasia is a condition in which normal medullary bone is replaced by an abnormal fibrous connective tissue proliferation in which new, nonmaturing bone is formed (Box 12-5). A genetic defect involving Gs-alpha proteins appears to underlie this process.

Etiology and Pathogenesis. The nature of this condition has not been firmly established. The name given to fibrous dysplasia was originally intended to indicate that the condition represented a dysplastic growth resulting from deranged mesenchymal cell activity or a defect in the control of bone cell activity. Genetic studies, however, have provided evidence that it may be better classified as a neoplastic process. Mutations of the Gs-alpha gene that transcribe transmembrane-signaling G proteins appear to be present in fibrous dysplasia. This genetic alteration may ultimately affect the proliferation and differentiation of fibroblasts/osteoblasts that make up these lesions.

Clinical Features. This disease most commonly presents as an asymptomatic, slow enlargement of the involved bone. Fibrous dysplasia may involve a single bone or several bones concomitantly. *Monostotic fibrous dysplasia* is the designation used to describe the process in one bone. *Polyostotic fibrous dysplasia* applies to cases in which more than one bone is involved. *McCune-Albright syndrome* consists of polyostotic fibrous dysplasia, cutaneous melanotic pigmentations (café-au-lait macules), and endocrine abnormalities. The most commonly reported endocrine disorder consists of precocious sexual development in girls. Acromegaly, hyperthyroidism, hyperparathyroidism, and hyperprolactinemia have also been described. *Jaffe-Lichtenstein syndrome* is characterized by multiple bone lesions of fibrous dysplasia and skin pigmentations.

Monostotic fibrous dysplasia is much more common than the polyostotic form, accounting for as many as 80% of cases. Jaw involvement is common in this form of the disease. Other bones that are commonly affected are the ribs and femur. Fibrous dysplasia occurs more often in the maxilla than in the mandible (Figure 12-6). Maxillary lesions may extend to involve the maxillary sinus, zygoma, sphenoid bone, and floor of the orbit. This form of the disease, with involvement of several adjacent bones, has been referred to as *craniofacial fibrous dysplasia*. The most common site of occurrence with mandibular involvement is in the body portion.

The slow, progressive enlargement of the affected jaw is usually painless and typically presents as a unilateral swelling. As the lesion grows, facial asymmetry becomes evident and may be the initial presenting complaint. The dental arch is generally maintained, although displacement of teeth, malocclusion, and interference with tooth eruption may occasionally occur. Tooth mobility is not seen.

This condition characteristically has its onset during the first or second decade of life. Rarely, the lesion presents later in life, although this may only reflect the insidious, asymptomatic nature of fibrous dysplasia. Monostotic fibrous dysplasia generally exhibits an equal gender distribution, and the polyostotic form tends to occur more commonly in females.

Fibrous dysplasia has a variable radiographic appearance that ranges from a radiolucent lesion to a uniformly radiopaque mass (Figure 12-7). The classic lesion has been described as having a radiopaque

---

Box 12-5 Fibrous Dysplasia

CLINICAL FEATURES

First and second decades (stabilizes at puberty and very slow growth thereafter)
Maxilla > mandible (one or more bones)
Ribs, femur, tibia also affected
Unilateral diffuse opacity
Asymptomatic; self-limiting
Serum laboratory values normal

HISTOPATHOLOGY

New fibrillar bone trabeculae
Few osteoblasts; no osteoclasts
Homogeneous pattern
Vascular matrix
No inflammatory cells

TREATMENT

Surgical recontouring for cosmetics (after growth spurt)
Regrowth in 25% of treated cases

>, More frequently affected than.

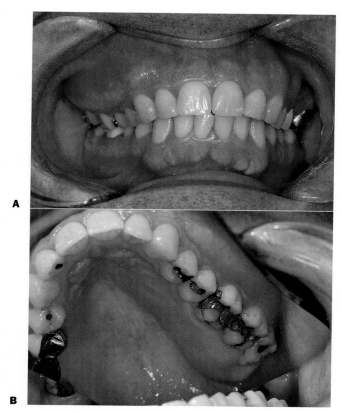

Figure 12-6 **A** and **B, Fibrous dysplasia** of the right maxilla demonstrating asymmetric expansion. **B** is mirror image.

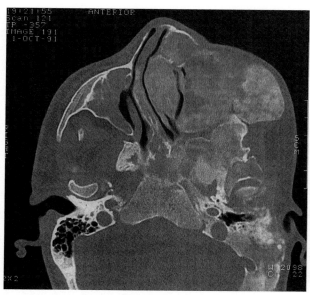

Figure 12-7 **Fibrous dysplasia** of the maxilla as demonstrated in a computed tomography (CT) scan.

change that imparts a "ground glass" or "peau d'orange" effect (Figure 12-8). This characteristic image, which is most identifiable on intraoral radiographs, is not, however, pathognomonic. Lesions of fibrous dysplasia may also present as unilocular or multilocular radiolucencies, especially in long bones. A third pattern, most commonly seen in patients with long-standing disease, is a mottled radiolucent and radiopaque appearance. Additional radiographic features that have been described include a fingerprint bone pattern and superior displacement of the mandibular canal in mandibular lesions.

An important distinguishing feature of fibrous dysplasia is the poorly defined radiographic and clinical margins of the lesion. The process appears to blend into the surrounding normal bone without evidence of a circumscribed border. In addition, these lesions are often elliptic as opposed to spheric.

Laboratory values for patients with monostotic fibrous dysplasia, specifically serum calcium, phosphorus, and alkaline phosphatase, are usually within normal ranges for patients with monostotic disease. However, these serum chemistry markers may be altered in patients with McCune-Albright syndrome.

Histopathology. Fibrous dysplasia consists of a slight to moderate cellular fibrous connective tissue stroma that contains foci of irregularly shaped trabeculae of immature bone (Figures 12-9 and 12-10). A relatively constant ratio of fibrous tissue to bone throughout a given lesion is characteristic. The fibroblasts exhibit uniform spindle-shaped nuclei, and mitotic figures are not seen. The bony trabeculae assume irregular shapes likened to Chinese characters, and they do not display any functional orientation. The bone is predominantly woven in type and appears to arise directly

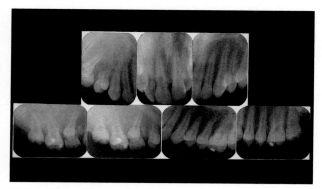

Figure 12-8 **Fibrous dysplasia** of the right maxilla causing a characteristic ground glass effect.

from the collagenous stroma without prominent osteoblastic activity. In a mature fibrous dysplasia lesion, lamellar bone may be found. Capillaries typically are prominent and uniformly distributed.

Differential Diagnosis. The primary differential consideration for fibrous dysplasia of the jaws is ossifying fibroma. As previously noted, clinical, radiographic, and microscopic features must be considered together in order to distinguish these processes. The well-circumscribed ossifying fibroma as compared with the diffuse fibrous dysplasia often serves as the differentiating factor. Additional features that aid in distinguishing these processes are listed in Box 12-6.

Chronic osteomyelitis may occasionally mimic the radiographic appearance of fibrous dysplasia. Inflam-

mation, often mild, is present in osteomyelitis and may be accompanied by symptoms that include tenderness, pain, or drainage. The slowly progressive, asymptomatic nature of fibrous dysplasia usually allows differentiation from malignant tumors of bone.

Treatment and Prognosis. After a variable period of prepubertal growth, fibrous dysplasia characteristically stabilizes, although a slow advance may be noted into adulthood. Small lesions may therefore require no treatment other than biopsy confirmation and periodic follow-up. Large lesions that have caused cosmetic or functional deformity may be treated by surgical recontouring. This procedure is generally deferred until after stabilization of the disease process. En bloc resections for complete removal are impractical and unnecessary, because the lesions are relatively large and poorly delineated.

Malignant transformation is a rare complication of fibrous dysplasia (fewer than 1% of cases) that has been described, usually in patients with the polyostotic type. Many of the patients reported on were treated with radiation therapy, suggesting a role for radiation in the transformation process, although malignant change has been documented in the absence of radiation treatment.

CEMENTOOSSEOUS DYSPLASIA

The term *cementoosseous dysplasia* refers to a disease process of the jaws for which the precise etiology is unknown. Cementoosseous dysplasia includes periapical cementoosseous dysplasia, focal cementoosseous dysplasia, and florid cementoosseous dysplasia—apparently similar disease processes dis-

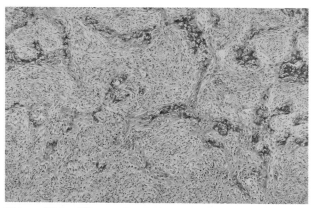

Figure 12-9 **Fibrous dysplasia** exhibiting fibroblastic matrix and uniform distribution of bony trabeculae (*purple*, not decalcified).

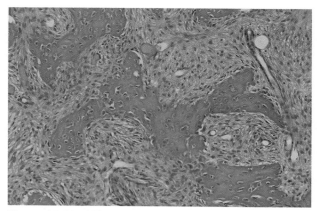

Figure 12-10 **Fibrous dysplasia** showing vascular fibroblastic matrix and irregular trabeculae of new bone.

Box 12-6 Fibrous Dysplasia vs. Ossifying Fibroma	
FIBROUS DYSPLASIA	**OSSIFYING FIBROMA**
First and second decades	Third and fourth decades
Maxilla > mandible	Mandible > maxilla
Diffuse opacity	Circumscribed
Self-limited	Continuous growth
One or more bones	One bone
Vascular matrix	Cellular fibrous matrix
Woven bone trabeculae	Bony islands and trabeculae
Stablizes at puberty	Not hormone related
Recontour for cosmetics	Excise

>, More frequently affected than.

tinguished on the basis of the extent of involvement of the affected portions of the jaws (see Chapter 11 for a comprehensive discussion). Cementoosseous dysplasia, ossifying fibroma, and fibrous dysplasia have been classified as fibroosseous lesions of the jaws. These fibroosseous diseases represent a diverse group of reactive, dysplastic, and neoplastic lesions characterized microscopically by the replacement of normal bone with a collagenous matrix containing trabeculae of immature bone and, in some instances, cementum-like material (see Boxes 12-1 and 12-2).

OSTEOBLASTOMA/OSTEOID OSTEOMA

Osteoblastoma is an uncommon primary lesion of bone that occasionally arises in the maxilla or the mandible (Box 12-7). *Osteoid osteoma* is thought to represent a smaller version of the same tumor, although some prefer to separate these lesions into two distinct entities. These are benign neoplasms of undetermined cause that may exhibit a seemingly rapid onset and cause pain. Clinically and histologically, they may be confused with osteosarcoma.

Clinical Features. The designation of *osteoblastoma* is used for lesions greater than 1.5 cm in diameter; the designation of *osteoid osteoma* is used for lesions less than 1.5 cm. These lesions arise most often in vertebrae and long bones and less commonly in the jaws and other craniofacial bones. The posterior tooth-bearing regions of the maxilla and mandible are the usual sites of jaw involvement (Figure 12-11). Lesions have been reported as arising in either medullary or periosteal sites. The bony cortices may be expanded and tender to palpation.

Most cases occur during the second decade, with 90% of lesions presenting before the age of 30 years. Males are affected more commonly than females, by a ratio of approximately 2 to 1.

Pain, often quite severe, is usually associated with osteoid osteomas and often with osteoblastomas. Localized swelling may occur alone or along with the pain. Symptomatology, including nocturnal pain, associated with osteoid osteoma is relieved by aspirin or nonsteroidal antiinflammatory drugs. This relief is less likely with osteoblastomas. The duration of signs or symptoms of osteoblastoma ranges from weeks to years.

Radiographically, lesions are well circumscribed and have a mixed lucent-opaque pattern. A thin radiolucency may be noted surrounding a variably calcified central tumor mass. Sclerosis of perilesional bone, a constant feature of osteoid osteoma, may be absent in osteoblastoma. Occasionally a peripheral sun ray pattern of new bone production may mimic osteosarcoma.

Histopathology. These lesions are composed of irregular trabeculae of osteoid and immature bone within a stroma containing a prominent vascular network (Figure 12-12). The bony trabeculae exhibit various degrees of calcification. Remodeling of the osseous tissue may be evident in the form of basophilic reversal lines. Several layers of plump, hyperchromatic osteoblasts typically line the bony trabeculae. Stromal cells are generally small and slender, although osteoblast-like cells and multinucleated giant cells may be noted in these areas.

Differential Diagnosis. Differential diagnosis considerations include cementoblastoma, ossifying fibroma, fibrous dysplasia, and osteosarcoma. Cementoblastoma can be differentiated from osteoblastoma because the former lesion arises from the surface of a tooth root and is fused to it. Ossifying fibroma is not painful and

---

Box 12-7 Osteoblastoma

Large counterpart of osteoid osteoma
 Osteoblastomas > 1.5 cm
 Osteoid osteomas 1.5 cm or less
50% are painful
Second decade is characteristic age
Circumscribed
Benign cellular (osteoblasts) neoplasm with new bone in scant fibrous stroma
Treatment by excision; few recurrences

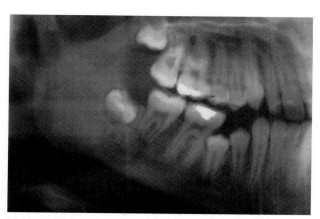

Figure 12-11 **Osteoblastoma** of the right mandible.

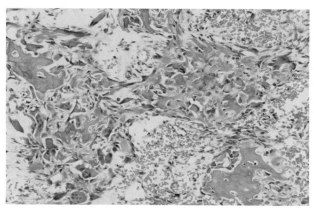

Figure 12-12 **Osteoblastoma** showing abundant prominent osteoblasts adjacent to new bone.

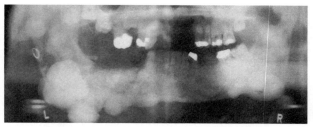

Figure 12-13 **Osteomas of Gardner's syndrome.**

microscopically does not have the numbers of osteoblasts seen in osteoblastoma/osteoid osteoma. Fibrous dysplasia has poorly defined radiographic margins and microscopically also does not have prominent osteoblasts.

The relatively rapid onset and the pain associated with some osteoblastomas necessitate differentiation from osteosarcoma. In biopsy specimens the hyperchromatic, large osteoblasts noted in osteoblastoma resemble the malignant cells of osteosarcoma. Cytologic atypia, abnormal mitotic figures, delicately calcified tumor osteoid, and a heterogeneous pattern, which are features of osteosarcoma, are not seen in osteoblastoma/osteoid osteoma.

Treatment and Prognosis. A conservative surgical approach (curettage or local excision) is curative in virtually all cases. In rare instances these tumors have been associated with a tendency to invade tissues locally and to recur subsequently. The term *aggressive osteoblastoma* has been suggested for such lesions, but most authorities believe that this is an unnecessary subclassification. Rare examples of malignant transformation of osteoblastoma have also been reported.

OSTEOMA

Osteomas are benign tumors that consist of mature, compact, or cancellous bone. Osteomas that arise on the surface of bone are referred to as *periosteal osteomas,* whereas those that develop centrally within bone are *endosteal osteomas.* Osteomas are relatively rare in the jaws. The cause of these lesions is unknown,

although trauma, infection, and developmental abnormalities have been suggested as contributing factors.

Clinical Features. Osteomas are most commonly identified during the second to fifth decades of life, and males are affected more often than females. Osteomas are usually solitary, except in patients with Gardner's syndrome.

Periosteal osteomas present clinically as asymptomatic, slow-growing, bony, hard masses. Asymmetry may be noted when lesions enlarge to sufficient proportion. Endosteal osteomas occurring within medullary bone may be discovered during routine radiographic examination as dense, well-circumscribed radiopacities, because extensive growth must take place before cortical expansion is evident. Osteomas may arise in the maxilla or mandible, as well as in facial and skull bones and within paranasal sinuses. Symptoms occasionally accompany these tumors. Headaches, recurrent sinusitis, and ophthalmologic complaints have been noted, depending on the lesion location.

Gardner's syndrome, inherited as an autosomal-dominant disorder, is characterized by intestinal polyposis, multiple osteomas, fibromas of the skin, epidermal and trichilemmal cysts, impacted permanent and supernumerary teeth, and odontomas (Figure 12-13). The genetic defect is found in a small region on the long arm of chromosome 5 (5q21), where the familial adenomatous polyposis (APC) gene resides. The majority of patients with Gardner's syndrome do not exhibit the complete spectrum of clinical disease expression. Osteomas associated with this syndrome may be found in the jaws (especially the mandibular angle) and also in facial and long bones. The intestinal polyps associated with Gardner's syndrome are commonly located in the colon and rectum. Significantly, the polyps, found microscopically to be adenomas, exhibit a very high

Box 12-8 Desmoplastic Fibroma

Young adults (younger than 30 years of age)
Bony counterpart of fibromatosis
Microscopic differential
    Odontogenic fibroma
    Odontogenic fibromyxoma
    Low-grade fibrosarcoma
    Follicular sac
Recurrence potential

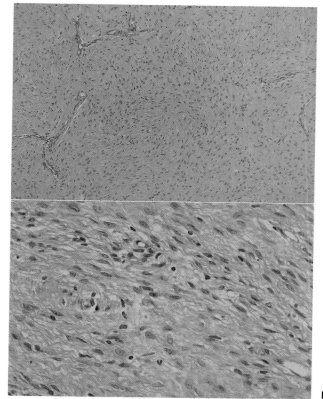

Figure 12-14 **A** and **B, Desmoplastic fibroma.** Note evenly distributed and benign-appearing fibroblasts in collagenous stroma.

rate of malignant transformation to invasive colorectal carcinoma.

Histopathology. Two distinct histologic variants of osteoma have been described. One form is composed of relatively dense, compact bone with sparse marrow tissue. The other form consists of lamellar trabeculae of cancellous bone with abundant fibrofatty marrow. Osteoblasts may be numerous, but osteoclasts are sparse.

Differential Diagnosis. Osteomas should be distinguished from exostoses of the jaws. Exostoses are bony excrescences on the buccal aspect of alveolar bone. These lesions are of reactive or developmental origin and are not thought to be true neoplasms. Osteoblastomas and osteoid osteomas, which might also be considered in a differential diagnosis, are likely to be painful and may exhibit a more rapid rate of growth than osteomas. Osteomas may also be confused radiographically with odontomas or focal sclerosing osteomyelitis.

Treatment and Prognosis. The treatment of osteomas is surgical excision. Lesions should also be excised for the purpose of establishing the diagnosis. In some instances periodic observation of small, asymptomatic osteomas is appropriate treatment. Osteomas do not recur following surgical removal.

DESMOPLASTIC FIBROMA

Desmoplastic fibroma is a benign, locally aggressive lesion of bone that can be considered the bony counterpart of fibromatosis (Box 12-8). The tumor appears usually in long bones and the pelvis but may occasionally affect the jaws. The cause of desmoplastic fibroma is unknown. The lesion usually exhibits locally aggressive clinical behavior, suggesting a neoplastic process. The potential role of genetic, endocrine, and traumatic factors in the pathogenesis of the lesion has led to speculation that it might represent an exuberant reactive proliferation.

Clinical Features. Most cases of desmoplastic fibroma of the jaws have occurred in patients under the age of 30 years, with a mean age of 14 years. There appears to be no gender predilection. The mandible, usually the body-ramus region, is affected more often than the maxilla. The lesions are slowly progressive and asymptomatic, eventually causing swelling of the jaw.

Radiographically, desmoplastic fibroma may be unilocular or multilocular. The radiographic margins may be either well demarcated or poorly defined. Cortical perforation and root resorption may be seen.

Histopathology. The lesion consists of interlacing bundles and whorled aggregates of densely collagenous tissue that contains uniform spindled and elongated fibroblasts (Figure 12-14). Some areas may exhibit hypercellularity with plumper fibroblast nuclei. However, cytologic atypia and mitotic figures are not found. Bone is not produced by lesional tissue.

Differential Diagnosis. Differential radiographic diagnostic considerations include odontogenic cysts, odontogenic tumors, and nonodontogenic lesions that typically occur in this age-group. The presence of aggressive features, such as cortical perforation, or local symptoms might suggest the possibility of a malignancy. In some cases histopathologic distinction between desmoplastic fibroma and well-differentiated fibrosarcoma may be difficult. The latter would exhibit greater cellularity, mitotic figures, and nuclear pleomorphism. Some similarities are noted histologically with central odontogenic fibroma, a nonaggressive lesion that contains odontogenic rests.

Treatment. Surgical resection of the lesion is generally reported as the treatment of choice. Curettage alone has been associated with a significant recurrence rate.

CHONDROMA

Chondroma is a benign cartilaginous tumor of unknown cause. Chondromas are rarely seen in the jaws, especially in comparison with their occurrence in other skeletal sites.

A chondroma commonly presents as a painless, slowly progressive swelling. The gradual expansion of the lesion rarely results in mucosal ulceration. Most lesions of the craniofacial complex arise in the nasal septum and ethmoid sinuses. Chondromas of the maxilla are most often found in the anterior region, where cartilaginous remnants of development are located. Mandibular chondromas have been noted in the body and symphysis areas, as well as in the coronoid process and the condyle. Chondromas occur with equal incidence in both genders, with the majority of tumors appearing before 50 years of age. The radiographic appearance of the chondroma is variable but often presents as an irregular radiolucent area. Foci of calcification may be evident within the radiolucent lesion.

The lesion consists of well-defined lobules of mature hyaline cartilage. The chondrocytes are small and contain single, regular nuclei. The degree of cellularity varies considerably from one area to another within the chondroma. The principal diagnostic problem rests in microscopically distinguishing chondroma from a well-differentiated chondrosarcoma.

Box 12-9 Central Giant Cell Granuloma

CLINICAL FEATURES

Most patients younger than 30 years of age; females affected more often than males
Lucency; mandible > maxilla; anterior jaw > posterior jaw
Recurrences unpredictable (10% to 50%)

HISTOPATHOLOGY

Benign fibroblast matrix (in cell cycle)
Giant cells variable (size, number, distribution)
Few to many mitotic figures
Cannot separate aggressive from nonaggressive lesions

TREATMENT

Traditional excision vs. medical management—calcitonin (osteoclast inhibition)

>, More frequently affected than.

The latter exhibits a heterogeneous pattern with atypical cartilage cells.

Chondromas are surgically excised, and recurrence is unusual. Any recurrence should be cause for reconsidering the original diagnosis in favor of the possibility of low-grade malignancy.

CENTRAL GIANT CELL GRANULOMA

Central giant cell granuloma (CGCG) is a benign proliferation of fibroblasts and multinucleated giant cells that occurs almost exclusively within the jaws (Box 12-9). The tumor typically presents as a solitary radiolucent lesion of the mandible or maxilla.

Etiology and Pathogenesis. Thought to represent a reparative response to intrabony hemorrhage and inflammation, CGCG was once regarded as a reactive lesion. However, because of its unpredictable and occasionally aggressive behavior, and because of its possible relationship to the giant cell tumor of long bones, CGCG is best classified as a benign neoplasm.

The primary tumor cells of CGCGs are fibroblasts. Secondary cells, which are microscopically the most prominent, are multinucleated giant cells. Accessory cells, seen in considerably smaller numbers, include macrophages, factor XIIIa+ dendrocytes, and endothelial cells. The fibroblasts make up the proliferative component of CGCGs, since they express proteins that are

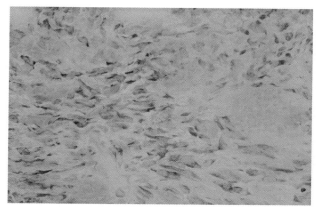

Figure 12-15 **Central giant cell granuloma** immunohistochemically stained for fibroblast-associated antigen. Note that stromal cells stain positive *(red)*.

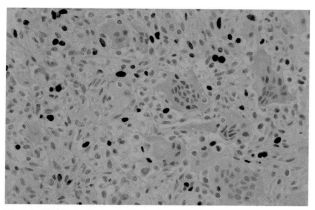

Figure 12-16 **Central giant cell granuloma** immunohistochemically stained for Ki-67 proliferation protein showing that proliferating cells are located in the stromal component.

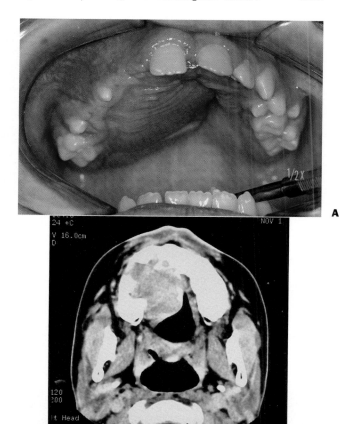

Figure 12-17 **Central giant cell granuloma.** Mass in right maxilla **(A)** is depicted in CT scan **(B).**

indicative of cells in the cell cycle. Tumor fibroblasts are also believed to be responsible for recruitment and retention of monocytes and subsequently for transformation into multinucleated giant cells (Figures 12-15 and 12-16).

Clinical Features. CGCG is an uncommon lesion and occurs less commonly than its relatively trivial peripheral counterpart. Lesions are found predominantly in children and young adults, with most cases (75%) presenting before 30 years of age. Females are affected more often than males, in a ratio of 2 to 1.

CGCG occurs almost exclusively in the maxilla and mandible, although isolated cases in facial bones and small bones of the hands and feet have been reported

(Figure 12-17). Lesions are seen more commonly in the mandible than in the maxilla (Figure 12-18). These lesions tend to involve the jaws anterior to the permanent molar teeth, with occasional extension across the midline. Rarely, lesions involve the posterior jaws, including the mandibular ramus and condyle.

CGCG typically produces a painless expansion or swelling of the affected jaw. Cortical plates are thinned; however, perforation with extension into soft tissues is uncommon. The radiographic features of GCGC consist of a multilocular or, less commonly, unilocular radiolucency of bone (Figure 12-19). The margins of the lesion are relatively well demarcated, often presenting a scalloped border. In some instances GCGC pursues a more aggressive clinical and radiographic course. These "aggressive" CGCGs may cause pain and exhibit rapid growth, root resorption, perforation of cortical bone, and recurrence.

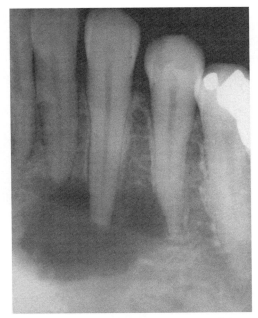

Figure 12-18   **Central giant cell granuloma** of the anterior mandible.

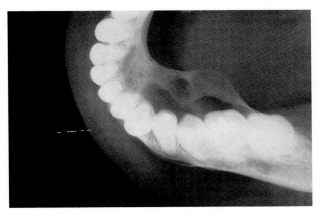

Figure 12-19   **Central giant cell granuloma** showing loculations and cortical expansion.

Histopathology. CGCG is composed of uniform fibroblasts in a stroma containing various amounts of collagen. Hemosiderin-laden macrophages and extravasated erythrocytes are usually evident, although capillaries are small and inconspicuous. Multinucleated giant cells are present throughout the connective tissue stroma, and they may be seen in patches or distributed evenly (Figures 12-20 and 12-21). Foci of osteoid may be present, particularly around the peripheral margins of the lesion.

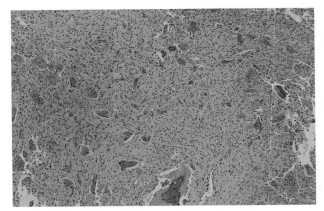

Figure 12-20   **Central giant cell granuloma** demonstrating characteristic patchy giant cell distribution in a fibroblastic matrix.

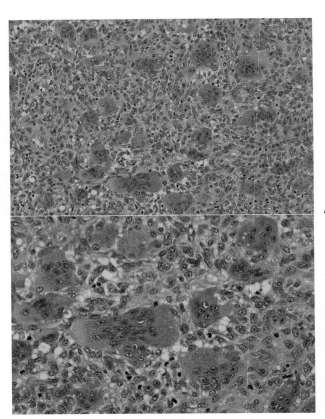

A

B

Figure 12-21   **A** and **B, Central giant cell granuloma.** Note cellular matrix and evenly distributed giant cells.

> **Box 12-10 Central Giant Cell Granuloma: Microscopic Differential**
>
> **HYPERPARATHYROIDISM**
>
> Elevated serum parathormone and alkaline phosphatase
> Multiple bone lesions; loss of lamina dura
>
> **ANEURYSMAL BONE CYST**
>
> Blood-filled sinusoids present
>
> **CHERUBISM**
>
> Symmetric lesions
> Family history
> Perivascular collagen cuffing

There are no microscopic features that distinguish aggressive CGCGs from nonaggressive ones. Numbers of mitotic figures, cellularity, giant cell numbers, giant cell nuclei numbers, and a giant cell pattern are not useful in predicting behavior or outcome.

Differential Diagnosis. The clinical differential diagnosis for a solitary or multilocular CGCG includes ameloblastoma, odontogenic myxoma, and odontogenic keratocyst. For patients in the characteristic young age range for CGCG, ameloblastic fibroma, ossifying fibroma, and adenomatoid odontogenic tumor might be added to this list.

The microscopic appearance of GCGC is virtually identical to that of the giant cell lesion associated with hyperparathyroidism (Box 12-10). This process must be differentiated on the basis of biochemical tests. Elevated serum levels of parathyroid hormone are indicative of primary hyperparathyroidism.

The giant cell tumor of (long) bone may exhibit histologic features similar to those of CGCG, although the former tends to have larger giant cells with more nuclei and a homogeneous pattern. Giant cell tumor is believed to rarely occur in the jaws, although differentiation from CGCG can be difficult.

Other giant cell–containing look-alikes or entities continuing multinucleated giant cells include aneurysmal bone cyst and cherubism. Diagnosis of aneurysmal bone cyst is made by the identification of sinusoidal blood spaces within the tumor mass. Cherubism is diagnosed on clinical pathologic grounds.

Treatment and Prognosis. Surgical management of these lesions is the treatment of choice. Excision or curettage of the tumor mass followed by removal of the peripheral bony margins results in a good prognosis and a low recurrence rate. A somewhat higher rate of recurrence has been reported in lesions arising in children and young teens. Lesions with aggressive clinical features also exhibit a tendency to recur, often necessitating more extensive surgical approaches, including resection. Intralesional injections of corticosteroids have been proposed as a nonsurgical method for management of these lesions, but results are varied and the rationale of this therapy is questionable. The use of exogenous calcitonin may have some merit in the treatment of aggressive lesions. Preliminary data suggest that lesions may stabilize or regress after several months of therapy. Recently the use of interferon alfa-2a has been proposed as an additional treatment modality on the basis of an antiangiogenic mode of action.

GIANT CELL TUMOR

Giant cell tumors are true neoplasms that arise most commonly in long bones, especially in the area of the knee joint. These tumors exhibit a wide spectrum of biologic behavior from benign to malignant. The relationship between this lesion and central giant cell granuloma is controversial. Most regard the giant cell tumor as a distinct entity from central giant cell granuloma, acknowledging the very rare occurrence of giant cell tumors within the jaws.

Giant cell tumors, although rare, have been reported in the jaws. Other sites of involvement in the head and neck include the sphenoid, ethmoid, and temporal bones. Giant cell tumors are most often seen in the third and fourth decades of life. Lesions exhibit slow growth and bone expansion, or they produce rapid growth, pain, or paresthesia. Radiographically, the giant cell tumor produces a radiolucent image.

Microscopically, this tumor is characterized by the presence of numerous multinucleated giant cells dispersed evenly among mononuclear fibroblasts (Figure 12-22). The nuclear morphology of both types of cells is virtually identical. Stromal cellularity is usually prominent, with minimal collagen production. Giant cells in giant cell tumors are usually larger and contain more nuclei than the corresponding cells of central giant cell granuloma. Significant variation is noted, however, such that any given lesion may present diagnostic difficulty because of considerable histologic overlap. Giant cell tumors may contain inflammatory cells and areas of necrosis while exhibiting a relative absence of hemorrhage and hemosiderin deposition.

Osteoid formation is also noted less often than in giant cell granulomas.

Surgical excision is the treatment of choice for giant cell tumors. These lesions exhibit a greater tendency to recur after treatment than do giant cell granulomas. Although too few cases have been reported in the jaws to predict recurrence rates, it is noteworthy that 30% of lesions in long bones recur after curettage.

HEMANGIOMA OF BONE

Hemangiomas of bone are rare intraosseous vascular malformations that, when seen in the jaws, can mimic both odontogenic and nonodontogenic lesions. Difficult-to-control hemorrhage is a notable complication of surgical intervention.

Clinical Features. More than half of the central hemangiomas of the jaws occur in the mandible, especially the posterior region. The lesion occurs approximately twice as often in females as in males. The peak age of discovery is the second decade of life.

A firm, slow-growing, asymmetric expansion of the mandible or maxilla is the most common patient complaint. Spontaneous gingival bleeding around teeth in the area of the hemangioma may also be noted. Paresthesia or pain is occasionally evident, as well as vertical mobility of involved teeth. Bruits or pulsation of large lesions may be detected with careful auscultation or palpation of the thinned cortical plates. Trophic effects of the hemangioma on adjacent hard and soft tissues are also common. Significantly, hemangiomas may be present without any signs or symptoms.

Radiographically, more than half of jaw hemangiomas occur as multilocular radiolucencies that have a characteristic soap bubble appearance (Figure 12-23). A second form of these lesions consists of a rounded, radiolucent lesion in which bony trabeculae radiate from the center of the lesion, producing angular loculations. Less commonly, hemangiomas appear as cystlike radiolucencies. The lesions may produce resorption of the roots of teeth in the area.

Histopathology. Hemangiomas of bone represent a proliferation of blood vessels (Figure 12-24). Most intrabony hemangiomas are of the cavernous type (large-caliber vessels). Fewer are of the capillary type (small-caliber vessels). Separation of hemangiomas into one of these two microscopic subtypes is, however, academic, since there is no difference in biologic behavior.

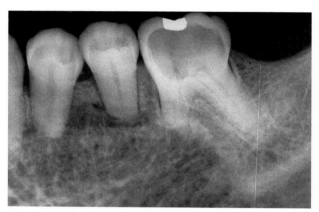

Figure 12-23 **Hemangioma of bone** showing honeycomb radiographic pattern with associated root resorption.

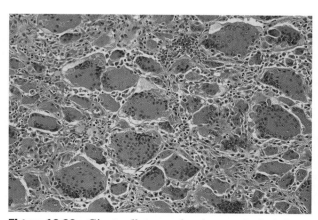

Figure 12-22 **Giant cell tumor** showing particularly large giant cells with abundant nuclei.

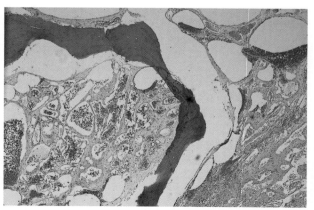

Figure 12-24 **Hemangioma of bone.** Note numerous vascular channels surrounded by trabecula of bone.

Differential Diagnosis. The differential diagnosis of multilocular hemangioma of bone includes ameloblastoma, odontogenic myxoma, odontogenic keratocyst, central giant cell granuloma, and aneurysmal bone cyst. A unilocular lesion may be easily confused with other cystic processes that occur within the jaws. Angiography often provides useful information in establishing the diagnosis of hemangioma.

Treatment and Prognosis. The most significant feature of hemangiomas of bone is that these lesions may prove life threatening if improperly managed. Extraction of teeth in an area involved by a central vascular lesion may result in potentially fatal bleeding. It is imperative to perform needle aspiration of any central lesion that potentially may be of vascular origin before performing a biopsy.

Methods used in the treatment of hemangioma of bone include surgery, radiation therapy, sclerosing agents, cryotherapy, and presurgical embolization techniques. The vascular supply of a given lesion, as well as its size and location, must be evaluated before the selection of a given treatment method.

LANGERHANS CELL DISEASE

Langerhans cell disease (LCD), also formerly known as *histiocytosis X* and *idiopathic histiocytosis*, is a disorder characterized by a proliferation of cells exhibiting phenotypic characteristics of Langerhans cells. The clinical manifestations of this process range from solitary or multiple bone lesions to disseminated visceral, skin, and bone lesions.

Historically, the term *histiocytosis X* was used to encompass three disorders: eosinophilic granuloma, Hand-Schüller-Christian syndrome, and Letterer-Siwe disease (Box 12-11). These entities were grouped together because of their similar microscopic appearance, despite the diverse manner of clinical disease expression. *Eosinophilic granuloma,* or *chronic localized LCD,* refers to solitary or multiple bone lesions only. *Hand-Schüller-Christian syndrome,* or *chronic disseminated LCD,* is a specific clinical triad of lytic bone lesions, exophthalmos, and diabetes insipidus. Many affected persons also exhibit lymphadenopathy, dermatitis, splenomegaly, or hepatomegaly. *Letterer-Siwe disease,* or *acute disseminated LCD,* is a malignant process characterized by a rapidly progressive, often fatal course. Widespread organ, bone, and skin involvement by the proliferative process in infants has been the common presentation.

Etiology and Pathogenesis. The etiology and pathogenesis of LCD remain obscure, although the cell of origin is now known (Box 12-12). Ultrastructural and immunohistochemical similarities have demonstrated that LCD tumor cells are similar to normal Langerhans cells that reside in epidermis and mucosa. How LCD develops from normal Langerhans cells or their precursor cells is unknown.

The acute form of this disease and some cases of the chronic forms are thought to represent a neoplastic transformation. Abnormalities of DNA content in the proliferative cells have been demonstrated in only a few cases of LCD, however. More recent investigations in a limited number of patients have demonstrated a clonal proliferation of Langerhans cells, supporting the concept of a neoplastic process. It has also been suggested that the disease may result from exuberant reaction to an unknown antigenic challenge. Evidence is emerging that some patients with LCD may exhibit defects in certain aspects of the cell-mediated arm of the immune system. A deficiency of suppressor T lymphocytes, as well as low levels of serum thymic factor, suggest the presence of a thymic abnormality in this disease. These immunologic defects may affect normal

---

Box 12-11 Langerhans Cell Disease: Classification

Eosinophilic granuloma (chronic localized): Solitary or multiple bone lesions
Hand-Schüller-Christian (chronic disseminated): Bone lesions, exophthalmos, diabetes insipidus
Letterer-Siwe (acute disseminated): Bone, skin, internal organs affected

---

Box 12-12 Langerhans Cell Disease

Proliferation of Langerhans cells
   Cells are CD1a+ and S-100+ positive
   Cells contain Birbeck granules (ultrastructure)
   Few macrophages (histiocytes) are present
Cause unknown
Any age; three variants
Radiograph shows punched-out noncorticated lesions or "floating teeth"
Several treatment options
Prognosis good to excellent; depends on form

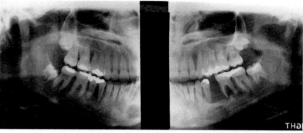

Figure 12-25 **Langerhans cell disease.** Note bilateral mandibular lesions.

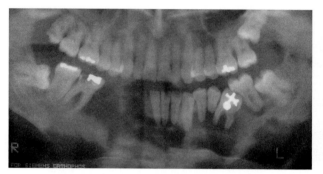

Figure 12-26 **Langerhans cell disease** resulting in marked destruction of the mandible. (Courtesy Dr. Jerry. R. Sorensen.)

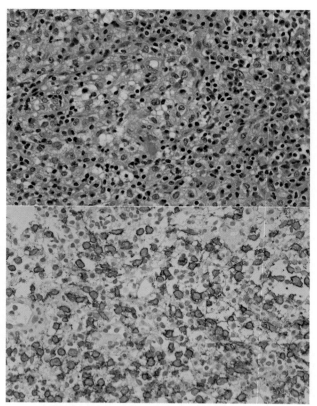

Figure 12-27 **Langerhans cell disease. A,** Lesion is composed of pale Langerhans cells, eosinophils, and other chronic inflammatory cells. **B,** Immunohistochemical stain for Langerhans cell–specific CD1a antigen shows positive staining *(brown)* of tumor cells.

regulatory mechanisms, with resultant Langerhans cell proliferation.

Clinical Features. LCD is generally a condition of children and young adults, but the age range extends to older adults. The monostotic and polyostotic forms of the disorder may affect virtually any bone of the body. The skull, mandible, ribs, vertebrae, and long bones are often involved. Oral changes may be the initial presentation in all forms of this disorder. Skin, mucosal, or bone involvement in the head and neck region was noted in more than 80% of children in one study. Tenderness, pain, and swelling are common patient complaints. Loosening of teeth in the area of the affected alveolar bone is a common occurrence. The gingival tissues are often inflamed, hyperplastic, and ulcerated. Oral mucosal lesions in the form of submucosal nodules, ulcers, and leukoplakia have also been described.

The jaws may exhibit solitary or multiple radiolucent lesions (Figures 12-25 and 12-26). The lesions often affect the alveolar bone, causing the teeth to appear as if they were floating in space. Bone lesions with a sharply circumscribed, punched-out appearance may also occur in the central aspect of the mandible or maxilla. These lesions are occasionally located exclusively in a periapical site, where they may mimic periapical inflammatory lesions. Jaw lesions may be accompanied by bone involvement elsewhere in the skeleton. Cervical lymphadenopathy, mastoiditis, and otitis media are head and neck manifestations that often present with multifocal involvement.

Histopathology. LCD is characterized by the proliferation of large cells with abundant cytoplasm, indistinct cell borders, and oval to reniform nuclei. These cells are most often arranged in sheets and may be admixed with various numbers of eosinophils and other inflammatory cells (Figure 12-27). A second population of macrophages is often evident. Multinucleated giant cells and foci of necrosis may also be noted. The ultrastructure of the tumor cells shows unique, rod-

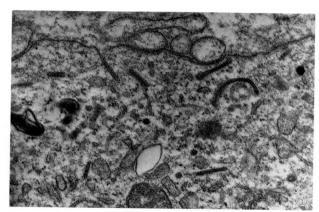

Figure 12-28 **Langerhans cell disease** electron micrograph of tumor cell cytoplasm exhibiting rod-shaped Langerhans cell (Birbeck) granules.

Box 12-13 Langerhans Cell Disease: Treatment

LOCALIZED DISEASE

Curettage
Radiation, low dose
Intralesional corticosteroid injection
Rare spontaneous regression

DISSEMINATED DISEASE

Immunosuppressive agents, corticosteroids

---

shaped cytoplasmic structures, which are identical to Birbeck granules, present in normal Langerhans cells (Figure 12-28). Immunohistochemical stains show that the tumor cells express CD1a antigen, S-100 protein, and human leukocyte antigens (HLA)-DR, which are also characteristic of normal Langerhans cells.

Differential Diagnosis. The classic presentation of LCD in the jaws often results in loosening or premature exfoliation of teeth and precocious eruption of permanent teeth. Under these conditions, a differential diagnosis should include juvenile or diabetic periodontitis, hypophosphatasia, leukemia, cyclic neutropenia, agranulocytosis, and primary or metastatic malignant neoplasms. Lesions located in a periapical site may be confused with a periapical cyst or granuloma; the presence of pulp vitality excludes this possibility.

Solitary radiolucent lesions in the central aspects of the jaws should be differentiated from odontogenic tumors and cysts. Numerous well-circumscribed radiolucencies may suggest multiple myeloma, although this occurs in a much older age-group. Histologic examination of tissue removed for a biopsy generally serves to distinguish this disorder from the other entities listed.

Treatment and Prognosis. The acute disseminated form commonly occurs during the first years of life and pursues a rapidly progressive course. The primary method of treatment involves the use of chemotherapeutic agents (Box 12-13). The disease may be fatal despite intensive treatment. Patients with a poor prognosis have been treated with allogeneic bone marrow transplantation with some success.

Disseminated visceral and bone involvement in somewhat older children often behaves in a more chronic fashion. Individual lesions may be effectively managed with surgical curettage or low-dose radiation therapy. Cytotoxic agents such as vincristine sulfate, cyclophosphamide, and methotrexate, often in conjunction with systemic corticosteroids, may be used for widespread or visceral involvement. The prognosis in this form of the disease is more optimistic, with half of the patients surviving for 10 to 15 years.

The localized form of LCD occurs in older children, adolescents, and young adults. These lesions may be treated successfully with vigorous surgical curettage, although intralesional corticosteroid injections and low-dose radiotherapy have been reported to be effective. Spontaneous regression of restricted disease has been reported, making treatment in some cases unnecessary. Involved teeth are generally sacrificed at the time of surgical therapy because of the absence of bony support. The prognosis for this form of the disorder is good. These patients must be evaluated for additional bone or visceral involvement, which is usually manifested within the first 6 months after detection of the original lesion. Long-term follow-up is necessary to rule out the possibility of recurrent disease.

TORI AND EXOSTOSES

Tori and exostoses are nodular protuberances of mature bone; their precise designation depends on the anatomic location. These lesions are of little clinical significance. They are nonneoplastic and rarely are a source of discomfort. The mucosa surfacing these lesions occasionally may be traumatically ulcerated, producing a slow-healing, painful wound or, less commonly, osteomyelitis. Surgical removal for the purpose of prosthetic rehabilitation may be necessary.

Etiology and Pathogenesis. The precise cause of these lesions remains obscure, although evidence has been presented to suggest that the torus may be an inherited condition. A simple dominant pattern of inheritance has been identified for palatal tori in a study of Venezuelan and Japanese populations. One investigator has indicated that both genetic and environmental factors determine the development of mandibular tori. The palatal torus is relatively prevalent in certain populations such as Asians, Native Americans, and the Inuit (Eskimos). The incidence in the general population of the United States is between 20% and 25%.

Mandibular tori are seen more commonly in certain groups such as blacks and some Asian populations. The overall incidence in the United States is estimated to be between 6% and 12%. The presence of mandibular tori was studied in patients with migraine headaches and temporomandibular disorders. A positive association suggested a possible role of parafunctional habits in the etiology of this condition.

The cause of exostoses is unknown. It has been suggested that the bony growths represent a reaction to increased or abnormal occlusal stresses of the teeth in the involved areas.

Torus Palatinus

Clinical Features. The palatal torus is a sessile, nodular mass of bone that presents along the midline of the hard palate (Figure 12-29). This lesion occurs in females twice as often as it does in males in some populations. The palatal torus usually appears during the second or third decade of life, although it may be noted at any age. The bony mass exhibits slow growth and is generally asymptomatic. These lesions are often present in a symmetric fashion along the midline of the hard palate. Tori have been noted to form various configurations such as nodular, spindled, lobular, or flat. Large tori may be evident on radiographs as diffuse radiopaque lesions.

Torus Mandibularis

Clinical Features. Mandibular tori are bony exophytic growths that present along the lingual aspect of the mandible superior to the mylohyoid ridge (Figure 12-30). These tori are almost always bilateral, occurring in the premolar region. Infrequently, a torus may be noted on one side only. These lesions are asymptomatic, exhibiting slow growth during the second and third decades of life.

Mandibular tori may arise as solitary nodules or as multiple nodular masses that appear to coalesce. A significant gender predilection is not evident. Curiously, mandibular and palatal tori do not often occur together in the same individual.

Exostoses

Clinical Features. Exostoses are multiple (or single) bony excrescences that occur less commonly than do tori. They are asymptomatic bony nodules that are present along the buccal aspect of alveolar bone (Figures 12-31 and 12-32). Lesions are noted most often in the posterior portions of both the maxilla and the mandible. Exostoses have been reported as rare occurrences following skin graft vestibuloplasty gingival grafts, as well as beneath the pontic of a fixed bridge.

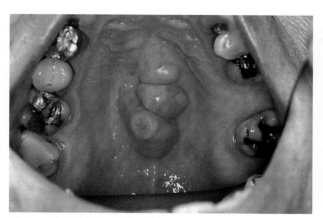

Figure 12-29 Torus palatinus.

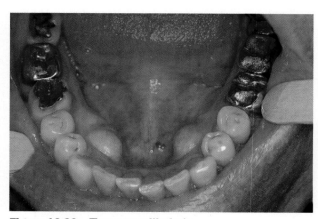

Figure 12-30 Torus mandibularis.

Histopathology. These lesions are composed of hyperplastic bone consisting of mature cortical and trabecular bone. The outer surface exhibits a smooth, rounded contour.

Treatment and Prognosis. Treatment of tori and exostoses is unnecessary unless it is required for prosthetic considerations or in cases of frequent trauma to the overlying mucosa. Recurrence after surgical excision is only rarely seen.

CORONOID HYPERPLASIA

Hyperplasia of the coronoid processes of the mandible is an uncommon condition that is often associated with limitation of mandibular motion.

Etiology and Pathogenesis. The cause of this process remains unknown. A history of trauma is present in many instances; however, the precise relationship

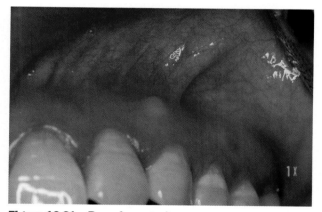

Figure 12-31   Buccal exostosis.

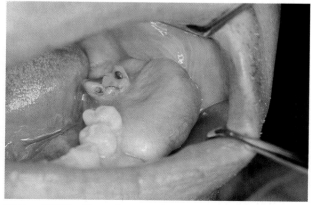

Figure 12-32   Buccal exostosis.

between the traumatic episode and the onset of coronoid enlargement has been difficult to establish. The coronoid enlargement appears to represent a hyperplastic process, although it has been suggested that the lesion may be neoplastic. Unilateral coronoid hyperplasia may be the result of a solitary osteochondroma; bilateral coronoid hyperplasia is apparently the result of a different process. The majority of cases have been reported in males, leading some investigators to suggest an X-linked inherited etiology. However, some cases have been reported in females, a finding that seems to preclude this possibility. Increased activity of the temporalis muscle with unbalanced condylar support has also been postulated as an etiologic factor.

Clinical Features. Hyperplasia of the coronoid processes is often bilateral, although unilateral enlargement has been noted. Bilateral coronoid hyperplasia typically results in limitation of mandibular movement, which is progressive over time.

The disorder is usually painless and, with a few exceptions, is not associated with facial swelling or asymmetry. Coronoid hyperplasia has been reported most often in young male patients. The age of onset is typically around puberty, although presentation for evaluation may be delayed for many years. Some cases have been noted, especially in females, before puberty and during adult life.

Enlarged and elongated coronoid processes are evident radiographically, although the general shape of the processes is usually normal. Unilateral coronoid hyperplasia often results in misshapen or mushroom-shaped coronoid processes on radiographs. Temporomandibular joint radiographs are unremarkable.

Histopathology. The enlarged coronoid processes consist of mature, hyperplastic bone. The bone may be partially covered by cartilaginous and fibrous connective tissue.

Differential Diagnosis. Bilateral coronoid hyperplasia rarely presents diagnostic difficulties. However, cases of unilateral coronoid hyperplasia must be differentiated from osseous and chondroid neoplasms.

Treatment and Prognosis. Treatment consists of surgical excision of the hyperplastic coronoid processes. Postoperative physiotherapy is also advocated. Long-term functional improvement has been variably successful as measured by an increase in mouth opening after surgical intervention. Recurrence has been rarely reported.

BIBLIOGRAPHY

Brannon RB, Fowler CB: Benign fibro-osseous lesions: a review of current concepts, *Adv Anat Pathol* 8(3):126-143, 2001.

Bridge JA: Cytogenetics and experimental models, *Curr Opin Oncol* 8:284-288, 1996.

Bunel K, Sindet-Pedersen S: Central hemangioma of the mandible, *Oral Surg Oral Med Oral Pathol* 75:565-570, 1993.

Candelere GA, Glorieux FH, Prud'homme J, et al: Increased expression of the C-fos proto-oncogene in bone from patients with fibrous dysplasia, *N Engl J Med* 332:1546-1551, 1995.

Cleveland DB, Goldberg KM, Greenspan JS, et al: Langerhans cell histiocytosis: report of three cases with unusual oral soft tissue involvement, *Oral Surg Oral Med Oral Pathol Oral Radiol Endod* 82:541-548, 1996.

Clifford T, Lamey PJ, Fartash L: Mandibular tori, migraine and temporomandibular disorders, *Br Dent J* 180:382-384, 1996.

Dal Cin P, Scoit R, Brys P et al: Recurrent chromosome aberrations in fibrous dysplasia of the bone: a report of the CHAMP study group: chromosomes and morphology, *Cancer Genet Cytogenet* 122:30-32, 2000.

Egeler RM, D'Angio GJ: Langerhans cell histiocytosis, *J Pediatr* 127:1-11, 1995.

Engel JD, Supancic JS, Davis LF: Arteriovenous malformation of the mandible: life-threatening complications during tooth extraction, *J Am Dent Assoc* 126:237-242, 1995.

Harris M: Central giant cell granulomas of the jaws regress with calcitonin therapy, *Br J Oral Maxillofac Surg* 31:89-94, 1993.

Haug RH, Hauer C, DeCamillo AJ, et al: Benign osteoblastoma of the mandible: report of a case, *J Oral Maxillofac Surg* 48:743-748, 1990.

Hegtvedt AK, Terry BC, Burkes EJ, et al: Skin graft vestibuloplasty exostosis: a report of two cases, *Oral Surg Oral Med Oral Pathol* 69:149-152, 1990.

Hopkins KM, Huttula CS, Kahn MA, et al: Desmoplastic fibroma of the mandible: review and report of two cases, *J Oral Maxillofac Surg* 54:1249-1254, 1996.

Kaban LB, Mulliken JR, Ezekowitz RA, et al: Antiangiogenic therapy of a recurrent giant cell tumor of the mandible with interferon alfa-2a, *Pediatrics* 103(6):1145-1149, 1999.

Kaplan I, Calderon S, Buchner A: Peripheral osteoma of the mandible: a study of 10 new cases and analysis of the literature, *J Oral Maxillofac Surg* 52:467-470, 1994.

Lucas DR, Unni KK, McLeod RA, et al: Osteoblastoma: clinicopathologic study of 306 cases, *Hum Pathol* 25:117-134, 1994.

Marie PJ, de Pollak C, Chanson P, et al: Increased proliferation of osteoblastic cells expressing the activating Gs alpha mutation in monostotic and polyostotic fibrous dysplasia, *Am J Pathol* 150:1059-1069, 1997.

Mascarello JT, Krous HF, Carpenter PM: Unbalanced translocation resulting in the loss of the chromosome 17 short arm in an osteoblastoma, *Cancer Genet Cytogenet* 69:65-67, 1993.

McLoughlin PM, Hopper C, Bowley NB: Hyperplasia of the mandibular coronoid process: an analysis of 31 cases and a review of the literature, *J Oral Maxillofac Surg* 53:250-255, 1995.

O'Malley M, Pogrel MA, Stewart JCB, et al: Central giant cell granulomas of the jaws: phenotype and proliferation-associated markers, *J Oral Pathol Med* 26:159-163, 1997.

Pammer J, Weninger W, Hulla H, et al: Expression of regulatory apoptotic proteins in peripheral giant cell granulomas and lesions containing osteoclast-like giant cells, *J Oral Pathol Med* 27:267-271, 1998.

Petrikowski CG, Pharoah MJ, Lee L: Radiographic differentiation of osteogenic sarcoma, osteomyelitis, and fibrous dysplasia of the jaws, *Oral Surg Oral Med Oral Pathol Oral Radiol Endod* 80:744-750, 1995.

Pogrel MA: The management of lesions of the jaws with liquid nitrogen cryotherapy, *J Calif Dent Assoc* 23:54-57, 1995.

Polandt K, Engels C, Kaiser E, et al: Gs alpha gene mutations in monostotic fibrous dysplasia of bone and fibrous dysplasia-like low-grade central osteosarcoma, *Virchows Arch* 439:170-175, 2001.

Riminucci M, Fisher LW, Shenker A, et al: Fibrous dysplasia of bone in the McCune-Albright syndrome, *Am J Pathol* 151:1587-1600, 1997.

Sakamoto A, Oda Y, Iwamoto Y, et al: A comparative study of fibrous dysplasia and osteofibrous dysplasia with regard to Gs alpha mutation at the Arg201 codon: polymerase chain reaction-restriction fragment length polymorphism analysis of paraffin-embedded tissues, *J Mol Diagn* 2:67-72, 2000.

Seah YH: Torus palatinus and torus mandibularis: a review of the literature, *Aust Dent J* 40:318-321, 1995.

Shapeero LG, Vanel D, Ackerman LV, et al: Aggressive fibrous dysplasia of the maxillary sinus, *Skeletal Radiol* 22:563-568, 1993.

Slootweg PJ, Muller H: Differential diagnosis of fibroosseous lesions: a histological investigation of 30 cases, *J Craniomaxillofac Surg* 18:210-214, 1990.

Slootweg PJ, Panders AK, Koopmans R, et al: Juvenile ossifying fibroma: an analysis of 33 cases with emphasis on histopathological aspects, *J Oral Pathol Med* 23:385-388, 1994.

Souza PEA, Paim JFO, Carvalhais JN, et al: Immunohistochemical expression of p53, MDM2, Ki-67 and PCNA in central giant cell granuloma and giant cell tumor, *J Oral Pathol Med* 28:54-58, 1999.

Stoll M, Freund M, Schmid H, et al: Allogeneic bone marrow transplantation for Langerhans cell histiocytosis, *Cancer* 66:284-288, 1990.

Takeuchi T, Takenoshita Y, Kubo K, et al: Natural course of jaw lesions in patients with familial adenomatosis coli (Gardner's syndrome), *Int J Oral Maxillofac Surg* 22:226-230, 1993.

Terry BC, Jacoway JR: Management of central giant cell lesions: an alternative to surgical therapy, *Oral Maxillofac Surg Clin North Am* 6:579-600, 1994.

Titgemeyer Cgrois N, Minkov M, et al: Pattern and course of single-system disease in Langerhans cell histiocytosis data from the DAL-HX 83- and 90-study, *Med Pediatr Oncol* 37:108-114, 2001.

Ueno H, Ariji E, Tanaka T, et al: Imaging features of maxillary osteoblastoma and its malignant transformation, *Skeletal Radiol* 23:509-512, 1994.

Waldron CA: Fibro-osseous lesions of the jaws, *J Oral Maxillofac Surg* 51:828-835, 1993.

Whitaker SB, Waldron CA: Central giant cell lesions of the jaws: a clinical, radiologic, and histopathologic study, *Oral Surg Oral Med Oral Pathol* 75:199-208, 1993.

Willman CL, Busque L, Griffith BB, et al: Langerhans'-cell histiocytosis (histiocytosis X): a clonal proliferative disease, *N Engl J Med* 331:154-160, 1994.

INFLAMMATORY JAW LESIONS

Osteomyelitis, by definition, is inflammation, not necessarily infection (by a microorganism), of bone and bone marrow. The term *osteitis* may be substituted for *osteomyelitis* to indicate inflammation of bone. In the mandible and maxilla most cases are related to a microbial (usually bacterial) infection that reaches the bone through nonvital teeth, periodontal lesions, or traumatic injuries. This, coupled with the patient's resistance factors, determines the clinical presentation, extent of the inflammatory process, and speed with

which the infection develops. The recognized subtypes of osteomyelitis are closely related and essentially represent differences in the etiologic agent and host response. The primary justification for separation of osteomyelitis into the various subtypes lies in the differences in treatment and prognosis for each. It is also important to be aware of clinical and radiographic presentations in making differential diagnoses of bone lesions.

PULPITIS

All the principles of inflammation that apply to any other body organ apply to lesions of the dental pulp. In addition, dental pulp has some unique features that make it unusually fragile and sensitive. First, it is encased by hard tissue (dentin/enamel) that does not allow for the usual swelling associated with the exudate of the acute inflammatory process. Second, there is no collateral circulation to maintain vitality when the primary blood supply is compromised. Third, biopsies and direct application of medications are impossible without causing necrosis of the entire pulp. Fourth, pain or increasing levels of sensitivity are the only signs that can be used to determine the severity of pulpal inflammation.

Because of referred pain and the lack of proprioceptors in the pulp, localizing the problem to the correct tooth can often be a considerable diagnostic challenge. Also of significance is the difficulty in relating the clinical status of a tooth to histopathology. Unfortunately, no reliable symptoms or tests consistently correlate the two. The level of pulpal inflammation is determined through a combination of clinical criteria. Results of electric, heat, cold, and percussion tests must be added to the patient history, clinical examination, and clinician experience to arrive at the most appropriate diagnosis for the correct tooth.

Generally, the more intense the pain and the longer the duration of symptoms, the greater the damage to the pulp. Severe symptoms usually indicate irreversible damage.

Etiology

In the dental pulp, inflammation is the response to injury, just as it is in any other organ. In addition, the pulp response includes stimulation of odontoblasts to deposit reparative dentin at the site to help protect the pulp. If the injury is severe, the result is, instead, necrosis of these cells.

Caries is the most common form of injury that causes pulpitis. The degree of damage depends on the rapidity and extent of hard tissue destruction. Entry of bacteria into the pulpal tissue through a carious lesion is not necessary for pulpitis to occur, but this appears to be an important factor in the intensification of the inflammatory response. Pulpal microbiology adjacent to carious dentin demonstrates a diverse flora, including gram-positive anaerobes and *Bacteroides* species with low numbers of lactobacilli. Operative dental procedures associated with cavity and crown preparations may also trigger an inflammatory response in the dental pulp. The heat, friction, chemicals, and filling materials associated with restoration of teeth are all potential irritants. It is well known that less damage occurs when a cooling water spray is used during tooth preparation than when no water is used. It is also well established that an insulating base (such as zinc oxide and eugenol under amalgam restorations) can provide significant protection of the pulp from irritating chemicals used in the preparation of nonmetallic restorative materials and from heat transferred through large metallic fillings.

Other types of injury that may trigger pulpitis are trauma, especially when it is severe enough to cause root or crown fracture, and periodontal disease that has extended to an apical or lateral root foramen.

Clinical and Histopathologic Features

Several detailed classifications of pulpitis that are based on histopathologic changes have been proposed. Because of the difficulty in correlating clinical features with microscopy, these schemes have proved to be of little practical value. Instead, most practitioners prefer a simple classification that is helpful in the clinical setting relative to treatment and prognosis (Table 13-1).

Focal Reversible Pulpitis. Focal reversible pulpitis is an acute, mild inflammatory pulpal reaction that typically follows carious destruction of a tooth or placement of a large metallic filling without an insulating base. It causes hypersensitivity to thermal and electric stimuli. The pain is mild to moderate and is typically intermittent. As the name implies, the changes are focal (subjacent to the injurious agent) and reversible if the cause is removed. Microscopically, the predominant feature is dilation and engorgement of blood vessels (hyperemia). Exudation of plasma proteins also occurs, but this is difficult to appreciate in microscopic sections.

Acute Pulpitis. The inflammatory response of acute pulpitis may occur as a progression of focal reversible pulpitis, or it may represent an acute exacerbation of an already-established chronic pulpitis. Pulpal damage may range in severity from simple acute inflammation marked by vessel dilation, exudation, and neutrophil chemotaxis to focal liquefaction necrosis (pulp abscess) to total pulpal suppurative necrosis. Constant, severe, tooth-associated pain is the usual presenting complaint. Pain is intensified with the application of heat or cold, although in cases in which liquefaction of the pulp has occurred, cold may in fact alleviate the symptoms. If there is an opening from the pulp to the oral environment, symptoms may be lessened because of the escape of the exudate that causes pressure on and chemical irritation of the pulpal and periapical nerve tissues.

TABLE 13-1　**Pulpitis and Periapical Diseases**			
	Pain	**Vitality Tests**	**Radiographs**
Reversible pulpitis	Mild	Reversible sensitivity to cold	No change
Acute pulpitis	Severe, constant	Hyperresponse to none	No change
Chronic pulpitis	Mild, intermittent	Reduced response	No change
Acute periapical abscess	Severe; pain on percussion	No response	No change
Periapical granuloma	None to slight	No response	Lucency
Periapical cyst	None to slight	No response	Lucency

In the early phases of acute pulpitis the tooth may be hyperreactive to electric stimulation, but as pulp damage increases, sensitivity is reduced until there is no response. Because the exudate is confined primarily to the pulp rather than the periapical tissues, percussion tests generally elicit a response that differs little from normal.

Chronic Pulpitis. Chronic pulpitis is an inflammatory reaction that results from long-term, low-grade injury or occasionally from quiescence of an acute process. Symptoms, characteristically mild and often intermittent, appear over an extended period. A dull ache may be the presenting complaint, or the patient may have no symptoms at all. As the pulp deteriorates, responses to thermal and electric stimulation are reduced. Microscopically, lymphocytes, plasma cells, and fibrosis appear in the chronically inflamed pulp. Unless there is an acute exacerbation of the chronic process, neutrophils are not evident.

Chronic Hyperplastic Pulpitis. This special form of chronic pulpitis occurs in the molar teeth (both primary and permanent) of children and young adults. The involved teeth exhibit large carious lesions that open into the coronal pulp chamber. Rather than undergoing necrosis, the pulp tissue reacts in a hyperplastic manner, producing a red mass of reparative granulation tissue that extrudes through the pulp exposure. This type of reaction is believed to be related to the open root foramen, through which a relatively rich blood supply flows.

Symptoms seldom occur, because there is no exudate under pressure, and there is generally no nerve tissue proliferating with the granulation tissue. Although the pulp tissue is viable, the process is not reversible and necessitates endodontic therapy or tooth extraction. The well-vascularized granulation tissue mass often becomes epithelialized, presumably by autotransplantation of epithelial cells from nearby mucosal surfaces.

Treatment and Prognosis

If the cause is identified and eliminated, focal reversible pulpitis should recede, returning the pulp to a normal state. If the inflammation progresses into an acute pulpitis with neutrophil infiltrates and tissue necrosis, recovery is unlikely regardless of attempts to remove the cause. Endodontic therapy or tooth extraction is the only treatment available at this stage.

With chronic pulpitis, pulpal death is the characteristic end result (Figure 13-1). Removal of the cause may slow the process or occasionally save the vitality of the pulp. Endodontic therapy or extraction is typically required. Chronic hyperplastic pulpitis is essentially an irreversible end stage that is treated with pulp extirpation and an endodontic filling or extraction.

PERIAPICAL ABSCESS

Etiology

Numerous sequelae may follow untreated pulp necrosis and are dependent on the virulence of the microorganisms involved and the integrity of the patient's overall defense mechanisms (Figure 13-2). From its origin in the pulp, the inflammatory process extends into the periapical tissues, where it may present as a

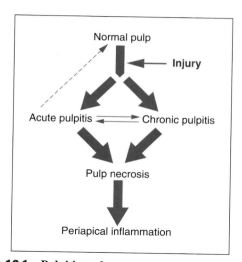

Figure 13-1 Pulpitis pathways.

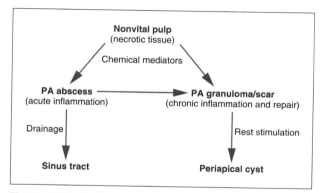

Figure 13-2 Pathogenesis of periapical inflammation.

granuloma or cyst (if chronic) or an abscess (if acute). Acute exacerbation of a chronic lesion may also be seen. The necrotic pulpal tissue debris, inflammatory cells, and bacteria, particularly anaerobes, all serve to stimulate and sustain the periapical inflammatory process.

Clinical Features

Patients with periapical abscesses typically have severe pain in the area of the nonvital tooth because of pressure and the effects of inflammatory chemical mediators on nerve tissue. The exudate and neutrophilic infiltrate of an abscess cause pressure on the surrounding tissue, often resulting in slight extrusion of the tooth from its socket. Pus associated with a lesion, if not focally constrained, seeks the path of least resistance and spreads into contiguous structures (Figures 13-3 to 13-5). The affected area of the jaw may be tender to palpation, and the patient may be hypersensitive to tooth percussion. The involved tooth is unresponsive to electric and thermal tests because of pulp necrosis.

Because of the rapidity with which this lesion develops, there is generally insufficient time for significant amounts of bone resorption to occur. Therefore radiographic changes are slight and are usually limited to mild radiographic thickening of the apical periodontal membrane space. However, if a periapical abscess develops as a result of acute exacerbation of a chronic periapical granuloma, a radiolucent lesion is evident. The *periapical granuloma* represents the result of chronic inflammation at the apex of a nonvital tooth. This is a sequela of pulp necrosis, which may develop through acute or low-grade chronic inflammation.

Notably, other, more serious conditions can occur in a periapical position (Box 13-1). A number of clinical clues may be present to alert the clinician that the periapical lesion may not be a simple dental granuloma (Box 13-2).

Histopathology

Microscopically, a periapical abscess appears as a zone of liquefaction composed of proteinaceous exudate, necrotic tissue, and viable and dead neutrophils (pus). Adjacent tissue containing dilated vessels and a neutrophilic infiltrate surrounds the area of liquefaction necrosis.

With chronicity, an abscess develops into a granuloma, which is composed of granulation tissue

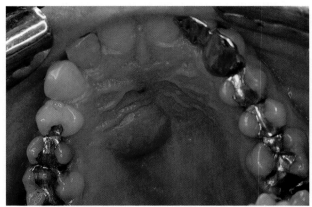

Figure 13-4 **Palatal abscess** representing extension of a periapical abscess.

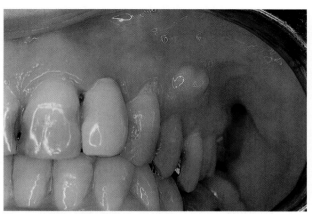

Figure 13-3 **Parulis (gingival abscess)** in maxillary mucosa and representing pus extension from a periapical abscess.

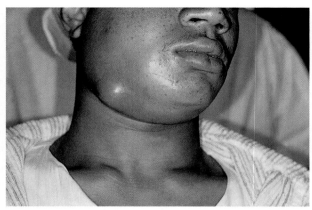

Figure 13-5 **Cutaneous abscess** related to extension from a mandibular periapical abscess.

and fibrous tissue infiltrated by variable numbers of neutrophils, lymphocytes, plasma cells, and macrophages. (NOTE: Periapical granuloma is to be distinguished from granulomatous inflammation, which is a distinctive type of chronic inflammation that is characteristic of certain diseases [e.g., tuberculosis, sarcoid, histoplasmosis] and features a predominance of macrophages and often multinucleated giant cells.) An acute flare of a periapical granuloma would show an abundant neutrophilic infiltrate in addition to granulation tissue and chronic inflammatory cells.

Box 13-1 Periapical Pathology

INFLAMMATORY

Periapical granuloma
Scar
Cyst
Chronic abscess
Actinomycosis

BENIGN

Traumatic bone cyst
Nasopalatine canal cyst
Langerhans cell disease
Adenomatoid odontogenic tumor
Periapical cementoosseous dysplasia
Ossifying fibroma

BENIGN, AGGRESSIVE

Odontogenic keratocyst
Calcifying odontogenic cyst
Central giant cell granuloma
Ameloblastoma
Calcifying epithelial odontogenic tumor
Myxoma

MALIGNANT

Metastasis
Lymphoma
Myeloma

Box 13-2 Noninflammatory Periapical Disease: Signs and Symptoms

Paresthesia or atypical pain
No relationship to periodontal ligament or lamina dura
Large lesions and lesions with ill-defined margins
Tooth vitality positive or equivocal

Treatment and Prognosis

Treatment of an acute periapical abscess requires observance of the standard principles of management of acute inflammation. Drainage should be established, either through an opening in the tooth itself or through the soft tissue surrounding the jaw if cellulitis has developed. Antibiotics directed against the offending organism are also required. Management must be thoughtful and skilled, because the consequences of delayed or inappropriate treatment can be significant and occasionally life threatening.

Spread of an abscess may be through one of several avenues. It may progress through the buccal cortical bone and gingival soft tissue, establishing a natural drain or sinus tract. The same type of situation may occur in the palate or skin; this depends on the original location of the abscess and the path of least resistance. If a drain is not established, the purulent exudate can cause an abscess or *cellulitis* in the soft tissues of the face, oral cavity, or neck. Cellulitis is an acute inflammatory process that is diffusely spread throughout the tissue rather than localized, as with an abscess. This variant is a result of infection by virulent organisms that produce enzymes that allow rapid spread through tissue. Bilateral cellulitis of the submandibular and sublingual spaces have been given the name *Ludwig's angina.*

A dangerous situation occurs when the acute infection involves major blood vessels, possibly resulting in bacteremia. Also, retrograde spread of the infection through facial emissary veins to the cavernous sinus may set up the necessary conditions for thrombus formation. *Cavernous sinus thrombosis* is an emergency situation that is often fatal.

Treatment of periapical granulomas and cysts is discussed in Chapter 10.

ACUTE OSTEOMYELITIS

Etiology

Acute inflammation of the bone and bone marrow of the mandible and maxilla results most often from extension of a periapical abscess. The second most common cause of acute osteomyelitis is physical injury, such as occurs with fracture or surgery. Osteomyelitis may also result from bacteremia.

Most cases of acute osteomyelitis are infectious. Almost any organism may be part of the etiologic picture, although staphylococci and streptococci are identified the most.

Clinical Features

Pain is the primary feature of this inflammatory process. Pyrexia, painful lymphadenopathy, leukocytosis, and other signs and symptoms of acute infection are also commonly present. Paresthesia of the lower lip occasionally occurs with mandibular involvement. In the development of a clinical differential diagnosis, the presence of this symptom should also suggest malignant mandibular neoplasms.

To be visible by conventional radiography, a lesion must have resorbed or demineralized approximately 60% of the bone. Therefore unless the inflammatory process has been present for some time, radiographic evidence of acute osteomyelitis is usually not present. With time, diffuse radiolucent changes begin to appear as more bone is resorbed and replaced by infection.

Histopathology

A purulent exudate occupies the marrow spaces in acute osteomyelitis. Bony trabeculae show reduced osteoblastic activity and increased osteoclastic resorption. If an area of bone necrosis occurs (sequestrum), osteocytes are lost and the marrow undergoes liquefaction.

Treatment

Acute osteomyelitis is usually treated with antibiotics and drainage. Ideally, the causative agent is identified, and an appropriate antibiotic is selected through sensitivity testing in the laboratory. Surgery may also be part of the treatment and ranges from simple sequestrectomy to excision with autologous bone replacement. Each case should be judged individually because of variations in disease severity, the organisms involved, and the patient's overall health.

CHRONIC OSTEOMYELITIS (CHRONIC OSTEITIS)

Etiology

Chronic osteomyelitis may be one of the sequelae of acute osteomyelitis (either untreated or inadequately treated), or it may represent a long-term, low-grade inflammatory reaction that never went through a significant or clinically noticeable acute phase (Box 13-3 and Table 13-2). In either event, acute and chronic osteomyelitis have many similar etiologic factors. Most cases are infectious, and as in most infections, the clinical presentation and course are directly dependent on the virulence of the microorganism involved and

---

Box 13-3   Chronic Osteomyelitis/Osteitis

DEFINITION

Inflammation of bone and bone marrow

CLINICAL FEATURES

Symptoms vary from mild to moderate pain
Exudate often not present
Radiographic image mottled; sclerosis typically occurs with time

HISTOPATHOLOGY

Low-grade lesions contain few inflammatory cells
May mimic (clinically and microscopically) benign fibroosseous lesions

---

TABLE 13-2   **Chronic Osteomyelitis: Types and Features**

	Etiology	Clinical Features	Radiographs	Treatment
Chronic osteomyelitis	Most infectious (bacteria)	Variable pain, swelling, drainage	Lucent or mottled pattern	Appropriate antibiotic, sequestrectomy
Chronic osteomyelitis with proliferative periostitis	Sequela of tooth abscess, extraction	Usually associated with lower molar; periosteum involved Children	Lucent or mottled pattern with concentric periosteal opacities	Tooth removal, antibiotics
Diffuse sclerosing osteomyelitis	Probably low-grade infection, pulpitis, periodontal disease	Occasional pain, swelling, drainage Mandible	Opacification throughout jaw	Antibiotics; find cause, if possible, and treat
Focal sclerosing osteitis	Low-grade focal bone irritation (e.g., pulpitis)	Asymptomatic; found on routine examination	Opaque mass, usually at root apex	Treat offending tooth

the patient's resistance. The anatomic location, immunologic status, nutritional status, patient's age, and presence of preexisting systemic factors, such as Paget's disease, osteopetrosis, or sickle cell disease, are other factors affecting the presentation and course.

Bone irradiated as part of head and neck cancer treatment is particularly susceptible to infection. Because of reduced vascularity and osteocyte destruction, osteoradionecrosis occurs in approximately 20% of patients who have undergone local tumoricidal irradiation. Secondary infection generally follows. Typical precipitating or triggering events include periapical inflammation resulting from nonvital teeth, extractions, periodontal disease, and fractures communicating with skin or mucosa.

Identification of a specific infectious agent involved in chronic osteomyelitis is usually difficult both microscopically and microbiologically. Sample error is significant, either because of small, difficult-to-reach bacterial foci or because of contamination of the lesion by resident flora. Previously taken antibiotics also reduce the chances of culturing the causative organism. Although an etiologic agent is often not confirmed, most investigators believe that bacteria (e.g., staphylococci, streptococci, *Bacteroides*, *Actinomyces*) are responsible for the vast majority of chronic osteomyelitis cases.

Clinical Features

The mandible, especially the molar area, is much more commonly affected than is the maxilla. This may relate, in part, to the more diffuse blood supply and the greater proportion of cancellous bone in the maxilla. Pain is usually present but varies in intensity, and it is not necessarily related to the extent of the disease. The duration of symptoms is generally proportional to the extent of the disease. Swelling of the jaw is a commonly encountered sign; loose teeth and sinus tracts are seen less often. Anesthesia is very uncommon.

Radiographically, chronic osteomyelitis appears primarily as a radiolucent lesion that may show focal zones of opacification. The lucent pattern is often described as moth-eaten because of its mottled radiographic appearance (Figures 13-6 and 13-7). Lesions may be very extensive, and margins are often indistinct.

Histopathology

The inflammatory reaction in chronic osteomyelitis can vary from very mild to intense. In mild cases micro-

scopic diagnosis can be difficult because of similarities to fibroosseous lesions such as ossifying fibroma and fibrous dysplasia. A few chronic inflammatory cells (lymphocytes and plasma cells) are seen in a fibrous marrow (Figure 13-8). Both osteoblastic and osteoclastic activity may be seen, along with irregular bony trabeculae—unlikely features of fibroosseous lesions. In advanced chronic osteomyelitis, necrotic bone (sequestrum) may be present, as evidenced by both necrotic marrow and necrotic osteocytes. Reversal lines reflect the waves of deposition and resorption of bone. Inflammatory cells are more numerous and osteoclastic activity more prominent than in mild cases.

Treatment

The basic treatment of chronic osteomyelitis centers around the selection of appropriate antibiotics and the proper timing of surgical intervention. Culture and sensitivity testing should be carried out. Combinations of antibiotics may, on occasion, be more suc-

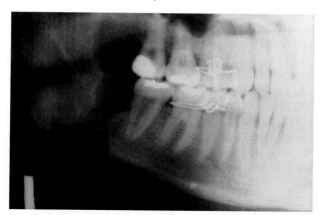

Figure 13-6 **Chronic osteomyelitis** in the region of third-molar extraction.

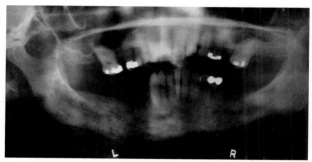

Figure 13-7 **Chronic osteomyelitis** of the mandible associated with periodontal disease. Note moth-eaten radiolucent appearance.

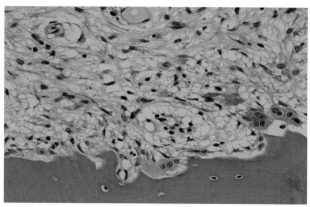

Figure 13-8 **Chronic osteomyelitis** showing fibrous marrow and osteoclastic resorption of resident bone.

cessful than single agents. The duration of antibiotic administration may also be relatively extended.

When a sequestrum develops, surgical removal appears to hasten the healing process. Excision of other nonvital bone, sinus tracts, and scar tissue has also been advocated. In cases in which the potential for pathologic fracture is significant, immobilization is required.

In recalcitrant cases of chronic osteomyelitis and most cases of osteoradionecrosis, the use of *hyperbaric oxygen* has provided significant benefit for patients. In difficult cases hyperbaric oxygen used in conjunction with antibiotics or surgery appears to be generally better than any of these methods used alone. The rationale for using hyperbaric oxygen is related to its stimulation of vascular proliferation, collagen synthesis, and osteogenesis. Contraindications include the presence of viral infections, optic neuritis, known residual or recurrent malignancies, and some lung diseases. The regimen typically used in this treatment adjunct involves placing a patient in a closed chamber with 100% oxygen at 2 atmospheres of pressure for 2 hours per day for several weeks. The elevated tissue oxygen levels achieved with this technique reach a limited maximum level by the end of therapy, but the effects appear to be long lasting. Specific hyperbaric oxygen protocols vary, however, with some advocating debridement or excision after hyperbaric oxygen therapy.

Chronic Osteomyelitis With Proliferative Periostitis (Garré's Osteomyelitis)

Etiology. Chronic osteomyelitis with proliferative periostitis, commonly known as Garré's osteomyelitis, is essen-tially a subtype of osteomyelitis that has a prominent periosteal inflammatory reaction as an additional component. It most often results from a periapical abscess of a mandibular molar tooth or an infection associated with tooth extraction or partially erupted molars. It is most common in children.

The eponym Garré's osteomyelitis has been applied to this condition after the author, Dr. K. Garré, who in 1893 described the clinical features of 72 patients with osteomyelitis. The disease he described was most common in the femur, with only three cases occurring in the jaws. In the absence of histologic and radiographic findings, which were unavailable at the time of the report, it is likely that Garré was describing a form of recalcitrant, acute osteomyelitis that occurred in both adults and children. It was not chronic osteomyelitis with proliferative periostitis. Therefore the term *Garré's osteomyelitis*, although widely used in reference to this condition, is inaccurate.

Clinical Features. This variety of osteomyelitis is uncommonly encountered. It has been described in the tibia, and in the head and neck area it is seen in the mandible. It typically involves the posterior mandible and is usually unilateral. Patients characteristically present with an asymptomatic bony, hard swelling with normal-appearing overlying skin and mucosa (Figure 13-9, *A*). On occasion, slight tenderness may be noted. This presentation necessitates the differentiation of this process from benign mandibular neoplasms. Radiographs and a biopsy provide a definitive diagnosis.

Radiographically, the lesion appears centrally as a mottled, predominantly lucent lesion in a pattern consistent with that of chronic osteomyelitis. The feature that provides the distinctive difference is the periosteal reaction. This, best viewed on an occlusal radiograph, appears as an expanded cortex, often with concentric or parallel opaque layers (Figure 13-9, *B*). Trabeculae perpendicular to the onionskin layers may also be apparent.

Histopathology. Reactive new bone typifies the subperiosteal cortical response. Perpendicular orientation of new trabeculae to redundant cortical bone is best seen under low magnification. Osteoblastic activity dominates in this area, and both osteoblastic and osteoclastic activity are seen centrally. Marrow spaces contain fibrous tissue with scattered lymphocytes and plasma cells. Inflammatory cells are often surprisingly scant, making microscopic differentiation from fibroosseous lesions a diagnostic challenge (Figure 13-9, *C* and *D*).

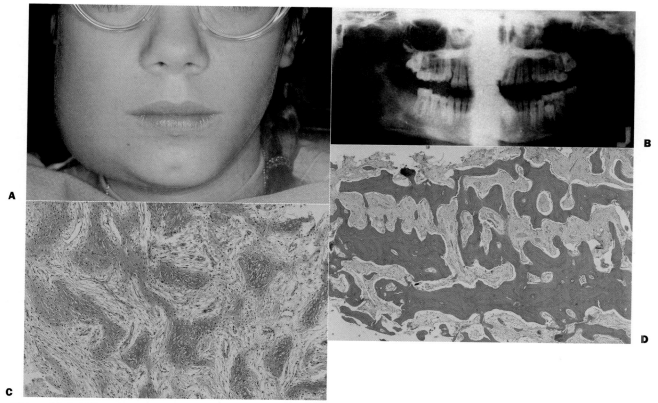

Figure 13-9 **Chronic osteomyelitis with proliferative periostitis (Garré's osteomyelitis)** of the right mandible (**A**). **B,** Note periosteal expansion in the radiograph. **C,** Tissue from the central mandible is minimally inflamed and has a fibroosseous appearance. **D,** Periosteal tissue shows sclerotic laminations.

Treatment. Identification and removal of the offending agent are of primary importance in chronic osteomyelitis with proliferative periostitis. Removal of the involved tooth is usually required. Antibiotics are generally included early in this treatment. The mandible then undergoes gradual remodeling without additional surgical intervention.

Diffuse Sclerosing Osteomyelitis

Etiology. Diffuse sclerosing osteomyelitis represents an inflammatory reaction in the mandible or maxilla, believed to be in response to a microorganism of low virulence. Bacteria are generally suspected as causative agents, although they are seldom specifically identified. Chronic periodontal disease, which appears to provide a portal of entry for bacteria, is important in the etiology and progression of diffuse sclerosing osteomyelitis. Carious nonvital teeth are less often implicated.

Clinical Features. This condition may be seen in any age, in either sex, and in any race, but it tends to occur most often in middle-aged black women. The disease is typified by a protracted chronic course with acute exacerbations of pain, swelling, and occasionally drainage.

Radiographically, this process is diffuse, typically affecting a large part of the jaw (Figures 13-10 and 13-11). The lesion is ill defined. Early lucent zones may appear in association with sclerotic masses. In advanced stages, sclerosis dominates the radiographic picture. Periosteal thickening may also be seen. Scintigraphy may be particularly useful in evaluating the extent of this condition.

Histopathology. The microscopic changes of this condition are inflammatory. Fibrous replacement of marrow is noted. A chronic inflammatory cell infiltrate and occasionally a neutrophilic infiltrate are also seen. Bony trabeculae exhibit irregular size and shape and may be lined by numerous osteoblasts. Focal osteoclastic activity is also present. The characteristic sclerotic

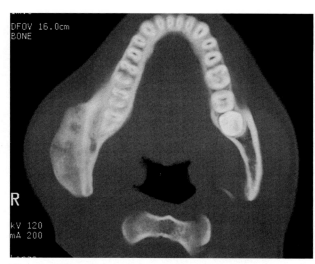

Figure 13-10 **Sclerosing osteomyelitis** of the right mandible in a computed tomography (CT) scan.

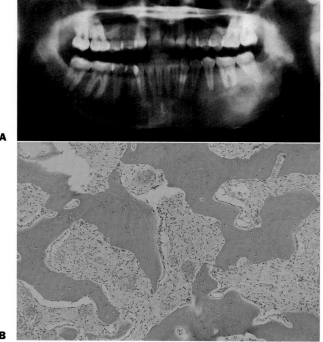

Figure 13-11 **A** and **B, Sclerosing osteomyelitis** of the left mandible. Biopsy specimen shows thick trabeculae, fibrous marrow, and scattered lymphocytes. (Courtesy Dr. Bruce A. Shapton.)

masses are composed of dense bone, often exhibiting numerous reversal lines.

Differential Diagnosis. Chronic sclerosing osteomyelitis shares many clinical, radiographic, and histologic features with florid osseous dysplasia. The two should be separated, because the former is an inflammatory/infectious process and the latter a bony dysplastic process. Treatment and prognosis are therefore dissimilar. Florid osseous dysplasia appears to be an extensive form of periapical cemental dysplasia and, unlike diffuse sclerosing osteomyelitis, may exhibit anterior periapical lesions and traumatic or simple bone cysts. Furthermore, florid osseous dysplasia is usually asymptomatic and appears as a fibroosseous lesion lacking an inflammatory cell infiltrate.

Treatment. The management of diffuse sclerosing osteomyelitis is problematic because of the relative avascular nature of the affected tissue and because of the large size of the lesion. Even with aggressive treatment, the course is protracted.

If an etiologic factor such as periodontal disease or a carious tooth can be identified, it should be eliminated. Antibiotics are the mainstay of treatment and are especially helpful during painful exacerbations. Surgical removal of the diseased area is usually an inappropriate procedure because of the extent of the disease. However, decortication of the affected site has resulted in improvement in some cases. Low-dose corticosteroids have also been used with some success. Hyperbaric oxygen therapy may prove to be a valuable adjunct. Recently treatment with pamidronate has shown promising results.

Focal Sclerosing Osteitis

Etiology. Focal sclerosing osteitis is a relatively common phenomenon that is believed to represent a focal bony reaction to a low-grade inflammatory stimulus. It is usually seen at the apex of a tooth with long-standing pulpitis. This lesion may occasionally be adjacent to a sound, unrestored tooth, suggesting that other etiologic factors such as malocclusion may be operative.

Synonyms for focal sclerosing osteitis include *focal sclerosing osteomyelitis, bony scar, condensing osteitis,* and *sclerotic bone.* The term *focal periapical osteopetrosis* has also been used to describe idiopathic lesions associated with normal, caries-free teeth.

Clinical Features. Focal sclerosing osteitis may be found at any age but is typically discovered in young adults. Patients are usually asymptomatic, and most lesions

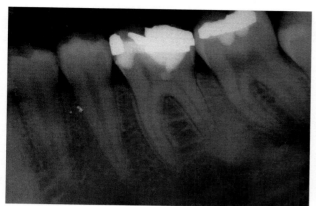

Figure 13-12 **Focal sclerosing osteitis** at the apex of first molar.

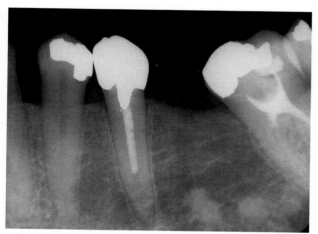

Figure 13-13 **Focal sclerosing osteitis.** Residual after tooth extraction.

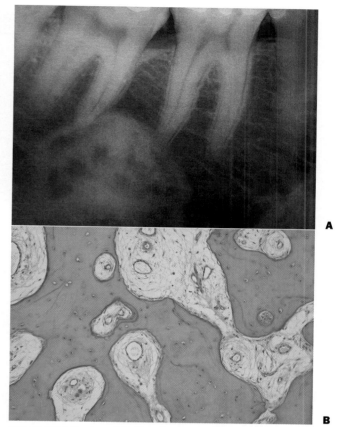

Figure 13-14 **A** and **B, Focal sclerosing osteitis.** Biopsy specimen shows dense sclerotic trabeculae and fibrous marrow with a few lymphocytes.

are discovered on routine radiographic examination. A majority are found at the apices of mandibular first molars, with a minority associated with mandibular second molars and premolars (Figure 13-12). When teeth are extracted, these lesions remain behind indefinitely (Figure 13-13).

Radiographically, one of several patterns may be seen (Figure 13-14). The lesion may be uniformly opaque; it may have a peripheral lucency with an opaque center; it may have an opaque periphery with a lucent center; or it may be composed of confluent or lobulated opaque masses.

Histopathology. Microscopically, these lesions are masses of dense sclerotic bone. Connective tissue is scant, as are inflammatory cells.

Differential Diagnosis. Differential diagnosis should include periapical cemental dysplasia, osteoma, complex odontoma, cementoblastoma, osteoblastoma, and hypercementosis. In most cases, however, diagnosis can be made with confidence on the basis of historical and radiographic features.

Treatment. Because it is believed to represent a physiologic bone reaction to a known stimulus, the lesion itself need not be removed. A biopsy might be contemplated to rule out more significant lesions that received serious consideration in the differential diagnosis. The inflamed pulp that stimulated the focal sclerosing osteomyelitis should be treated. The decision about whether the tooth should be restored, treated endodontically, or extracted should be made on a case-by-case basis according to findings.

BIBLIOGRAPHY

Brook I, Frazier E, Gher M: Aerobic and anaerobic microbiology of periapical abscess, *Oral Microbiol Immunol* 6:123-125, 1991.

Epstein J, van der Meij E, McKenzie M, et al: Postradiation osteonecrosis of the mandible, *Oral Surg Oral Med Oral Pathol Oral Radiol Endod* 83:657-662, 1997.

Hahn C, Falkler W, Minah G: Microbiological studies of carious dentin from human teeth with irreversible pulpitis, *Arch Oral Biol* 36:147-153, 1991.

Kim S: Neurovascular interactions in the dental pulp in health and inflammation, *J Endod* 16:48-53, 1990.

Marx RE, Carlson ER, Smith BR, et al: Isolation of *Actinomyces* species and *Eikenella corrodens* from patients with chronic diffuse sclerosing osteomyelitis, *J Oral Maxillofac Surg* 52:26-33, 1994.

Soubrier M, Dubost JJ, Ristori JM, et al: Pamidronate in the treatment of diffuse sclerosing osteomyelitis of the mandible, *Oral Surg Oral Med Oral Pathol Oral Radiol Endod* 92:637-640, 2001.

Wood RE, Nortje CJ, Grotepass F, et al: Periostitis ossificans versus Garré's osteomyelitis. I. What did Garré really say? *Oral Surg Oral Med Oral Pathol* 65(6):773-777, 1988.

Malignancies of the Jaws

Richard J. Zarbo, DMD, MD, and Eric R. Carlson, DMD, MD

Malignant nonodontogenic tumors of the jaws, both primary and metastatic, are rare in comparison with tumors arising in the surrounding soft tissues. Despite the infrequent occurrence of these entities, a diagnosis of a malignant jaw tumor has serious prognostic implications, often signaling a treatment plan requiring major therapeutic intervention. Generally, this group of lesions causes sign and symptoms that are often highly suggestive of intrabony malignancy (Box 14-1). Tumors discussed in this chapter are those arising from the hard tissues (osteosarcoma and chondrosarcoma) and those involving the marrow cavity of the mandible and maxilla (Ewing's sarcoma, Burkitt's lymphoma, plasma cell neoplasias, and metastatic carcinoma).

OSTEOSARCOMA

Osteosarcomas account for approximately 20% of all sarcomas and, after plasma cell neoplasia, are the most common primary bone tumors. Approximately 5% of osteosarcomas occur in the jaws, with an incidence of approximately 1 case in 1.5 million persons per year (Box 14-2). Osteosarcomas arise in several clinical settings, including preexisting bone abnormalities such as *Paget's disease, fibrous dysplasia, giant cell tumor, multiple osteochondromas, bone infarct, chronic osteomyelitis,* and *osteogenesis imperfecta.* Some osteosarcomas have also been preceded by radiation therapy to the affected bone for unrelated or antecedent disease. The vast majority of osteosarcomas involve the tubular long bones, especially those adjacent to the knee. Osteosarcomas can also be classified by their site of origin into (1) the conventional type, arising within the medullary cavity; (2) juxtacortical tumors, arising from the periosteal surface; and (3) extraskeletal osteosarcomas, arising rarely in soft tissue.

The molecular mechanism associated with osteosarcoma pathogenesis appears to be related to mutations or amplifications of one or more genes. Alterations in *p53, Rb* (retinoblastoma), *CDK4* (cyclin-dependent kinase 4), *MDM2* (murine double minute 2), *c-fos, c-myc,* and *SAS* (sarcoma amplified sequence) genes have all been cited as contributing to osteosarcoma development. Protein expression of the defective/amplified genes results in loss of control of cell proliferation and differentiation (see also the discussion on pathogenesis of squamous cell carcinoma in Chapter 2).

Clinical Features. Conventional osteosarcomas involving the mandible and maxilla display a slight predilection for males (60%). Although the peak incidence of osteosarcomas of the skeleton occurs in the second decade, those arising in the jaws present 1 to 2 decades later, with a mean age of 35 years (range 8 to 85 years). The mandible is more commonly affected than the maxilla by a ratio of 1.7 to 1. The majority (60%) of mandibular osteosarcomas arise in the body of the

---

Box 14-1 Malignancy in the Jaws: Signs and Symptoms

Paresthesia
Pain
Loose teeth, vertical mobility, premature loss
Tooth resorption more likely than displacement
Rapid growth
Acquired malocclusion
Radiographic changes
    Uniformly widened periodontal membrane space
    Ill-defined lesion

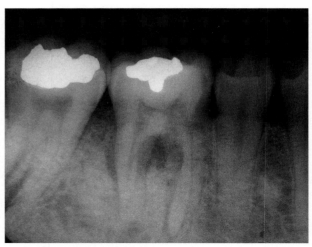

Figure 14-1   **Osteosarcoma** surrounding the roots of first molar tooth. Note widened periodontal ligament.

Box 14-2 Osteosarcoma of the Jaws

ETIOLOGY

No known risk factors
Genes that may be altered—*p53, Rb, CDK4, MDM2, c-fos, c-myc, SAS*

CLINICAL FEATURES

Swelling, pain, paresthesia, periodontal ligament invasion
Mean age—35 years; age range from 10 to 85 years
Males and females equally affected; mandible > maxilla

HISTOPATHOLOGY

Malignant cells producing osteoid
Well differentiated
Chondroblastic osteosarcoma most common subtype

TREATMENT

Resection to multimodality; good prognosis

>More frequently affected than.

---

mandible; the remaining sites of predilection include the symphysis, angle of the mandible, ascending ramus, and temporomandibular joint. In the maxilla there is a nearly equal incidence of tumors involving the alveolar ridge and maxillary antrum, with few affecting the palate.

Osteosarcomas involving the jaws present most commonly with swelling and localized pain. In some cases there may be loosening and displacement of teeth, as well as paresthesia due to involvement of the inferior alveolar nerve. Maxillary tumors display similar clinical symptoms but may cause paresthesia of the infraorbital nerve, epistaxis, nasal obstruction, or eye problems such as proptosis and diplopia. Mucosal ulceration is usually not seen until late-stage disease. The average duration of symptoms is 3 to 4 months before diagnosis.

The radiographic appearance of conventional intramedullary osteosarcoma can be quite variable, reflecting the degree of calcification. There appears to be little relationship between the radiographic pattern and the histologic subtype of osteosarcoma. Early osteosarcomas that involve the alveolar process may be characterized by localized widening of the periodontal ligament space of one or two teeth (Figures 14-1 and 14-2). The widened space results from tumor invasion of the periodontal ligament and resorption of the surrounding alveolar bone (Figure 14-3). Advanced tumors can be visualized as "moth-eaten" radiolucencies or irregular, poorly marginated radiopacities. The majority of these neoplasms have mixed radiographic features. A characteristic sun ray or sunburst radiopaque appearance due to periosteal reaction may be seen in jaw lesions but is not diagnostic of osteosarcoma (Figure 14-4).

Histopathology. Histologically, all osteosarcomas have a sarcomatous stroma in common that directly produces tumor osteoid (Figure 14-5). Variable histologic patterns dominate and have been designated as *chondroblastic* (most common) (Figure 14-6), *osteoblastic,* and *fibroblastic* (Figure 14-7). An additional variant, designated as *telangiectatic,* that displays multiple aneurysmal blood-filled spaces lined by malignant cells rarely occurs in the head and neck region.

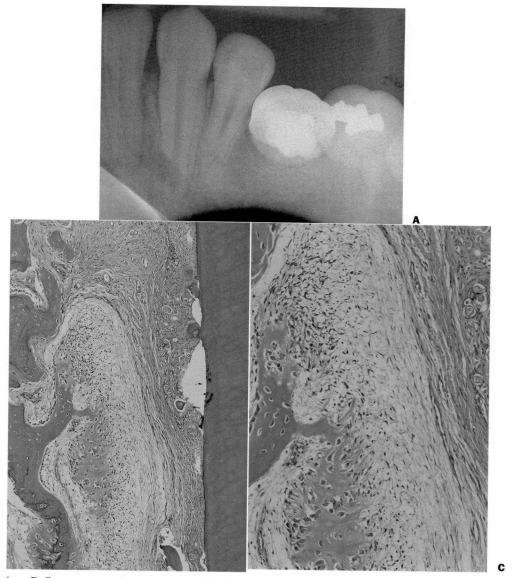

Figure 14-2 **A** to **C, Osteosarcoma** between a mandibular lateral incisor and a canine. Note slight widening of periodontal ligaments of both teeth. **B** and **C,** Surgical specimen shows a malignant bone-producing neoplasm occupying the periodontal ligament space. The tooth is to the right, and alveolar bone is to the left.

Central low-grade osteosarcoma is a recently described variant that may involve the jaws. Histologically, it resembles fibrous dysplasia because of the minimally atypical spindle cell proliferation with occasional mitotic figures and bone spicules. Unlike fibrous dysplasia, the radiographic appearance is usually that of an invasive intramedullary growth with poor margination and cortical destruction. Also unlike fibrous dysplasia, the proliferation permeates bone marrow, may extend through the periosteum, and may invade

soft tissues. Recurrent tumor or long-standing lesions convert to conventional high-grade osteosarcoma.

All histologic variants reflect the multipotentiality of the neoplastic mesenchymal cells in producing osteoid, cartilage, and fibrous tissue. Such histologic subclassification, however, bears no prognostic significance. However, patients with high-grade lesions have a poorer prognosis compared with those with low-grade lesions. Chondroblastic osteosarcomas are the most common histologic type (50%) occurring in

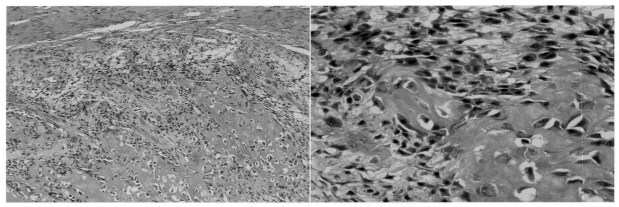

A   B

Figure 14-3   **A** and **B, Osteosarcoma** composed of atypical cells in association with tumor bone.

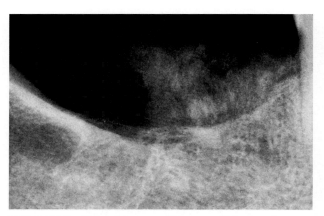

Figure 14-4   **Osteosarcoma** of the mandible showing a sunburst pattern of tumor bone radiating from the alveolar ridge.

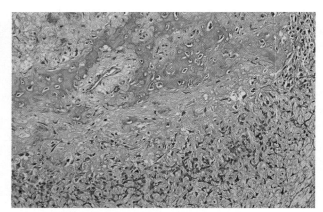

Figure 14-5   **Osteosarcoma** exhibiting a partially myxoid microscopic appearance.

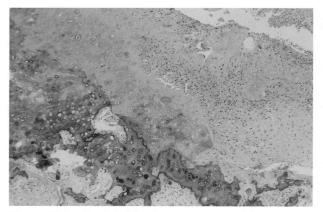

Figure 14-6   **Chondroblastic osteosarcoma.** Note cartilage and bone at lower left.

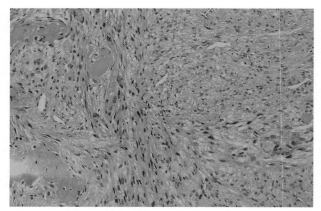

Figure 14-7   **Fibroblastic osteosarcoma** composed of spindled tumor cells and small islands of tumor bone.

Figure 14-8 **Jaw sarcoma treatment. A,** Axial computed tomography (CT) scan of a large fibrosarcoma of the mandible with extension into the lateral pharynx. **B,** Tumor resection required wide margins, including sacrifice of the condyle. Appropriate sacrifice of surrounding anatomic barriers allows for negative margins on the specimen. **C,** The specimen radiograph confirms the inclusion of acceptable linear bony margins with the specimen.

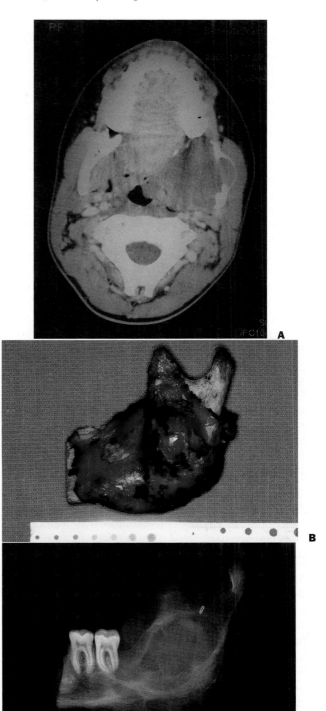

the jaws, although osteoblastic histologic variants predominate in the skeleton. Most osteosarcomas of the mandible tend to be lytic (40%); those in the maxilla are often osteoblastic (50%).

Differential Diagnosis. The uniform widening of the periodontal ligament space of involved teeth appears to be characteristic for early osteosarcoma that involves the alveolus. However, this focal radiographic defect may also have been seen with other malignancies surrounding teeth. Uniform widening of periodontal ligament spaces surrounding all teeth may be seen in scleroderma. Moth-eaten radiolucencies are common to other malignancies, chronic osteomyelitis, and several benign neoplasms. A sclerotic radiographic appearance may be seen with some metastatic carcinomas and in the calcifying epithelial odontogenic tumor, which is also often associated with an impacted tooth.

The histologic diagnosis hinges on finding the malignant cells producing osteoid. Many jaw osteosarcomas are predominantly chondroblastic, however, and may be misdiagnosed as chondrosarcoma. Osteosarcomas with a predominant fibroblastic component may be misdiagnosed as fibrous dysplasia, fibrosarcoma, or malignant fibrous histiocytoma of bone.

Management The management of sarcomas of the facial skeleton involves both surgery and chemotherapy. Surgical management of osteosarcoma of the mandible, however, is the mainstay of therapy and possesses numerous characteristics similar to the management of carcinomas of the jaws, with some notable differences. The similarities include the required attention to surrounding anatomic barriers with their appropriate sacrifice (Figure 14-8). Invasion of the anatomic barriers surrounding any head and neck tumor may be assessed by physical examination and/or special imaging studies. When a small sarcoma originates within the medullary component of the mandible, cortical bone is the first anatomic barrier the tumor encounters that forestalls its growth. Once the cortical bone is violated, the less robust periosteum is subsequently encountered. With continued growth, muscle, mucosa, and skin ultimately become invaded by the malignancy. The general approach to malignant tumor surgery of the head and neck is that at least one uninvolved anatomic barrier margin be included on the tumor specimen as part of the en bloc resection. This practice allows better analysis of tumor margins. The main difference between resection of carcinoma in bone compared with resection of sarcomas lies in the recommended linear bony margin. Whereas carcinomas may be resected with a 2-cm linear margin in bone, it is generally recommended that sarcoma resections include a 3-cm margin. Attention to proper anatomic barrier sacrifice, as well as the inclusion of the recommended linear bony margin, enhances the potential for long-term palliation or cure of patients with sarcomas of the jaws.

Although sarcomas were traditionally managed surgically, it is now recognized that chemotherapy plays an important role in most, if not all, patients with these tumors. Chemotherapy may be administered preoperatively (neoadjuvant chemotherapy) or postoperatively (adjuvant chemotherapy). Indications for neoadjuvant chemotherapy include the following:

- The elimination of micrometastases or macrometastases
- Reduction of the primary tumor size
- Induction of partial or complete tumor necrosis
- Increased likelihood of tumor-free margins at the time of ablative surgery

Most studies indicate that intramedullary sarcomas of the jawbones show no response to radiation therapy.

The principles of management of sarcomas of the jaws are consistent for all subtypes of sarcoma. Moreover, the management of all variants of osteosarcoma, including low-grade osteosarcoma, postradiation osteosarcoma, intramedullary osteosarcoma, and juxtacortical osteosarcoma, are identical. Studies demonstrate that conservative management of those sarcomas with an otherwise inherently better prognosis than others will lead to local recurrence and increase the tendency for distant metastasis. These two scenarios are associated with greatly diminished survival rates, thereby justifying aggressive surgical management from the onset.

Prognosis. Overall, 5-year survival rates of 25% to 40% are reported for jaw osteosarcomas. Patients with mandibular tumors generally fare better than patients with maxillary tumors. As with most malignant jaw tumors, initial radical surgery results in a superior survival rate of 80% as compared with a 25% survival rate with local or conservative surgery. Osteosarcomas of the jaws commonly recur (40% to 70%), with a metastatic rate of 25% to 50%. Osteosarcomas are more likely to metastasize to lung and brain than to regional lymph nodes. Once the disease has become metastatic, the mean survival time is 6 months. Nearly 80% of patients dying of the disease do so within the first 2 years. Local recurrences and isolated metastatic deposits are treated by surgical excision and chemotherapy.

PAROSTEAL OSTEOSARCOMA

In contrast to the central intramedullary osteosarcomas, juxtacortical (parosteal and periosteal) osteosarcomas arise at the periphery of bone at the periosteal surface, with distinct clinical, histologic, and radiographic features, as well as a different biologic behavior. Juxtacortical osteosarcomas are uncommon neoplasms that account for approximately 5% of all osteosarcomas of the skeleton; they are rarely seen in the jaws. Most juxtacortical osteosarcomas arising in the jaws are the biologically low-grade parosteal subtype or, rarely, the periosteal subtype.

Parosteal osteosarcoma occurs over a wide age range, with a peak incidence at 39 years (Figures 14-9 and 14-10). When the long bones are affected, there is a female predominance (3 to 2), but when the jaws are affected, there is a male predominance. This variant of juxtacortical osteosarcoma most commonly involves the distal femoral metaphysis. The tumor presents as a slow-growing swelling or palpable mass, often accompanied by a dull, aching sensation. Radiographically, the tumor is often radiodense and attached to the external surface of bone by a broad sessile base. It is often more radiodense at the base than at the periphery. The broad pedicle is not continuous radiographically with the underlying marrow cavity. A radiolucent clear space, corresponding to the periosteum, can often be identified between the tumor and the underlying cortex.

Histologically, parosteal osteosarcomas are well differentiated and characterized by a spindle cell stroma with minimal atypia and rare mitotic figures separating irregular trabeculae of woven bone (Figure 14-11). The periphery is less ossified than the base; it may have a lobulated cartilaginous cap, or it may be ir-

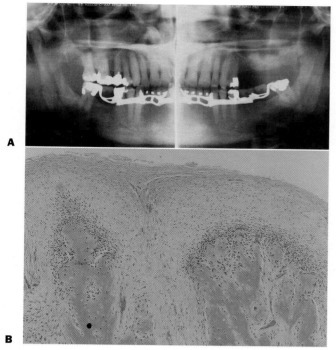

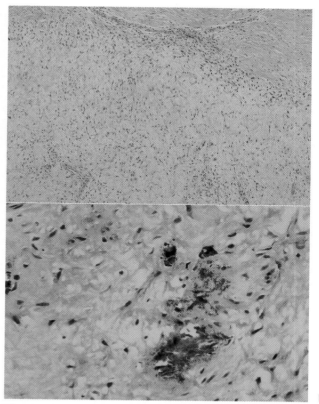

Figure 14-9 **A** and **B, Parosteal osteosarcoma** of the left maxilla. Biopsy specimen shows a pale peripheral myxoid zone overlying a cellular zone and tumor osteoid.

Figure 14-11 **A** and **B, Parosteal osteosarcoma** exhibiting a myxoid microscopic appearance with foci of atypical calcification of irregular osteoid **(B).**

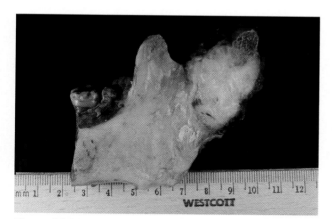

Figure 14-10 **Parosteal osteosarcoma.** Gross specimen shows a white mass covering the ramus and condyle.

regular because of linear extensions into soft tissue. Medullary involvement is unusual at initial presentation, but approximately 20% of tumors, especially recurrent ones, exhibit invasion of the underlying bone. This does not seem to affect the prognosis adversely. The bland histologic appearance of paro-steal osteosarcoma raises the possibility of osteoma, osteochondroma, and exostosis.

PERIOSTEAL OSTEOSARCOMA

Periosteal osteosarcoma occurs much less often than does parosteal osteosarcoma. It has a 2-to-1 male predominance and a peak age of occurrence of 20 years. These tumors commonly involve the upper tibial metaphysis. They are rarely seen in the jaws.

The radiographic appearance of periosteal osteosarcoma is distinct from that of parosteal osteosarcoma. The cortex of involved bone is radiographically intact and sometimes thickened, with no tumor involvement of the underlying marrow cavity. The tumor is most often radiolucent, corresponding to its predominantly cartilaginous component, and has a more poorly defined periphery. On occasion, a periosteal reaction in the form of Codman's triangle may be noted, as well as variably sized perpendicular calcified spicules of bone radiating from the cortex. Overall, the periosteal osteosarcoma tumor matrix is not as radiographically dense or homogeneous as that of the parosteal osteosarcoma.

Histologically, periosteal osteosarcoma is composed of lobules of poorly differentiated malignant cartilage; it often shows central ossification. The malignant cartilage and osteoid appear to radiate from an intact cortex. The osteoid present in this variant is fine and lacelike, and it is found in the chondroid islands among intervening malignant spindle cells. These histologic features can be identical to those of intramedullary osteosarcomas; therefore radiographic correlation is necessary to make this diagnosis. The malignant cytologic features also distinguish this variant of juxtacortical osteosarcoma from the parosteal type. In periosteal osteosarcoma, there is typically minimal tumor infiltration into cortical bone without medullary involvement. This feature helps differentiate this lesion from a chondroblastic intramedullary osteosarcoma that has permeated the cortex and formed a soft tissue mass.

The juxtacortical osteosarcoma must be completely removed by either en bloc resection or radical excision. A significant local recurrence rate can be expected if the underlying cortical bone is not removed with these lesions. The overall 5-year survival rate for juxtacortical osteosarcomas of the skeleton is 80%. In one series of juxtacortical osteosarcomas, pulmonary metastases developed in 13% of patients with parosteal osteosarcomas and in 22% of patients with periosteal osteosarcomas. Overall, the survival rate for juxtacortical osteosarcomas is superior to that of conventional intramedullary osteosarcomas. However, it is not known whether juxtacortical osteosarcomas of the jaws are substantially different in biologic behavior from those occurring in long bones. Meaningful conclusions comparing the treatment and prognosis of parosteal and periosteal osteosarcomas in the jaws cannot be made because of the few cases reported and the various methods of treatment used (curettage, local excision, and radical resection).

CHONDROSARCOMA

Chondrosarcomas arising in the mandible and maxilla are extremely rare and have accounted for approximately 1% of chondrosarcomas of the entire body. The appearance of benign chondrogenic tumors in the jaws is also rare. The histologic distinction between a benign chondroma and a low-grade chondrosarcoma is not well defined, and clinical experience dictates that well-differentiated chondrogenic neoplasms in the jaws be considered potentially malignant and handled accordingly.

Clinical Features. Chondrosarcomas more often involve the maxillofacial area (60%) than the mandible (40%). Lesions arising in the maxilla usually involve the anterior region (lateral incisor–canine region) and the palate. Mandibular chondrosarcomas occur most often in the premolar and molar regions, symphysis, coronoid process, and occasionally the condylar process. There is no distinct gender predilection. Chondrosarcomas predominate in adulthood and old age. Although the mean age of occurrence of chondrosarcomas is 60 years, almost half of the jaw lesions have arisen in the third and fourth decades of life.

The most common signs are a painless swelling and expansion of the affected bones, resulting in loosening of teeth or ill-fitting dentures. Pain, visual disturbances, nasal signs, and headache may result from extension of chondrosarcomas from the jaw bones to contiguous structures.

The radiographic appearance of chondrosarcoma varies from moth-eaten radiolucencies that are solitary or multilocular to diffusely opaque lesions (Figure 14-12). Many chondrosarcomas contain mottled densities corresponding to areas of calcification and ossification. Localized widening of the periodontal ligament space may also be seen in chondrosarcoma. Computed tomography (CT) visualization of cartilaginous neoplasms appears to be superior in defining the peripheral extent of the tumor compared with panoramic or flat-plate radiographs. A multilocular radiographic appearance may suggest a differential diagnosis of ameloblastoma, central giant cell granuloma, odontogenic myxoma, and keratocyst, whereas other patterns may suggest metastatic carcinoma, osteosarcoma, and calcifying epithelial odontogenic tumor.

Histopathology. The histologic appearance of chondrosarcomas is variable (Figure 14-13). Most of these tumors arising in the jaws are well differentiated. The prognostic significance of the pathologic grading of chondrosarcomas is well established. The incidence of metastatic disease has been shown to be 0%, 10%, and 70% for chondrosarcomas of histologic grade I, grade II, and grade III, respectively. Grade I chon-

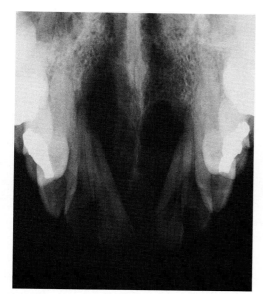

Figure 14-12 **Chondrosarcoma** of the anterior maxilla.

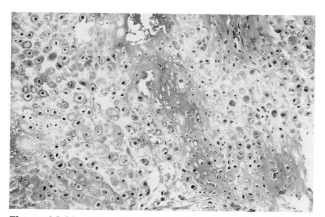

Figure 14-13 **Chondrosarcoma** showing a sheet of atypical cartilage.

drosarcomas often have a lobular architecture; they range from proliferations resembling benign cartilage to those with increased numbers of chondrocytes in a chondroid to myxomatous stroma. Grade II tumors often have a myxoid stroma with enlarged chondrocyte nuclei displaying occasional mitotic figures. Increased cellularity is often noted at the periphery of the cartilaginous lobules. Grade III chondrosarcomas are markedly cellular, often with a spindle cell component. Mitotic figures may be numerous.

Differential Diagnosis. The histologic differential diagnosis of chondrosarcoma may include benign chondroma,

which is rare in the jaws and should be considered only if the lesion is a small, incidental finding. The histology more commonly evokes the possibility of the chondroblastic variant of osteosarcoma, which accounts for nearly 50% of the osteosarcomas in the jaws. This latter entity is recognized when adequate tissue sampling reveals foci of malignant osteoid formation. In addition, chondroid areas of pleomorphic adenoma arising in overlying soft tissues may mimic cartilaginous tumors of bone. Chondromyxoid fibroma is a rare, benign neoplasm of bone that may resemble chondrosarcoma because of the presence of large atypical cells; however, it has a distinctly lobulated appearance with a prominent myxoid element and focal calcifications. Synovial chondromatosis involving the temporomandibular joint may also simulate chondrosarcoma.

Treatment and Prognosis. Because chondrosarcomas are radioresistant neoplasms, wide local or radical surgical excision is the treatment of choice. Therefore the location of the primary lesion and the adequacy of surgical resection (tumor-free margins) are of prime prognostic significance for chondrosarcomas of the jaws. In addition, the pathologic grade of chondrosarcoma is indicative of its innate biologic behavior and propensity for metastasis. The most common cause of death due to chondrosarcomas of the jaws is uncontrolled local recurrence and extension into adjacent vital structures. Metastasis, more common with high-grade chondrosarcomas, is generally to lung or bone. The usual clinical course of chondrosarcomas is long, with recurrences not uncommonly occurring 5 years or even 10 to 20 years after therapy. The 5-year survival rate for chondrosarcomas of the jaws (15% to 20%) appears to be poorer than that for chondrosarcomas in other body sites.

Mesenchymal Chondrosarcoma

Mesenchymal chondrosarcoma is a rare form of chondrosarcoma that is both histologically distinct and clinically unique compared with chondrosarcomas arising in bone. Chromosomal translocations (chromosomes 13 and 21) have been reported in skeletal and extraskeletal mesenchymal chondrosarcomas.

As many as one third of mesenchymal chondrosarcomas arise in soft tissue. Those that arise in bone show a predilection for the maxilla, mandible, and ribs. In one series of 15 mesenchymal chondrosarcomas of bone, one third occurred in the jaws. Most tumors arise between the ages of 10 and 30 years, with a nearly equal gender distribution. This presentation is distinctly different from other forms of chondrosarcoma that occur with a mean age of 60 years.

Similar to the situation with the other malignant neoplasms discussed, pain and, at times, swelling are the usual presenting symptoms. The radiologic appearance is of a lytic lesion that may be ill defined or sharply defined. Most contain stippled or large areas of calcification.

The characteristic histologic appearance of mesenchymal chondrosarcoma is that of anaplastic small cell malignancy containing zones of readily identifiable and often well-formed malignant cartilage. The undifferentiated small cell proliferation resembles Ewing's sarcoma and often displays a hemangiopericytoma-like growth pattern. It has been suggested that the small cell undifferentiated proliferation represents precartilaginous mesenchyme.

Appropriate sampling of these tumors demonstrates a bimorphic proliferation of undifferentiated small cells alternating with areas of cartilage. The latter finding distinguishes mesenchymal chondrosarcoma from similar-appearing Ewing's sarcoma, hemangiopericytoma, and even synovial sarcoma.

Mesenchymal chondrosarcoma is a highly malignant neoplasm that requires radical or wide surgical excision. Like other chondrosarcomas, it is relatively radioresistant. The 5-year survival rate is 50%, and the 10-year survival rate is 20%. The prognosis for jaw lesions is somewhat better. In addition to local recurrence, mesenchymal chondrosarcomas show a significant rate of distant metastases, often to lung and bone. Detection of metastatic disease in survivors may be delayed until 12 to 22 years after treatment of the primary tumor.

EWING'S SARCOMA AND PRIMITIVE NEUROECTODERMAL TUMOR

Ewing's sarcoma has been a highly lethal round cell sarcoma that was first described by James Ewing in 1921. The cause is unknown, the cell of origin uncertain, and even the multipotentiality of antigenic expression controversial. Ewing's sarcoma is related to the primitive neuroectodermal tumor (PNET), sharing a common karyotype translocation t(11;12) (q24;q12) in approximately 90% of these tumors. This translocation results in juxtaposition of the ENS and the FLI-

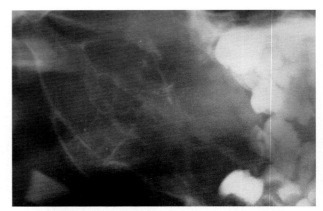

Figure 14-14   **Ewing's sarcoma** of the mandibular ramus in a 4-year-old boy.

1 genes. Ewing's sarcoma accounts for approximately 6% of all malignant bone tumors. Approximately 4% of Ewing's sarcomas have arisen in the bones of the head and neck, with 1% occurring in the jaws. Most involve the bones of the lower extremity or pelvis. When the jaws are involved, the predilection is for the ramus of the mandible, with few cases reported in the maxilla. Because Ewing's sarcoma has a propensity to metastasize to other bones, the possibility that jawbone involvement represents metastatic disease from another skeletal site should always be considered.

Clinical Features. Ninety percent of Ewing's sarcomas occur between the ages of 5 and 30 years, and more than 60% affect males (Figure 14-14). The mean age of occurrence for primary tumors involving the bones of the head and neck is 11 years. Pain and swelling are the most common presenting symptoms. Involvement of the mandible or maxilla may result in facial deformity, destruction of alveolar bone with loosening of teeth, and mucosal ulcers. Radiographic findings in the jaws are nonspecific and may simulate an infectious process, as well as a malignant process. The most characteristic appearance is that of a moth-eaten destructive radiolucency of the medullary bone and erosion of the cortex with expansion. A variable periosteal onionskin reaction may also be seen. A significant number of patients also have a soft tissue mass.

Histopathology. With an adequate biopsy specimen, Ewing's sarcoma is recognized microscopically as a proliferation of uniform, closely packed cells that may be compartmentalized by fibrous bands. The round to oval nuclei have finely dispersed chromatin and inconspicuous nucleoli (Figure 14-15). The cytoplasm char-

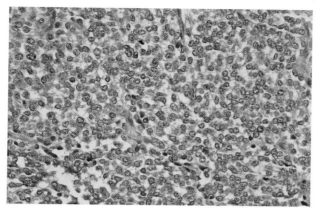

Figure 14-15 **Ewing's sarcoma** demonstrating characteristic round cell cytologic morphology.

acteristically stains with the periodic acid–Schiff stain, indicating the presence of glycogen. Although glycogen staining by this technique is helpful in diagnosis, some otherwise histologically acceptable cases of Ewing's sarcoma have yielded negative results. In addition, other tumors that mimic Ewing's sarcoma may contain glycogen.

Differential Diagnosis. Microscopically, Ewing's sarcoma is sufficiently undifferentiated or anaplastic that its appearance is readily simulated by other so-called small round cell tumors common to childhood and adolescence. This differential diagnosis includes lymphoma/leukemia, metastatic neuroblastoma, mesenchymal chondrosarcoma, small cell osteosarcoma, and although rare for this age-group, metastatic carcinoma. Routine light microscopy can often be used to discriminate between these similar-appearing neoplasms, but electron microscopy or immunohistochemistry must often be used to reach a conclusive diagnosis. By electron microscopy, the cells of Ewing's sarcoma are characterized by pools of cytoplasmic glycogen, sparse organelles, and rare primitive intercellular junctions. By immunohistochemistry, all Ewing's sarcomas contain abundant vimentin intermediate filaments. The presence of other classes of intermediate filaments has been demonstrated in frozen tissue specimens. Both PNETs and Ewing's sarcomas lack morphologic evidence of neural morphologic differentiation, but they share a high level of expression of the CD99 antigen (MIC-2 gene product) detected by antibodies 12 E7, HBA 71, or O13.

Treatment and Prognosis. The highly malignant nature of this sarcoma is reflected in its propensity for metasta-

sis, especially to lungs, other bones, and lymph nodes. Multiple-method treatment protocols, involving surgery or radiation for local control and chemotherapy for systemic micrometastases, have dramatically improved the formerly dismal 10% 5-year survival rate. With these newer intensive therapies, 80% 2-year disease-free survival rates and 60% 5-year actuarial survival rates have been reported. Clinical features associated with a poor prognosis include presentation before age 10 years, the presence of metastatic disease, systemic symptoms, a high erythrocyte sedimentation rate, an elevated serum lactate dehydrogenase value, and thrombocytosis. In addition, the site of involvement appears to be of prognostic significance in Ewing's sarcomas—patients with mandibular tumors are noted to have a more favorable overall survival time than those with any other bone site of origin.

BURKITT'S LYMPHOMA

Burkitt's lymphoma (see also Chapter 9) is a high-grade non-Hodgkin's lymphoma that is endemic in Africa and occurs only sporadically in North America and Western Europe. It was first recognized in 1958 by Dennis Burkitt in Uganda as a jaw malignancy occurring with high frequency in African children. By 1961, further reports demonstrated the distinctive clinical and pathologic features of this tumor, by then confirmed to be a malignant lymphoma. Subsequently, nonendemic forms of Burkitt's lymphoma were recognized in the United States. The endemic and sporadic forms of Burkitt's lymphoma are histologically and immunophenotypically identical. Clinical differences exist, however, between the endemic and sporadic forms.

Both sporadic and endemic forms of Burkitt's lymphoma are characterized by a translocation of the distal part of chromosome 8 to chromosome 14. The former is the site of the *c-myc* oncogene, and the latter, the immunoglobulin heavy-chain locus. This translocation may be directly involved in the enhanced tumor cell proliferation of Burkitt's lymphoma, which has been shown to have the highest proliferation rate of any neoplasm in humans, with a potential doubling time of 24 hours and a growth fraction of nearly 100%.

Clinical Features. In Africa, lymphoma accounts for 50% of all childhood malignancies, but it constitutes only 6% to 10% of childhood malignancies in the United States and Europe. Whereas the endemic form of

Burkitt's lymphoma has a peak incidence between 3 and 8 years of age and a 2-to-1 male predominance, the sporadic form affects a slightly older age-group, with a mean age of 11 years, and has no gender predilection. The overwhelming majority (77%) of cases of sporadic Burkitt's lymphoma occur in whites.

Endemic Burkitt's lymphoma typically involves the mandible, maxilla, and abdomen, with extranodal involvement of the retroperitoneum, kidneys, liver, ovaries, and endocrine glands. The incidence of jaw tumors in endemic Burkitt's lymphoma is related to the age of the patient, with 88% of those younger than 3 years of age and only 25% of those older than 15 years of age showing jaw involvement. Involvement of the jaws is relatively uncommon in the sporadic form of this disease, occurring in approximately 10% of cases. The sporadic Burkitt's lymphoma presents most often as an abdominal mass involving the mesenteric lymph nodes or ileocecal region, often with an intestinal obstruction. Involvement of the retroperitoneum, gonads, and other viscera occurs less often. Although predominantly an extranodal disease, involvement of cervical lymph nodes or bone marrow has also been noted. A notable difference between the endemic and nonendemic forms of Burkitt's lymphoma is that the Epstein-Barr virus genome can be detected in 95% of the endemic cases but in only 10% of sporadic cases.

When the mandible and maxilla are involved, the initial focus is usually in the posterior region, more commonly in the maxilla than in the mandible (Figure 14-16). The tumors in the sporadic form appear more localized, whereas in the endemic form, they more commonly involve all four quadrants. The usual signs associated with jaw lesions are an expanding intra-oral mass and mobility of teeth. Pain and paresthesia are occasionally present. In addition to a facial mass, in the sporadic disease, toothache is a common complaint, as is paresthesia of the lip. Burkitt's lymphoma has also been noted to invade the dental pulp, especially in developing teeth. Radiographically, a moth-eaten, poorly marginated destruction of bone is observed (Figure 14-17). The cortex may be expanded, eroded, or perforated, with soft tissue involvement.

Histopathology. Burkitt's lymphoma is a neoplastic B-cell proliferation that contains cell-surface B-lineage differentiation antigens and monoclonal surface immunoglobulin. The proliferation is extremely monomorphic, composed of medium-sized lymphocytes with round nuclei and three to five small basophilic nucleoli. Throughout the lymphoid proliferation are numerous scattered macrophages containing nuclear debris, contributing to the so-called starry sky appearance (Figure 14-18). Immunohisto-

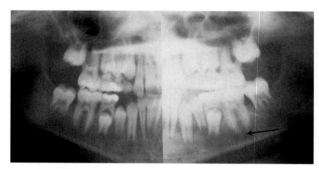

Figure 14-17 **Burkitt's lymphoma** presenting as a periapical radiolucency (mandibular left first molar). The patient also had a numb lip.

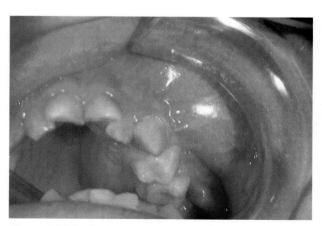

Figure 14-16 **Burkitt's lymphoma** of the left maxilla.

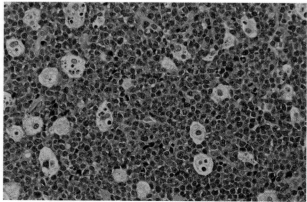

Figure 14-18 **Burkitt's lymphoma** exhibiting starry sky effect. Pale cells are tingible body macrophages.

chemical stain for Ki-67 protein shows almost all cells in cell cycle—a feature that can be useful in diagnosis. The histologic differential diagnosis includes other subtypes of non-Hodgkin's lymphoma, undifferentiated carcinoma and sarcoma, metastatic neuroblastoma, and acute leukemia.

Treatment and Prognosis. Burkitt's lymphoma was at one time invariably fatal within 4 to 6 months of diagnosis. However, because of its high proliferation rate, Burkitt's lymphoma has proved to be extremely sensitive to combination chemotherapy and is therefore potentially curable. The endemic and sporadic forms of Burkitt's lymphoma show similar complete response rates to chemotherapy, with similar rates of relapse and survival. With combination chemotherapy the overall 2-year survival rate is 55%, with a range of 80% for low-stage disease and 40% for advanced-stage disease.

PLASMA CELL NEOPLASMS

Multiple Myeloma

Plasma cell neoplasms (see also Chapter 9) are derived from bone marrow stem cells of B-lymphocyte lineage, and they are functionally differentiated in their ability to produce and secrete immunoglobulin. Because these tumors are derived from a single neoplastic clone, they are associated with the production of monoclonal immunoglobulin components, with the immunoglobulin light chain restricted to either the kappa or the lambda type. These tumors may present in soft tissue as extramedullary plasmacytoma, in bone as a solitary lytic lesion known as plasmacytoma of bone, or most commonly, as part of the multifocal disseminated disease multiple myeloma. Eighty percent of extramedullary plasmacytomas involve the head and neck region, with a predilection for the nasopharynx, nasal cavity, paranasal sinuses, and tonsils. The tumors have also been reported in the gingiva, palate, floor of the mouth, and tongue. Solitary plasmacytoma of bone is rare in the jaws; it more commonly appears in the ileum, femur, humerus, thoracic vertebrae, and skull. Multiple myeloma is a disease of the hematopoietic marrow–bearing bone of the skeleton, but 70% to 95% of affected individuals have also had radiographic involvement of the bones of the maxilla or mandible (Box 14-3).

Clinical Features. Rarely encountered before the fifth decade of life, multiple myeloma appears at a mean age of 63 years. It has a slight male predominance.

Involvement of the jaws may be asymptomatic or may produce pain, swelling, expansion, numbness, mobility of teeth, or pathologic fracture. Rarely is there an associated soft tissue mass. Some patients may exhibit weakness, weight loss, anemia, and hyperviscosity syndromes. Approximately 10% of patients with multiple myeloma develop *systemic amyloidosis*, a condition associated with other systemic diseases (Box 14-4) (see also discussion on multiple myeloma in Chapter 9). Eighty-five percent of patients with multiple myeloma have abnormal results of a skeletal radiographic survey. Although the remaining patients have an apparently normal radiographic series, they demonstrate plasmacytosis on marrow aspirate or a biopsy specimen.

The most common peripheral blood abnormality is anemia with rouleau formation and, rarely, circulating plasma cells. The production of monoclonal immunoglobulin components by the neoplastic plasma cells results in an excess of abnormal protein that circulates in serum and can often be detected in urine.

Box 14-3 Multiple Myeloma

ORIGIN

B-lymphocyte malignancy; monoclonal population; abnormal monoclonal immunoglobulin produced

CLINICAL AND LABORATORY FEATURES

Types—multiple, solitary, extramedullary
Patients over 50 years of age
Pain, swelling, numbness
Weight loss, weakness, anemia, bleeding, infection, amyloidosis (10%)
Punched-out skeletal lesions
Bence Jones protein (light chains) in urine
M protein in serum

TREATMENT

Chemotherapy; poor prognosis

Box 14-4 Amyloidosis

Occurs in 10% of myeloma patients
May also appear secondary to chronic disease (e.g., rheumatoid arthritis, chronic osteomyelitis, chronic renal failure)
Kidney, heart, gastrointestinal tract, liver, spleen commonly affected
Oral lesions seen in tongue (macroglossia), gingiva

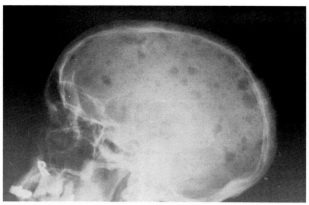

Figure 14-19   **Multiple myeloma** of the skull as punched-out radiolucencies.

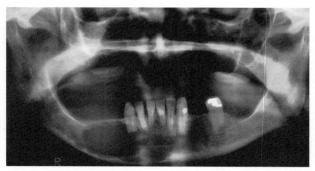

Figure 14-20   **Multiple myeloma** presenting as a radiolucency of the mandible. (Courtesy Dr. Steven Rowan.)

On serum protein electrophoresis, most patients with myeloma are found to have a decreased quantity of normal immunoglobulin and an abnormal monoclonal immunoglobulin protein peak, known as an *M spike*. The immunoglobulin is usually of the IgG or IgA class, with a monoclonal light-chain component. Some plasma cell neoplasms may secrete only a monoclonal light chain. These monoclonal immunoglobulin components can be demonstrated by immunoelectrophoresis of both serum and urine in approximately 95% of patients with myeloma. Urinary monoclonal light chains, so-called Bence Jones proteinuria, may be detected in approximately 50% of patients with myeloma. Two percent of myeloma cases are nonsecretory, although monoclonal immunoglobulin may be demonstrated within plasma cell cytoplasm by the immunoperoxidase method.

The radiographic appearance of myeloma can vary. Typically seen are multiple sharply punched-out but noncorticated radiolucent areas of bone destruction in the jaws and in many of the hematopoietic marrow–containing bones of the skeleton (Figures 14-19 and 14-20). Plasma cell tumors in the jaws may be expansile and on rare occasions may be osteosclerotic. The finding of a solitary plasma cell tumor in the jaws is more often a manifestation of systemic disease than a manifestation of a solitary plasmacytoma of bone.

Histopathology. Histologically, all clinical manifestations of plasma cell tumors are similar. Tumors are composed of a monotonous proliferation of neoplastic plasma cells that may display a wide range of differentiation, from mature-appearing plasma cells to less well differentiated forms resembling immunoblastic large cell lymphomas. The abundant plasma cells within bone marrow can be distinguished from the plasma cells of chronic osteomyelitis or periapical granuloma by the associated proliferation of small vessels and fibroblasts with admixed neutrophils and macrophages in the reactive lesions. In addition, with the immunoperoxidase technique a monoclonal intracytoplasmic immunoglobulin light chain can be demonstrated in nearly all plasma cell neoplasms, whereas reactive plasma cell infiltrates are uniformly polyclonal (Figure 14-21).

Differential Diagnosis. Although the punched-out lytic appearance is characteristic, the radiographic differential diagnosis of these jaw lesions includes other malignant neoplasms of the jaws, such as metastatic carcinoma, lymphoma, and Langerhans cell disease. Therefore diagnosis must be confirmed by a biopsy specimen or aspirate. Histologically, very poorly differentiated plasma cell neoplasms may simulate other relatively undifferentiated malignant neoplasms, such as lymphoma, leukemia, undifferentiated carcinoma, metastatic malignant melanoma, and neuroblastoma. These entities can be distinguished by immunoperoxidase detection of the leukocyte common antigen in lymphomas/leukemias, cytokeratin in carcinomas, S-100 protein and melanoma-associated antigens in melanoma, and neuron-specific enolase in neuroblastoma. Plasma cell tumors do not express these antigens, but express CD79a antigen.

Treatment and Prognosis. Most patients with myeloma die of infection or, less commonly, of renal failure, disseminated myeloma, cardiac complications, or hematologic complications of hemorrhage or thrombosis. Multiple myeloma is treated with chemotherapeutic alkylating agents and steroids, with local radiation directed to painful bone lesions. Newer therapeutic

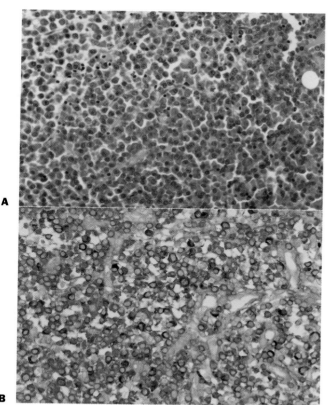

Figure 14-21 **Multiple myeloma. A,** Sheet of atypical plasma cells. **B,** With the use of immunohistochemistry, all cells stained positive *(brown)* for lambda light chains, demonstrating monoclonality of the tumor (cells were negative for kappa light chains).

regimens (none curative) have included combination chemotherapy, bone marrow transplantation, and the biologic response modifier interferon-alpha as maintenance therapy. The overall median survival time is related to the stage of disease and ranges from more than 60 months in patients with low stage I disease to 23 months in those presenting with high stage III disease. Indicators of prognosis correlate with the myeloma cell burden and include the hemoglobin level, serum calcium level, serum and urine M-component, degree of bone involvement, and creatinine levels indicative of renal failure.

Solitary Plasmacytoma of Bone

Like multiple myeloma, solitary plasmacytoma of bone is a disease of adulthood, with a mean age of 50 years at presentation and a predominance in men. Solitary plasmacytomas rarely occur in the jaws, but when they do, they are often located in the angle of the mandible. For a diagnosis of solitary plasmacytoma to be established, a radiologic bone survey and random bone marrow aspirate and biopsy specimen should reveal no evidence of plasmacytosis in other areas of the body. However, 30% to 75% of cases of solitary plasmacytoma of bone eventually progress to multiple myeloma. It is not possible to predict which patients will develop disseminated disease and which will not. As with multiple myeloma, the clinical symptoms include pain, swelling, and pathologic fracture.

Radiographically, solitary plasmacytoma is a well-defined lytic lesion that may be multilocular, resembling the appearance of central giant cell granuloma. Solitary plasmacytomas may destroy the cortical bone and spread into adjacent soft tissue. Unlike those with multiple myeloma, patients with solitary plasmacytoma of bone have a normal peripheral blood picture and a normal differential and clinical chemistry profile. In up to 25% of cases of solitary plasmacytoma of bone, a monoclonal immunoglobulin can be demonstrated in serum or urine. Biopsy material of solitary plasmacytoma of bone reveals a histologic appearance identical to that of multiple myeloma, with a monotonous proliferation of neoplastic plasma cells producing monoclonal immunoglobulin components.

Solitary plasmacytoma of bone is treated primarily by local radiotherapy. Accessible lesions may be surgically excised, followed by radiation therapy. Ten percent to 15% of patients have local recurrence of the solitary plasmacytoma, and small numbers of patients may develop an additional solitary plasmacytoma of bone. Although a significant proportion of cases progress to multiple myeloma, the overall survival time of patients with solitary plasmacytoma is 10 years, in contrast to the 20-month mean survival time of patients initially diagnosed with multiple myeloma. This appears to indicate that many solitary plasmacytomas are biologically low-grade, but slowly progressive, forms of multiple myeloma.

METASTATIC CARCINOMA

The most common malignancy affecting skeletal bones is metastatic carcinoma. However, metastatic disease to the mandible and maxilla is unusual; it is estimated that 1% of malignant neoplasms metastasize to these sites (Box 14-5). Approximately 80% of these metastases are to the mandible, 14% to the maxilla, and 5% to both jaws. Occasionally, metasta-

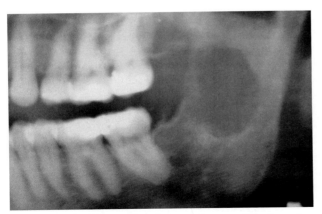

Figure 14-22   **Metastatic adenocarcinoma of the breast** to the mandibular ramus.

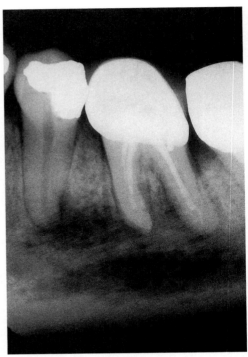

Figure 14-23   **Metastatic adenocarcinoma of the breast** to the mandibular body.

> **Box 14-5 Malignancies Most Likely to Metastasize to the Jaws**
>
> Breast carcinoma
> Lung carcinoma
> Prostate adenocarcinoma
> Colorectal carcinoma
> Renal cell carcinoma

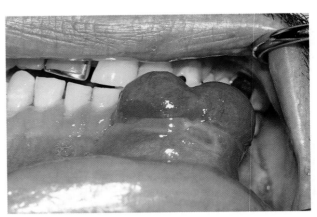

Figure 14-24   **Metastatic cancer** (undetermined primary site) to the gingiva.

tic deposits are seen in the gingiva with a clinical appearance that simulates pyogenic granuloma. In adults metastases to the jaws most commonly originate from primary carcinomas of the breast in women and of the lung in men. Other common primary sites in decreasing order of frequency are the prostate, gastrointestinal tract, kidney, colon, and rectum. In children neuroblastoma of adrenal glands is the most common primary site in the first decade of life, but bone malignancies are the most common primary site in the second decade of life. Jawbone metastasis may be the first sign of malignancy in as many as 30% of cases.

Clinical Features. Individuals likely to be affected by metastatic carcinoma to the jaws are in the older age-groups, most in the fifth to seventh decades of life, with an average age of 45 years, reflecting the greater prevalence of malignancy in this population. The mechanism of spread to the jaws is usually hematogenous from the primary visceral neoplasm or from lung metastases. Within the jaw, the premolar-molar region, the angle, and the body of the mandible are more com-

monly involved by metastatic disease (Figures 14-22 to 14-24). Bone pain, loosening of teeth, lip paresthesia, bone swelling, gingival mass, and pathologic fracture may be clinically evident.

Most jaw metastases appear radiographically as poorly marginated, radiolucent defects. Some metastatic carcinomas, notably prostate and thyroid, are often

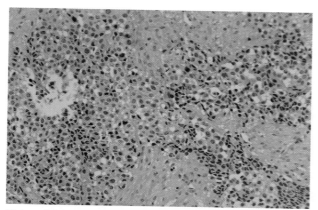

Figure 14-25 **Metastatic breast cancer** excised from a mandibular radiolucency.

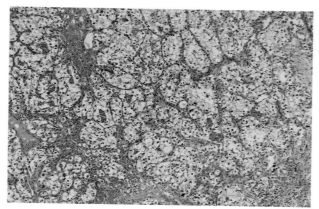

Figure 14-26 **Metastatic renal clear cell carcinoma** excised from a periapical radiolucency.

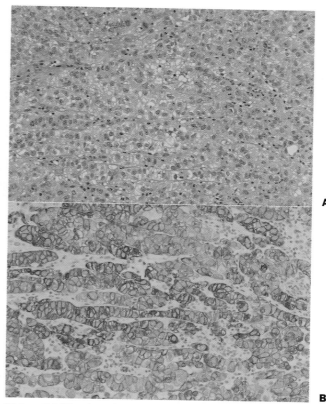

Figure 14-27 **A** and **B, Metastatic lung cancer** presenting as a mandibular radiolucency. **B,** Immunohistochemical stain for CK7 (cytokeratin 7) was helpful in determining the source of the primary lesion.

characterized by an osteoblastic process. Although the appearance of osteomyelitis is also a moth-eaten radiolucency, it rarely expands the cortical bone.

Histopathology. The histologic appearance of metastatic carcinoma can be extremely variable, reflecting the tumor type and grade of tumor differentiation (Figures 14-25 to 14-27). A prominent desmoplastic stromal response is often present. The diagnosis of metastatic carcinoma in difficult cases can be verified with an immunoperoxidase stain for cytokeratin, which is present in all carcinoma cells. In addition, immunoperoxidase staining to identify tissue-specific markers such as prostate-specific antigen, prostatic alkaline phosphatase, thyroglobulin, or calcitonin can indicate a primary origin in the prostate or thyroid gland. Antibodies to tumor type–specific antigens that are reactive in formalin-fixed, paraffin-embedded material and capable of pointing to a primary site in the lung, breast, colon, or kidney are becoming increasingly available. It is anticipated that with advances in monoclonal antibody development, this technique will be very useful in identifying carcinomas of unknown metastatic origin.

Differential Diagnosis. The differential diagnosis of intrabony, poorly differentiated carcinoma includes anaplastic sarcoma, lymphoma, and amelanotic melanoma. The very rare primary intraosseous carcinoma of probable odontogenic origin is considered in Chapter 11. The presence of cytokeratin within the tumor cells is diagnostic of carcinoma. Immunoperoxidase stains for the leukocyte common antigen verify a diagnosis of lymphoma/leukemia, whereas immunoreactivity with melanoma-associated antigens and S-100 protein indicates a diagnosis of melanoma. Although many of these sophisticated diagnostic techniques can be used to identify the nature of an anaplastic neoplasm, there is no substitute for an accurate medical history and physical examination, especially in the diagnosis of metastatic carcinoma.

Treatment and Prognosis. Metastatic carcinoma of the jaws requires further workup to identify the primary site and to stage the degree of metastatic involvement. This is useful in identifying whether the jaw metastasis represents a solitary focus or, as is often the case, is merely the clinical sign of disseminated skeletal disease. A single focus may be treated by surgical excision or chemoradiotherapy. Generalized skeletal metastases are usually an ominous event and are treated palliatively. The prognosis for patients with metastatic carcinoma of the jaws is grave, with a dismal 10% 5-year survival rate and more than two thirds of patients dying within a year.

BIBLIOGRAPHY

OSTEOSARCOMA

Bennett JH, Thomas G, Evans AW, et al: Osteosarcoma of the jaws: a 30-year retrospective review, *Oral Surg Oral Med Oral Pathol Oral Radiol Endod* 90:323-333, 2000.

Gadwal SR, Gannon FH, Fanburg-Smith JC, et al: Primary osteosarcoma of the head and neck in pediatric patients, *Cancer* 91:598-605, 2001.

Ha PK, Eisele DW, Frassica FJ, et al: Osteosarcoma of the head and neck: a review of the Johns Hopkins experience, *Laryngoscope* 109:964-969, 1999.

Kurt A-M, Unni KK, McLeod RA, et al: Low-grade intraosseous osteosarcoma, *Cancer* 65:1418-1428, 1990.

Longhi A, Benassi MS, Molendini L, et al: Osteosarcoma in blood relatives, *Oncol Rep* 8:131-136, 2001.

Lopes MA, Nikitakis NG, Ord RA, et al: Amplification and protein expression of chromosome 12q13-15 genes in osteosarcomas of the jaws, *Oral Oncol* 37:566-571, 2001.

Okada K, Frassica FJ, Sim FH, et al: Parosteal osteosarcoma: a clinicopathological study, *J Bone Joint Surg Am* 76A:366-378, 1994.

Ragazzini P, Gamberi G, Benassi MS, et al: Analysis of SAS gene and CDK4 and MDM2 proteins in low-grade osteosarcoma, *Cancer Detect Prevent* 23:129-136, 1999.

Raymond AK: Surface osteosarcoma, *Clin Orthop Rel Res* 270:140-148, 1991.

Wunder JS, Eppert K, Burrow SR, et al: Co-amplification and overexpression of CDK4, SAS, and MDM2 occurs frequently in human parosteal osteosarcomas, *Oncogene* 18:783-788, 1999.

CHONDROSARCOMA

Hackney F, Aragon S, Aufdemorte T, et al: Chondrosarcoma of the jaws: clinical findings, histopathology and treatment, *Oral Surg Oral Med Oral Pathol* 71:139-143, 1991.

Naumann S, Krallman PA, Unni KK, et al: Translocation der(13;21)(q10;q10) in skeletal and extraskeletal mesenchymal chondrosarcoma. *Mod Pathol* 15:572-576, 2002.

Saito K, Unni KK, Wollan PC, et al: Chondrosarcoma of the jaw and facial bones, *Cancer* 76:1550-1558, 1995.

Vencio EF, Reeve CM, Unni KK, et al: Mesenchymal chondrosarcoma of the jaw bones: clinicopathologic study of 19 cases, *Cancer* 82:2350-2355, 1998.

EWING'S SARCOMA

de Alava E, Gerald WL: Molecular biology of the Ewing's sarcoma/primitive neuroectodermal tumor family, *J Clin Oncol* 18:204-213, 2000.

Delattre O, Zucman J, Melot T, et al: The Ewing family of tumors—a subgroup of small-round-cell tumors defined by specific chimeric transcripts, *N Engl J Med* 331:294-299, 1994.

Sandberg AA, Bridge JA: Updates on cytogenetics and molecular genetics of bone and soft tissue tumors: Ewing sarcoma and peripheral primitive neuroectodermal tumors, *Cancer Genet Cytogenet* 123:1-26, 2000.

West DC: Ewing sarcoma family of tumors, *Curr Opin Oncol* 12:323-329, 2000.

PLASMA CELL NEOPLASMS

Falk RH, Comenzo RL, Skinner M: The systemic amyloidosis, *N Engl J Med* 337:898-909, 1997.

Oken MM: Multiple myeloma: prognosis and standard treatment, *Cancer Invest* 15:57-64, 1997.

METASTATIC CARCINOMA

Campbell F, Herrington CS: Application of cytokeratin 7 and 20 immunohistochemistry to diagnostic pathology, *Curr Diagn Pathol* 7:113-122, 2001.

Chu P, Wu E, Weiss LM: Cytokeratin 7 and cytokeratin 20 expression in epithelial neoplasms: a survey of 435 cases, *Mod Pathol* 13:962-972, 2000.

Hirshberg A, Leibovich P, Buchner A: Metastatic tumors to the jawbones: analysis of 390 cases, *J Oral Pathol Med* 23:337-341, 1994.

METABOLIC AND GENETIC DISEASES

METABOLIC CONDITIONS

Paget's Disease

Paget's disease, or osteitis deformans, is a chronic, slowly progressive bone condition of undetermined cause (Box 15-1). An unproven theory of an infec-tious cause, such as the measles virus, has been raised on the basis of ultrastructural alterations of osteoclastic nuclei within pagetic bone. Paget's disease generally progresses through several stages that include an initial resorptive phase, followed by a vascular phase, and eventually by a sclerosing phase.

Clinical Features. Paget's disease is a hyperactive bone turnover state that typically occurs in patients older than 50 years of age. It is relatively common and has been reported to occur in 3% to 4% of the middle-aged population and in as many as 10% to 15% of the elderly. In approximately 14% of cases a positive family history can be elicited. Paget's disease has a 3-to-2 male predilection, and it seems to occur more often in patients of Northern European descent.

The most common sites of involvement include the pelvis, skull, tibia, vertebrae, humerus, and sternum. The jaws are affected in approximately 20% of patients, with the maxilla involved twice as often as the mandible (Figure 15-1). At initial presentation, symptoms often relate to deformity or pain in the affected bone(s). Bone pain is described as deep and aching. A per-ception of elevated skin temperature over the affected bone is often noted due to the hypervascularity of the underlying bone. Neurologic complaints—including headache, auditory or visual disturbances, facial paraly-sis, vertigo, and weakness—may be related, in large part, to narrowing of the skull foramina, resulting in compression of vascular and neural elements. Approx-imately 10% to 20% of patients are asymptomatic and are incidentally diagnosed after radiographic or lab-oratory studies are performed for unrelated problems.

Classically, dental patients who wear complete den-tures may complain of newly acquired poor prosthetic adaptation and function as the maxilla symmetrically enlarges. The alveolar ridge ultimately widens, with a relative flattening of the palatal vault. When teeth

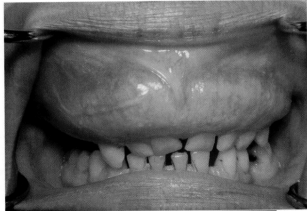

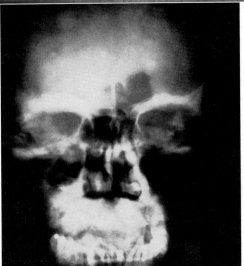

> ## Box 15-1 Paget's Disease
>
> A progressive metabolic disturbance of many bones; unde-
> termined cause
> Commonly affects the spine, femurs, cranium, pelvis, and
> sternum
> Adults, typically older than 50 years of age
> Symptoms—bone pain, headache, altered vision and
> hearing, facial paralysis, vertigo
> Oral signs
>   Bilateral, symmetric jaw enlargement—15% of all patients
>   with Paget's disease; maxilla > mandible
>   Acquired diastemas, ill-fitting denture, patchy opacities,
> hypercementosis
> Oral complications
>   Early—bleeding following jaw surgery
>   Late—jaw fracture, osteomyelitis
>
> >, Affected more frequently than.

Figure 15-1   **A** and **B, Paget's disease** of the maxilla. Note uniform, symmetric enlargement in **A** and opacification of the maxilla and skull in **B.**

are present, increased spacing, as well as loosening, is noted. In severe cases, continued enlargement of the maxilla or mandible can make closure of the lips difficult or impossible.

The classic radiographic findings in the late stage of Paget's disease are due to bony sclerosis providing a patchy radiopaque pattern described as resembling cotton wool. In the jaws this pattern of bone change may be associated with hypercementosis or resorption of tooth roots, loss of lamina dura, and obliteration of the periodontal ligament space (Figures 15-2 and 15-3).

Histopathology. In the initial resorptive phase, random overactive osteoclastic bone resorption is evident. Resorbed bone is replaced by vascularized connective tissue in company with prominent osteolysis and osteogenesis. Bone eventually develops a dense mosaic pattern as a result of reversal lines in increasingly sclerotic bone, as osteoclasts give way to osteoblasts (Figures 15-4 and 15-5).

The laboratory can provide important information about the diagnosis of Paget's disease. Serum calcium and serum phosphate levels are normal in the presence of markedly elevated alkaline phosphatase levels. The intense osteoblastic activity in this metabolically active bone is believed to be responsible for the elevated alkaline phosphatase levels. The amount of bone resorption may be correlated to increases in urinary calcium and hydroxyproline levels.

Treatment. The primary indicator for therapeutic intervention is patient discomfort. Elevation of alkaline

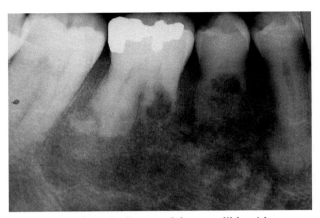

Figure 15-2   **Paget's disease** of the mandible with associated root resorption.

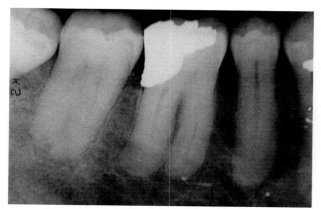

Figure 15-3 **Paget's disease** of the mandible with associated hypercementosis.

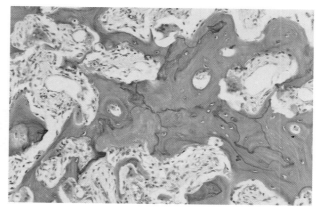

Figure 15-5 **Paget's disease** showing a mosaic bone pattern with reversal lines and prominent capillaries.

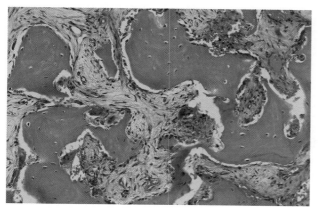

Figure 15-4 **Paget's disease** with fibrotic marrow and numerous osteoblasts and osteoclasts.

> ### Box 15-2 Hyperparathyroidism
>
> Primary hyperparathyroidism—parathyroid adenoma, adenocarcinoma, hyperplasia
> Secondary hyperparathyroidism—compensatory hyperplasia for low serum calcium levels due to renal failure, malabsorption, or vitamin D deficiency
> Elevated serum parathormone (PTH), calcium, and alkaline phosphatase levels and decreased phosphate levels
> Kidney stones, metastatic calcification, osteoporosis, fibroblastic/giant cell tumors of bone, neurologic alterations, arrhythmias, polyuria

phosphatase levels to twice normal levels is also an indication for treatment. Therapy is essentially symptomatic, with analgesics used for pain control. The use of calcitonin or bisphosphonate as parathormone antagonists has been effective. Both suppress bone resorption and deposition, as reflected in a reduction in the biochemical indices, including alkaline phosphatase and urinary hydroxyproline levels. A 50% reduction in either index constitutes a good therapeutic response.

Paget's disease is a slowly progressive disorder, but it is seldom fatal. Relief of symptoms, in particular bone pain, with orally administered bisphosphonates is beneficial. Complications include skeletal deformity, weakened bones, neurologic deficits, and pathologic fracture. Heart failure may also be an important complication of Paget's disease as a consequence of the hypervascular bone. In the early vascular phase, bleeding following any type of bone surgery (e.g., tooth extraction) can be problematic. In a small percentage of cases malignant transformation into osteosarcoma may occur. Depending on the series reported, this has ranged from 1% to 15%.

Hyperparathyroidism

Hyperparathyroidism may be one of three types: primary, secondary, or hereditary (Box 15-2). Rarely, hyperparathyroidism may be associated with a Noonan-type syndrome, a complex, autosomal-dominant inherited trait comprising short stature, unusual facies, mental retardation, and cardiac defects.

Primary hyperparathyroidism is characterized by hypersecretion of parathyroid hormone from one or more hyperplastic parathyroid glands (3%), a parathyroid adenoma (90%), or less commonly, an adenocarcinoma (3%). Characteristic abnormal laboratory findings are elevated parathormone levels and elevated calcium and alkaline phosphatase levels resulting from parathormone stimulation of osteoclast-mediated bone resorption, from decreasing calcium excretion in the kidneys, and from increased intestinal resorption.

Secondary hyperparathyroidism occurs as a compensatory response to hypocalcemia, as may be found in renal failure, in patients undergoing renal dialysis, and in those with intestinal malabsorption syndromes. In these patients there is a reduction in vitamin D_3, which is activated in the kidney. Vitamin D_3 is required for calcium absorption and metabolism. The hereditary form has been shown to be an autosomal-dominant condition mapped to chromosome 1q21–q31, the location of the HRPT2 endocrine tumor gene.

Clinical Features. The disease spectrum of primary hyperparathyroidism ranges from asymptomatic cases (diagnosed by routine serum calcium determinations) to severe cases manifesting as lethargy and occasionally coma. The incidence increases with age and is greater in postmenopausal women. Early symptoms include fatigue, weakness, nausea, anorexia, arrhythmias, polyuria, thirst, depression, and constipation. Bone pain and headaches are often reported.

Several clinical features are associated with the primary form of this disease, classically described as "stones, bones, groans, and moans." Lesions of the kidneys, skeletal system, gastrointestinal tract, and nervous system are responsible for this syndrome complex. The renal component includes the presence of renal calculi or, more rarely, nephrocalcinosis associated with hypercalcemia.

Gastrointestinal manifestations include peptic ulcer secondary to the increase in gastric acid, pepsin, and serum gastrin levels. Rarely, pancreatitis may develop secondary to obstruction of the smaller pancreatic ducts by calcium deposits.

Neurologic manifestations may become evident when serum calcium levels are very high, exceeding 16 to 17 mg/dl. In such instances coma or parathyroid crisis may occur. Loss of memory and depression are common, and rarely, true psychosis may appear. Some of the neurologic findings may be attributed to calcium deposits in the brain.

Severe osseous changes (called, in the past, *osteitis fibrosa cystica*) are the result of significant bone demineralization, with fibrous replacement producing radiographic changes that appear cystlike. In the jaws these lesions resemble central giant cell granuloma

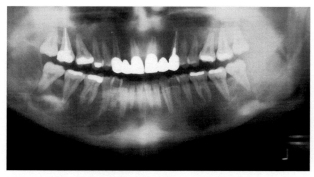

Figure 15-6   **Hyperparathyroidism** producing numerous mandibular radiolucencies.

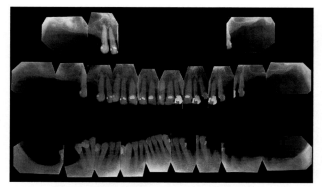

Figure 15-7   **Hyperparathyroidism** resulting in loss of lamina dura.

microscopically. Less obvious radiographic changes may include an osteoporotic appearance of the mandible and maxilla, reflecting a more generalized resorption (Figure 15-6). Loosening of the teeth may also occur, as well as corresponding obfuscation of trabecular detail and overall cortical thinning. Partial loss of lamina dura is seen in a minority of patients with hyperparathyroidism (Figure 15-7). Pulpal obliteration, with complete calcification of the pulp chamber and canals, has been reported in association with secondary hyperparathyroidism.

Histopathology. The bone lesions of hyperparathyroidism, although not specific, are important in establishing the diagnosis. The bony trabeculae exhibit osteoclastic resorption, as well as the formation of osteoid trabeculae by large numbers of osteoblasts. In these areas a delicate fibrocellular stroma contains numerous multinucleated giant cells. Accumulations of hemosiderin and extravasated red blood cells also are noted. As a result, the tissues may appear reddish brown, accounting for the term *brown tumor.* The lesions are microscopically identical to central giant cell granulomas.

Treatment. Management of primary hyperparathyroidism is aimed at eliminating the parathyroid pathology and monitoring the fall in C-terminal parathyroid hormone concentration. Surgery is the treatment of choice in most instances because it offers the best opportunity for long-term cure. Treatment of secondary hyperparathyroidism due to increased parathyroid function resulting from chronic renal failure is aimed at management of kidney disease. The dental and oral considerations in this form of hyperparathyroidism are similar to those in the primary form of the disease.

Hyperthyroidism

Hyperfunction of the thyroid gland, or hyperthyroidism, encompasses several conditions or diseases. This condition is characterized by excessive amounts of the thyroid hormones triiodothyronine (T_3) and thyroxine (T_4) or by increased levels of thyroid-stimulating hormone (TSH) and associated hypermetabolism. In adults hyperthyroidism occurs with an incidence of 3 cases per 10,000 population per year, with a distinct female preponderance of approximately 5 to 1.

The most common disorder leading to clinical hyperthyroidism is Graves' disease, accounting for 70% to 85% of all cases. The exact cause of this particular process is obscure but appears to be related to the production of abnormal thyroid stimulator (long-acting thyroid stimulator [LATS]), which differs chemically and functionally from TSH. LATS is able to bind the thyroid-TSH receptors in preference to TSH and remain bound for prolonged periods. The LATS substance is an immunoglobulin G (IgG) produced by B lymphocytes, which is capable of inducing thyroid hyperplasia and increasing iodine uptake by the thyroid, free of any pituitary gland influence. Thyrotoxicosis may also result from excess stimulation of the thyroid gland via the hypothalamic pituitary axis or by secretion of thyroid hormone from ectopic, endogenous, or exogenous sources.

Heat intolerance, hyperhidrosis, and palmar erythema are common findings. Fine motor tremor and muscle weakness, palpitations, diarrhea, anxiety, weight loss, and menstrual dysfunction are also commonly encountered. Patients may complain of an

---

> **Box 15-3 Oral Manifestations of Hyperparathyroidism, Hyperthyroidism, and Hypophosphatasia**
>
> *Hyperparathyroidism:* Multiple jaw lucencies (giant cell lesions); loss of lamina dura; pulp calcification
> *Hyperthyroidism:* Premature exfoliation and eruption of teeth; osteoporosis
> *Hypophosphatasia:* Premature loss of teeth; reduced cementum and dentin; short roots; large pulps

---

altered complexion and thinning, brittle hair. Ocular changes include upper lid retraction and so-called lid lag on normal blinking. The bright-eyed stare that often results from upper lid retraction may be further accentuated by exophthalmos. Pretibial myxedema and acropachy may be found in patients with Graves' disease.

Cardiac manifestations are among the earliest and most consistent features of this disease. The increased metabolic activity places greater demand on the cardiovascular system; accordingly, increases in stroke volume, pulse rate, and cardiac output are usually observed.

Although the oral manifestations of this condition are not specific, they are consistent (Box 15-3). In children premature or accelerated exfoliation of deciduous teeth and the concomitant rapid eruption of permanent teeth are often noted. In adults osteoporosis of the mandible and maxilla may be found. On occasion, patients may complain of a burning tongue, as well as other, nonspecific symptoms. Of interest is a reported threefold increase in the incidence of dental erosion in these patients in comparison with euthyroid control subjects.

Treatment consists of thyroid-suppressive drug therapy or radioactive iodine administration, which essentially inactivates the hyperfunctional thyroid tissue. Thyroid-suppressive drugs include thiocarbamides such as propylthiouracil and methimazole. These drugs inhibit iodine oxidation and iodination of tyrosyl residues—two steps in the synthesis of thyroid hormones. Surgical therapy remains an option, although the potential for inadvertent parathyroid gland removal and subsequent hypoparathyroidism is a risk.

Of clinical importance is the need to reduce stress to minimize the risk of precipitating a thyroid crisis in patients with poorly controlled disease. The use of

---

Box 15-4 Hypothyroidism

Delayed skeletal and dental development
Sexual immaturity
Edema of face, eyes, lips, tongue
Mental lethargy
Skin changes—dry, cold, scaly
Slow pulse
Fatigue, lethargy
Anemia—microcytic, hypochromic

---

certain drugs such as epinephrine and atropine is contraindicated because they may precipitate a thyroid storm, which is a life-threatening state of thyroid hormone–induced hypermetabolism.

Hypothyroidism

Hypothyroidism is a systemic condition that is caused by reduced production of thyroid hormone. This results from a number of factors that include congenital defect, iodine deficiency goiter, autoimmune (Hashimoto's) thyroiditis, diseases of the pituitary and hypothalamus, and idiopathic causes. The common result of these etiologic factors is cretinism when the condition occurs in children and myxedema when it occurs in adults.

The key clinical features are listed in Box 15-4. Diagnosis is based on the history, physical examination, and determination of serum levels of TSH and T_4. TSH is decreased when the disease arises directly or primarily within the thyroid glands, and T_4 is decreased when the disease has an origin that is primary or secondary to the thyroid. Treatment is based on gradual replacement with synthetic and natural thyroid hormone preparations.

Hypophosphatasia

Hypophosphatasia represents a deficiency of alkaline phosphatase. This hereditary disorder is transmitted in an autosomal-recessive manner. Of dental significance is that this unusual genetic metabolic disease is one of the main causes of premature loss of the primary dentition. (Other conditions in which premature tooth exfoliation may be seen include cyclic neutropenia, idiopathic histiocytosis, juvenile periodontitis, acrodynia, rickets, and Papillon-Lefèvre syndrome.) Although the primary dentition is nearly exclusively involved, adolescent and adult patients with this condition may also experience dental abnormalities, including reduced marginal alveolar bone, abnormal root cementum, focal areas of dentin resorption, altered mineralization of coronal dentin, and large coronal pulp chambers of the molar dentition.

The chief clinical features of hypophosphatasia include enlarged pulp chambers of the primary teeth, alveolar bone loss with a predisposition for the anterior portion of the mandible and maxilla, and hypoplasia or aplasia of cementum over the root surface. Root development may be deficient, especially toward the apex. The crowns of the involved teeth demonstrate rickets-type changes, which are chiefly characterized by hypoplastic enamel defects. Enamel hypoplasia, increased pulp spaces, and premature tooth exfoliation are present in the permanent and primary dentitions. The dental abnormalities are a result of inadequate formation of both dentin and cementum.

Long bones show inadequate levels of mineralization with abnormally wide osteoid seams. Serum chemistry studies indicate a reduction in alkaline phosphatase levels, with concomitant urinary findings of detectable phosphoethanolamine. Tissue levels of alkaline phosphatase are likewise decreased in this disorder.

Four clinical types of hypophosphatasia have been recognized:

1. A congenital type has a 75% rate of neonatal mortality.
2. An early infantile type appears within the first 6 months of life, with a mortality rate of 50%. Renal calcinosis, as well as a risk of cranial synostosis, delayed motor development, and premature loss of teeth, may accompany this disease.
3. A late infantile or childhood type begins between 6 and 24 months of age. Skeletal findings tend to be less pronounced, but abnormalities of long bone structures, including irregular ossifications at the metaphysis, may be observed, along with rickets-type changes at the costochondral junctions. Of importance in this form of the disease is premature loss of the anterior primary teeth, often the first sign of the illness.
4. The adult type, although distinctly uncommon, is characterized by bone pain, pathologic fractures, and a childhood history of rickets.

No successful treatment is known, apart from controlling the hypercalcemia resulting from the hypophosphatasia. Large doses of vitamin D have occasionally produced partial improvement, although hypercalcemia and soft tissue calcinosis may result from such an approach. Genetic counseling of the family, as well as early diagnosis, is of great value.

Infantile Cortical Hyperostosis

Infantile cortical hyperostosis, or Caffey's disease, is a self-limited, short-lived proliferative bone disease of undetermined etiology. It is characterized by cortical thickening of various bones, most commonly the mandible (80% of cases) and less commonly the clavicles, long bones, maxilla, ribs, and scapulae. Pain, fever, and hyperirritability may precede or develop concurrently with the swelling. From 75% to 90% of cases demonstrate mandibular involvement, typically over the angle and ascending ramus symmetrically. Sporadic cases of infantile cortical hyperostosis almost always show mandibular involvement, with familial cases demonstrating such involvement approximately 60% of the time.

In addition to the osseous changes, swelling of the overlying soft tissues usually occurs. There are no gender, racial, or geographic predilections. The characteristic age of onset is usually by the seventh month of life, with the average age of onset being 9 weeks.

Radiographically, an expansile hyperostotic process is visible over the cortical surface, with rounding or blunting of the mandibular coronoid process. Initially, the hyperostotic element is separated from the underlying bone by a thin radiolucent line.

Diagnosis may be facilitated by the use of technetium (^{99m}Tc) scans, which are often positive before routine radiographic detection is made. Laboratory findings that are also helpful in establishing the diagnosis include an elevated erythrocyte sedimentation rate, increased phosphatase levels, anemia, leukocytosis, and occasionally thrombocytopenia or thrombocytosis.

Infantile cortical hyperostosis is usually a self-limiting process, with treatment generally directed at supportive care. Systemic corticosteroids and nonsteroidal antiinflammatory drugs have been used with some success. This disease has a tendency to follow an uneven though predictable course, with relapses and remissions possible. During such recurrences or relapses, the use of nonsteroidal antiinflammatory drugs has been recommended to control symptoms and halt progression of the disease, suggesting that prostaglandins may have a role in the etiology. The resolution phase ranges from 6 weeks to 23 months, with an average duration of 9 months. Radiographic and histologic resolution may take up to several years, with a generally excellent prognosis despite the possibility of recurrences and occasional residual effects, such as severe malocclusion and mandibular asymmetry.

Phantom Bone Disease

Phantom bone disease, also known as massive osteolysis, Gorham's disease, or vanishing bone disease, is an unusual process characterized by posttraumatic or spontaneous slow, progressive, localized destruction of bone. It is a nonneoplastic condition characterized by a proliferative vascular and connective tissue response. The fibrovascular tissue may completely replace the involved bone, but the mechanism of bone destruction and resorption is unknown. This is a rare entity of unknown cause, with fewer than 150 cases reported since its initial description in 1838. The process has been described in virtually every bone in the body, with 15 cases reported in the maxillofacial region.

No ethnic or gender predilection has been noted. There appears to be no genetic basis for transmission. Various studies, including metabolic, endocrine, and neurologic tests, have not been helpful in determining the cause of phantom bone disease.

In most patients the disease develops before the fourth decade of life, although it has been described in patients ranging from 18 months to 72 years of age. The onset of the disease is insidious; pain is usually not a feature unless there is concomitant pathologic fracture of the involved bone. Progressive atrophy of the affected bone resulting in significant deformity constitutes a useful diagnostic sign of massive osteolysis. Although most cases involve a single bone, the disease may also be polyostotic, usually affecting contiguous bones. This disease is progressive but variable—over time, the bone may completely disappear, or it may spontaneously stabilize. Significant regeneration has not been reported.

The earliest radiographic sign of the disease has been reported to be one or more intermedullary subcortical radiolucencies of variable size, usually with indistinct margins and thin radiopaque borders. In time, these foci enlarge and coalesce, eventually involving the cortex. A characteristic tapering ultimately occurs when long bones are affected.

Laboratory studies fail to show biochemical abnormalities. Microscopically, replacement of bone by connective tissue with many dilated capillaries and anastomosing vascular channels is noted. As the disease progresses, dissolution of both medullary and cortical bone is seen. A fibrotic band, thought to represent residual periosteum, persists.

There is no effective treatment for phantom bone disease, although moderate doses of radiation therapy (40 to 45 Gy in 2-Gy fractions) have resulted in good outcomes with few long-term complications. Limited success has been obtained with bone grafts and implants.

Acromegaly

Acromegaly is a rare condition with a prevalence of approximately 50 to 70 cases per million population and an incidence of 3 cases per million per year. This disease is characterized by bony and soft tissue overgrowth and metabolic disturbances. These changes occur secondary to chronic hypersecretion of growth hormone subsequent to the closure of the epiphyseal plates. If hypersecretion occurs before epiphyseal closure, gigantism results.

Etiology. The cause in more than 90% of cases is hypersecretion of growth hormone from a benign pituitary adenoma, subsequent to epiphyseal closure. The pituitary tumor may occasionally produce prolactin along with growth hormone (somatomedin C) or other hormones, including TSH or adrenocorticotropic hormone (ACTH). Such adenomas, although most common in the pituitary gland itself, may also arise in ectopic locations along the migration path of tissue from Rathke's pouch. In general, growth hormone levels correlate proportionally to the size of the adenoma, as well as to the overall severity of the disease.

Clinical Features. Acromegaly presents most often in the fourth decade, with an even gender distribution and no racial or geographic predominance. This disorder is of insidious onset, with diagnosis often delayed for many years. Younger patients have more aggressive tumors and develop clinically recognizable acromegaly more rapidly.

Clinical signs and symptoms result from the local effects of the expanding pituitary mass and the effects of excess growth hormone secretion (Figure 15-8). Affected individuals present with hyperhidrosis; coarse body hair; muscle weakness; paresthesia, especially carpal tunnel syndrome; dysmenorrhea; and decreased libido or impotence. Sleep apnea, hypertension, and heart disease are also encountered. Skin tag formation is common and may be a marker for colonic polyps. In the facial bones and the jawbones, new periosteal

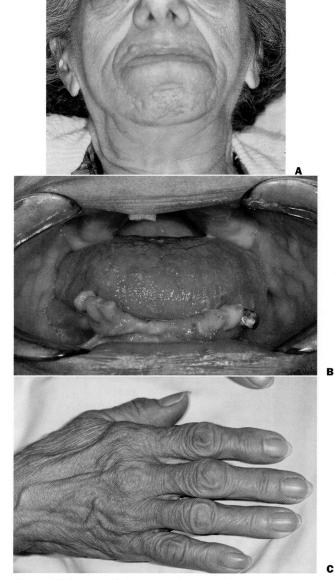

Figure 15-8   **A** to **C, Acromegaly** of the jaw and hand.

bone formation may be seen, as well as cartilaginous hyperplasia and ossification. The resultant orofacial changes include frontal bossing, nasal bone hypertrophy, and relative mandibular prognathism or prominence. Enlargement of the paranasal sinuses, as well as secondary laryngeal hypertrophy, produces a rather deep, resonant voice, which is typical of acromegaly. Overall coarsening of the facial features is noted, secondary to connective tissue hyperplasia.

Oral manifestations include enlargement of the mandible and maxilla, with secondary separation of teeth due to alveolar overgrowth. Condylar hyperplasia with concomitant bone formation at the anterior portion of the mandible and a distinct increase in the gonial angle produces a rather typical dental malocclusion and prognathism. A complete posterior crossbite is a common finding in such a circumstance. Thickened oral mucosa, increased salivary gland tissue, macroglossia, and prominent lips are also noted in most instances. It has been reported that with the concomitant changes in mandibular structure, marked alterations in the diameter of the inferior alveolar canal, myofascial pain dysfunction syndrome, and speech abnormalities may result. The demonstration of growth hormone levels that are nonsuppressible by glucose loading is diagnostic. Computed tomography or magnetic resonance imaging of the sella turcica may help confirm the diagnosis of acromegaly-associated tumor. Radioimmunoassay studies of somatomedin C may be used as a routine screening test.

Treatment. Treatment relates to normalization of growth hormone levels, with concomitant preservation of normal pituitary function. Associated causes of death include hypertension, diabetes, pulmonary infections, and cancer. The most commonly used treatment is transsphenoidal surgery; a rapid therapeutic response is usually noted. Conventional radiotherapy to this area during a 4- to 6-week period carries a 70% rate of normalization of pituitary function, although hypopituitarism may be an unfavorable sequela. Current medical therapy uses bromocriptine (a dopamine agonist) or octreotide as adjunctive agents but not as the primary modality.

Successful management may be reflected in reversal of soft tissue abnormalities, although many of the facial deformities may persist. In such instances corrective oral and maxillofacial surgery may be indicated, including mandibular osteotomy and partial glossectomy.

GENETIC ABNORMALITIES

Cherubism

Cherubism is a benign hereditary condition of the maxilla and/or mandible, usually found in children by 5 years of age (Box 15-5). The term *cherubism* has been used to describe patients with cherubic facies of marked fullness of the jaws and cheeks and upwardly gazing eyes. Cherubism usually occurs as an autosomal-dominant disorder, with 100% penetrance

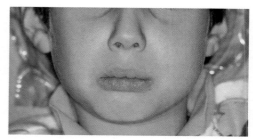

Figure 15-9 **Cherubism** resulting in fullness of the maxilla.

Box 15-5 Cherubism

Autosomal-dominant condition
Self-limiting; stabilizes after puberty
Symmetric (bilateral), asymptomatic swelling of the jaws
"Soap bubble" radiolucencies
Microscopically is a giant cell lesion
  Characteristic perivascular collagen condensation sometimes present

---

in males and 50% to 75% penetrance in females, with a 2-to-1 male predominance. Sporadic cases have also been reported.

Clinical Features. The mandibular angle, ascending ramus, retromolar region, and posterior maxilla are most often affected. The coronoid process can also be involved, but the condyles are always spared. The vast majority of cases occur only in the mandible. The bony expansion is most often bilateral, although unilateral involvement has been reported. The specific gene maps to chromosome 4p16.3, which encodes the SH3-binding protein, SH3 BP2.

Patients typically have a painless symmetric enlargement of the posterior region of the mandible, with expansion of the alveolar process and ascending ramus. The clinical appearance may vary from a barely discernible posterior swelling of a single jaw to marked anterior and posterior expansion of both jaws, resulting in masticatory, speech, and swallowing difficulties (Figures 15-9 and 15-10). Intraorally, a hard, nontender swelling can be palpated in the affected area.

With maxillary disease, involvement of the orbital floor and anterior wall of the antrum occurs. Superiorly directed pressure on the orbit results in an increas-

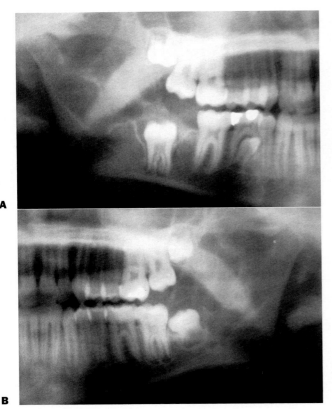

A

B

Figure 15-10   Cherubism of the right **(A)** and left **(B)** mandibular rami.

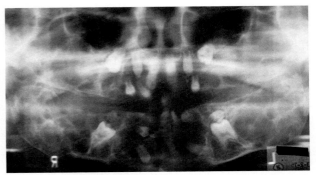

Figure 15-11   **Cherubism** of all four quadrants in an 8-year-old boy.

ing prominence of the sclera and the appearance of upturned eyes. The palatal vault may be reduced or obliterated. Maxillary involvement usually results in the greatest deformity. All four quadrants of the jaws may be simultaneously involved with this painless process of bony expansion (Figure 15-11). Premature exfoliation of the primary dentition may occur as early as 3 years of age. Displacement of developing tooth follicles results in poor development of selective permanent teeth and ectopic eruption or impaction. Permanent teeth may be missing or malformed, with the mandibular second and third molars most often affected. Significant malocclusions can be anticipated even with unifocal involvement.

Submandibular and upper cervical lymphadenopathy are common, although reactive regional lymphadenopathy, particularly of submandibular lymph nodes, usually subsides after 5 years of age. Intelligence is unaffected. Serum calcium and phosphorus levels are within normal limits, but alkaline phosphatase levels may be elevated.

Radiographic surveys may provide the only signs of disease. The radiographic lesions characteristically appear as numerous well-defined multilocular radiolucencies of the jaws. The borders are distinct and divided by bony trabeculae. Seen in the mandible are expansion and thinning of the cortical plate with occasional perforation; displacement of the inferior alveolar canal may be noted. An occlusal radiograph of the maxilla may give a soap bubble–like picture with maxillary antrum obliteration. Unerupted teeth are often displaced and appear to be floating in the cyst-like spaces.

Histopathology. Histologically, the lesions are composed of a vascularized fibrous stroma containing multinucleated giant cells, resembling central giant cell granuloma (Figure 15-12). Mature lesions exhibit a large amount of fibrous tissue and fewer giant cells. A distinctive feature that is often present is eosinophilic perivascular cuffing of collagen surrounding small capillaries throughout the lesion.

Treatment and Prognosis. The prognosis is relatively good, particularly if the disease is limited to only one jaw—especially the mandible. After a rapid pace of bone expansion, the disease is usually self-limiting and regressive. Radiographic evidence of the condition tends to persist. Although it is generally accepted that spontaneous regression begins at puberty, with relatively good resolution by age 30, no long-term follow-up of spontaneous resolution has been documented. Surgical intervention must be based on the need to improve function, prevent debility, and satisfy aesthetic considerations. If necessary, conservative curettage of the lesion with bone recontouring may be performed.

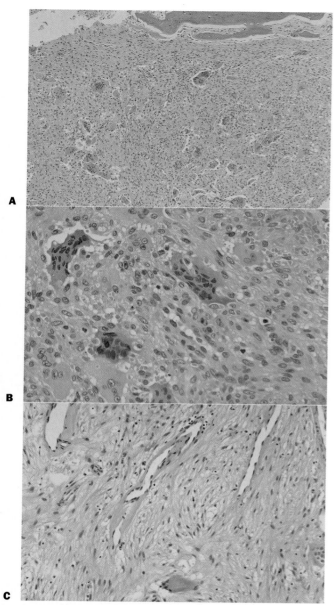

Figure 15-12 **A** to **C, Cherubism** biopsy specimen showing multinucleated giant cells in fibroblastic stroma. Note eosinophilic perivascular cuffing in **C.**

Osteopetrosis

Osteopetrosis, also known as Albers-Schönberg disease, is an uncommon hereditary bone condition characterized by a generalized symmetric increase in skeletal density and defective bone resorption. It can be divided into three clinical groups. The infantile-malignant form is autosomal recessive in nature and

is fatal within the first 2 to 3 years of life in the absence of treatment. An intermediate autosomal-recessive type is nonfatal but clinically aggressive, with onset usually within the first decade. An autosomal-dominant form is the least severe form, with full life expectancy but with considerable morbidity secondary to orthopedic alterations.

The characteristic feature of osteopetrosis is an absence of physiologic bone resorption due to reduced osteoclastic activity. The lack of bone resorption and remodeling results in accumulation of bone mass and manifests itself in skeletal disturbances, including sclerosis of bone marrow, decreased hematopoietic activity, and growth retardation. In mice with phenotypic features of osteopetrosis, the genetic abnormality resides in the granulocyte-macrophage colony-stimulating factor (GM-CSF). This abnormality has not been identified in humans.

Clinical Features. Bone pain is the most common symptom. Cranial nerve compression may result in blindness, deafness, anosmia, ageusia, and sometimes facial paralysis. Normal cortical and cancellous bone is replaced by a dense, poorly structured bone that is fragile and has a propensity for pathologic fracture.

Delayed dental eruption is due to bony ankylosis, absence of alveolar bone resorption, and the formation of pseudoodontomas during apicogenesis. Premature exfoliation may be due to a defect in the periodontal ligament.

The clinically benign adult form of osteopetrosis may not be diagnosed until the third or fourth decade. Optic and facial nerve impairment is often present as a result of narrowing of the cranial foramina and the resultant pressure on the nerves. The first sign of the disease often is pathologic fracture.

Dental findings include delayed eruption, congenitally absent teeth, unerupted and malformed teeth, and enamel hypoplasia (Figure 15-13). Decreased alveolar bone production, defective and abnormally thickened periodontal ligament, and marked mandibular prognathism have been reported. An elevated caries index may be secondary to enamel hypoplasia. This has serious implications because of the propensity for the development of osteomyelitis resulting from inadequate host response because of the diminished vascular component of osteopetrotic bone. Osteomyelitis is a serious complication of the disease; it occurs most often in the mandible and occasionally in the maxilla, scapula, and extremities.

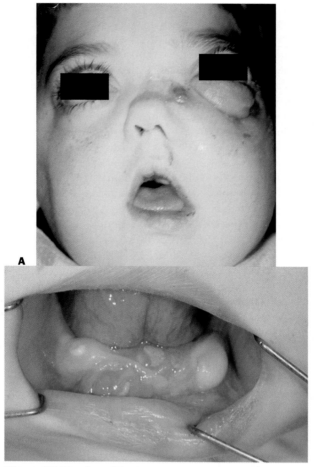

A

B

Figure 15-13 **A** and **B, Osteopetrosis** in a child. Note infraorbital draining sinuses due to secondary osteomyelitis, and note malformed teeth in an irregular jaw.

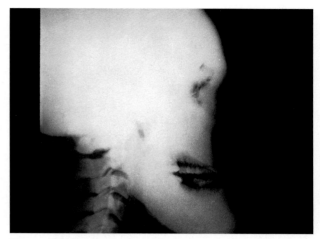

Figure 15-14 **Osteopetrosis** showing sclerotic change in the jaws and skull.

Radiographic findings are characteristic of this disease (Figure 15-14). The classic bone-within-bone radiographic presentation is due to a defect in metaphyseal bone remodeling resulting in greatly thickened cortices and medullary space obliteration. Skeletal density generally is greatly increased because of a uniform diffuse sclerosing of all bones. The mandible is less often involved than are other bones. Loss of the distinct interface between cortical and medullary bone appears, along with clubbing of the long bones with transverse peripheral banding.

Histopathology. Osteopetrosis is histologically characterized by normal production of bone with absence of physiologic bone resorption. The pattern of endochondral bone formation is disrupted, with a decrease in osteoclastic function and a compensatory increase in the number of osteoclasts. This results in failure to develop normal lamellar structure in the bone and an absence of definable marrow cavities. Biopsy specimens of endochondral bone exhibit a core of calcified cartilage surrounded by bone matrix.

Treatment and Prognosis. The prognosis for infantile osteopetrosis is poor, with patients rarely surviving adolescence. Recent medical advances designed to increase osteoclast differentiation and activity using high-dose calcitriol have proved to be helpful. Bone marrow transplantations in the severe childhood or malignant forms of this disease have been performed in an effort to provide monocyte precursors of osteoclasts.

Death results from secondary infection or anemia. The adult variety is more variable and insidious. Bone involvement is similar to the infantile recessive type but is usually less severe. The diagnosis often is not made until a pathologic fracture occurs. The differential diagnosis should include osteomalacia, Paget's disease, hyperparathyroidism, acromegaly, and malignant bone disease.

Osteogenesis Imperfecta

Osteogenesis imperfecta represents a genetically heterogeneous group of heritable defects of connective tissue. Classically, this condition or syndrome may include fragile bones, blue sclerae, ligament laxity, hearing loss, and dentinogenesis imperfecta. Some affected patients exhibit extreme bone fragility with numerous fractures and die during the perinatal period; others suffer only mild bone fragility and live a normal life span. Clinical presentation and severity are extremely variable. Patients with osteogenesis imperfecta are classified according to their clinical and radiographic manifestations, as well as by inheritance pattern. Four distinct types have been identified: two inherited as autosomal-dominant traits, one inherited as an autosomal-recessive trait, and one inherited as both an autosomal-dominant and autosomal-recessive trait. The presence of numerous long bone fractures early in life with dentinogenesis imperfecta, blue sclerae, or both, is sufficient to establish the diagnosis. Early hearing loss in a patient or a member of a family with a history of fragile bones is highly suggestive of the disorder.

Biochemical findings suggest that osteogenesis imperfecta syndromes are a result of inborn errors of collagen metabolism. Most forms of the disease are believed to be caused by mutations in the structural genes for the collagen protein (COL 1A2 gene). The primary biochemical defect in most cases appears to involve the biosynthesis of type I collagen. The heterogeneity of these defects is at least in part explained by the more than 400 mutations in 6 of the 19 identified forms of collagen. More specifically, genetic mutations have been identified for both pro-alpha chains of type I procollagen in this disease.

Clinical Features. Osteogenesis imperfecta type I is characterized by osteoporosis, bone fragility, blue sclerae, and conductive hearing loss in adolescents and adults. Fractures may be present at birth in 10% of patients or may commence during infancy or childhood. There is considerable variability in the age of onset, frequency of fractures, and degree of skeletal deformity. Generally, birth weight and height are normal. Mild short stature is postnatal in onset and relates to the degree of involvement of the limbs and spine. Long bone deformities tend to be mild, with bowing of the limbs and angulation deformities occurring at previous fracture sites. Progressive kyphoscoliosis is seen in 20% of adults and may be severe. Hearing impairment, which usually begins in the second decade of life, is present in 35% of adults. Dentinogenesis imperfecta (see Chapter 16) is present in some patients with osteogenesis imperfecta type I.

Osteogenesis imperfecta type II is a lethal syndrome, with half of all patients stillborn. It has an autosomal-recessive mode of transmission, although spontaneous cases have been reported. It is characterized in infancy by low birth weight, short stature, and broad thighs extending at right angles to the trunk. The limbs are short, curved, and grossly deformed. The skin is thin and frail and may be torn during delivery. Cranial vault ossification is lacking, and the facies is notable for hypotelorism: a small beaked nose and a triangular shape. Defects in skeletal ossification lead to extreme bone fragility and frequent fractures, even during delivery. Dental abnormalities have been found, including atubular dentin with a lacework of argyrophilic fiber structures, an absence of predentin, and an abundance of argyrophilic fibers in the coronal pulp.

Osteogenesis imperfecta type III is a rare disorder characterized in neonates by severe bone fragility, multiple fractures, and progressive skeletal deformity. The sclerae are blue at birth, but the color normalizes with age; adolescents and adults exhibit normal sclera coloration. Childhood mortality is high because of cardiopulmonary complications, and the prognosis is poor because of severe kyphoscoliosis. Individuals with type III disease exhibit the shortest stature of all patients with osteogenesis imperfecta. Dentinogenesis imperfecta is found in some patients with osteogenesis imperfecta type III.

Osteogenesis imperfecta type IV is a dominantly inherited osteopenia leading to bone fragility, without the other classic features associated with the osteogenesis imperfecta syndromes. The sclerae are bluish at birth only. Onset of fractures ranges from birth to adulthood, and the skeletal deformities are extremely variable. Bowing of the lower limbs at birth may be the only feature of this syndrome, and progressive deformities of the long bones and vertebral column may occur without fractures. Spontaneous improvement often occurs with puberty. Dentinogenesis imperfecta is seen in some patients with osteogenesis imperfecta type IV. The incidence of hearing impairment in adults is low.

Treatment and Prognosis. There is no specific treatment for this condition. Management of fractures may be a significant orthopedic challenge. Rehabilitation and physical therapy for recurrent fractures, limb deformities, and kyphoscoliosis are suggested. Middle ear surgery may correct hearing loss. With the onset of puberty, the severity of this problem often lessens. When dentinogenesis imperfecta is present, management is focused around the preservation of the teeth. Generally, the primary dentition is more problematic. To prevent wear and improve aesthetic appearance, full crown coverage may be necessary.

Because of the wide variation in clinical expression, the prognosis ranges from very good (dominant form) to very poor (recessive form). Genetic counseling is essential, and patient support groups may provide needed emotional support to affected individuals and their families.

Cleidocranial Dysplasia

Cleidocranial dysplasia is notable for aplasia or hypoplasia of the clavicles, characteristic craniofacial malformations, and the presence of numerous supernumerary and unerupted teeth.

Etiology and Pathogenesis. Cleidocranial dysplasia is transmitted by an autosomal-dominant mode of inheritance with high penetrance and variable expressivity. A recessive form has been reported in two families. About one third of cases are sporadic and appear to represent new mutations. It occurs with equal frequency among males and females; there is no racial predilection. Most patients with the disorder are of normal intelligence. Studies involving a large kindred of more than 1000 people in South Africa have isolated the origin of this disorder to the short arm of chromosome 6 (a microdeletion defect). Studies have identified a transcription factor (CBFA1) as being causative in this disorder.

Intramembranous and endochondral bones in the skull are affected, resulting in a sagittally diminished cranial base, transverse enlargement of the calvarium, and delayed closure of the fontanels and sutures. Hydrocephalic pressure on unossified regions of the skull, especially the fontanels, causes biparietal and frontal bossing and extension of the cranial vault. The deficiency of the clavicles is responsible for the long appearance of the neck and the narrow shoulders. The combined abnormalities of the middle third of the face and the dental alveolar complex result in the characteristic facial appearance.

Delayed or failed eruption of the teeth has been associated with lack of cellular cementum. It has been postulated that failure of cementum formation may be due to mechanical resistance to eruption by the dense alveolar bone overlying the unerupted teeth. The formation of supernumerary teeth is due to incomplete or severely delayed resorption of the dental lamina, which is reactivated at the time of crown completion of the normal permanent dentition.

Clinical Features. The clinical appearance of cleidocranial dysplasia is so distinct that it is pathognomonic.

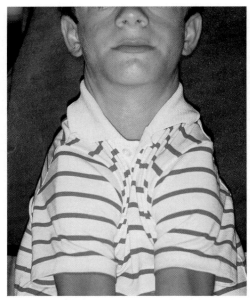

Figure 15-15   Cleidocranial dysplasia in a patient able to approximate his shoulders because of hypoplastic clavicles.

The stature is mildly to moderately shortened, with the neck appearing long and narrow and the shoulders markedly drooped. Complete or partial absence of clavicular calcification, with associated muscle defects, results in hypermobility of the shoulders, allowing for variable levels of approximation in an anterior plane (Figure 15-15).

The head is large and brachycephalic. Patients have pronounced frontal, parietal, and occipital bossing. The facial bones and paranasal sinuses are hypoplastic, giving the face a small and short appearance. The nose is broad based, with a depressed nasal bridge. Ocular hypertelorism is often present. The entire skeleton may be affected, with defects of the pelvis, long bones, and fingers. Hemivertebrae and posterior wedging of the thoracic vertebrae may contribute to the development of kyphoscoliosis and pulmonary complications.

Maxillary hypoplasia gives the mandible a relatively prognathic appearance, although some patients may show variable mandibular prognathism because of an increased length of the mandible in conjunction with a short cranial base. The palate is narrow and highly arched, and there is an increased incidence of submucosal clefts and complete or partial clefts of the palate involving the hard and soft tissues. Nonunion of the symphysis of the mandible is seen.

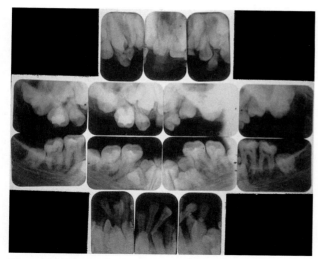

Figure 15-16 **Cleidocranial dysplasia** showing unerupted and supernumerary teeth.

The formation, maturation, and eruption of the deciduous dentition are usually normal. Extreme delay in physiologic root resorption occurs, however, and the result is prolonged exfoliation of primary teeth. Eruption of the permanent dentition is severely delayed, and many teeth fail to erupt. Unerupted supernumerary teeth are often present in all regions (Figure 15-16). They develop on completion of normal crown formation in the permanent dentition lingual and occlusal to the normal unerupted crown. Only one supernumerary tooth per normal tooth is generally noted. The overretention of deciduous teeth, failure of eruption of permanent teeth, numerous supernumerary teeth, and maxillary hypoplasia result in severe malocclusion.

Radiographic findings of clinical significance pertain to the abnormalities of the craniofacial region, dentition, clavicles, and pelvis. Radiographs of the skull classically exhibit patent fontanels and wormian bones, broad and anomalous cranial sutures, and underdeveloped paranasal sinuses. The clavicles may be aplastic unilaterally or bilaterally, or they may be hypoplastic, appearing as small fragments attached to the sternum or acromial process. The mandible and maxilla contain many unerupted and supernumerary teeth, which are often malpositioned.

Treatment. There is no specific treatment for patients with cleidocranial dysplasia. Genetic counseling is most important. Protective headgear may be recommended while fontanels remain patent. The current mode of therapy for the dental anomalies combines early surgical intervention with orthodontic therapy. Extraction of supernumerary teeth and overretained primary teeth, when the root formation of succedaneous teeth is greater than 50%, is followed by surgical exposure of unerupted teeth and orthodontic treatment. Early surgical exposure of unerupted teeth has resulted in stimulation of cementum formation and eruption of the dentition with normal root formation. Orthognathic surgery for correction of the dental-facial deformity, postsurgical orthodontics, and prosthetics can be anticipated.

Crouzon's Syndrome (Craniofacial Dysostosis)

Crouzon's syndrome is characterized by variable cranial deformity, maxillary hypoplasia, and shallow orbits with exophthalmos and divergent strabismus. The character of the cranial deformity depends on the sutures affected, the degree of involvement, and the sequence of sutural fusion. Increased interpupillary distance and exophthalmos are constant features of Crouzon's syndrome and develop in early childhood as a result of premature synostosis of the coronal suture. Systemic complications include mental retardation, hearing loss, speech and visual impairment, and convulsions.

Etiology and Pathogenesis. Craniofacial dysostosis is inherited in an autosomal-dominant mode, with complete penetrance and variable expressivity. About one third of the cases reported arise spontaneously. The genetic abnormality is thought to be a missense mutation in the fibroblast growth factor receptor 2 (FGFR2) gene. The severity of expression of the disease increases in successive siblings, with the youngest child most severely affected.

Craniosynostosis results when premature fusion of the cranial sutures occurs. The cause is not known, but premature closure of these sutures can initiate changes in the brain secondary to increased intracranial pressure.

The deformities of the cranial bones and orbital cavities are the result of the fusion of sutures and increased intracranial pressure. Underdevelopment of the supraorbital ridges and overgrowth of the sphenoid wing result in small and shallow orbits. Exophthalmos and reduced orbital volume are the result. Hypertelorism is accentuated by a downward and forward displacement of the ethmoid plate. Abnormalities of the bony orbit account for several functional ocular abnormalities. Severe distortion of the cranial base leads to reduced maxillary growth and nasopharyngeal hypoplasia with potential upper airway restriction.

Clinical Features. Patients with Crouzon's syndrome have a characteristic facies that is often described as frog-like. Midface hypoplasia and exophthalmos are striking. Patients have relative mandibular prognathism, with the nose resembling a parrot's beak. The upper lip and philtrum are usually short, and the lower lip often droops. The cranial deformity is dependent on which sutures are involved. Proptosis with strabismus and orbital hypertelorism is common. Optic nerve damage occurs in 80% of cases.

Oral findings include severe maxillary hypoplasia, resulting in a narrowing of the maxillary arch and a compressed, high-arched palate. Bilateral posterior lingual crossbites are common. Premature posterior occlusion as a result of the inferiorly positioned maxilla results in an anterior open bite.

Radiographs of the skull reveal obliterated suture lines with obvious bony continuity. A hammered-silver appearance is often seen in regions of the skull where compensatory deformity cannot occur. Lordosis of the cranial base is apparent on lateral skull projections, and angular deformities with vertical sloping of the anterior cranial fossa can be visualized. A large calvarium with hypoplasia of the maxilla, shallow orbits, and a relatively large mandible is common.

Treatment and Prognosis. The age of onset and the degree of craniosynostosis influence the severity of the complications, which range from craniofacial dystrophy to hearing loss, speech and visual impairment, and mental retardation. With a high degree of suspicion, the condition is often identifiable at birth. Ultrasonic prenatal diagnosis of exophthalmos has been reported. Early recognition is essential to guide growth and development of the face and cranium. Surgical intervention may be necessary if exophthalmos is progressive, optic nerve damage or visual acuity is impaired, evidence of developing mental deficiency is noted, or intracranial pressure continues to rise. Treatment includes the surgical placement of artificial sutures to allow growth of the brain while minimizing intracranial pressure and secondary calvarial deformities. Orthodontic treatment with subsequent orthognathic surgical intervention has been successful in managing the concomitant dentofacial deformity.

Treacher Collins Syndrome (Mandibulofacial Dysostosis)

Treacher Collins syndrome primarily affects structures developing from the first branchial arch, but it also involves the second branchial arch to a minor degree. Individuals have a convex facial profile with a prominent nose and retrusive chin. It is generally a bilateral anomaly with a characteristic facies, including downward sloping of the palpebral fissures, colobomas of the lower eyelid, mandibular and midface hypoplasia, and deformed pinnas (Figure 15-17).

Etiology and Pathogenesis. Treacher Collins syndrome is transmitted by an autosomal-dominant mode of inheritance, although about half of the cases are due to spontaneous mutation. The genetic mutation is thought to be a balanced translocation in the 5q32–33.2 region. The gene has a high degree of penetrance, but variable expressivity is common. Affected siblings are

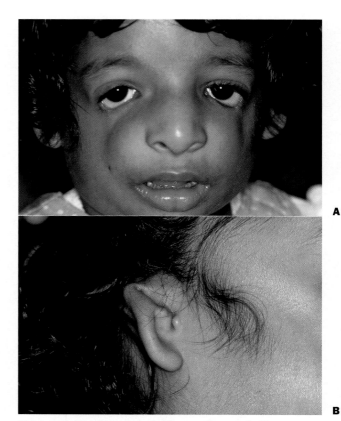

Figure 15-17   Treacher Collins syndrome. A, Note sloping palpebral fissures and colobomas of the lower eyelids. **B,** Microtia and preauricular hair extension.

remarkably similar, and the syndrome becomes progressively more severe in succeeding generations. This disorder is relatively rare, with an incidence between 0.5 and 10.6 cases per 10,000 births.

It is believed that the embryologic and morphologic defects that result in the phenotypic expression of this syndrome begin as early as the sixth to seventh embryonic week. A defect in the stapedial artery during embryogenesis may be responsible for the anatomic deficits seen. Stapedial artery dysfunction gives rise to defects of the stapes and incus and the first arch vessels supplying the maxilla. Failure of the inferior alveolar artery to develop an ancillary vascular supply gives rise to mandibular abnormalities. Improper orientation and hypoplasia of the mandibular elevator muscles, resulting from an aplastic or hypoplastic zygomatic arch, may also be contributory.

Mandibular retrognathia and midface vertical excess may be accentuated by the pull of abnormally oriented mandibular elevator muscles, causing a backward rotation in the mandibular growth pattern. The syndrome seems to be limited to defects of the bones and soft tissue of the face. Vascularization of the posterior portion of the second visceral arch by the stapedial artery seems unimpaired.

Clinical Findings. Treacher Collins syndrome is a manifestation of combined developmental anomalies of the second and, mainly, first branchial arches. It includes various degrees of hypoplasia of the mandible, maxilla, zygomatic process of the temporal bone, and external and middle ear. Abnormalities of the medial pterygoid plates and hypoplasia of the lateral pterygoid muscles are common. Right-to-left asymmetry of the deformities is generally seen. In the fully expressed syndrome the facial appearance is characteristic and is often described as birdlike or fishlike.

Notched or linear colobomas of the outer third of the lower eyelids are found in 75% of patients. The lower eyelashes are absent medial to the colobomas in about 50% of patients. Antimongoloid obliquity, or downward slanting of the palpebral fissures, is striking.

Congenital atresia of the external auditory canal and microtia are often present. The ears are low set, with deformed, crumpled, or absent pinnae. Middle ear defects include fibrous bands of the long process of the incus, malformed and fixed stapes and malleus, and accompanying conductive hearing loss. Ear tags and blind fistulas are often located between the pinna and the commissures of the mouth.

Atypical hair growth in the shape of a tonguelike process extends from the hairline toward the cheeks. Other associated anomalies such as skeletal deformities and facial clefts may be concomitant.

Oral findings include cleft palate in about 30% of patients and macrostomia in 15% of patients. A high-arched palate and dental malocclusion consisting of apertognathia and widely separated and displaced teeth are common. Severe mandibular hypoplasia is most characteristic. The underdeveloped zygomaticomaxillary complex leads to a clinically severe midface deficiency.

Treacher Collins syndrome is notable for characteristic radiographic findings, including downward sloping floors of the orbits, a peaked bony nasal contour, an aplastic or hypoplastic zygomatic process of the temporal bone, and an obtuse mandibular angle. Lateral cephalograms demonstrate antigonial notching and a broad curvature of the mandible. The peculiar broad and concave nature of the inferior border of the mandible is characteristic and helps distinguish this condition from other syndromes involving the mandible. The condyle and coronoid processes are often flattened or aplastic.

Treatment and Prognosis. Treatment is directed at correction or reconstruction of the existing deformities. Neutralization of conductive hearing loss through surgery and hearing aids is helpful. Ophthalmologic surgery to correct eye deformities by orbital reconstruction is often performed. Extensive orthodontic treatment before orthognathic surgical reconstruction of the mandible and maxilla can be anticipated.

Pierre Robin Syndrome

The clinical presentation of micrognathia, glossoptosis, and high-arched or cleft palate in neonates has been termed *Pierre Robin syndrome*. This malformation complex can occur as an isolated finding or as a component of various syndromes or developmental anomalies. The mandibular retrognathia and hypoplasia is considered the primary malformation. Respiratory and feeding problems are prevalent and may result in episodic airway obstruction, infant hypoxia, malnutrition, and failure to thrive.

Etiology and Pathogenesis. The incidence of Pierre Robin syndrome is 5.3 to 22.7 per 100,000 births, with 39%

of infants exhibiting no additional abnormalities. Of the remaining infants, 25% have known syndromes, and 36% have one or more anomalies that are not part of a known syndrome. A candidate gene for this syndrome has been identified at 2q32.3–q33.2 and contributes to the syndrome as the result of an unbalanced reciprocal translocation with 21q32.3–q33.21. This candidate gene has not yet been fully characterized.

Fetal malposition and interposition of the tongue between the palatal shelves have long been considered the etiologic catalysts for palatal deformity and micrognathia. Arrest of mandibular development may prevent descent of the tongue and failure of palatal shelf elevation and fusion. Evidence suggests that the primary defect may be due to genetically influenced metabolic growth disturbances of the maxilla and mandible rather than to mechanical obstruction by the tongue during embryogenesis. Organogenetic differences lead to the variable presentation of micrognathia and cleft palate.

Clinical Features. Infants present with severe micrognathia and mandibular hypoplasia. A U-shaped cleft palate is a common but not constant feature, and in some instances the palate is highly arched. Glossoptosis is the result of the retropositional attachment of the genioglossus muscle because of the retrognathic mandible. The geniohyoid muscle is foreshortened, so that support to the hyoid bone and strap muscles of the larynx is also compromised.

Treatment and Prognosis. Respiratory and feeding problems are common in the immediate postnatal and neonatal periods. Constant medical supervision may be necessary to prevent airway obstruction and hypoxia, cor pulmonale, gastroesophageal reflux, bronchopneumonia, and exhaustion. In most cases conservative repositioning of the infant and frequent prone positioning are sufficient to prevent upper airway obstruction, by making optimal use of the effects of gravity during resting and feeding. Continuous pulse oximetry and apnea monitoring are prudent during the neonatal period. In severe cases with chronic upper airway obstruction and failure to thrive, intraoral or nasal pharyngeal airway placement, some surgical form of tongue and lip adhesion, and even tracheostomy as a last resort may be considered. Feeding infants with mandibular hypoplasia requires expertise and patience. Nasogastric feeding tubes may be required. After the first few months of life, mandibular growth and improved control of tongue musculature result in significant abatement of symptoms.

The growth of the mandible is remarkable during the first 4 years of life, and a normal profile is often achieved between 4 and 6 years of age. Some patients have a residual mild mandibular retrognathia requiring treatment later in life.

Marfan's Syndrome

Marfan's syndrome is a heritable disorder of connective tissue, characterized by abnormalities of the skeletal, cardiovascular, and ocular systems. It is currently estimated that 23,000 Americans have Marfan's syndrome. Diagnosis is problematic because of the extreme variability of clinical expression. The disorder is notable for a number of sudden catastrophic deaths that have occurred in affected (undiagnosed) athletes.

Etiology and Pathogenesis. Marfan's syndrome is an inherited autosomal-dominant disorder that affects 1 in 10,000 individuals. There are no ethnic, racial, or gender predilections. The condition exhibits complete but extremely variable penetrance, with the offspring of an affected individual having a 50% chance of acquiring the disorder. Approximately 15% to 35% of cases arise spontaneously as a result of gamete gene mutation in the ovum or sperm; a greater number occur with increasing paternal age. Diagnosis is currently based on characteristic abnormalities of the musculoskeletal, ocular, and cardiovascular systems and a positive family history. Because most features progress with age, the diagnosis is often more obvious in older persons. The gene for Marfan's syndrome has been located on chromosome 15 and will provide for diagnostic testing in pairs at risk. Recent studies involving factors responsible for assisting in microfibril formation have identified the gene for fibrillin (FBN1) as the disease-causing gene in this disorder. The Marfan gene is believed to produce a change in one of the proteins that provides strength to a component of connective tissue, probably collagen.

Clinical Features. Patients characteristically possess a tall, slender stature with relatively long legs and arms, large hands with long fingers, and loose joints. The arms, legs, and digits are disproportionately long compared with the patient's trunk. Chest deformities include a protrusion or indentation of the breast bone (pectus carinatum or pectus excavatum, respectively). The normal thoracic kyphosis is often absent, leading to a straight back. Various degrees of scoliosis are present. Oral findings include a narrow, high-arched palate and dental crowding. The face appears long and narrow.

The cardiovascular system is affected in nearly all persons. Mitral valve prolapse, as a result of myxomatous change, occurs in 75% to 85% of affected patients, and a small percentage develop mitral regurgitation. There is cystic medionecrosis of the aorta, resulting in ascending aortic dilation, aortic regurgitation, and heart failure. A significant consequence of this change to the media layer of the aorta is progressive dissection, which may lead to aneurysms and placing patients at great risk for death.

Ocular findings include dislocation of the lens (ectopia lentis), which occurs in half of these patients. The most common eye anomaly, however, is myopia (nearsightedness). Retinal detachment occurs infrequently, but it is more prevalent after lens removal.

Treatment and Prognosis. Morbidity and mortality are directly related to the degree of connective tissue abnormality in the involved organ systems. The cardiovascular abnormalities of ascending aorta dilation and mitral valve prolapse, subluxation of the lens of the eye, chest cavity deformities and scoliosis, and the potential for pneumothorax are serious prognostic indicators.

Treatment of patients with Marfan's syndrome consists of annual medical examinations with a cardiovascular emphasis, frequent ophthalmologic examination, scoliosis screening, and echocardiography. Physical activity often is restricted and redirected in an attempt to protect the aorta.

Antibiotic prophylaxis has been recommended for infective endocarditis, regardless of the clinical evidence of valvular disease. Beta-blockers such as propranolol are often used to reduce aortic stress and have been shown to significantly reduce both the rate of aortic dilation and the risk of serious complications. Mortality has been drastically reduced with the use of composite grafts to replace the aortic valve and the region containing the aortic aneurysm. The prognosis for untreated aneurysms of the ascending aorta is extremely poor.

Ehlers-Danlos Syndrome

Ehlers-Danlos syndrome is an uncommon inherited disorder of connective tissue, clinically characterized by joint hypermobility, skin hyperextensibility, and fragility. The clinical manifestations of the disease are due to inherited defects in collagen metabolism. In addition to the skin and joint anomalies, severe cardiovascular and gastrointestinal complications may occur and coexist.

The condition has been classified into eight variants. The periodontal form (Ehlers-Danlos syndrome type VIII) is characterized by rapidly progressing periodontal disease resulting in complete tooth loss by the second or third decade of life.

Etiology and Pathogenesis. Various subtypes of Ehlers-Danlos syndrome are inherited as autosomal-dominant, autosomal-recessive, and X-linked traits. The clinical presentations of the recessively inherited forms are more severe.

At least 10 subtypes of Ehlers-Danlos syndrome have been classified on the basis of genetic, biochemical, and clinical characteristics. For instance, in the potentially lethal type IV variant, mutations in the gene for type III procollagen have been identified. Mutations in the lysyl hydrolase gene are associated with the type XI variant, whereas types VIIa and VIIb are related to type I collagen gene mutations.

From a clinical standpoint, defects in type III collagen formation are associated with spontaneous rupture of the aorta or intestines, tissues rich in type III collagen. Deficiencies in collagen hydroxylysine are secondary to depressed levels of lysyl hydroxylase. Others may have a defect in collagen metabolism, preventing the conversion of procollagen to collagen. Also, a disorder of copper metabolism has been noted in some patients.

Clinical Features. Classic clinical features include marked hyperelasticity of the skin and extreme laxity of the joints. The skin may be stretched for several centimeters, but when released, it resumes its former contours. Skin manifestations include a velvety appearance with a high degree of fragility and a tendency toward bruising. Minor trauma may produce ecchymoses, bleeding, and large, gaping wounds with poor healing tendencies and "cigarette paper" scar formation, which is especially evident on the forehead and lower legs and over pressure points. Other cutaneous findings include molluscoid pseudotumors, redundant skin on the palms and soles, and subcutaneous lipid-containing cysts, which may calcify.

Articular hypermobility is variable. It may be of sufficient severity to cause spontaneous dislocation of the joints. Extreme joint laxity leads to genu recurvatum (back knee), flat feet, habitual joint dislocation, kyphoscoliosis, and other skeletal deformities.

Patients may have severe cardiovascular, gastrointestinal, and pulmonary manifestations. Cardiovascular anomalies include dissecting aortic aneurysm, mitral valve prolapse, and rupture of major blood vessels. The majority of patients have a bleeding diathesis that may consist of a tendency to bruise or that may be severe, with hematoma formation and bleeding from the nose, gut, lungs, and urogenital tract.

Rupture of the bowel and bladder may occur. Pulmonary problems include spontaneous pneumothorax and respiratory impairment secondary to chest wall deformities. Hernias, gastrointestinal diverticula, and ocular defects may be encountered.

Orofacial features include a narrow maxilla, flattened midface, and wide nasal bridge. Other facial findings include hypertelorism, epicanthal folds, a hollowed appearance of the eyes, and scarring of the forehead and chin. Fragility of gingival and mucosal tissues may be problematic. The incidence of temporomandibular joint dysfunction is increased as a result of profound laxity of the joint, contributing to hypermobility and dislocation. Marked extensibility of the tongue, enabling contact with the tip of the nose, has been described.

Dental findings include deep anatomic grooves and excessive cuspal height of the molars and premolars. Stunted or dilacerated roots and the presence of freefloating coronal pulp stones secondary to alteration and calcification of intrapulpal vascular structures have been noted. Irregular composition of dentinal tubules, denticles, and enamel hypoplasia are often seen.

Treatment and Prognosis. The prognosis is dependent on the severity of the systemic manifestations. The cardiovascular status of all patients should be evaluated and closely monitored. Sudden death in youth or early adult life may occur as a result of dissecting aneurysms and ruptured arteries.

Surgical intervention must be tempered in light of connective tissue fragility. Joint ligament repair is often unsuccessful because of suture failure. Wound healing is usually delayed, and prolonged bleeding may occur after injury. Osteoarthritis is a common complication in patients with repeated dislocations.

Down Syndrome (Trisomy 21)

Down syndrome is a common and easily recognizable chromosome aberration. The incidence is reported to be 1 in 600 to 1 in 700 live births; however, more than half of the affected fetuses spontaneously abort during early pregnancy. Approximately 10% to 15% of all institutionalized patients have Down syndrome.

Most cases of trisomy 21 (94%) are caused by nondisjunction, resulting in an extra chromosome. The remaining patients with Down syndrome have various chromosome abnormalities. The translocation type occurs in 3%, mosaicism occurs in 2%, and rare chromosome aberrations make up the remaining 1% of cases. The incidence of this condition rises with increasing maternal age.

Etiology and Pathogenesis. Possible etiologies for Down syndrome include undetected mosaicism in a parent, repeated exposure to the same environmental insult, genetic predisposition to nondisjunction, an ovum with an extra chromosome 21, or a preferential survival in utero of trisomy 21 embryos and fetuses with increasing maternal age. Parents of any age who have had one child with trisomy 21 have a significant risk (about 1%) of having a similarly affected child—a risk of recurrence equivalent to that affecting births to a mother older than age 45 years. No racial, social, economic, or gender predilections have been identified.

Clinical Features. Patients with Down syndrome present with numerous characteristic clinical findings and various common systemic manifestations (Figure 15-18). A number of common phenotypic findings in children with Down syndrome have been identified; these can assist in establishing a diagnosis.

Various degrees of mental retardation exist in all patients with Down syndrome. Most mildly affected individuals are highly functioning and are able to perform well in a workshop environment. Dementia affects about 30% of patients with Down syndrome, and early aging is common. After age 35, nearly all individuals develop the neuropathologic changes analogous to those found in Alzheimer's disease, although 70% exhibit no clinically detectable behavioral changes. These two disorders have many neuropathologic and neurochemical similarities, and an increased risk for Down syndrome has been found in families with a predilection for Alzheimer's disease.

In Down syndrome the skull is brachycephalic, with a flat occiput and prominent forehead. A third or fourth fontanel is present, and all the fontanels are large and have extended patency. Sagittal suture separation greater than 5 mm is present in 98% of affected individuals. Frontal and sphenoid sinuses are absent, and the maxillary sinus is hypoplastic in more than 90% of patients. Midface skeletal deficiency is quite marked, with ocular hypotelorism, a flattened nasal bridge, and relative mandibular prognathism.

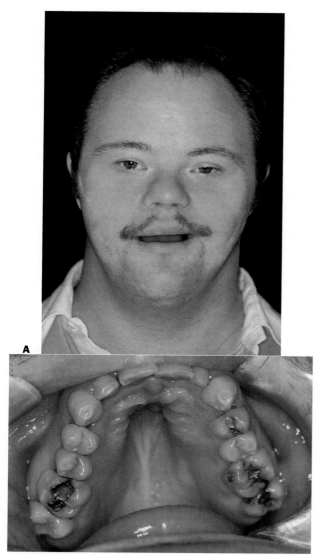

Figure 15-18 **A** and **B,** Down syndrome facies. Note high-arched palate with decreased width and length in **B.**

The eyes are almond shaped, with upward-slanting palpebral fissures, epicanthic folds, and Brushfield's spots of the iris often noted. Other ocular anomalies include convergent strabismus, nystagmus, refractive errors, keratoconus, and congenital cataracts.

Congenital heart disease is present in 30% to 45% of all patients with Down syndrome. Anomalies include atrioventricular communication, partial endocardial cushion abnormalities, and ventricular septal defects. A study revealed a 50% prevalence of mitral valve prolapse; one third of these patients had negative auscultatory findings. Tetralogy of Fallot, patent ductus arteriosus, and secundum atrial septal defects are seen less often.

It appears that T-cell and probably B-cell function is aberrant, with some affected children being more susceptible to infectious diseases. Respiratory tract infections are extremely common. Thyroid dysfunction occurs in upward of 50% of all patients. There is also an increased incidence of acute lymphocytic leukemia and hepatitis B antigen carrier status.

Skeletal problems include hypoplasia of the maxilla and sphenoid bones, rib and pelvic abnormalities, hip dislocation, and patella subluxation. Of particular concern is the presence of atlantoaxial instability in 12% to 20% of persons with Down syndrome, as a result of the increased laxity of the transverse ligaments between the atlas and the odontoid process. Delay in recognizing this condition may result in irreversible spinal cord damage, which might occur during manipulation of the neck in patients undergoing dental therapy or general anesthesia.

Oral manifestations of Down syndrome are common. The tongue is often fissured, and macroglossia is usually relative to the small oral cavity, although true macroglossia is possible. An open-mouth posture is common because a narrow nasopharynx and hypertrophied tonsils and adenoids cause upper airway compromise. A protruding tongue and habitual mouth breathing result in drying and cracking of the lips. Palatal width and length are significantly decreased, and a bifid uvula and cleft lip and palate are occasionally observed. Elevated concentrations of sodium, calcium, and bicarbonate ion have been demonstrated in parotid saliva.

The dentition exhibits a number of characteristic anomalies, and periodontal disease is prevalent. The incidence of dental caries, however, appears to be no greater than in normal individuals. Considering the existence of poor oral hygiene, this may reflect the greater buffering capacity of the saliva or the ability to control dietary intake in institutional and home settings. The defective immune system and neutrophil motility defect directly contribute to rampant and precocious periodontal disease.

Eruption of both the primary and the permanent dentitions is delayed in 75% of cases. Abnormalities in eruption sequence occur often. Hypodontia occurs in both dentitions, and microdontia is often seen. Developmental tooth anomalies, including crown and root malformations, are often present. Almost 50% of patients with Down syndrome exhibit three or more dental anomalies. Enamel hypocalcification occurs in about 20% of patients.

Occlusal disharmonies consisting of mesiocclusion due to a relative prognathism, posterior crossbites, apertognathia, and severe crowding of the anterior teeth are common. Posterior crossbites are of maxillary basal bone origin, whereas anterior open bites are due to dental-alveolar discrepancies.

Treatment and Prognosis. Infants with Down syndrome that includes significant congenital heart disease have a poor prognosis. Causes of death commonly include cardiopulmonary complications, gastrointestinal malformations, and acute lymphoblastic leukemia.

Recent technologic advances in cardiovascular diagnosis have brought about a marked improvement in the prognosis. Newborns require chest x-ray studies, electrocardiograms, echocardiograms, and subsequent pediatric cardiac consultation if cardiovascular anomalies are detected.

Regular ophthalmologic and audiologic follow-ups are extremely important. They can intercept early visual and hearing problems that may affect learning and development. Detection of atlantoaxial instability may prevent a catastrophic spinal injury.

Dental therapy is directed at prevention of dental caries and periodontal disease. Frequent follow-up and institution of stringent home care regimens are critical. Highly functioning children may be candidates for orthodontic intervention and subsequent maxillofacial surgery, if required. Guidelines established by the American Heart Association for antibiotic prophylaxis should be followed for those patients with congenital heart disease.

Hemifacial Atrophy

Hemifacial atrophy is a rare disorder that represents a progressive unilateral atrophy of the face. It may occasionally affect other regions on the same side of the body. The cause of this condition is totally unknown, although trauma, dysfunction of the peripheral nervous system, infection, and genetic abnormalities have been suggested.

Hemifacial atrophy typically appears during young adulthood. The most common early sign is a painless cleft or furrow near the midline of the face. The condition involves both soft tissue and bone of the affected side. Orally, the tongue, lips, and salivary glands may show hemiatrophy. Developing teeth may show incomplete root development and delayed eruption. Uni-

lateral involvement of the brain, ears, larynx, esophagus, diaphragm, and kidneys has been reported. Various associated ophthalmologic conditions are often encountered.

Progressive hemifacial atrophy associated with contralateral jacksonian epilepsy, trigeminal neuralgia, and changes in the eyes and hair is known as *Romberg's syndrome*. Unilateral atrophy of the upper lip with visible exposure of the maxillary teeth on the affected side is characteristic in moderately and severely involved cases.

The differential diagnosis should include facial hypoplasia, scleroderma, fat necrosis, and oculoauriculovertebral-related disorders. The distinction between Romberg's syndrome and localized scleroderma is often difficult and depends on the absence or presence of skin pigmentation and other inflammatory changes.

Hemifacial Hypertrophy

Congenital hemihypertrophy is a rare disorder characterized by gross body asymmetry. It may be simple, limited to a single digit; segmental, involving a specific region of the body; or complex, encompassing half the body. The enlargement is usually unilateral, although limited bilateral crossover does occur. All tissues in the region of abnormal growth may be involved, but a selective number of tissues are occasionally affected. Histologically, it has been determined that there is an actual increase in the number of cells present rather than an increase in cell size. It classically presents as a unilateral, localized overgrowth of the facial soft tissues, bones, and teeth (Figure 15-19).

Etiology and Pathogenesis. Gross asymmetry has been found in 1 in 86,000 patients, with a 3-to-2 female preponderance. In males involvement of the right side is more common. Almost all cases appear to be sporadic. There are equal numbers of segmental and complex forms, with neither side of the body exhibiting a greater incidence of involvement. Wilms' tumor is the most common neoplasm reported in association with hemihypertrophy.

Multiple etiologic factors have been implicated in the development of hemihypertrophy, including anatomic and functional vascular or lymphatic abnormalities, endocrine dysfunction, an altered intrauterine environment, central nervous system disturbances, chromosome abnormalities, and asymmetric cell division. Etiologic heterogeneity may be responsible for

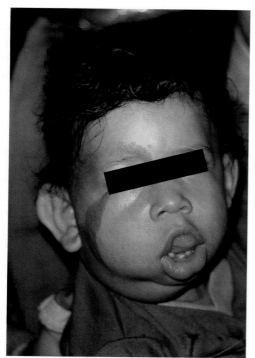

Figure 15-19 **Hemifacial hypertrophy** as part of epidermal nevus syndrome.

the varied clinical presentation, affecting single or multiple systems, and the degree of tissue involvement.

Clinical Features. The varieties and complexities of hemihypertrophy have resulted in a wide range of reported dentofacial findings. In some patients the face is involved solely, but unilateral facial enlargement is often associated with hypertrophy of a portion of the body. The tissues involved are often not affected uniformly, accentuating the variable clinical presentation.

Craniofacial findings include asymmetry of the frontal bone, maxilla, palate, mandible, alveolar process, condyles, and associated overlying soft tissue. The skin may be thickened, with excessive secretions by sebaceous and sweat glands and hypertrichosis. The pinnae are often remarkably enlarged. Unilateral enlargement of one of the cerebral hemispheres may be responsible for mental retardation in 15% to 20% of patients and for the occurrence of seizure disorders.

The oral findings are quite striking, affecting the dentition and tongue to a significant degree. The tongue is unilaterally hyperplastic and often distorted in appearance, with a distinct midline demarcation. The fungiform papillae are usually enlarged and resemble soft polypoid excrescences. Dysgeusia has been reported. Intraoral soft tissues are thickened and anatomically enlarged, often being described as overabundant and lying in soft, velvety folds.

Dental findings include abnormalities in crown size and root size and shape, as well as precocious development and eruption. The permanent canines, premolars, and first molars are most often enlarged. When the primary dentition is affected, abnormalities are limited to the second molars and, less commonly, the canines. Unilateral macrodontia approaches but does not exceed a 50% increase in crown dimension in mesiodistal and buccolingual diameters. Root size and shape are proportionately enlarged or uncommonly shortened, and premature apical development is usual. The primary teeth on the affected side calcify, erupt, and exfoliate sooner than the contralateral teeth. Eruption of the affected permanent teeth by age 4 or 5 years has been reported.

Dental malocclusions are common because of asymmetric growth of the maxilla, mandible, and alveolar process and abnormalities of tooth morphology and eruption patterns. Midline deviations, severely canted occlusal planes, and open bites are common.

Lateral and posterior-anterior cephalograms demonstrate pronounced bony asymmetry and facial bone hypertrophy, as well as evidence of hypertrophied soft tissues, such as tonsillar enlargement. Root anomalies, crown enlargement, and evidence of premature eruption are easily identifiable by panoramic or periapical radiography.

Differential Diagnosis. The diagnosis of true congenital hemifacial hypertrophy rests on the presence of unilateral hypertrophy of the craniofacial structures and associated soft tissue, including the dentition. Perception of contralateral dissimilarity may be difficult and often subjective, resulting in delayed diagnosis of congenital hemifacial hypertrophy in the infant. Angioosteohypertrophy (Klippel-Trénaunay-Weber syndrome) can be ruled out by the absence of an overlying cutaneous nevus flammeus. Neurofibromatosis may cause gross enlargement of the soft tissue and skeleton of half the face, but it does not affect tooth size or the eruption sequence. Lymphangioma and hemangioma are characterized by soft tissue enlargement; they do not affect tooth morphology. Acromegaly produces symmetric bilateral jaw enlargement. Fibrous dysplasia, craniofacial dysostosis, and chronic inflammatory diseases should also be ruled out.

Congenital hemifacial hypertrophy has been reported concomitantly with conductive hearing loss, seizure disorders, and Wilms' tumor. Other syndromes and conditions that produce soft and hard tissue hypertrophy and asymmetry include Russell's (or Russell-Silver) syndrome, congenital lymphedema, arteriovenous aneurysms, multiple exostoses, and facial tumors of childhood.

Treatment and Prognosis. During infancy and childhood, patients should be examined frequently to facilitate early identification of potential neoplasms involving the liver, adrenal glands, and kidneys. Growth and development should be observed closely for evidence of mental impairment or abnormalities of sexual development.

Abnormalities during the mixed dentition phase relate to tooth size–arch size discrepancies and abnormalities in the eruption sequence. Asymmetric growth of the craniofacial complex and dental alveolus require early orthodontic intervention, including space maintenance, minor tooth movement, and functional appliances. Surgical reconstruction of hard and soft tissue anomalies to improve function and aesthetics must be anticipated.

The common association of congenital hemihypertrophy with vascular anomalies, embryonal neoplasms, and mental retardation requires a multidisciplinary team of dental and medical specialists.

Clefts of the Lip and Palate

Clefts of the lip and palate are commonly encountered congenital anomalies that often result in severe functional deficits of speech, mastication, and deglutition. The prevalence of associated congenital malformations, as well as learning disabilities secondary to hearing deficits, is often increased.

Generally, clefts of the lip and palate are classified into four major types: (1) cleft lip, (2) cleft palate, (3) unilateral cleft lip and palate, and (4) bilateral cleft lip and palate. Other clefts of the lip and mouth include lip pits, linear lip indentations, submucosal clefts of the palate, bifid uvula and tongue, and numerous facial clefts extending through the nose, lips, and oral cavity. Clefting deformities are extremely variable in character; they may range from furrows in the skin and mucosa to extensive cleavages involving muscle and bone. A combination of cleft lip and palate is the most common clefting deformity seen.

Etiology and Pathogenesis. Cleft lip and palate account for approximately 50% of all cases, whereas isolated cleft lip and isolated cleft palate each occur in about 25%

of cases. The incidence of cleft lip and cleft palate has been reported to be 1 in 700 to 1000 births, with variable racial predilection. Isolated cleft palate is less common, with an incidence of 1 in 1500 to 3000 births. Cleft lip with or without cleft palate is more common in males, and cleft palate alone is more common in females.

The majority of cases of cleft lip or cleft palate, or both, can be explained by the multifactorial threshold hypothesis. The multifactorial inheritance theory implies that many contributory risk genes interact with one another and the environment and collectively determine whether a threshold of abnormality is breached, resulting in a defect in the developing fetus. Multifactorial or polygenic inheritance explains the transmission of isolated cleft lip or palate, and it is extremely useful in predicting occurrence risks of this anomaly among family members of an affected individual.

Disruption of normal patterns of facial growth, including deficiencies of any of the facial processes, may lead to maldevelopment of the lips and palate. Cleft lip generally occurs at about the sixth to seventh week in utero; it is a result of failure of the epithelial groove between the medial and the lateral nasal processes to be penetrated by mesodermal cells.

Cleft palate is a result of epithelial breakdown at about the eighth week of embryonic development, with ingrowth failure of mesodermal tissue and lack of lateral palatal segment fusion. Most embryologists believe that true tissue deficiencies exist in all clefting deformities and that actual anatomic structures are absent. Various degrees of cleft lip and palate may occur, ranging from mild notching of the vermilion border or bifid uvula to severe bilateral complete clefts of the lip, alveolus, and entire palate.

Clinical Features. The Veau system of classification for cleft lip and palate is widely used by clinicians; it helps to describe the variety of lip and palatal clefts seen. The system classifies cleft lip and cleft palate separately into four major categories, with emphasis on the degree of clefting present.

Cleft lip may vary from a pit or small notch in the vermilion border to a complete cleft extending into the floor of the nose (Figures 15-20 to 15-22). Using the Veau classification, a class I cleft of the lip is a unilateral notching of the vermilion border that does not extend into the lip. If the unilateral notching of the vermilion extends into the lip but does not involve the floor of the nose, it is designated as a class II cleft.

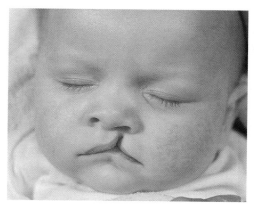

Figure 15-20 Cleft lip.

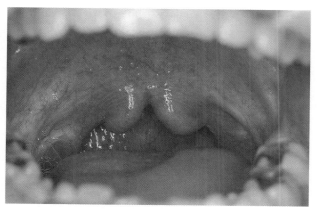

Figure 15-22 Cleft (bifid) uvula.

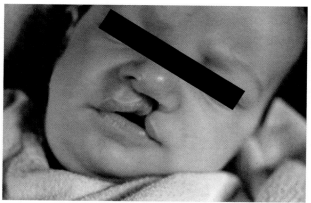

Figure 15-21 **Complete unilateral cleft** extending through the alveolus and into the floor of the nose.

Class III lip clefts are unilateral clefts of the vermilion border extending through the lip into the floor of the nose. Any bilateral cleft of the lip, exhibiting incomplete notching or a complete cleft, is classified as a class IV cleft.

Clefting deformities of the palate can also be divided into four clinical types using the Veau system. A cleft limited to the soft palate is a class I palatal cleft. Class II clefts are defects of the hard and soft palate; they extend no farther than the incisive foramen and therefore are limited to the secondary palate only. Clefts of the secondary palate may be complete or incomplete. A complete cleft includes the soft and hard palate, extending to the incisive foramen. An incomplete cleft involves the velum and a portion of the hard palate, not extending to the incisive foramen. Complete unilateral clefts extending from the uvula to the incisive foramen in the midline and the alveolar process uni-

laterally are designated as class III palatal clefts. Class IV clefts are complete bilateral clefts involving the soft and hard palate and the alveolar process on both sides of the premaxilla, leaving it free and often mobile.

Submucosal clefts are not included in this system of classification, but they can be identified clinically by the presence of a bifid uvula, palpable notching of the posterior portion of the hard and soft palate, and the presence of a zona pellucida (a thin, translucent membrane) covering the defect.

Clefts of the soft palate, including submucosal clefts, are often associated with velopharyngeal incompetence or eustachian tube dysfunction. Recurrent otitis media and hearing deficits are common complications. Palatal pharyngeal incompetence results from failure of the soft palate and pharyngeal wall to make contact during swallowing and speech, thus preventing the necessary muscular seal between the nasopharynx and the oropharynx. Speech is often characterized by air emission from the nose and has a hypernasal quality.

The prevalence of dental anomalies associated with cleft lip and palate is remarkable. Abnormalities of tooth number, size, morphology, calcification, and eruption have been well described. Both deciduous and permanent dentitions may be affected. The lateral incisor in the vicinity of the cleft is often involved, but teeth outside the cleft area exhibit developmental defects to a greater degree than is seen in unaffected patients.

The incidence of congenitally missing teeth is high, especially among deciduous and permanent maxillary lateral incisors adjacent to the alveolar cleft. The prevalence of hypodontia increases directly with the severity of the cleft. Complete unilateral and bilateral alveolar clefts are often associated with supernumerary teeth as well, usually the maxillary lateral incisors. Tooth formation is often delayed, and enamel hypoplasia, microdontia or macrodontia, and fused teeth are often seen.

Treatment and Prognosis. The prognosis is dependent on the severity of the clefting disorder. Aesthetic considerations and hearing and speech deficits often result in significant developmental problems.

Treatment is chronologically sequenced and often requires a multidisciplinary team concept because of the extensive nature of the problem and its impact on the child and the immediate family. Craniofacial or cleft palate teams are made up of dental, medical, and surgical specialists, with the assistance of allied health professionals in social services, child development, and hearing and speech therapy.

Generally, cleft lip repair is accomplished during early infancy when the child is stable, weighs at least 10 pounds, and has hemoglobin levels of 10 mg/dl. Cheiloplasty is often required later in life. Orthodontic or surgically placed orthopedic devices are being used in infants to guide the dentoalveolar segments into normal anatomic relationships and facilitate plastic surgical closure. Closure of soft palate defects with sliding or pharyngeal flaps by 1 year of age is often recommended to promote normal speech development. Palatal obturators are often fabricated for infants who have cleft palate disorders and who are having difficulty feeding or are regurgitating food or liquids through the nasal cavity. Early audiologic and speech evaluation is highly recommended, and hearing aids are often indicated to prevent associated learning problems in children who have cleft palate and frequent episodes of otitis media. Chronic otitis media and associated low-frequency hearing loss are results of improper orientation of the eustachian tubes and inserting muscles, resulting in middle ear fluid stasis and retrograde infection.

Preventive dental services are extremely important, because an intact dentition is the foundation for future orthodontic therapy. Treatment is often required to correct developmental dental defects. Orthodontic treatment is sometimes initiated during the primary dentition to correct unilateral and bilateral posterior maxillary crossbites and to retract an anteriorly displaced premaxillary segment.

Once into the mixed dentition phase of development, conventional orthodontic therapy is initiated to establish a normal maxillary arch form. This is often done in preparation for an autogenous bone graft (commonly iliac crest) to the alveolar cleft to reestablish maxillary arch continuity. It is recommended that the grafting procedure be performed when root formation of the unerupted permanent tooth associated with the alveolar defect (usually the maxillary canine) has reached one-quarter to one-half completion. These teeth have been shown to successfully erupt passively or mechanically through the graft site, consolidating the arch, preserving the graft, and reestablishing alveolar competence.

Further orthodontic treatment, followed by orthognathic surgery, is often required for those patients with significant dentofacial deformities. Frequent plastic surgical procedures to correct the aesthetics and function of the vermilion border, lip, philtrum, and nose can be anticipated.

Fragile X Syndrome

It has long been recognized that of mentally deficient in the general population, more men than women are affected. The large percentage of mentally disabled males and historical documentation of families with affected male and unaffected female children are highly suggestive of an X-linked inheritance pattern. Since the report in 1943 of a family with 11 severely retarded males delivered to an apparently unaffected mother, multiple case reports have identified a syndrome (fragile X syndrome) characterized by X-linked mental retardation, macroorchidism, and a characteristic phenotypic presentation.

Etiology and Pathogenesis. The fragile X syndrome, believed to account for 30% to 50% of all families with X-linked mental retardation, takes its name from an identifiable fragile site on the X chromosome that is a reliable diagnostic marker. It is now recognized that X-linked mental retardation may be as common as Down syndrome in males; it accounts for approximately 25% of all mentally disabled males, with an incidence of 0.3 to 1 affected child per 1000 male births. The finding of 20% to 30% of female carriers with various degrees of mental retardation may be explained by lyonization or random inactivation of one of the X chromosomes.

The family history remains the primary tool for recognition of patients with X-linked mental retardation. In the fragile X syndrome, specific cytogenetic studies can aid in the diagnosis. In affected males 4% to 50% (median, 20%) of cells exhibit the chromosome change—an abnormal secondary constriction near the terminal end of the long arm (q) of the X chromosome. This segment is often broken and has been termed the *fragile site*. In 50% of female carriers the fragile X chromosome cannot be detected at all. Abnormalities of speech have also been noted in the fragile X syndrome, and it has been theorized that major genes related to verbal function are located on the X chromosome and are disrupted at the fragile site. Recent genetic and biochemical studies have isolated a specific nucleotide alteration. This involves an expanded CGG repeat at one end (5′) of the FMR1 gene, which in turn is related to a methylation step in the production of FMR protein. Degrees of altered methylation by way of FMR gene product may help explain the range of clinical findings.

Clinical Features. The classic clinical presentation is that of a mentally retarded male with postpubescent macroorchidism, large ears, prognathism, and a long, narrow face with a high forehead and prominent supraorbital ridges (Figure 15-23). Other findings include hyperextensible joints, mitral valve prolapse, cleft palate, and an association with Pierre Robin syndrome. Patients have a characteristic repetitive jocular speech and may exhibit hyperactive behavior or autism. The characteristic speech pattern, termed *cluttering,* is hurried and presents as repetitive sentences that come out in a rush. The hands are often large and fleshy, and the iris may be pale. Hand biting has been reported. Oral findings include a high-arched palate, prominent lateral palatine ridges, anterior and posterior dental crossbites, and increased occlusal attrition. A high-normal birth weight is common, and an increased head circumference during infancy and childhood is noted.

The degree of mental retardation is variable, even among affected siblings. Results of testicular biopsies and endocrine function tests are found to be within normal limits.

Treatment and Prognosis. The significance of identification of X-linked retardation in families cannot be over-

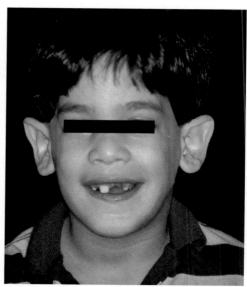

Figure 15-23 **Fragile X syndrome,** consisting of mental retardation, a long narrow face, and large ears.

emphasized. Because the syndrome is inherited as an X-linked trait and the fragile X site can be identified in 30% to 50% of families with X-linked mental retardation, early diagnosis and genetic counseling are imperative.

Fragile X syndrome screening of the mentally retarded population has proved to be cost-effective. Genetic counseling of families with positive histories may help to advise potential or proven carriers of the risks of bearing an affected child. The only reliable means of prenatal diagnosis currently is by examination of fetal chromosomes. There is no method of excluding carrier status in females who do not express the fragile X chromosome.

Mitral valve prolapse has been reported to occur in as many as 80% of males affected with this syndrome, supporting the need for definitive cardiac evaluation before dental therapy.

BIBLIOGRAPHY

METABOLIC CONDITIONS

Bernstein RM, Zaleske DJ: Familial aspects of Caffey's disease, *Am J Orthop* 24:777-781, 1995.

Carrillo R, Morales A, Rodriguez-Peralto JL, et al: Benign fibroosseous lesions in Paget's disease of the jaws, *Oral Surg Oral Med Oral Pathol* 71:588-592, 1991.

Dickson GR, Hamilton A, Hayes D, et al: An investigation of vanishing bone disease, *Bone* 11:205-210, 1990.

Dunbar SF, Rosenberg A, Mankin H, et al: Gorham's massive osteolysis: the role of radiation therapy and a review of the literature, *Int J Radiol Oncol Biol Phys* 26:491-497, 1993.

Ezzat S, Forster MJ, Berchtold P, et al: Acromegaly: clinical and biochemical features in 500 patients, *Medicine* 73:233-240, 1994.

Freedy RM, Bell KA: Massive osteolysis (Gorham's disease) of the temporomandibular joint, *Ann Otol Rhinol Laryngol* 101:1018-1020, 1992.

Houston MS, Hay ID: Practical management of hyperthyroidism, *Am Fam Physician* 41:909-916, 1990.

Kanzler A, Farmand M, DiGiacomi B, et al: Pathologic changes in the face and skull in acromegaly, *Swiss Dent J* 13:35-44, 1992.

Melmed S: Acromegaly, *N Engl J Med* 322:966-977, 1990.

Merkow RL, Lane JM: Paget's disease of bone, *Orthop Clin North Am* 21:171-189, 1990.

Olsson A, Matsson L, Blomquist HK, et al: Hypophosphatasia affecting the permanent dentition, *J Oral Pathol Med* 25:343-347, 1996.

Parisien M, Silverberg SJ, Shane E, et al: Bone disease in primary hyperparathyroidism, *Endocrinol Metab Clin North Am* 19:19-34, 1990.

Petti GH Jr: Hyperparathyroidism, *Otolaryngol Clin North Am* 23:339-355, 1990.

Piatelli A: Symmetrical pulpal obliteration in mandibular first molars, *J Endod* 18:515-516, 1992.

Reginster JY, Lecont MP: Efficacy and safety of drugs for Paget's disease of bone, *Bone* 17(suppl 5):485S-488S, 1995.

Szabo J, Heath B, Hill VM, et al: Hereditary hyperparathyroidism-jaw tumor syndrome: the endocrine gene HRPT2 maps to chromosome 1q21-q31, *Am J Hum Genet* 56:944-950, 1995.

Thomas DW, Tate RJ, Shepherd JP: Paget's disease of bone: current concepts in pathogenesis and treatment, *J Oral Pathol Med* 23:12-16, 1994.

Thometz JG, DiRaimiondi CA: A case of recurrent Caffey's disease treated with naproxen, *Clin Orthop* 323:304-309, 1996.

van Damme PA, Mooren RE: Differentiation of multiple giant cell lesions, Noonan-like syndrome and (occult) hyperparathyroidism, *Int J Oral Maxillofac Surg* 23:32-36, 1994.

GENETIC ABNORMALITIES

Augarten A, Sagy M, Yahav J, et al: Management of upper airway obstruction in Pierre Robin syndrome, *Br J Oral Maxillofac Surg* 28:105-108, 1990.

Bull MJ, Givan DC, Sadove AM, et al: Improved outcome in Pierre Robin syndrome: effect of multidisciplinary evaluation and management, *Pediatrics* 86:294-301, 1990.

de Vries BB, Jansen CC, Duits AA, et al: Variable FMR1 gene methylation of large expansions leads to variable phenotype in three males from one fragile X family, *J Med Genet* 33:1007-1010, 1996.

Felix R, Hofstetter W, Cecchini MG: Recent developments in the understanding of osteopetrosis, *Eur J Endocrinol* 134:143-156, 1996.

Fraser FC: The genetics of cleft lip and cleft palate, *Am J Hum Genet* 22:336-352, 1970.

Fridrich KL, Fridrich HH, Kempf KK, et al: Dental implications in Ehlers-Danlos syndrome, *Oral Surg Oral Med Oral Pathol* 69:431-435, 1990.

Gluckman E: Bone marrow transplantation in children with hereditary disorders, *Curr Opin Pediatr* 8:42-44, 1996.

Gorlin RJ, Cohen MM, Levin LS: *Syndromes of the head and neck,* ed 3, New York, 1990, Oxford University Press.

Jacenko O: *c-fos* and bone loss: a proto-oncogene regulator osteoclast lineage determination, *Bioassays* 17:277-281, 1995.

Jensen BL, Kreiborg S: Development of the dentition in cleidocranial dysplasia, *J Oral Pathol Med* 19:89-93, 1990.

Jones JE, Friend GW: Cleft orthotics and obturation, *Oral Maxillofac Surg Clin North Am* 3:517-529, 1991.

Kainulainen K, Pulkkinen L, Savolainen A, et al: Location on chromosome 15 of the gene defect causing Marfan syndrome, *N Engl J Med* 323:935-939, 1990.

Kivirikko KI: Collagens and their abnormalities in a wide spectrum of diseases, *Ann Med* 25:113-126, 1993.

Loesch DZ, Hay DA, Mulley J: Transmitting males and carrier females in fragile X—revisited, *Am J Med Genet* 51:392-399, 1994.

Mundlos S, Otto F, Mulliken JB, et al: Mutations involving the transcription factor CBFA1 cause cleidocranial dysplasia, *Cell* 89:773-779, 1997.

Mundy GR: Cytokines and local factors which affect osteoclast function, *Int J Cell Cloning* 10:215-222, 1992.

Nunn JH, Durning P: Fragile X (Martin Bell) syndrome and dental care, *Br Dent J* 168:160, 1990.

Prockop DJ, Kivirikko KI: Collagens: molecular biology, diseases, and potentials for therapy, *Annu Rev Biochem* 64:403-434, 1995.

Prockop DJ, Kuivaniemi H, Tromp G: Molecular basis of osteogenesis imperfecta and related disorders of bone, *Clin Plast Surg* 21:407-413, 1994.

Ramesar RS, Greenberg J, Martin R, et al: Mapping of the gene for cleidocranial dysplasia in historical Cape Town (Arnold) kindred and evidence for locus homogeneity, *J Med Genet* 33:511-514, 1996.

Ranalli DN, Guzman R, Schmutz JA: Craniofacial and intraoral manifestations of congenital hemifacial hyperplasia: report of case, *ASDC J Dent Child* 57:203-208, 1990.

Reinhardt DP, Chalberg SC, Sakai LY: The structure and function of fibrillin, *Ciba Found Symp* 192:128-143, 1995.

Richardson A, Deussen FF: Facial and dental anomalies in cleidocranial dysplasia: a study of 17 cases, *Int J Pediatr Dent* 4:225-231, 1994.

Rousseau F, Heitz D, Biancalana V, et al: Direct diagnosis by DNA analysis of the fragile X syndrome of mental retardation, *N Engl J Med* 325:1673-1681, 1991.

Spengler DE: Staging in cleft lip and palate habilitation, *Oral Maxillofac Surg Clin North Am* 3:489-499, 1991.

Tiegs RD: Heritable metabolic and dysplastic bone diseases, *Endocrinol Metab Clin North Am* 19:133-173, 1990.

Tiziani V, Reichenberger E, Buzzo CL, et al: The gene for cherubism maps to chromosome 4p16, *Am J Hum Genet* 65(1):158-166, 1999.

Trummer T, Brenner R, Just W, et al: Recurrent mutations in the COL1A2 gene in patients with osteogenesis imperfecta, *Clin Genet* 59(5):338-342, 2001.

Ueki Y, Tiziani V, Santanna C, et al: Mutations in the gene encoding c-abl-binding protein SH3 BP2 cause cherubism, *Nat Genet* 28(2):125-126, 2001.

Ulseth JO, Hestnes A, Stovner LJ, et al: Dental caries and periodontitis in persons with Down syndrome, *Special Care Dent* 11:71-74, 1991.

Ward LM, Lalic L, Roughly PJ, et al: Thirty three novel COL1A1 and COL1A2 mutations in patients with osteogenesis imperfecta types I-IV, *Hum Mutat* 17(5):434-439, 2001.

Yeswell HN, Pinnell SR: The Ehlers-Danlos syndromes, *Semin Dermatol* 12:229-240, 1993.

ABNORMALITIES OF TEETH

ALTERATIONS IN SIZE

Microdontia

In generalized microdontia all teeth in the dentition appear smaller than normal. Teeth may actually be measurably smaller than normal, as in pituitary dwarfism, or they may be relatively small in comparison with a large mandible and maxilla.

In focal, or localized, microdontia a single tooth is smaller than normal. The shape of these microdonts is also often altered with the reduced size. This phenomenon is most commonly seen with maxillary lateral incisors in which the tooth crown appears cone or peg shaped, prompting the designation *peg lateral* (Figure 16-1). An autosomal-dominant inheritance pattern has been associated with this condition. Peg laterals are of no significance other than cosmetic appearance. The second most commonly seen microdont is the maxillary third molar, followed by supernumerary teeth (Figure 16-2).

Macrodontia

Generalized macrodontia is characterized by the appearance of enlarged teeth throughout the dentition. This may be absolute, as seen in pituitary gigantism, or it may be relative owing to a disproportionately small maxilla and mandible. The latter results in crowding of teeth and possibly an abnormal eruption pattern because of insufficient arch space.

Focal, or localized, macrodontia is characterized by an abnormally large tooth or group of teeth. This relatively uncommon condition is usually seen with mandibular third molars. In the rare condition known as *hemifacial hypertrophy,* teeth on the affected side are abnormally large compared with the unaffected side.

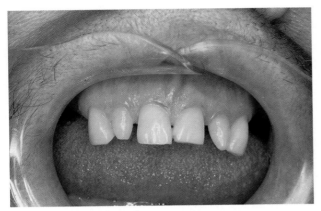

Figure 16-1   Peg laterals.

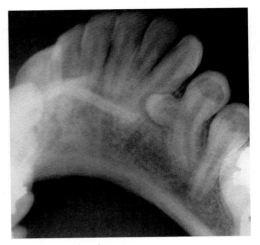

Figure 16-3   Gemination.

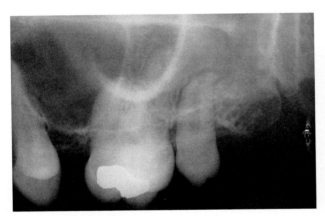

Figure 16-2   Microdont.

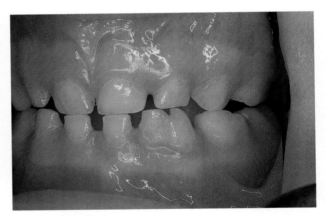

Figure 16-4   Fusion.

ALTERATIONS IN SHAPE

Gemination

Gemination is the fusion of two teeth from a single enamel organ (Figure 16-3). The typical result is partial cleavage, with the appearance of two crowns that share the same root canal. Complete cleavage, or twinning, occasionally occurs, resulting in two teeth from one tooth germ. Although trauma has been suggested as a possible cause, the cause of gemination is unknown. These teeth may be cosmetically unacceptable and may cause crowding.

Fusion

Fusion is the joining of two developing tooth germs, resulting in a single large tooth structure (Figures 16-4 and 16-5). The fusion process may involve the entire length of the teeth, or it may involve the roots only, in which case cementum and dentin are shared. Root canals may also be separate or shared. It may be impossible to differentiate fusion of normal and supernumerary teeth from gemination. The cause of this condition is unknown, although trauma has been suggested.

Concrescence

Concrescence is a form of fusion in which the adjacent, already-formed teeth are joined by cementum (Figure 16-6). This may take place before or after eruption of teeth and is believed to be related to trauma or overcrowding. Concrescence is most commonly seen in association with the maxillary second and third molars. This condition is of no significance,

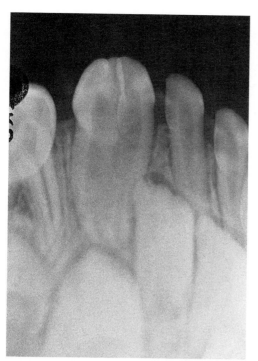

Figure 16-5 Fusion.

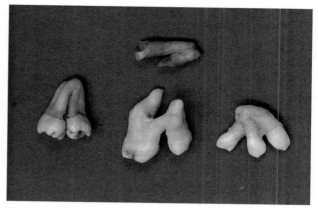

Figure 16-6 Concrescence.

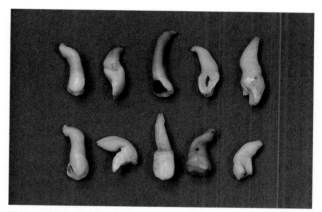

Figure 16-7 Dilaceration.

unless one of the teeth involved requires extraction. Surgical sectioning may be required to save the other tooth.

Dilaceration

Dilaceration is an extraordinary curving or angulation of tooth roots (Figure 16-7). The cause of this condition has been related to trauma during root development. Movement of the crown or of the crown and part of the root from the remaining developing root may result in sharp angulation after the tooth completes development. Hereditary factors are believed to be involved in a small number of cases. Eruption generally continues without problems. However, extraction may be difficult. Obviously, if root canal fillings are required in these teeth, the procedure is challenging.

Dens Invaginatus

Also known as dens in dente or tooth within a tooth, dens invaginatus is an uncommon tooth anomaly that represents an exaggeration or accentuation of the lingual pit (Figures 16-8 and 16-9).

This defect ranges in severity from superficial, in which only the crown is affected, to deep, in which both the crown and the root are involved. The permanent maxillary lateral incisors are most commonly involved, although any anterior tooth may be affected. Bilateral involvement is commonly seen. The cause of this developmental condition is unknown. Genetic factors are believed to be involved in only a small percentage of cases.

Because the defect cannot be kept free of plaque and bacteria, dens invaginatus predisposes the tooth to early decay and subsequent pulpitis. Prophylactic filling of the pit is recommended to avoid this complication. Because the defect may often be identified on radiographic examination before tooth eruption, the patient can be prepared in advance of the procedure. In cases in which pulpitis has led to nonvitality, endodontic procedures may salvage the affected tooth.

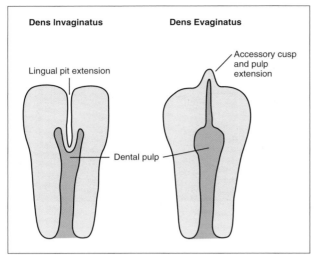

Figure 16-8   Morphology of dens invaginatus and dens evaginatus.

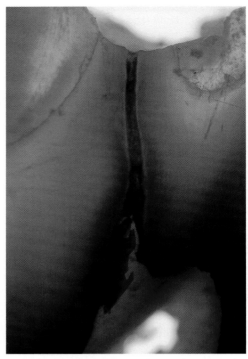

Figure 16-10   **Dens evaginatus.** Ground section showing pulpal extension through dentin to the surface of a worn occlusal cusp.

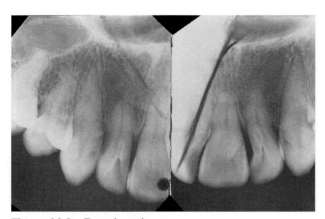

Figure 16-9   **Dens invaginatus.**

Dens Evaginatus

Dens evaginatus is a relatively common developmental condition affecting predominantly premolar teeth (Leung's premolars) (Figure 16-10). It has been reported almost exclusively in Asians, Inuits, and Native Americans. The defect, which is often bilateral, is an anomalous tubercle, or cusp, located in the center of the occlusal surface. Because of occlusal abrasion, the tubercle wears relatively quickly, causing early exposure of an accessory pulp horn that extends into the tubercle. This may result in periapical pathology in young, caries-free teeth, often before completion of root development and apical closure, making root canal fillings more difficult. Judicious grinding of the

opposing tooth or the accessory tubercle to stimulate secondary dentin formation may prevent the periapical sequelae associated with this defect.

Taurodontism

Taurodontism is a variation in tooth form in which teeth have elongated crowns or apically displaced furcations, resulting in pulp chambers that have increased apical-occlusal height (Figure 16-11). Because this abnormality resembles teeth in bulls and other ungulates, the term *taurodontism* was coined. Various degrees of severity may be seen, but subclassifications that have been developed to describe them appear to be of academic interest only. Taurodontism may be seen as an isolated incident, in families, and in association with syndromes such as Down syndrome and Klinefelter's syndrome; it was also seen in the now extinct Neanderthals. Although taurodontism is generally an uncommon finding, it has been reported to have a relatively high prevalence in Eskimos, and it has been reported to be as high as 11% in a Middle Eastern population. Other than a possible relationship to other genetically determined abnormalities, tau-

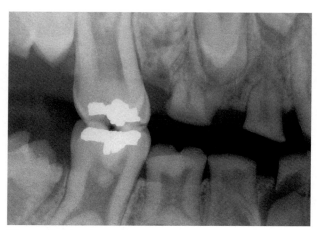

Figure 16-11   Taurodontism.

rodontism is of little clinical significance. No treatment is required.

Supernumerary Roots

Accessory roots are most commonly seen in mandibular canines, premolars, and molars (especially third molars). They are rarely found in upper anterior teeth and mandibular incisors. Radiographic recognition of an extraordinary number of roots becomes important when extractions or root canal fillings are necessary.

Enamel Pearls

Droplets of ectopic enamel, or so-called enamel pearls, may occasionally be found on the roots of teeth (Figure 16-12). They occur most commonly in the bifurcation or trifurcation of teeth but may appear on single-rooted premolar teeth as well. Maxillary molars are more commonly affected than are mandibular molars. These deposits are occasionally supported by dentin and rarely may have a pulp horn extending into them. This developmental disturbance of enamel formation may be detected on radiographic examination. It is generally of little significance except when located in an area of periodontal disease. In such cases it may contribute to the extension of a periodontal pocket because a periodontal ligament attachment would not be expected and hygiene would be more difficult.

Attrition, Abrasion, Erosion

Attrition is the physiologic wearing of teeth as a result of mastication. It is an age-related process and varies from one individual to another. Factors such as diet,

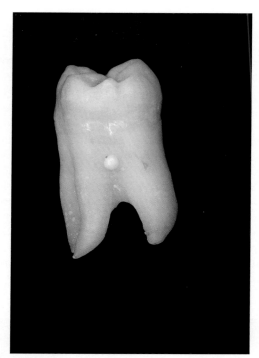

Figure 16-12   Enamel pearl.

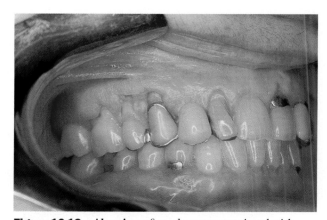

Figure 16-13   **Abrasion** of tooth roots associated with toothbrushing.

dentition, jaw musculature, and chewing habits can significantly influence the pattern and extent of attrition.

Abrasion is the pathologic wearing of teeth as a result of an abnormal habit or abnormal use of abrasive substances orally (Figures 16-13 and 16-14). Pipe smoking, tobacco chewing, aggressive toothbrushing, and use of abrasive dentifrices are among the more common causes. The location and pattern of abrasion are directly dependent on the cause, with so-called toothbrush abrasion along the cementoenamel junction an easily recognized pattern.

Erosion is the loss of tooth structure from a non-bacterial chemical process (Figure 16-15). Most commonly, acids are involved in the dissolution process from either an external or an internal source. Externally, the acid may be found in the work environment (e.g., battery manufacturing) or in the diet (e.g., citrus fruits and acid-containing soft drinks). The internal source of acid is most probably from regurgitation of gastric contents. This may be seen in any disorder in which chronic vomiting is a part. Self-induced vomiting, as a component of bulimia or, less commonly, anorexia nervosa, has become an increasingly important cause of dental erosion and other oral abnormalities. The pattern of erosion associated with vomiting is usually generalized tooth loss on the lingual surfaces of maxillary teeth. However, all surfaces may be affected, especially in individuals who compensate for fluid loss by excessive intake of fruit juices. In many cases of tooth erosion no cause is found.

ALTERATIONS IN NUMBER

Anodontia

Absence of teeth is known as *anodontia*. This condition is further qualified as complete anodontia, when all teeth are missing; as partial anodontia or hypodontia, when one or several teeth are missing (Figure 16-16); as pseudoanodontia, when teeth are absent clinically because of impaction or delayed eruption; or as false anodontia, when teeth have been exfoliated or extracted. Partial anodontia is relatively common. Congenitally missing teeth are usually third molars, followed by second premolars and maxillary lateral incisors.

Traditionally, hypodontia has been thought to be the result of a single dominant gene. More recent evidence using two multiple threshold models has shown that hypodontia better fits a polygenic (caused by both environmental and genetic factors) rather than a single major gene model. The prevalence of any type of hypodontia in the general population is 4.6%, and there is no significant difference between males and females. The prevalence of maxillary lateral incisor absence is 2.1% and is significantly lower in males than in females. The prevalence of absence of the second premolars is 1.9% for the general population, with no significant difference between males and females. These findings suggest that different forms of hypodontia may be caused by, or be associated with, different

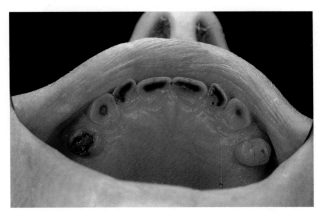

Figure 16-14   **Abrasion** of teeth associated with cigar chewing.

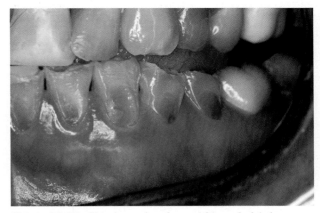

Figure 16-15   **Erosion** related to acid in soft drinks.

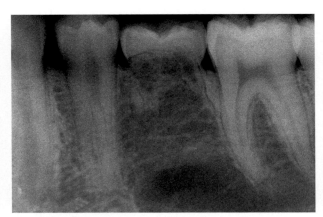

Figure 16-16   **Anodontia** of a permanent second premolar with ankylosis of an erupted primary molar.

gene loci or genetic factors. However, the gene responsible for oligodontia or hypodontia has not yet been located.

Complete anodontia is rare but is often associated with a syndrome known as *hereditary ectodermal dysplasia,* which is usually transmitted as an X-linked recessive disorder. Partial anodontia is more typical of this syndrome, however (Figures 16-17 and 16-18). The few teeth that are present are usually conical.

Impaction

Impaction of teeth is a common event that most often affects the mandibular third molars and maxillary cuspids. Less commonly, premolars, mandibular cuspids, and second molars are involved. It is rare to see impactions of incisors and first molars. Impaction occurs because of obstruction from crowding or from some other physical barrier. It may occasionally be due to an abnormal eruption path, presumably because of unusual orientation of the tooth germ. *Ankylosis,* the fusion of a tooth to surrounding bone, is another cause of impaction. This usually occurs in association with erupted primary molars. It may result in impaction of a subjacent permanent tooth. The reason for ankylosis is unknown, but it is believed to be related to periapical inflammation and subsequent bone repair. With the focal loss of the periodontal ligament, bone and cementum become inextricably mixed, causing fusion of the tooth to alveolar bone.

Supernumerary Teeth

Extra, or supernumerary, teeth in the dentition most probably result from continued proliferation of the permanent or primary dental lamina to form a third tooth germ (Figure 16-19). The resulting teeth may have a normal morphology or may be rudimentary and miniature. Most are isolated events, although some may be familial and others may be syndrome associated (Gardner's syndrome and cleidocranial dysplasia). Supernumerary teeth are found more often in the permanent dentition than in the primary dentition and are much more commonly seen in the maxilla than in the mandible (10 to 1). The anterior midline of the maxilla is the most common site, in which case the supernumerary tooth is known as a *mesiodens* (Figures 16-20 and 16-21). The maxillary molar area (fourth molar or paramolar) is the second most common site. The significance of supernumerary teeth is that they occupy space. When they are impacted,

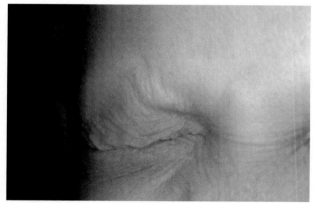

Figure 16-18 **Hereditary ectodermal dysplasia** resulting in lack of hair (including eyebrows and eyelashes) and poorly developed sweat glands.

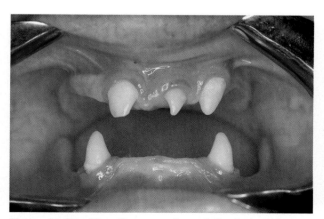

Figure 16-17 **Hereditary ectodermal dysplasia** with **partial anodontia (hypodontia).**

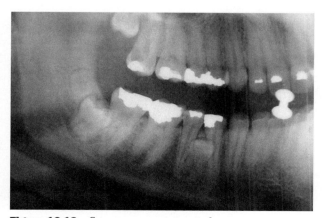

Figure 16-19 **Supernumerary premolar.**

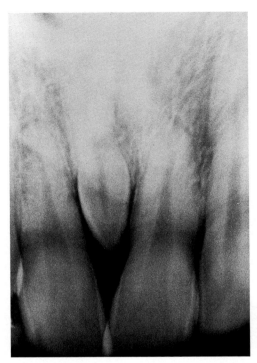

Figure 16-20 Mesiodens.

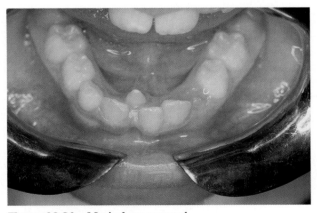

Figure 16-21 **Mesiodens** erupted.

they may block the eruption of other teeth, or they may cause delayed eruption or maleruption of adjacent teeth. If supernumerary teeth erupt, they may cause malalignment of the dentition, and they may be cosmetically objectionable.

Supernumerary teeth appearing at the time of birth, known as *natal teeth,* are believed to be a rare event. More commonly seen are prematurely erupted deciduous teeth, usually mandibular central incisors. Not to be confused with either of these phenomena is the appearance of the common gingival or dental lamina cysts of the newborn.

Supernumerary teeth appearing after the loss of the permanent teeth are known as *postpermanent dentition.* This is generally regarded as a rare event. Most teeth appearing after extraction of the permanent teeth are believed to arise from eventual eruption of previously impacted teeth.

DEFECTS OF ENAMEL

Environmental Defects of Enamel

During enamel formation, ameloblasts are susceptible to various external factors that may be reflected in erupted teeth. Metabolic injury, if severe enough and long enough, can cause defects in the quantity and shape of enamel or in the quality and color of enamel. Quantitatively defective enamel, when of normal hardness, is known as *enamel* hypoplasia (Figures 16-22 and 16-23). Qualitatively defective enamel, in which normal amounts of enamel are produced but are hypomineralized, is known as *enamel hypocalcification* (Figure 16-24). In this defect the enamel is softer than normal. The extent of the enamel defect is dependent on three conditions: (1) the intensity of the etiologic factor, (2) the duration of the factor's presence, and (3) the time at which the factor occurs during crown development. The factors that lead to ameloblast damage are highly varied, although the clinical signs of defective enamel are the same.

Etiologic factors may occur locally, affecting only a single tooth, or they may act systemically, affecting all teeth in which enamel is being formed. Local trauma or abscess formation can adversely affect the ameloblasts overlying a developing crown, resulting in enamel hypocalcification or hypoplasia. Affected teeth may have areas of coronal discoloration, or they may have actual pits and irregularities. This is most commonly seen in permanent teeth in which the overlying deciduous tooth becomes abscessed or is physically forced into the enamel organ of the permanent tooth. The resulting hypoplastic or hypocalcified permanent tooth is sometimes known as *Turner's tooth.*

For systemic factors to have an effect on developing permanent teeth, they must generally occur after birth and before the age of 6 years. During this time the crowns of all permanent teeth (with the exception of the third molars) develop. Because most enamel defects affect anterior teeth and first molars, systemic

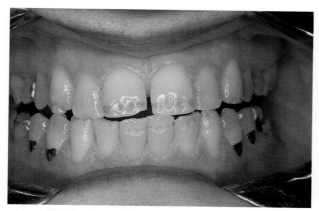

Figure 16-22 Enamel hypoplasia.

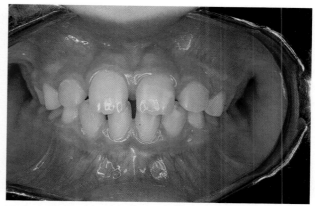

Figure 16-24 Enamel hypocalcification (Turner's tooth).

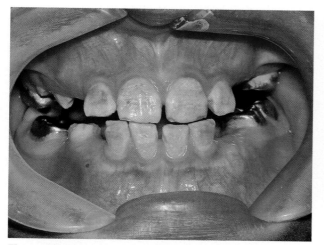

Figure 16-23 Enamel hypoplasia believed to be caused by childhood rickets.

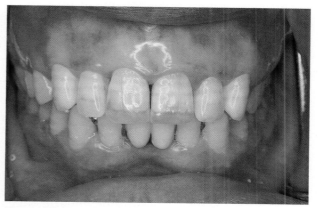

Figure 16-25 Fluorosis.

factors occur predominantly during the first 18 months of life. Primary teeth and possibly the tips of first permanent molars and permanent central incisors may reflect ameloblast dysfunction occurring in utero, since these are the teeth undergoing enamel calcification during this period. The specific causes of systemically induced enamel defects are often obscure but are usually attributed to childhood infectious diseases. This, however, has not been well substantiated with research data. Other cited causes of enamel hypoplasia or hypocalcification include nutritional defects such as rickets, congenital syphilis, birth trauma (neonatal line in primary teeth), fluoride, and idiopathic factors. The enamel hypoplasia that may be seen with congenital syphilis is rather characteristic. The in utero infection by *Treponema pallidum* affects the developing permanent incisors and first molars. Affected incisors, also known as *Hutchinson's incisors,* are tapered incisally and are notched centrally on the incisal edge. Affected molars, also known as *mulberry molars,* show a lobulated or crenated occlusal surface.

Ingestion of drinking water containing fluoride at levels greater than 1 part per million during the time crowns are being formed may result in enamel hypoplasia or hypocalcification, also known as *fluorosis* (Figures 16-25 and 16-26). Endemic fluorosis is known to occur in areas where the drinking water contains excessive naturally occurring fluoride. As with other causative agents, the extent of damage is dependent on the duration, timing, and intensity or concentration. Mild to moderate fluorosis ranges clinically from white enamel spots to mottled brown-and-white discolorations. Severe fluorosis appears as pitted, irregular, and discolored enamel. Although fluoride-induced enamel hypoplasia or hypocalcification is caries resistant, it may be cosmetically objectionable, making aesthetic dental restorations desirable.

Amelogenesis Imperfecta

Amelogenesis imperfecta is a heterogeneous group of similar-appearing hereditary disorders of enamel formation that affects both dentitions (Table 16-1). Most cases of amelogenesis imperfecta fall into one of two major types: *hypoplastic* or *hypocalcified* (Figures 16-27 to 16-29). A third type, known as *hypomaturation,* has been added to the list. Numerous subtypes of the three major groups are also recognized; these are based on different inheritance patterns, clinical appearances, and radiographic images.

The hereditary patterns range from autosomal dominant or recessive to X-linked dominant or recessive. Most cases of amelogenesis imperfecta are inherited as an autosomal-dominant trait, but the hypoplastic type is inherited as an X-linked dominant trait. Differences in manifestations between males and females in the hypoplastic forms are based on the Lyon phenomenon, in which each cell of a female randomly inactivates one or another of the genes on its X chromosome. Affected males may have a very thin, smooth enamel layer, whereas females may have thicker enamel with vertical grooves. The protein defect is thought to affect amelogenin, which is involved in enamel mineralization. The locus for amelogenin has been localized to the distal portion of the short (p) arm of the X chromosome. Refining the location further, the locus has been assigned to a 5-kilobase (5000 base pairs) area on chromosome Xp22.3–p22.1. The genetic abnormality may involve a deletion of up to five of the seven exons coding for the gene, although some cases show variable deletion sizes. Therefore the phenotype of amelogenesis imperfecta is complex, reflecting the complex pattern of genetic alterations.

In the *hypoplastic* type of amelogenesis imperfecta, teeth erupt with insufficient amounts of enamel, ranging from pits and grooves in one patient to complete absence (aplasia) in another. Because of reduced enamel thickness in some cases, abnormal contour and absent interproximal contact points may be evident. In the hypocalcified type, the quantity of enamel is normal, but it is soft and friable, so that it fractures and wears readily. The color of the teeth varies from tooth to tooth and patient to patient—from white opaque to yellow to brown. Teeth also tend to darken with age as a result of exogenous staining. Radiographically, enamel appears reduced in bulk, often showing a thin layer over occlusal and interproximal surfaces. Dentin and pulp chambers appear normal. Other than cosmetic restoration, no treatment is necessary. Although the enamel is soft and irregular, teeth are not caries prone.

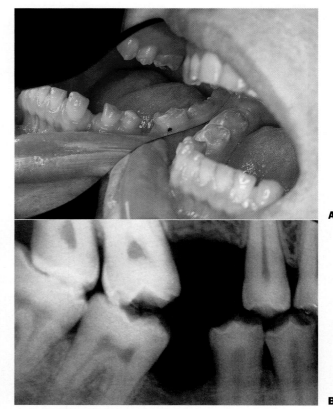

A

B

Figure 16-27   **A and B, Amelogenesis imperfecta,** hypoplastic type.

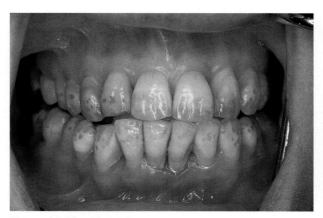

Figure 16-26   **Fluorosis.**

TABLE 16-1 **Hereditary Conditions of Teeth**

	Amelogenesis Imperfecta	Dentinogenesis Imperfecta	Dentin Dysplasia
Heredity	Many patterns	Autosomal dominant	Autosomal dominant
Teeth affected	All teeth, both dentitions	All teeth, both dentitions	All teeth, both dentitions
Tooth color	Yellow	Yellow	Normal
Tooth shape	Smaller, pitted	Extreme occlusal wear	Normal
X-ray findings	Normal pulps/dentin; reduced enamel	Obliterated pulps, short roots, bell crowns	Obliterated pulps, periapical cysts/granulomas
Systemic manifestations	No	Osteogenesis imperfecta occasionally	No
Treatment	Full crowns	Full crowns	None; early tooth loss

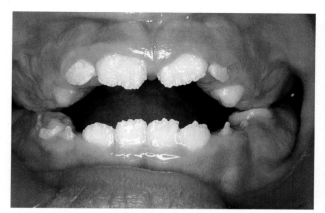

Figure 16-28 **Amelogenesis imperfecta,** hypoplastic type.

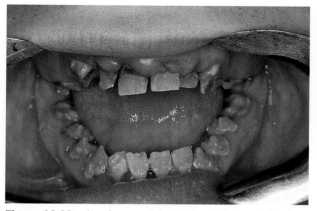

Figure 16-29 **Amelogenesis imperfecta,** hypocalcified type.

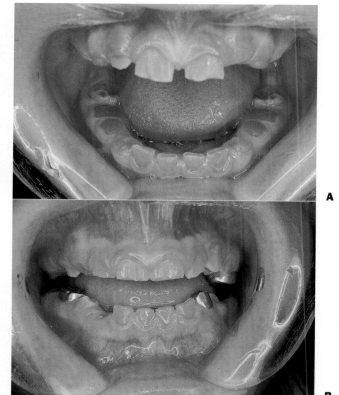

A

B

Figure 16-30 **Dentinogenesis imperfecta. A** and **B,** Brothers.

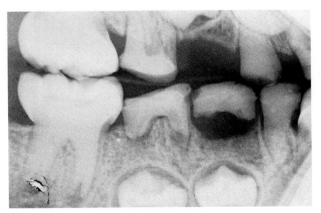

Figure 16-31 Dentinogenesis imperfecta.

DEFECTS OF DENTIN

Dentinogenesis Imperfecta

Dentinogenesis imperfecta is an autosomal-dominant trait with variable expressivity (Figures 16-30 and 16-31). It affects dentin of both the primary and the permanent dentitions. Because of the clinical discoloration of teeth, this condition has also been known as (hereditary) *opalescent dentin.*

Dentinogenesis imperfecta has been divided into three types. In type I, in which the dentin abnormality occurs in patients with concurrent osteogenesis imperfecta, primary teeth are more severely affected than permanent teeth. In type II, patients have only dentin abnormalities and no bone disease. In type III, or the Brandywine type (discovered in a triracial population in Brandywine, Maryland), only dental defects occur. This type is similar to type II, but with some clinical and radiographic variations. Features of type III that are not seen in types I and II include multiple pulp exposures, periapical radiolucencies, and a variable radiographic appearance.

Dentinogenesis imperfecta has an autosomal-dominant pattern of inheritance. Cosegregation between this condition and localized juvenile periodontitis in certain families indicated that the genetic loci were separate but perhaps closely linked. With the use of the genetic mapping technique known as chromosome walking, it was concluded that the type I locus was located on chromosome 4 at position q13 to q21. A deficiency of dentin phosphoprotein was suggested as a causative factor, given that the locus for this protein was thought to be near the dentinogenesis imperfecta gene. However, later studies have shown that the gene for dentin phosphoprotein is not located on chromosome 4, excluding it as a candidate. Osteopontin, a bone glycoprotein, is also expressed in dentin. However, there is no association between a type of polymorphism at the osteopontin locus and dentinogenesis imperfecta type II.

Clinically, all three types share numerous features. In both dentitions the teeth exhibit an unusual translucent, opalescent appearance with color variation from yellow-brown to gray. The entire crown appears discolored because of the abnormal underlying dentin. Although the enamel is structurally and chemically normal, it fractures easily, resulting in rapid wear. The enamel fracturing is believed to be due to the poor support provided by the abnormal dentin and possibly in part to the absence of the microscopic scalloping normally seen between dentin and enamel that is believed to help mechanically lock the two hard tissues together. Overall tooth morphology is unusual for its excessive constriction at the cementoenamel junction, giving the crowns a tulip or bell shape. Roots are shortened and blunted. The teeth do not exhibit any greater susceptibility to caries, and they may in fact show some resistance because of the rapid wear and absence of interdental contacts.

Radiographically, types I and II exhibit identical changes. Opacification of dental pulps occurs because of continued deposition of abnormal dentin. The short roots and the bell-shaped crowns are also obvious on radiographic examination. In type III the dentin appears thin and the pulp chambers and root canals extremely large, giving the appearance of thin dentin shells—hence, the previous designation of *shell teeth.*

Microscopically, the dentin of teeth in dentinogenesis imperfecta contains fewer, but larger and irregular, dentinal tubules. The pulpal space is nearly completely replaced over time by the irregular dentin. Enamel appears normal, but the dentinoenamel junction is smooth instead of scalloped.

Treatment is directed toward protecting tooth tissue from wear and toward improving the aesthetic appearance of the teeth. Generally, fitting with full crowns at an early age is the treatment of choice. Despite the qualitatively poor dentin, support for the crowns is adequate. These teeth should not be used as abutments, because the roots are prone to fracture under stress.

Dentin Dysplasia

Dentin dysplasia is another autosomal-dominant trait that affects dentin (Figures 16-32 and 16-33). This is a rare condition that has been subdivided into type I

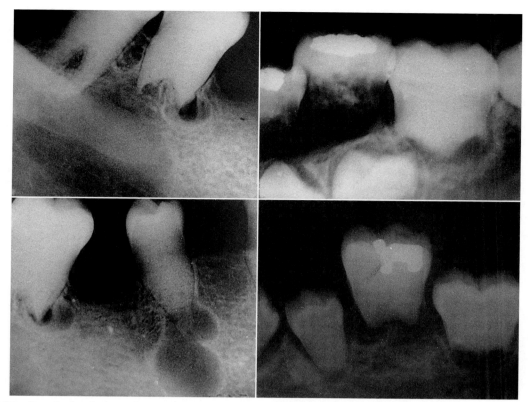

Figure 16-32   Dentin dysplasia. Note obliterated pulps, short roots, and periapical lesions.

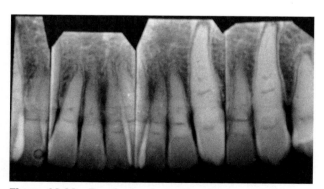

Figure 16-33   Dentin dysplasia. Note horizontal ribbons (chevrons) of dental pulp.

(radicular type) and a more rare type II (coronal type) that varies slightly in its clinical presentation. In dentin dysplasia type II the color of the primary dentition is opalescent and the permanent dentition is normal; in type I both dentitions are of normal color. The coronal pulps in type II are usually large (thistle tube appearance) and are filled with globules of abnormal dentin. Also, periapical lesions are not a regular feature of type II, as they are of type I.

Clinically, the crowns in dentin dysplasia type I appear to be normal in color and shape. Premature tooth loss may occur because of short roots or periapical inflammatory lesions. Teeth show greater resistance to caries than do normal teeth.

Radiographically, in dentin dysplasia type I, roots appear extremely short and pulps are almost completely obliterated. Residual fragments of pulp tissue appear typically as horizontal lucencies (chevrons). Periapical lucencies are typically seen; they represent chronic abscesses, granulomas, or cysts. In dentin dysplasia type II, deciduous teeth are similar in radiographic appearance to those in type I, but permanent teeth exhibit enlarged pulp chambers that have been described as thistle tube in appearance.

Microscopically, the enamel and the immediately subjacent dentin appear normal. Deeper layers of dentin show atypical tubular patterns, with amorphous, atubular areas and irregular organization. On the pulpal side of the normal-appearing mantle of dentin, globular or nodular masses of abnormal dentin are seen.

Treatment is directed toward retention of teeth for as long as possible. However, because of the short roots and periapical lesions, the prognosis for prolonged retention is poor. This dental condition has not been associated with any systemic connective tissue problems.

DEFECTS OF ENAMEL AND DENTIN

Regional Odontodysplasia

Regional odontodysplasia is a dental abnormality that involves the hard tissues that are derived from both epithelial (enamel) and mesenchymal (dentin and cementum) components of the tooth-forming apparatus (Figures 16-34 and 16-35). The teeth in a region or quadrant of the maxilla or mandible are affected to the extent that they exhibit short roots, open apical foramina, and enlarged pulp chambers. The thinness and poor mineralization quality of the enamel and dentin layers have given rise to the term *ghost teeth*.

The permanent teeth are affected more than the primary teeth, and the maxillary anterior teeth are affected more than other teeth. Eruption of the affected teeth is delayed or does not occur.

The cause of this rare dental abnormality is unknown, although numerous etiologic factors have been suggested, including trauma, nutritional deficiencies, infections, metabolic abnormalities, systemic diseases, local vascular compromise, and genetic influences.

Because of the poor quality of the affected teeth, their removal is usually indicated. The resulting edentulous zone can then be restored with a prosthesis or implant.

ABNORMALITIES OF DENTAL PULP

Pulp Calcification

Pulp calcification is a rather common phenomenon that occurs with increasing age for no apparent reason (Figures 16-36 and 16-37). There appears to be no relation to inflammation, trauma, or systemic disease. Pulp calcification may be of microscopic size or may be large enough to be detected radiographically. Calcifications may be either diffuse (linear) or nodular (pulp stones). The diffuse, or linear, deposits are typically

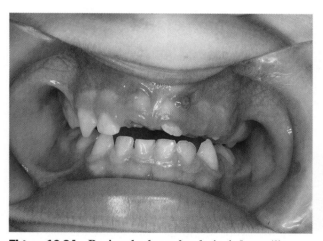

Figure 16-34   **Regional odontodysplasia,** left maxilla.

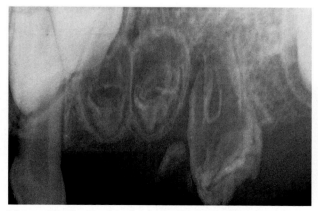

Figure 16-35   **Regional odontodysplasia** (ghost teeth).

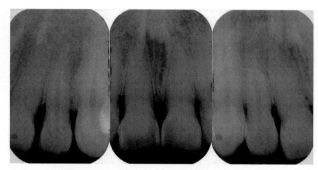

Figure 16-36   **Pulp calcification,** diffuse.

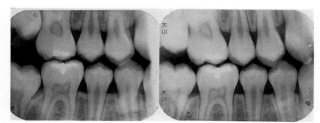

Figure 16-37   **Pulp calcification.** Pulp stones are evident in the molars.

found in the root canals and generally are parallel to the blood vessels. Pulp stones are usually found in the pulp chamber. When they are composed predominantly of dentin, they are referred to as *true denticles;* when they represent foci of dystrophic calcification, they are referred to as *false denticles.* Pulp stones are occasionally subdivided into attached and free types, depending on whether they are incorporated into the dentin wall or are surrounded by pulpal tissue.

Pulp stones appear to have no clinical significance. They are not believed to be a source of pain and are not associated with any form of pulpitis. They may, however, be problematic during endodontic therapy of nonvital teeth.

Internal Resorption

Resorption of the dentin of the pulpal walls may be seen as part of an inflammatory response to pulpal injury, or it may be seen in cases in which no apparent trigger can be identified (Figures 16-38 and 16-39). The resorption occurs as a result of the activation of osteoclasts or dentinoclasts on internal surfaces of the root or crown. Resorption lacunae, containing these cells and chronic inflammatory cells, are seen. Reversal lines may also be found in the adjacent hard

tissue, indicating attempts at repair. In time, the root or crown is perforated by the process, making the tooth useless.

Any tooth may be involved, and usually only a single tooth is affected, although cases in which more than one tooth is involved have been described. In advanced cases teeth may appear pink because of the proximity of pulp tissue to the tooth surface. Until root fracture or communication with a periodontal pocket occurs, patients generally have no symptoms.

The treatment of choice is root canal therapy before perforation. Once there is communication between pulp and periodontal ligament, the prognosis for saving the tooth is very poor. The process occasionally may spontaneously stop for no apparent reason.

External Resorption

Resorption of teeth from external surfaces may have one of several causes (Figures 16-40 to 16-44). This change may be the result of an adjacent pathologic process, such as (1) chronic inflammatory lesions, (2) cysts, (3) benign tumors, or (4) malignant neoplasms. The pathogenesis of external resorption from these causes has been related to the release of chemical mediators, increased vascularity, and pressure. External resorption of teeth may also be seen in association with (1) trauma, (2) reimplantation or transplantation of teeth, and (3) impactions. Trauma that causes injury to or necrosis of the periodontal ligament may initiate resorption of tooth roots. This trauma may be from a single event, from malocclusion, or from excessive orthodontic forces. Because reimplanted and transplanted teeth are nonvital and have no sur-

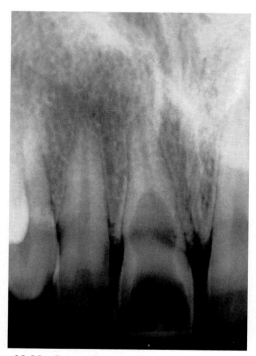

Figure 16-38 Internal resorption.

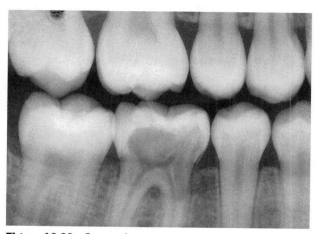

Figure 16-39 Internal resorption.

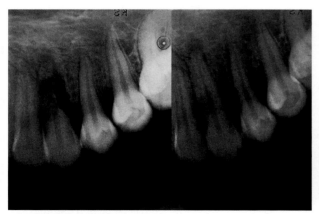

Figure 16-40 **External resorption.**

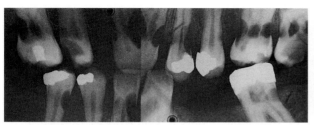

Figure 16-41 **External resorption,** cervical area.

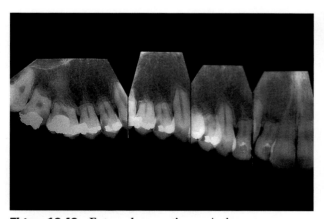

Figure 16-42 **External resorption,** apical.

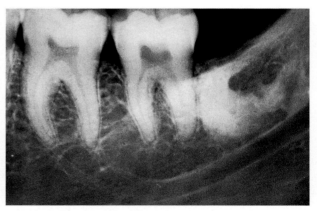

Figure 16-43 **External resorption** of an impacted tooth.

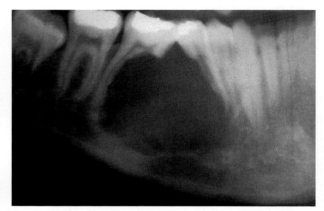

Figure 16-44 **External resorption** induced by a central giant cell granuloma.

rounding viable periodontal ligament, they are eventually resorbed and replaced by bone. This is basically a natural physiologic process in which the calcified collagen matrix of the tooth serves as a framework for the deposition of new, viable bone. Impacted teeth, when they impinge or exert pressure on adjacent teeth, may cause root resorption of the otherwise normally erupted tooth. Impacted teeth themselves may occasionally undergo resorption. The cause of

this phenomenon is unknown, although it is believed to be related to a partial loss of the protective effect of the periodontal ligament or reduced enamel epithelium.

Finally, external resorption of erupted teeth may be idiopathic. This may occur in one or more teeth. Any tooth may be involved, although molars are least likely to be affected. One of two patterns may be seen. In one, resorption occurs immediately apical to the cementoenamel junction, mimicking a pattern of caries associated with xerostomia. In external resorption, however, the lesions occur on root surfaces below the gingival epithelial attachment. In the other pattern of external resorption the process starts at the tooth apex and progresses occlusally.

External resorption is a particularly frustrating type of dental abnormality for both patients and practitioners because there is no plausible or evident explanation for the condition and no effective treatment. Over an extended clinical course, resorption eventually causes loss of the affected tooth.

ALTERATIONS IN COLOR

Exogenous Stains

Stains on the surface of teeth that can be removed with abrasives are known as *exogenous* or *extrinsic stains.* The color change may be caused by pigments in dietary substances (e.g., coffee, "betel" areca nut, tobacco) or by the colored by-products of chromogenic bacteria in dental plaque. Chromogenic bacteria are believed to be responsible for brown, black, green, and orange stains observed predominantly in children. Brown and black stains are typically seen in the cervical zone of teeth, either as a thin line along the gingival margin or as a wide band. This type of stain is also often found on teeth adjacent to salivary duct orifices. Green stain is tenacious and is usually found as a band on the labial surfaces of the maxillary anterior teeth. Blood pigments are thought to contribute to the green color. Orange or yellow-orange stains appear on the gingival third of teeth in a small percentage of children. These are generally easily removed.

Endogenous Stains

Discoloration of teeth resulting from deposits of systemically circulating substances during tooth development is defined as *endogenous* or *intrinsic staining.*

Systemic ingestion of *tetracycline* during tooth development is a well-known cause of endogenous staining of teeth (Figure 16-45). Tetracycline binds calcium and therefore is deposited in developing teeth and bones. The drug's bright yellow color is reflected in the subsequently erupted teeth. The fluorescent property of tetracycline can be demonstrated with an ultraviolet light in clinically erupted teeth. With time, the tetracycline oxidizes, resulting in a color change from yellow to gray or brown with the loss of its fluorescent quality. Because tetracycline can cross the placenta, it may stain primary teeth if taken during pregnancy. If it is administered between birth and age 6 or 7 years, permanent teeth may be affected. Only a small minority of children given tetracycline for various bacterial diseases, however, exhibit clinical evidence of discoloration. Staining is directly proportional to the age at which the drug is administered and the dose and duration of drug usage.

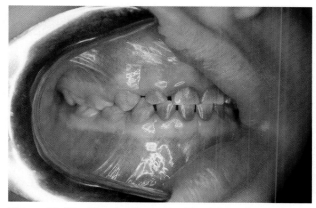

Figure 16-45   Tetracycline stain. Note the yellow color (tetracycline) of the posterior teeth and the gray color of the anterior teeth, in which there has been oxidation of endogenous tetracycline.

The significance of tetracycline staining lies in its cosmetically objectionable appearance. Because other, equally effective antibiotics are available, tetracycline should not be prescribed for children younger than 7 years of age except in unusual circumstances.

It should be noted that minocycline, a semisynthetic derivative of tetracycline, can stain the roots of adult teeth. It may also stain skin and mucosa in a diffuse or patchy pattern (see Chapter 5).

Rh incompatibility (erythroblastosis fetalis) has been cited as a cause of endogenous staining in primary teeth. Because of red blood cell hemolysis resulting from maternal antibody destruction of fetal red blood cells, blood breakdown products (bilirubin) are deposited in developing primary teeth. The teeth appear green to brown. Treatment is not required, because only primary teeth are affected.

Congenital porphyria, one of several inborn errors of porphyrin metabolism, is also a potential cause of endogenous pigmentation. This autosomal-recessive trait is also associated with photosensitivity, vesiculobullous skin eruptions, red urine, and splenomegaly. Teeth may appear red to brown because of deposition of porphyrin in the developing teeth. Affected teeth fluoresce red with ultraviolet light.

Liver disease, *biliary atresia* and *neonatal hepatitis,* may produce discoloration of the primary dentition. In biliary atresia the teeth may assume a green discoloration; a yellowish brown color is noted in cases of neonatal hepatitis. This is secondary to the deposition or incorporation of bilirubin in developing enamel and dentin.

BIBLIOGRAPHY

Ahlquist M, Grondahl H: Prevalence of impacted teeth and associated pathology in middle-aged and older Swedish women, *Community Dent Oral Epidemiol* 19:116-119, 1991.

Aine L, Backstrom MC, Maki R, et al: Enamel defects in primary and permanent teeth of children born prematurely, *J Oral Pathol Med* 29:403-409, 2000.

Alvesalo L, Varrela J: Taurodontism and the presence of an extra Y chromosome: study of 47 XYY males and analytical review, *Hum Biol* 63:31-38, 1991.

Chapple JR, Nunn JH: The oral health of children with clefts of the lip, palate, or both, *Cleft Palate Craniofac J* 38:525-528, 2001.

Dankner E, Harari D, Rotstein I: Dens evaginatus of anterior teeth: literature review and radiographic survey of 15,000 teeth, *Oral Surg Oral Med Oral Pathol Oral Radiol Endod* 81:472-475, 1996.

Dong J, Gu TT, Simmons D, et al: Enamelin maps to human chromosome 4q21 within the autosomal dominant amelogenesis imperfecta locus, *Eur J Oral Sci* 108:353-358, 2000.

Kurisu K, Tabata MJ: Human genes for dental anomalies, *Oral Dis* 3:223-228, 1997.

Peck S, Peck L, Kataja M: Mandibular lateral incisor-canine transposition, concomitant dental anomalies, and genetic control, *Angle Orthod* 68:455-466, 1998.

Rajpar MH, Harley K, Laing K, et al: Mutation of the gene encoding enamel-specific protein, enamelin, causes autosomal-dominant amelogenesis imperfecta, *Hum Mol Genet* 10:1673-1677, 2001.

Sandor GKB, Carmichael RP, Coraza L, et al: Genetic mutations in certain head and neck conditions of interest to the dentist, *J Can Dent Assoc* 67(10):577-584, 2001.

Seow WK: Enamel hypoplasia in the primary dentition: a review, *ASDC J Dent Child* 58:441-452, 1991.

Thesleff I: Genetic basis of tooth development and dental defects, *Acta Odontol Scand* 58:191-194, 2000.

Uyeno DS, Lugo AL: Dens evaginatus: a review, *ASDC J Dent Child* 63:328-332, 1996.

Vaikuntam J, Tatum NB, McGuff HS: Regional odontodysplasia: review of the literature and report of a case, *J Clin Pediatr Dent* 21:35-40, 1996.

Vastardis H: The genetics of human tooth agenesis: new discoveries for understanding dental anomalies, *Am J Orthod Dentofacial Orthop* 117:650-656, 2000.

Wright J, Robinson C, Shoe R: Characterization of the enamel ultrastructure and mineral content in hypoplastic amelogenesis imperfecta, *Oral Surg Oral Med Oral Pathol* 72:594-601, 1991.

Wright JT: Normal formation and development defects of the human dentition, *Pediatr Clin North Am* 47:975-1000, 2000.

Wright JT, Hall KI, Yamauche M: The enamel proteins in human amelogenesis imperfecta, *Arch Oral Biol* 42:149-159, 1997.

COMMON SKIN LESIONS OF THE HEAD AND NECK

Ginat Wintermeyer Mirowski, DMD, MD, and Todd W. Rozycki, MD

Macules and Patches
  Vitiligo
  Ephelides (Freckles)
  Café-au-Lait Macules
  Solar Lentigo (Liver Spot)
  Melasma (Mask of Pregnancy)
  Erysipelas
  Telangiectasia
  Petechiae, Purpura, and Ecchymoses
Papules and Plaques
  Acrochordon (Skin Tag)
  Fibrous Papule
  Angiofibroma (Adenoma Sebaceum)
  Neurofibroma
  Syringoma
  Molluscum Contagiosum
  Sebaceous Hyperplasia
  Xanthelasma
  Milia
  Solar (Senile) Comedones (Favre-Racouchot Syndrome)
  Nevomelanocytic Nevi (Moles)
  Cutaneous Melanoma
  Seborrheic Keratosis
  Acne
  Perioral Dermatitis
  Folliculitis
  Furuncle
  Miliaria

  Granuloma Faciale
  Hemangioma
  Morbilliform Drug Eruptions
  Lichen Planus
  Varix
Nodules
  Keratoacanthoma
  Basal Cell Carcinoma
  Squamous Cell Carcinoma
Wheals
  Urticaria (Hives)
  Angioedema
Papulosquamous Dermatoses
  Actinic Keratoses (Solar Keratoses)
  Seborrheic Dermatitis
  Psoriasis
  Atopic Dermatitis
  Keratosis Pilaris
  Pityriasis Rosea
  Warts (Verruca Vulgaris and Flat Warts)
Vesicles/Bullae/Pustules
  Herpes Simplex Infection
  Varicella-Zoster Infection
  Contact Dermatitis
  Impetigo
  Rosacea
  Erythema Multiforme
  Pemphigus Vulgaris

Erosions/Fissures/Ulcers/Scars

> **Perlèche**
>
> **Burns**
>
> **Keloid**

Connective Tissue Diseases

> **Dermatomyositis**
>
> **Lupus Erythematosus**
>
> **Scleroderma**

MACULES AND PATCHES

A macule is defined as a well-circumscribed, flat, discolored area approximately 0.5 cm in diameter. It may be brown, red, blue, white, yellow, or pink. A larger, flat, discolored area is a patch (Box 17-1).

Vitiligo

Vitiligo is an autoimmune condition characterized by loss of melanocytes and pigment from affected tissues. Vitiligo occurs at any age and in both men and women. The clinical course is unpredictable. Spontaneous repigmentation may occur but is rare. Toxic destruction of melanocytes after chemical exposure has occasionally been noted.

Clinical Features. Depigmented macules and patches have relatively distinct and possibly hyperpigmented margins. Perioral and periocular tissues are preferentially affected, as are the nape of the neck and areas of repeated trauma, such as the knees, elbows, and hands (Figures 17-1 and 17-2).

> ### Box 17-1 Dermatology Terms
>
> *Macule:* Flat, circumscribed, discolored area ~0.5 cm.
> *Patch:* Larger flat, discolored area.
> *Papule:* Raised bump <0.5 cm.
> *Plaque:* Elevated plateau >0.5 cm.
> *Nodule:* Elevated, circumscribed lesion >0.5 cm.
> *Wheal:* Transient papule/plaque caused by vascular fluid leakage.
> *Papulosquamous:* Papules with scaling.
> *Vesicle:* Fluid-filled blister <0.5 cm.
> *Bulla:* Fluid-filled blister >0.5 cm.
> *Pustule:* Circumscribed collection of pus ranging from 0.1 to 2 cm.
> *Erosion:* Loss of epidermis.
> *Fissure:* Shallow linear cracks.
> *Ulcers:* Loss of epidermis with dermal damage.

Treatment. Treatment is difficult and may center on the use of cosmetic products such as tanning creams and cosmetic cover-ups of affected areas or depigmentation of normal adjacent skin. Sunscreens with a sun protection factor of 15 or greater should be used to prevent both sunburns and future skin cancers. Patients only rarely respond to topical steroids. Topical or systemic psoralens and ultraviolet light (PUVA) therapy may be effective but requires months of treatment. Autologous minigrafts may accelerate repigmentation.

Ephelides (Freckles)

Ephelides are small (less than 0.5 cm), tan to brown, discrete macules on sun-exposed skin.

Clinical Features. Ephelides are found on the nose, cheeks, dorsal surface of the arms, and upper trunk of fair individuals with red-blond hair.

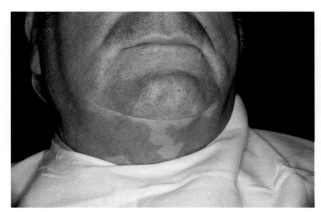

Figure 17-1 Vitiligo of the face.

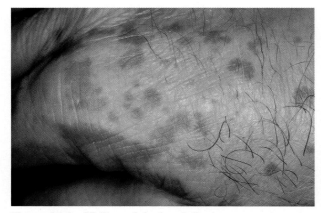

Figure 17-2 **Vitiligo of the hand.** Dark areas represent normal skin color for this patient.

Histopathology. In ephelides, melanocytes are approximately one-third less abundant than in normal skin; however, they contain a greater number of melanosomes, which also tend to be large, elongated, or rod shaped.

Treatment. No treatment is indicated. Sun avoidance and sun protection (SPF ≥15) will help to fade these macules and prevent new ones from forming. Trichloroacetic acid is occasionally used to peel off a few at a time; results are variable.

Café-au-Lait Macules

See Chapter 5.

Solar Lentigo (Liver Spot)

A solar lentigo is a benign, irregularly shaped, hyperpigmented macule. Solar lentigines tend to be larger and darker than ephelides.

Clinical Features. These discrete macules occur in skin that has been chronically exposed to the sun; however, unlike freckles, which tend to fade when protected from solar exposure, solar lentigines persist (Figures 17-3 and 17-4). Lentigines are associated with other signs of chronic sun exposure, such as depigmented macules, actinic purpura, and actinic keratoses. Although lentigines are benign, any lentigo that enlarges or develops increased pigmentation, localized thickening, or a highly irregular border should be evaluated for melanoma. Perioral lentigines are associated with Addison's disease, Peutz-Jeghers syndrome, and Laugier-Hunziker syndrome.

Histopathology. Lentigines contain a marked increase in melanocyte density, increased pigmentation of the basal cell layer and adjacent keratinocytes, and elongation of rete ridges. Melanophages may be present in the upper dermis.

Treatment. Most normal-appearing solar lentigines do not require treatment. If any underlying pathologic change is suspected, a biopsy is required, with possible excision pending final diagnosis. Cosmetic ablation may be performed with cryotherapy (liquid nitrogen), laser vaporization, or topical tretinoin.

Melasma (Mask of Pregnancy)

Melasma is an acquired pigmentation, commonly noted in pregnancy and in women taking birth control pills; 10% of cases are seen in males. Sunlight seems to have an important role in the development and darkening of melasma. Melasma occurring during pregnancy usually disappears several months after delivery; however, discontinuing oral contraceptives rarely eliminates melasma even 5 years after discontinued use. The infrequency of melasma in postmenopausal women receiving estrogen replacement therapy indicates that estrogen alone is not the etiologic agent.

Clinical Features. Melasma is characterized by well-demarcated, symmetric, brown to grayish patches on the face. It has a predilection for the cheeks, forehead, and upper lip.

Histopathology. Three types of melasma are seen histologically: (1) epidermal type, (2) dermal type, and (3) mixed type. All types show an increase in the number

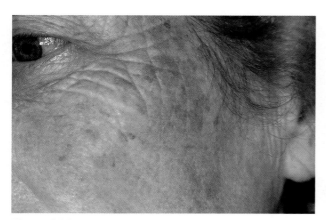

Figure 17-3 **Lentigines** of the face.

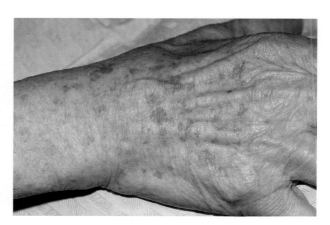

Figure 17-4 **Lentigines** of the hand.

and activity of melanocytes, as well as increased transfer of melanosomes. In epidermal melasma, melanin is also increased in the basal and suprabasal layers. In dermal melasma, melanin-laden macrophages are found in the mid and upper dermis.

Treatment. Wood's lamp evaluation of epidermal melasma (positive) versus dermal melasma (negative) is an aid in treatment considerations. Epidermal melasma may be treated with bleaching agents such as 2% to 4% hydroquinone and the concomitant use of strong sunscreens and topical tretinoin cream at night. Dermal melasma does not respond to treatment.

Erysipelas

Erysipelas is an acute superficial cellulitis characterized by marked lymphatic vessel involvement. It is due to group A streptococci in children or group B streptococci in neonates. Rarely, *Staphylococcus aureus* may be responsible.

Clinical Features. Erysipelas occurs in infants, young children, and the elderly. A small break in the skin with subsequent contamination with streptococci is the typical precedent. A recent history of an upper respiratory tract infection with streptococci is often elicited. Erysipelas presents as bright to dusky red, warm, shiny skin that is often indurated and edematous. The sharply demarcated, advancing raised border may be painful. The bridge of the nose and one or both cheeks are often affected; the process usually stops at the beard or hairline. Patients present with a high fever, general malaise, and a leukocytosis of 15,000 cells/mm³ or greater. Complications such as abscess formation, necrotizing fasciitis, and septicemia are rare but may occur after inadequate therapy or in immunocompromised patients.

Histopathology. The epidermis is usually unaffected. Marked edema and lymphatic dilation are noted in the dermis, with a diffuse, mostly neutrophilic infiltrate extending throughout the dermis and occasionally into the subcutaneous fat. Gram stain reveals streptococci in the tissue and lymphatics.

Treatment. Uncomplicated erysipelas is often a self-limited process, remaining confined to the lymphatics and subcutaneous tissues and subsiding over 7 to 10 days. Antibiotic therapy shortens this process; however, more than a week may be required for more complete resolution. Recurrences are common.

Telangiectasia

Telangiectasias are permanently dilated dermal blood vessels that appear as red or violaceous threads in different patterns (Figure 17-5). They occur in many cutaneous and systemic conditions, including sun-damaged skin, CREST syndrome (*c*alcinosis, *R*aynaud's, *e*sophageal constriction, *s*clerodactyly, and *t*elangiectasias), systemic lupus erythematosus (SLE), rosacea, cirrhosis, hereditary hemorrhagic telangiectasia, and pregnancy, as well as following radiation therapy. They are only cosmetic problems, and bleeding occurs very rarely. Spider angiomas, one type of telangiectatic pattern, are often treated either by electrodesiccation of the central arteriole or by laser ablation. In general, telangiectasias are not treated.

Petechiae, Purpura, and Ecchymoses

Petechiae are tiny, well-circumscribed macules that represent punctate hemorrhages in the dermis. Conditions in which petechiae may occur include gonococcemia, meningococcemia, amyloidosis, and various leukocytoclastic vasculitides. Petechiae disappear after the underlying disease process has ceased.

Purpura are circumscribed intradermal deposits of hemorrhage that measure more than 0.1 to 5.0 cm in diameter. Purpura may accompany platelet abnormalities, Rocky Mountain spotted fever, scurvy, or trauma.

Ecchymoses, or bruises, are large dermal hemorrhages that occur most often after blunt trauma (Figure 17-6) but may be due to platelet dysfunction or amyloidosis. They are red to purple initially but in time exhibit red, yellow, and green colors as the extravasated blood is degraded.

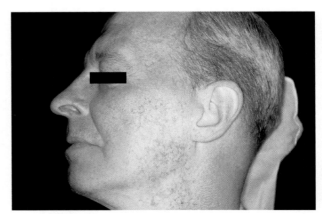

Figure 17-5   **Telangiectasias,** postradiation.

PAPULES AND PLAQUES

A papule is a raised bump that measures up to 0.5 cm in diameter. A plaque is an elevated, plateaulike area that measures greater than 0.5 cm and may be formed by the confluence of multiple papules.

Acrochordon (Skin Tag)

Acrochordons are soft, flesh-colored, pedunculated benign skin tumors. Acrochordons may have irregular or smooth surfaces. They occur around the eyelids, neck, and axillae and remain asymptomatic unless the pedicle twists, resulting in infarction. The stalk is composed of loose collagen fibers and dilated capillaries. Skin tags may be removed by snipping with curved iris scissors, or they may be destroyed with the use of electrocautery or cryotherapy.

Fibrous Papule

Clinical Features. Fibrous papules are dome-shaped, firm, flesh-colored papules with a broad base; they occasionally are pedunculated (Figure 17-7). These occur in middle age and affect both genders equally.

Histopathology. The epidermal changes observed include hyperkeratosis with a slight degree of hypergranulosis and flattened epithelial ridges. The primary alterations are within the dermis (i.e., hyperplastic collagen and spindle-shaped or stellate multinucleated cells). Collagen bundles are coarse and are often arranged vertically toward the superficial aspects of the dermis. Blood vessels are usually increased in number and dilated.

Treatment. Treatment is surgical in nature. Curettage followed by cautery of the surgical bed generally prevents recurrence.

Angiofibroma (Adenoma Sebaceum)

Angiofibromas occur as solitary papules or as part of the triad (mental deficiency, epilepsy, and multiple angiofibromas of the face) of tuberous sclerosis, an autosomal-dominant syndrome.

Clinical Features. Angiofibromas appear as small (0.1 to 0.3 cm), flesh-colored, brown or reddish, smooth, shiny papules on both sides of the nose, on the medial cheeks, and extending slightly down the nasolabial folds.

Histopathology. Angiofibromas are indistinguishable histologically from solitary fibrous papules of the face. The epidermis is normal in architecture, the papillary dermis is absent, there is considerable dermal fibrosis (with collagen fibers running perpendicular to the epidermis), and capillaries are dilated. In the papillary dermis, stellate, glialike cells and occasional multinucleated giant cells are present. The sebaceous glands are generally atrophic.

Treatment. Shave excision is often curative; however, when many lesions are present, as in tuberous sclerosis, dermabrasion or laser treatment may be helpful. Recurrence is common.

Neurofibroma

Figure 17-8; see also Chapter 7.

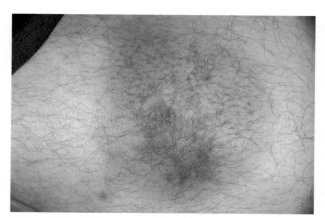

Figure 17-6   **Ecchymosis** of the thigh.

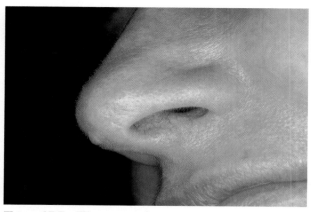

Figure 17-7   **Fibrous papule.**

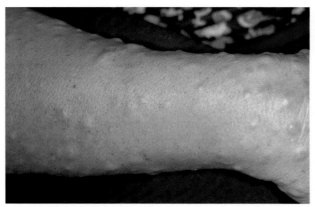

Figure 17-8   **Neurofibromas,** forearm.

Syringoma

Syringoma is a benign tumor that represents an adenoma of intraepidermal eccrine ducts.

Clinical Features. Clinically, numerous firm, flesh-colored to yellowish papules, 0.2 to 0.4 cm in diameter, are found under the eyelids and on the cheeks, axillae, pubic area, and abdomen. Hormonal influences have been postulated because they proliferate at puberty and women are more commonly affected. Syringomas proliferate and increase in size during pregnancy and premenstrually.

Histopathology. The epidermis may show keratin-filled ductal lumina with occasional keratohyalin-containing cells. In the papillary dermis are many small, cystic ducts and solid epithelial strands embedded in a fibrous stroma. Some of the ducts may have small, commalike excrescences that may give them the appearance of tadpoles.

Treatment. These tumors have no malignant potential but are disfiguring and may be removed for purely cosmetic reasons by electrodesiccation, curettage, or excision.

Molluscum Contagiosum

Molluscum contagiosum is a common viral skin disease that presents as discrete white/skin-colored, umbilicated papules. The etiologic agent is a large DNA poxvirus. The clinical presentation and treatments depend on the age and immune status of the host. Molluscum contagiosum is transmitted by direct contact and ultimately involutes spontaneously, with an associated mild inflammatory reaction and ten-

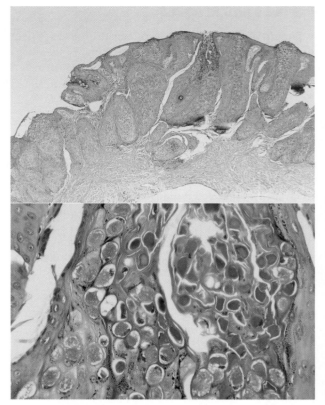

Figure 17-9   **A** and **B, Molluscum contagiosum.** Note viral inclusions (molluscum bodies) in **B.**

derness. In immunosuppressed individuals *Cryptococcus neoformans* may present as umbilicated papules that clinically resemble molluscum contagiosum.

Clinical Features. In healthy children 1 to 50 or more papules may be noted on the skin. These develop 2 to 3 months after the initial inoculation and are typically asymptomatic. The lesions have a predilection for the neck, trunk, eyelids, and anogenital area. Dozens or even hundreds of such lesions can be seen in immunosuppressed individuals of all ages, in whom spontaneous involution does not occur.

Histopathology. A striking characteristic of the epidermis in molluscum lesions is the appearance of a widened epithelial ridge as great as six times normal (Figure 17-9). Intracytoplasmic inclusions, called *molluscum bodies* or *Henderson-Patterson bodies*, are noted in infected cells and extend toward the surface, eventually completely obliterating the epithelium. These inclusions are pathognomonic.

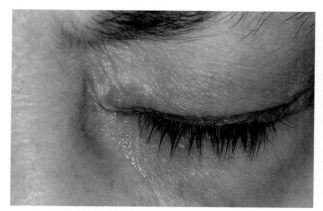

Figure 17-10 Xanthelasma.

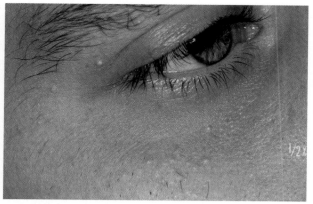

Figure 17-11 Milia.

Treatment. Molluscum contagiosum often resolves spontaneously. Treatment may shorten the duration of the disease, as well as reduce the chance for autoinoculation and transmission to others. Curettage followed by minimal electrocautery or cryotherapy with liquid nitrogen or dry ice may be effective at decreasing the size and number of lesions. In immunocompromised individuals the lesions are particularly recalcitrant to all treatments.

Sebaceous Hyperplasia

Clinical Features. Sebaceous hyperplasia presents as small (0.1 to 0.3 cm), soft, yellow, slightly umbilicating papules on the face or forehead of middle-aged or older persons.

Histopathology. Usually noted is a single enlarged sebaceous gland composed of many lobules grouped around a central dilated duct. The sebaceous glands usually are fully mature, but there may be more than one peripheral row of undifferentiated cells that possess very little lipid.

Treatment. Treatment is removal of the elevated portion of the papule by a shave biopsy, curettage, electrodesiccation, or treatment with trichloroacetic acid. Oral isotretinoin is dramatically effective, but side effects limit its usefulness.

Xanthelasma

Clinical Features. Xanthelasma presents as yellow papules and plaques or macules that may or may not be associated with hyperlipidemia. The upper eyelids are the predominant sites, and the lesions are not associated with hyperlipoproteinemia (Figure 17-10).

Histopathology. Histologically, foam or xanthoma cells, which are macrophages that have ingested lipid material, are present within the superficial dermis and are surrounded by fibrous connective tissue.

Treatment. No treatment is indicated; however, excision or the sequential application of trichloroacetic acid may be used for cosmetic purposes. Xanthelasma may recur.

Milia

Milia are small (0.1 to 0.2 cm) white cysts of the upper segment of the hair follicle (Figure 17-11). No treatment is necessary. Milia may be removed for cosmetic considerations by incising the overlying epidermis and gently extracting the cyst contents.

Solar (Senile) Comedones (Favre-Racouchot Syndrome)

Numerous open, dilated, and cystic blackheads characterize solar comedones. They are found in elderly individuals in whom the facial skin (especially lateral to the eyes) exhibits extensive sun damage.

Histopathology. The surrounding epidermis appears normal, but the dermis may have variable solar elastosis. Characteristically seen are dilated pilosebaceous openings with distended, horn-filled hair follicles. Sebaceous gland atrophy with rare inflammation occurs because the comedones are open.

Nevomelanocytic Nevi (Moles)

Nevomelanocytic nevi are flat or slightly raised, light brown to brown-black papules measuring 0.1 to 0.6 cm (Figures 17-12 and 17-13). Nevi are rare at birth and usually appear after the age of 2 years. After childhood, some flat nevi change into compound nevi (elevate). Dysplastic nevi are asymmetric moles with irregular borders and characteristic histologic features. Individuals with numerous large, dysplastic nevi are at a higher risk for melanoma. Degeneration of nevi into melanoma is exceedingly rare. Epidemiologic studies have found that many nonfreckling, lighter-skinned individuals and light-skinned blacks may have nevi. Clearly, removing all cutaneous moles is an impossible and inappropriate task. However, if a particular mole exhibits transformation or is irritated, removal with pathologic evaluation is indicated. Microscopically, clusters of melanocytes are found at the dermal-epidermal junction, in the dermis, or both in the dermis and at the junction of the dermis and epidermis.

Spitz nevus (benign juvenile melanoma) is a type of cutaneous nevus that is a worrisome-appearing benign tumor of children and young adults. Its clinical and histologic appearance is similar to that of melanoma. These nevi are hairless, red to reddish brown, dome-shaped papules or nodules with a verrucous or smooth surface. Most Spitz nevi measure less than 0.6 cm. They are usually solitary but occasionally are numerous, appearing suddenly on the face and lower extremities. Microscopically, differentiation between Spitz nevus and melanoma may be difficult. Architecturally, Spitz nevi are symmetric and resemble nevi with compound, junctional, or intradermal patterns. The epidermis is often hyperplastic and has elongated rete ridges; permeation of the epidermis by nevus cells is usually slight. Cytologically, large spindle-shaped and epithelioid cells differentiate Spitz nevi from other nevi and most melanomas. Maturation of the cells, with increasing depth and uniformity of cells from one side to the other, is also an important differentiating feature. Mitoses are found in approximately one half of Spitz nevi; however, atypical mitoses are not common. Spitz nevi should be removed for histologic examination because they cannot be differentiated from melanoma on a purely clinical basis, especially at or beyond puberty.

Blue nevus is an aggregate of melanin-producing cells in the dermis. These nevi appear blue because melanin deep in the dermis absorbs long-wavelength light, and blue is reflected to the observer (Tyndall effect). Blue nevi generally have no malignant potential. They appear as small (less than 1.0 cm), well-circumscribed, dome-shaped blue to black papules on the hands, feet, and head. They may be congenital but are most commonly acquired by late childhood. Microscopically, the dermis contains elongated, wavy, dendritic, melanin-containing cells whose processes extend in bundles parallel to the epidermis. The cells may extend to the subcutaneous fat or approach the epidermis. Small, unchanging blue nevi in adults require no therapy. If a blue lesion suddenly appears, enlarges, or exceeds 1.0 cm, it must be removed for histologic examination to rule out melanoma.

Cutaneous Melanoma

The incidence of melanomas of the skin has been increasing during the past several years. Melanoma

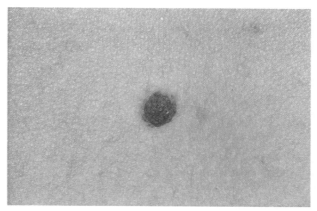

Figure 17-12   Nevomelanocytic nevus, back.

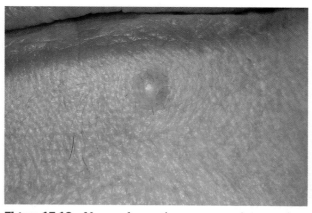

Figure 17-13   Nevomelanocytic nevus, nonpigmented.

now represents approximately 2% of all cancers (excluding basal cell and squamous cell carcinomas of the skin). Predisposing risk factors include a positive family history, light natural pigmentation, and acute intermittent exposure to sunlight, especially in childhood. Most melanomas arise de novo. The best indicator of prognosis is the microscopic depth of invasion of the tumor. This may be measured with a relatively subjective assessment using Clark's levels (1 to 5) or with an objective determination known as *Breslow's measurement.* With Breslow's measurement the thickness of the primary lesion is measured with a microscope ocular micrometer, from the top of the granular layer to the deepest tumor cell. Thinner neoplasms have a better prognosis. Generally, the larger the lesion and the greater the spread, the poorer the prognosis.

Clinical Features. Approximately 20% of all melanomas occur on the head and neck (Figure 17-14). Melanomas are characterized by two growth phases: a horizontal and a vertical phase. Melanomas are classified into three predominant types according to their clinical features. *Superficial spreading melanomas* account for approximately 60% of all melanomas. Nodular melanomas account for 30%, and lentigo maligna melanomas account for 10% of melanomas. A *superficial spreading melanoma* advances across the skin, producing an irregular patch of various colors. Neoplastic cells are found in nests at the epidermal-dermal junction and extend laterally from the center of the lesion. In this prolonged horizontal, or *radial growth phase,* the lesion may be designated microscopically as melanoma in situ. Treatment during the radial or in situ growth phase yields excellent results.

A vertical growth phase is signaled by the appearance of clusters of neoplastic cells within the underlying dermis. The lesion develops metastatic potential

that significantly affects the prognosis. *Nodular melanoma* has only a vertical (invasive) growth phase and thus exhibits a poorer prognosis. *Nodular melanoma* presents as darkly pigmented papules or nodules that may ulcerate or may exhibit rapid growth. Neoplastic melanocytes are found in both the dermis and the epidermis.

Lentigo maligna melanoma occurs predominantly on sun-exposed skin of the elderly. Its radial growth phase may last as long as 25 or 30 years. Clinically, lentigo maligna melanoma appears as a flat, irregularly pigmented patch with ill-defined margins. The prognosis is generally considered excellent until the lesion enters a vertical phase.

Treatment. Surgical excision remains the treatment of choice for all types of melanomas. Generally, 1-cm margins are recommended for thin lesions and 2- to 3-cm margins are recommended for thicker lesions. Elective dissection of regional lymph nodes is a controversial issue but is more likely to be performed with excision of thicker neoplasms. Chemotherapy, immunotherapy, and radiation therapy may be added to the treatment regimen.

Seborrheic Keratosis

Seborrheic keratosis is a benign epidermal proliferation. An increased prevalence is noted from middle age to the later years. The cause is unknown.

Clinical Features. Seborrheic keratoses may present as solitary lesions, but multiple lesions are commonly found (Figures 17-15 and 17-16). Plaques range from light brown to black, with sharp, delineated margins. Clinically, seborrheic keratoses have a greasy-feeling

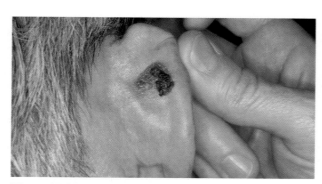

Figure 17-14 Melanoma.

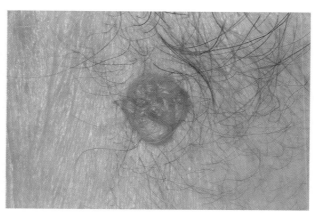

Figure 17-15 Seborrheic keratosis.

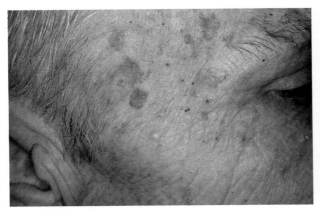

Figure 17-16   Seborrheic keratosis and comedones.

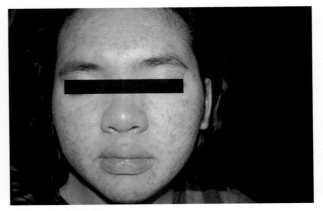

Figure 17-17   Acne.

keratotic crust that is loosely attached. A stuck-on quality is typical. The surface may be rough or warty because of tightly aggregated fine fissures or clefts. During the early phases of development, seborrheic keratoses may be flat, with a dull or matte surface quality that is similar in appearance to solar or simple lentigines. Seborrheic keratoses may be mistaken for pigmented basal cell carcinoma or nodular melanoma.

Histopathology. Seborrheic keratoses show a wide range of histologic variation. Many microscopic subtypes may be seen in the same lesion; common features include hyperkeratosis, acanthosis, and papillomatosis. A biphasic hyperplasia of both the epidermis and the supporting papillary dermis is noted. Small keratotic pseudocysts or horn cysts appear as a result of invagination of the stratum corneum. A mild chronic inflammatory cell infiltrate can be found in the dermis, occasionally producing a lichenoid pattern. In irritated lesions small whorls of prematurely keratinizing cells known as *squamous eddies* are seen.

Treatment. No treatment is indicated. If lesions become cosmetically objectionable, removal is advised. Curettage with superficial electrocautery of the base, cryotherapy, or electrosurgery may be used.

Acne

Acne is a chronic skin condition of the pilosebaceous apparatus. The face, neck, and trunk are commonly affected. Acne may range in severity from trivial to disfiguring (conglobata form) and may have a profound impact on the psychologic outlook of affected individuals. The cause appears to be multifactorial, and treatment regimens are directed toward these various factors.

At least three major, interrelated contributing events appear to initiate acne: (1) follicular hyperkeratosis, (2) follicular bacterial proliferation, and (3) increased sebum production. Hyperkeratosis of the follicular epithelium leads to follicular plugging, which in turn produces the primary lesion, a *comedo*. A noninflamed collection of keratin, sebum, and bacteria that does not communicate with the surface is a *closed comedo* (whitehead), whereas an *open comedo* (blackhead) communicates with the skin surface. Oxidation of pigment causes the lesion to appear black.

Propionibacterium acnes, a diphtheroid, is a gram-negative resident of the pilosebaceous unit. *P. acnes* proliferates, especially with follicular plugging, and produces lipases that act on triglycerides, a major component of sebum, resulting in the formation of free fatty acids that diffuse into the perifollicular tissues, where they act as irritants and inflammatory stimuli. *P. acnes* also produces enzymes and chemical mediators that promote follicular and perifollicular inflammation. Increased production of sebum appears to have a major role in the cause of acne because sebum acts as a substrate for *P. acnes*. Increased sebum production occurs predominantly through the stimulation of sebaceous glands by androgens and, in part, by progestins. Chronic mechanical trauma, stress, and drugs such as birth control pills, corticosteroids, lithium, cyclosporine, phenytoin, and barbiturates may exacerbate acne. Cosmetics may promote comedogenesis. Genetic influences also have been noted.

Clinical Features. The face, neck, back, and trunk are commonly affected by acne (Figure 17-17). Comedones may become inflamed, resulting in pustules. Healing of larger, deeper nodules or cysts may result in pitted or depressed scars, hypertrophic scars, or keloids. Hypopigmentation or hyperpigmentation may also be seen.

Treatment. Topical measures are recommended for mild to moderate disease; systemic medications (with or without topical agents) are recommended for severe or recalcitrant acne. Therapeutic measures are generally targeted at the major etiologic components. Topical treatments include the use of benzoyl peroxide preparations, antibiotics, or both. The antikeratinizing agent retinoic acid (tretinoin) may be effective when used alone or in combination with other topical agents. Systemic antibiotics such as erythromycin, clindamycin, tetracycline, and trimethoprim-sulfamethoxazole are effective in reducing bacterial numbers and inflammation. Oral 13-*cis*-retinoic acid (isotretinoin) can be particularly effective in controlling nodulocystic acne. However, isotretinoin is associated with significant side effects that include cheilitis, dry skin, elevation of serum triglyceride and cholesterol levels, elevation of liver enzymes, pseudotumor cerebri, and most important, high teratogenicity. Patient education, to keep expectations realistic and compliance high, must be part of the patient treatment package.

Perioral Dermatitis

Perioral dermatitis is an inflammatory eruption characterized by periorificial papules and pustules. The use of topical steroids predisposes to this acneiform eruption, although tartar control dentifrices have also been implicated. Women between the ages of 15 and 45 years are predominantly affected, although it is occasionally seen in children and in men.

Clinical Features. Perioral dermatitis usually presents as a symmetric eruption consisting of tiny papules, microvesicles, or small pustules around the nasal alae and the mouth and on the chin (Figure 17-18). The eruption may also be seen in the glabellar and eyelid regions. These changes are superimposed on a diffuse or patchy erythematous base associated with variable degrees of scaling. A highly characteristic feature is the appearance of a narrow margin of normal skin between the vermilion and the eruption.

Histopathology. Epidermal changes tend to be relatively mild and include slight acanthosis, spongiosis, and

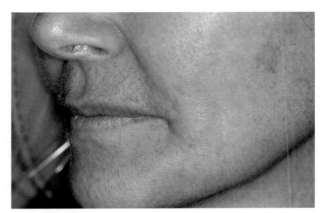

Figure 17-18 **Perioral dermatitis.**

parakeratosis. Scattered throughout the dermis is a mild inflammatory cell infiltrate of lymphocytes, plasma cells, and macrophages.

Treatment. If sensitizing agents are identified, withdrawal of these should be curative. To prevent rebound due to discontinuation of topical steroids, the application of 1% hydrocortisone for a short time has proved to be beneficial in some cases. A short course of systemic antibiotics (for 1 to 2 months) may be necessary for acute control, but topical antibiotics (metronidazole) are the mainstay of treatment.

Folliculitis

Folliculitis, or inflammation of the hair follicle, may be due to various factors. Infection with *Staphylococcus* and *Candida* is a common cause. Pseudofolliculitis barbae, or razor bumps, is a foreign-body reaction to ingrown hairs and is more prevalent in African-Americans. Dermatophyte infection of the hair follicles may produce a similar picture and should be considered in the differential diagnosis. Candidal infection most often involves perioral hairs and is accompanied by flaking of the skin. Bacterial infection may occur after injury, abrasion, or occlusive steroid treatment and is usually due to *Staphylococcus*. However, follicular infection with dermatophytes can occur, although it is usually limited to the beard and mustache areas. Bacterial cultures, Gram staining, or potassium hydroxide preparations may be helpful in diagnosis.

Clinical Features. Folliculitis is manifested as a painless or slightly tender pustule with surrounding erythema.

Histopathology. Pustules show considerable perifollicular infiltrate of neutrophils or lymphocytes, with occasional necrosis of the hair follicle and perifollicular epidermis. Follicular pus collections are noted. Pseudofolliculitis barbae usually demonstrates hair growth back into the epidermis, with resulting neutrophilic infiltrate.

Treatment. The cause dictates the treatment. If razor irritation is suspected, postponement of shaving, later use of hydrating lubricants, and the use of new razors is recommended. Warm, wet compresses or oral antibiotics may be useful. Fungal infection with *Candida* or dermatophytes should be treated with appropriate systemic antifungals.

Furuncle

The furuncle, or boil, is a deep, painful, fluctuant inflammatory nodule that is preceded by staphylococcal folliculitis. Furuncles occur in areas of heavy perspiration or friction, such as the face, neck, axillae, and buttocks.

Clinical Features. A furuncle is a firm, tender, erythematous nodule. Rupture may occur spontaneously, with extrusion of pus and sometimes a necrotic core.

Histopathology. Perifollicular necrosis with many neutrophils and fibrinoid material is identified, and a large abscess is located in the subcutaneous tissue. A Gram stain reveals gram-positive cocci, and the cultures are positive for *S. aureus.*

Treatment. Moist heat application may decrease pain and promote drainage. Incisional drainage may be required, as well as oral antibiotics if the lesions are accompanied by fever, are difficult to eradicate, or are complicated by cellulitis. Rarely, furuncles may result in bacteremia. Squeezing furuncles located around the lips and nose may seed the cavernous sinus via the facial and angular emissary veins.

Miliaria

Miliaria, or heat rash, is a dermatologic condition that occurs in predisposed individuals after exercise or heat exposure. It is due to obstruction of the intraepidermal portion of eccrine ducts, with subsequent leakage of sweat into the surrounding tissue and an inflammatory response. Three distinct types are noted, depending on the histologic level of leakage: miliaria crystallina, miliaria rubra, and miliaria profunda.

Clinical Features. Miliaria crystallina is characterized by small, asymptomatic, superficial papules or vesicles ("dewdrops") that often occur after an insult to the horny layer, such as in a sunburn. Miliaria rubra, or prickly heat, develops in skin covered by clothing as a result of obstruction of the eccrine duct deeper in the epidermis. This eruption is pruritic, or prickly, with papulovesicles surrounded by erythema. Anhidrosis and heat intolerance can occur. Miliaria profunda most often develops in people in tropical climates, particularly after several episodes of miliaria rubra. In this case the occlusion occurs at the dermal-epidermal junction. The lesions are white to flesh-colored papules and are not pruritic. Anhidrosis can be severe.

Histopathology. Miliaria crystallina is characterized by intracorneal or subcorneal vesicles in continuity with the underlying eccrine ducts, with a neutrophilic infiltrate at the periphery of the vesicle. The surrounding epidermis is spongiotic, and the papillary dermis is edematous. In miliaria rubra, spongiotic vesicles in the spiny layer are continuous with sweat ducts. Spongiosis and a lymphocytic infiltrate of the periductal area are usually noted. Miliaria profunda is similar to miliaria rubra but involves the lower epidermis and the upper dermis.

Treatment. Treatment is supportive and includes allowing air to circulate, control of fever, and application of a camphor-menthol–containing lotion to relieve the itching.

Granuloma Faciale

Granuloma faciale is a cutaneous lesion of unknown cause; however, some immunofluorescence data have suggested that it is immune complex mediated. No systemic involvement is noted.

Clinical Features. The lesions of granuloma faciale classically are asymptomatic soft, brown-red papules, plaques, or nodules. They range in size from a few millimeters to several centimeters. They occasionally become annular and are made worse or darkened after exposure to sunlight. These granulomas are seen primarily in middle life and are more common in men and in Caucasians. Granuloma faciale does not ulcerate, but telangiectasias may occur on its surface.

Histopathology. The epidermis is unaffected. A dense, mostly neutrophilic infiltrate is found in the dermis and occasionally extending into the subcutaneous tissue. A grenz zone (unaffected border) separates the infiltrate from the epidermis. Immunofluorescence studies have shown deposition of immunoglobulin

(IgG, IgM), complement, and fibrin around vessels and at the dermal-epidermal junction.

Treatment. Granuloma faciale is notoriously resistant to treatment and has a high rate of recurrence. Radiation, cryotherapy, cauterization, and systemic corticosteroids all provide unpredictable control of these lesions. Surgical removal and dermabrasion have shown better results, but recurrence is still likely.

Hemangioma

See Chapter 4.

Morbilliform Drug Eruptions

Morbilliform, or maculopapular, eruptions are the most common of the drug-induced reactions. Although any drug may be implicated, antibiotics are the most likely class of medications to cause morbilliform eruptions. New medications are highly suspicious.

Clinical Features. The eruption presents as symmetric erythematous, blanching macules and papules that may become confluent. The eruption appears on the trunk or on areas of physical trauma, at any time from less than a week after starting treatment until several weeks after discontinuing the drug. Patients may experience involvement of mucous membranes (erythema, lichenoid change), mild fever, or pruritus. The major differential diagnosis is that of viral exanthems; laboratory findings are nonspecific and generally unrewarding. However, if fever and eosinophilia are associated with the eruption, the drug should be discontinued and the patient evaluated for evidence of liver toxicity, as is encountered in the phenytoin (Dilantin) hypersensitivity syndrome.

Histopathology. Some vacuolation of the dermal-epidermal junction may be observed. A variable, mainly perivascular infiltrate of lymphocytes and sometimes eosinophils is characteristic. Occasionally noted are papillary edema and fibrinoid deposition.

Treatment. The eruption often disappears or decreases in severity despite ongoing use of the causative agent. Discontinuation of the offending agent is curative; however, the eruption may not disappear for several weeks. Further support measures include topical steroids and antihistamines.

Lichen Planus

See Chapter 3.

Varix

See Chapter 4.

NODULES

A nodule is an elevated, circumscribed, solid lesion that measures more than 0.5 cm.

Keratoacanthoma

See Chapter 6.

Basal Cell Carcinoma

Basal cell carcinoma is the most prevalent cancer of the skin, and it is also the most prevalent cancer of the head and neck. The lesion is most often encountered in older patients on non–hair-bearing skin. Men are more commonly affected than women, presumably because of greater cumulative sun exposure. This malignancy arises from basal cells of the skin. The vast majority of basal cell carcinomas occur on sun-exposed skin. Except in very rare instances, basal cell carcinoma does not occur on mucous membranes.

Individuals at increased risk for the development of basal cell carcinoma are those with lighter natural skin pigmentation, those with a long history of chronic sun exposure, and those with one of several predisposing hereditary syndromes. Among the latter is nevoid basal cell carcinoma syndrome, in which individuals have multiple odontogenic keratocysts, skeletal abnormalities, and numerous basal cell carcinomas.

Clinical Features. Basal cell carcinoma presents as an indurated pearly papule or nodule with telangiectatic vessels coursing over its surface (Figures 17-19 and 17-20). With time, the center of the tumor becomes ulcerated and crusted. If untreated, the tumor exhibits a slow but relentless locally destructive nature. Other clinical forms may on occasion be seen. The pigmented form of basal cell carcinoma presents in a manner similar to that of the noduloulcerative type, with the addition of melanin pigmentation within or at the periphery. The superficial form presents as a scaly erythematous lesion flush with the skin surface, occasionally appearing as an atrophic scarlike process. The fibrosing form of basal cell carcinoma presents as an indurated yellowish plaque that may be slightly depressed or flat, resembling a slow or insidiously enlarging scar in the absence of trauma. Because basal

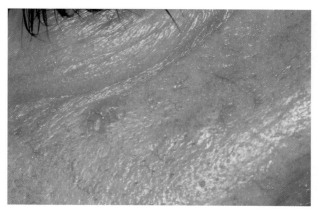

Figure 17-19   Basal cell carcinoma.

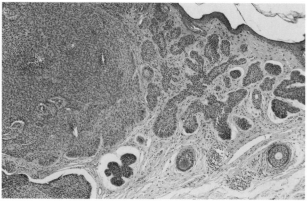

Figure 17-21   **Basal cell carcinoma.** Note solid tumor *(left)* and nested tumor *(right).*

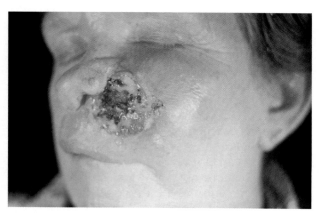

Figure 17-20   Basal cell carcinoma.

cell carcinomas are generally slow growing and rarely metastatic, the prognosis is very good.

Histopathology. In basal cell carcinomas, nests and cords of cuboidal cells arise from the region of the epidermal basal cells (Figure 17-21). The neoplastic cells around the periphery of the invading nests and strands are usually palisaded and often columnar. In some infiltrative basal cell carcinomas, tiny infiltrative nests are found in a fibroblastic stroma. This has been described as an aggressive growth pattern and may portend a more aggressive clinical course.

Treatment. Various surgical procedures (standard scalpel surgery, cryosurgery, electrosurgery, Mohs' microscopically guided surgery) and irradiation can be used to treat basal cell carcinoma. The type of treatment depends on the size and location of the neoplasm, as well as the experience and training of the clinician.

Squamous Cell Carcinoma

In the vast majority of cases squamous cell carcinoma of the face and lower lip arises from epidermal keratinocytes that have been damaged by sunlight. Unlike basal cell carcinoma, this neoplasm has a significant potential to metastasize to regional lymph nodes and beyond. As with basal cell carcinoma, several factors contribute to the etiology of squamous cell carcinoma; however, the chief factor remains repeated and chronic damage caused by sunlight. The highest incidence is noted in fair-skinned individuals after long-term exposure to sunlight. In addition, carcinogens such as tars, oils, and arsenicals; exposure to x-rays; and the presence of skin diseases that cause scarring, such as severe burns and discoid lupus erythematosus (DLE), also predispose to malignant transformation of the epithelium.

Clinical Features. The clinical course is insidious, evolving over months to years. A central ulcer with slightly raised indurated margins and surrounding erythema eventually forms. Lesions may occasionally appear as verrucous growths, papules, or plaques. Areas of the face most commonly affected include the lower lip, tip of the ear, forehead, and infraorbital/nasal bridge region (Figure 17-22). Lesions are firm and indurated, reflecting tumor infiltration of adjacent tissues.

Lesions that arise within solar keratoses are less aggressive than those arising de novo or in some sun-protected locations. Squamous cell carcinomas arising in sites of irradiation, burns, or chronic degenerative skin disorders are more aggressive than their sun-exposure counterparts. A squamous cell carcinoma arising in solar cheilitis tends to invade and metasta-

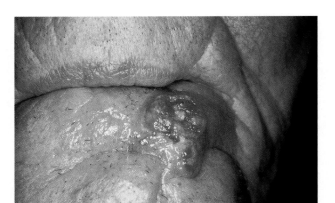

Figure 17-22 Squamous cell carcinoma.

size at an earlier point than its counterpart in sun-damaged skin. Intraoral squamous cell carcinomas are far more aggressive than cutaneous tumors.

Histopathology. This tumor consists of atypical keratinocytes that invade the dermis and beyond. As with intraoral squamous cell carcinoma, cytologic features include an increased nuclear-cytoplasmic ratio, nuclear hyperchromatism, individual cell keratinization, tumor giant cells, atypical mitotic figures, and an increased mitotic rate.

Treatment. The mainstay of therapy remains excision. The mode of excision, however, depends on the size and location of the lesion. Larger carcinomas may be treated with wide excision, often with reconstructive grafts, or irradiation therapy. Microscopically directed surgery (Mohs' surgery) may be used because of its advantage in tissue conservation. The overall 5-year cure rate for squamous cell carcinoma of the skin is approximately 90%.

WHEALS

A wheal is a transient papule or plaque formed by serum exudation into the dermis. Wheals are produced by vasodilation and fluid leakage secondary to histamine release from mast cells and basophils.

Urticaria (Hives)

Clinical Features. Urticaria, or wheals, may be erythematous or white; they may be of any size; and they usually are pruritic. Urticaria may be caused by a reaction to foods, insect venom, infections, drugs, systemic

disease, and physical stimuli. Physical hives include dermographism and cholinergic, solar, and cold urticaria.

Histopathology. Histopathologic features include dermal edema, dilated venules, and swelling of endothelial cells, without many inflammatory cells. In chronic lesions the edema may be accompanied by a mixed inflammatory cell infiltrate.

Treatment. Avoidance of the precipitating factor with the use of antihistamines and possibly corticosteroids or epinephrine for severe or refractory cases is curative. A skin biopsy and further workup for internal disease may occasionally be necessary.

Angioedema

See Chapter 2.

PAPULOSQUAMOUS DERMATOSES

Actinic Keratoses (Solar Keratoses)

Actinic keratoses are epithelial changes noted typically in light-complexioned individuals who have had long-term exposure to sunlight. A small percentage of these lesions develop into squamous cell carcinoma. Outdoor workers and individuals participating in extensive outdoor recreation are particularly prone to the development of actinic keratoses.

Clinical Features. Oval plaques, usually less than 1 cm in diameter, are typically found on the forehead, cheeks, temples, lower lip, ears, and lateral portions of the neck (Figure 17-23). The color may vary from yellow-brown to red, and the texture is usually rough and sandpaper-like.

Histopathology. Common to the many actinic keratosis microscopic subtypes are nuclear atypia, an increased nuclear-cytoplasmic ratio, and atypical proliferation of basal cells. The dermis generally contains a lymphocytic inflammatory cell infiltrate. Elastotic or basophilic change of collagen and irregular clumps of altered elastic fibers and regenerated collagen are noted in these areas.

Treatment. Individual actinic keratoses may be treated with cryotherapy. However, in patients with confluent actinic keratoses, the therapeutic mainstay is topical application of 5-fluorouracil. Additional treatment modalities include curettage and surgical excision. For

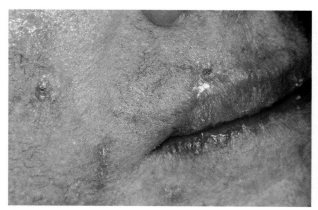

Figure 17-23 Actinic keratosis.

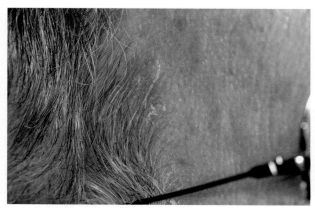

Figure 17-24 Seborrheic dermatitis, erythematous scale.

lesions that are indurated or nodular or that demonstrate marked inflammation, a biopsy to rule out invasive squamous cell carcinoma is necessary.

Seborrheic Dermatitis

Seborrheic dermatitis is a chronic waxing and waning papulosquamous eruption of unknown etiology. It is more common in individuals of northern European or Celtic background. Seborrheic dermatitis can also be seen in individuals with zinc deficiency, those receiving hyperalimentation, and those with Parkinson's disease or in an immunosuppressed state.

Clinical Features. The onset of seborrheic dermatitis is gradual, usually with symptoms of pruritus, and is often increased with perspiration. Worsening during winter months is typical. Commonly affected is the scalp, followed by the eyelid margins, nasolabial folds, cheeks, forehead, and eyebrows (Figure 17-24). At times, otitis externa may be the presenting manifestation of this reaction.

Seborrheic dermatitis may present within the first few weeks of life but more commonly appears between 20 and 50 years of age. Males are more commonly affected. Affected areas may appear yellowish red to gray to white. Dry, scaling macules or papules of various sizes and with diffuse margins are often present. Lesions tend to assume nummular (coin-shaped) or polycyclic (clustered or coalesced circular arrays) patterns. In contrast, scalp psoriasis tends to be sharply circumscribed and raised, with a silvery scale that is more compact.

Histopathology. The early lesions of seborrheic dermatitis are characterized by widely dilated superficial blood vessels with corresponding edema within the papillary dermis and a sparse perivascular lymphocytic infiltrate. The epidermis exhibits a slight degree of focal spongiosis. On the surface a scale or crust containing neutrophils is noted at the follicular ostia. Later, follicular plugging, crusts at the infundibular ostia, spongiosis, and superficial perivascular round cell infiltrates are noted. Chronic lesions tend to be psoriasiform.

Treatment. Conservative therapy is recommended, especially in mild cases. Recurrences and remissions are characteristic. The use of topical steroids or systemic or topical ketoconazole provides significant benefit.

Psoriasis

Psoriasis is a common skin disease affecting 2% of the population. It is of unknown cause but is strongly linked to heredity. Triggering factors include systemic infections, stress, and drugs. Psoriasis appears to be an immunoregulatory disorder in which epidermal changes are related to a defect in the control of keratinocyte proliferation. The hyperproliferative state of the affected epidermis produces a turnover rate that is as much as eight times greater than normal.

Clinical Features. Psoriasis occurs at any age but most commonly appears during young adult life. It is a chronic disease that may persist throughout life, with periods of exacerbation and remission. Various triggers, such as trauma, infection, and stress, may precipitate new episodes. The development of psoriatic lesions following trauma of normal-appearing skin is known as *Koebner's reaction* or *phenomenon.*

The basic skin lesion of psoriasis is a well-defined erythematous plaque covered by silvery scales (Figure

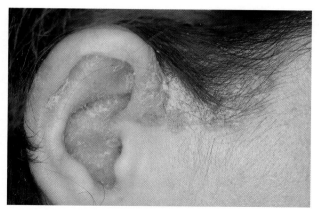

Figure 17-25 Psoriasis.

17-25). When the scales are removed, small pinpoint bleeding is seen because of increased vascularity under focal areas of epidermal thinning, the so-called *Auspitz sign*. Oral lesions of psoriasis are rare. Geographic tongue has also been listed as an oral manifestation of psoriasis; this may simply be a coincidental finding.

In a small percentage of psoriatic patients a seronegative polyarthritis may be identified. The temporomandibular joint may occasionally be one of the joints involved in this process. Pain and restricted motion are encountered with erosion of the condyle.

Histopathology. Because of the hyperproliferative nature of psoriasis, epithelial hyperplasia due to acanthosis and parakeratosis is seen. Connective tissue papillae contain lymphocytes and prominent capillaries covered by thinned epithelium. Neutrophils are usually found in the epithelium, often in aggregates between epithelial cells, producing microabscesses that are called *Munro microabscesses*.

Treatment. A wide variety of drugs are available for the treatment of cutaneous psoriasis. The drug or combination of drugs used depends on the clinician's training and experience and the patient's response. Topical preparations (tars, anthralin, and corticosteroids), systemic agents (methotrexate and retinoids), and photochemotherapy (PUVA) all have their advantages and proponents.

Atopic Dermatitis

Atopic dermatitis (AD) is a chronic, relapsing inflammatory condition affecting all age-groups; infants, children, and adolescents are predominantly affected. A personal or family history of AD, eczema, asthma, hay fever, or sinusitis is usually elicited. AD has a female predominance and often an association with an elevated serum IgE level.

Clinical Features. AD is characterized by periods of exacerbation and remission. AD presents as small follicular, erythematous papules associated with considerable pruritus. However, these may enlarge and become lichenified or may evolve into vesicles or bullae. In infants AD predominates on the face. As afflicted children mature, AD tends to affect flexural skin. In older children and adults AD involves the antecubital and popliteal fossae and the sides of the neck.

Histopathology. The epidermis exhibits mild spongiosis and parakeratosis in the early phases of AD, with lymphocytes and histiocytes scattered around the superficial vascular plexus. AD of longer duration is marked by elongation of the rete ridges, hyperkeratosis, and wedge-shaped hypergranulosis with areas of developing parakeratosis. Spongiosis and cellular infiltrates are less prominent. Eosinophils are less common in AD than in allergic contact dermatitis.

Treatment. Treatment of AD is usually empirical, and decisions about treatment are based on the skin findings at a specific time. Eliminating irritating factors and using topical steroids temporarily can improve follicular eczema. When lichenified, AD does not resolve unless the chronic irritant or trauma is eliminated. Treating with hydration and water trapping with hydrophobic agents is helpful. Histamine receptor (types 1 and 2) blocking agents may also provide benefit in preventing and controlling the associated pruritus. Recently treatment with tacrolimus and pimecrolimus have proved promising.

Keratosis Pilaris

Keratosis pilaris is a very common asymptomatic and persistent skin condition associated with AD. Areas typically affected include the lateral aspects of the arms, the thighs, the buttocks, and the face. Keratosis pilaris is more severe in the winter months.

Clinical Features. Discrete, keratotic, follicular papules are surrounded by a rim of erythema.

Histopathology. The orifice and upper portion of the follicular infundibulum are blocked and dilated by an orthokeratotic plug of keratin. A twisted villous hair may be trapped within the plug. A mild mononuclear cell infiltrate is often present in the surrounding dermis.

Treatment. A lubricating cream may help to smooth the rough skin; keratolytic agents such as lactic acid lotions or salicylic acid may also be used. Retinoic acid may be of benefit in severe cases.

Pityriasis Rosea

Pityriasis rosea (PR) is an acute, self-limited dermatitis that follows a distinctive course. PR affects females more often than males, occurs from late childhood to middle age, and is of unknown cause. Although PR has many similarities to viral exanthems, no infective agent has been isolated. PR-like rashes have also been described after initiation of treatment with drugs such as barbiturates, bismuth, and angiotensin-converting enzyme inhibitors, but these rashes tend to show some atypia when compared with classic PR. PR is often preceded by a prodrome with symptoms of fever, malaise, loss of appetite, nausea, and joint pain.

Clinical Features. The primary plaque, or herald patch, is a round or oval salmon-colored, peripherally scaling plaque that is seen in the majority of cases. It is commonly located on the trunk. The secondary eruption appears simultaneously or up to several weeks later. Either small plaques that resemble miniature versions of the primary plaque or small erythematous papules on the trunk, neck, or back characterize PR. The herald patch and the eruption may occur at the same time. They appear in a Christmas tree pattern on the back because they lie in skin cleavage lines. The secondary eruption reaches its peak within 2 weeks, lasts for 2 to 10 weeks, and is variably pruritic.

Histopathology. In the secondary lesions, spongiosis due to intracellular edema, variable acanthosis, focal parakeratosis, and exocytosis of lymphocytes are noted in the epidermis. A dermal lymphoid infiltrate with eosinophils or macrophages and erythrocyte extravasation in the dermis is seen. The herald patch has similar, but amplified, findings.

Treatment. Because PR is self-limited, active therapy usually is not needed. Irritants should be minimized, with severe itching treated with zinc oxide, calamine lotion, or oral antihistamines. In more severe cases topical corticosteroids or even a short course of oral corticosteroids may be useful.

Warts (Verruca Vulgaris and Flat Warts)

Verruca vulgaris, the common wart, is caused by human papillomavirus (HPV) (Figure 17-26). Many subtypes of HPV are responsible. They appear as firm, circumscribed, verrucous papules or nodules on the hands, face, or scalp. Any skin site may be affected, including the lips and oral mucosa. Warts show hyperkeratosis, acanthosis, and papillomatosis. Also seen are foci of koilocytic cells (vacuolated cells) in the stratum malpighii, focal areas of parakeratosis, and clumped keratohyaline granules. Most warts regress spontaneously within 2 years. Treatment for warts is nonspecific destruction; various destructive methods include cryotherapy, salicylates, and excision. Cimetidine has been reported to be effective in children.

Flat warts are flat, smooth papules that typically measure 0.2 to 0.4 cm. They are usually flesh colored or hyperpigmented and have minimal scale. The dorsal aspects of the hands and the face are commonly involved sites. Like other warts, flat warts are caused by HPV, specifically subtypes 3 and 10. These subtypes have not been associated with malignant transformation. The epidermis shows hyperkeratosis, acanthosis, and slight elongation of rete ridges but no papillomatosis or parakeratosis. The cells of the granular layer often have diffuse vacuolation with basophilic nuclei. The dermis appears normal. Treatment is often difficult and frustrating. Results often depend on the modality used. These include the application of dry ice, liquid nitrogen, caustic agents, or retinoic acid.

VESICLES/BULLAE/PUSTULES

Vesicles, bullae, and pustules represent a circumscribed collection of fluid within or just beneath the epithelium. Vesicles measure up to 0.5 cm, whereas bullae measure greater than 0.5 cm in diameter. Pustules are circumscribed collections of pus (leukocytes and

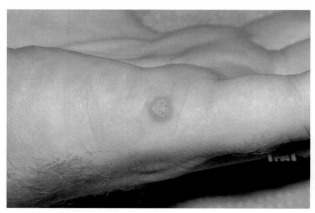

Figure 17-26 Verruca vulgaris.

serum) that vary in size from 0.1 to 2 cm. Pustules may be primary or secondary lesions.

Herpes Simplex Infection

See Chapter 1.

Varicella-Zoster Infection

See Chapter 1.

Contact Dermatitis

Contact dermatitis (CD) is a spongiotic dermatitis that is a reaction to environmental substances. CD may be classified as irritant or allergic CD. Irritant CD is a nonallergic inflammation of the skin caused by direct toxic effects of irritants. Toxic chemicals include alkalis, detergents, and organic solvents. Even repeated wetting and drying is very irritating. Allergic CD is a delayed-type hypersensitivity reaction that is precipitated by specific antigens that include *Rhus* (poison ivy, oak, and sumac), nickel, rubber, preservatives in cosmetics, and topical medications.

Clinical Features. Allergic and irritant CD are not always clinically distinguishable. CD may present as simple dryness, cracking, or erythema but may be vesicular, necrotic, or ulcerative (Figure 17-27). The reaction depends on the type of chemical, its concentration, the mode of exposure, local barriers, and the body site. Allergic CD may present 24 to 72 hours after exposure to the antigen as pruritic, erythematous vesicles and papules. Sharply demarcated reaction patterns are diagnostic of an allergic CD and represent the exact shape of the offending substance.

Histopathology. The histologic pattern of irritant CD ranges from the spongiotic changes of allergic CD to extensive ulceration. Necrosis, often into the dermis, neutrophilic infiltration, and acantholysis are much more common in irritant CD than in the allergic form. In early allergic CD, the epidermis is spongiotic, and vesicles, if present, may contain Langerhans cells. Eosinophils are often present in the dermal infiltrate and areas of spongiosis. Continued exposure to the antigen may eventually produce lichen simplex chronicus.

Treatment. Diagnosis and identification of the offending compound by history or by testing for delayed hypersensitivity reaction (patch testing) is the first step in managing suspected allergic CD. In both allergic and irritant dermatitis, subsequent avoidance of the offending substance is required, and desensitization for the antigenic substance may be beneficial if it is identified.

Impetigo

Impetigo is an acute superficial bacterial infection of the skin. This superficial infection of the skin is due to group A streptococci, *S. aureus,* or a mixture of the two. Complications associated with impetigo are unusual. Nonetheless, glomerulonephritis can occur with some strains of streptococci. In the vast majority of cases, however, impetigo clears rapidly with proper therapy.

Clinical Features. This infection, common in children and adolescents, is highly contagious and spreads readily within the home, school, or institution. The initial lesion is a small vesicle on the face, extending periorally and along the base of the nose (Figure 17-28). As vesicles rupture, crusts form and pus appears. Autoinoculation produces spread to other sites. Areas affected are pruritic and typically measure from 1 to 3 cm. Central healing is noted as the lesions progress centrifugally (polycyclic pattern). In the perioral region, impetigo may be confused with recurrent or secondary herpes simplex virus (HSV) infections.

Treatment. Antibiotics are required to treat impetigo. Penicillinase-stable antibiotics may be necessary if *Staphylococcus* is an etiologic agent. New generations of potent topical antibiotics such as mupirocin are also clinically effective.

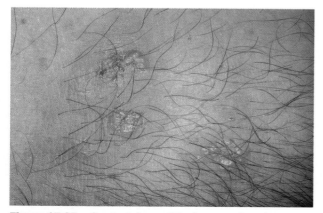

Figure 17-27 **Contact dermatitis** due to poison ivy.

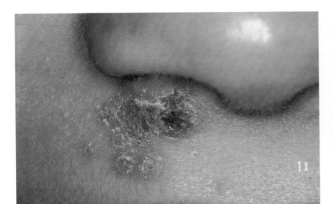

Figure 17-28 Impetigo.

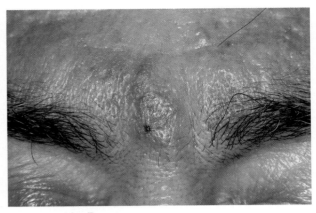

Figure 17-29 Rosacea.

Rosacea

Rosacea represents an inflammatory process that involves the infundibular portion of the hair follicles with various levels of severity. The specific cause of rosacea is unknown, but several factors can influence the evolution of this condition. An underlying vasomotor instability that is worsened by the intake of hot beverages, alcohol, and hot or spicy foods is believed to be involved. Environmental factors such as extreme temperatures and sunlight can also exacerbate this condition. Vasodilator drugs can produce flushing and worsen the condition. Rosacea may develop in association with the use of topical corticosteroid medications, sometimes called *steroid rosacea*. Topically applied potent preparations initially produce vasoconstriction. On discontinuation of this therapy, however, rebound vasodilation takes place and often worsens the underlying condition.

Clinical Features. Rosacea is characterized by facial erythema with or without an overlying papular/pustular eruption (Figure 17-29). Comedones of acne are absent. Distribution is over the central portion of the face, especially the cheeks, nose, and chin. The condition usually begins in the fourth decade of life and may occur later in women in association with menopause. The eyes may also be involved, with attendant symptoms of conjunctivitis, blepharitis, and keratitis.

Severe and long-standing cases of rosacea may result in the formation of bulbous, greasy, and hypertrophic lesions of the nose. This condition, known as *rhinophyma*, occurs particularly in men older than 40 years of age (Figure 17-30). The nasal tip and alae are usually involved by persistent lymphedema and sebaceous

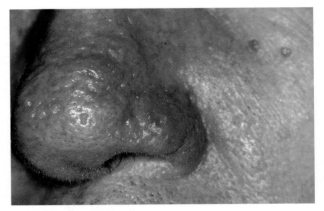

Figure 17-30 Rhinophyma.

gland hyperplasia, resulting in the clinical appearance of extremely dilated follicles containing large plugs of keratin and sebaceous material.

Histopathology. Rosacea is essentially a follicular inflammatory process that progresses to a suppurative folliculitis and ultimately to a granulomatous form with associated dermatitis. Epithelioid granulomas may form. In rhinophyma, massive sebaceous gland hyperplasia and associated infundibular cysts are seen. Cysts tend to rupture or leak into the surrounding dermis, causing a granulomatous response and suppuration.

Treatment. The mainstay of therapy remains systemic tetracycline and topical metronidazole. Patients are urged to avoid heat, cold, sunlight, alcohol, coffee, and spicy foods. Rhinophyma management is surgical.

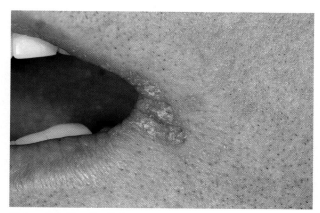

Figure 17-31   Perlèche.

Erythema Multiforme

See Chapter 2.

Pemphigus Vulgaris

See Chapter 1.

EROSIONS/FISSURES/ULCERS/SCARS

Erosions, fissures, ulcers, and scars all represent focal destruction of cutaneous tissue. Erosions are defined as loss of the epidermis only. Erosions heal without scar formation. Ulcers are defined as epidermal loss and dermal damage. Cutaneous ulcers heal with scar formation. Scars are permanent alterations in the appearance of skin and are due to damage and collagenous repair of the skin.

Perlèche

Perlèche, or angular cheilitis, is inflammation and atrophy of the skin folds at the angles of the mouth. This may be due to excessive lip licking, thumb sucking, or sagging of facial skin in edentulous or elderly persons. Prolonged contact with saliva results in maceration, with possible secondary infection by *Candida* or staphylococci.

Clinical Features. The skin at the angles of the mouth has erythematous fissures, often with exudate and crust (Figure 17-31). Further licking to moisten the inflamed area exacerbates the problem.

Treatment. Treatment consists of applying antimicrobial creams, followed by low-potency steroid creams, until the symptoms resolve. Protective lip balm may help prevent recurrence.

Burns

The skin is burned on exposure to extremes of heat, with severity depending on the temperature, skin thickness, and duration of exposure. Thermal damage to the skin causes coagulation necrosis, enzymatic inactivation, and capillary damage.

Clinical Features. Healing is slow, with considerable scarring. *First-degree* burns are superficial burns that appear soft and hyperemic without blister formation. Healing occurs without scarring. *Second-degree* burns may be superficial or deep and involve the dermis to some extent. *Third-degree* burns involve full-thickness destruction of the skin with extensive scar formation that almost always requires grafting.

Histopathology. *First-degree* burns show intraepidermal edema and occasionally superficial necrosis. In *second-degree* burns, variable epidermal necrosis, blister formation, and epidermal edema are noted. Superficial necrosis of dermal collagen may be observed. *Third-degree* burns are characterized by full-thickness necrosis of the epidermis and dermis. Scars show homogeneous collagen and loss of skin appendages.

Treatment. Treatment depends on the type of burn and exceeds the scope of this chapter.

Keloid

Clinical Features. Keloids are hyperplastic scars that persist or enlarge over the course of one to several years. These lesions are often tender, painful, or hyperesthetic, especially early in development. They are commonly located on the shoulder, chest, or head but may occur anywhere, usually after injury. Keloids are more common in African-Americans.

Histopathology. The epidermis may be flattened, and adnexal structures or elastic fibers may be few. In the dermis, nodules of hypereosinophilic collagen are arranged in thick, compacted bands.

Treatment. Treatment includes surgical removal, steroid injections, cryotherapy, or silicone gel sheeting. Recurrences are very common.

CONNECTIVE TISSUE DISEASES

Dermatomyositis

Dermatomyositis is one of the major systemic inflammatory diseases of connective tissue. It is manifested as an inflammatory myopathy with characteristic cutaneous findings. Dermatomyositis is an uncommon disease with characteristic dual peaks of occurrence: one in childhood and one in late middle age. Systemic manifestations of dermatomyositis include proximal symmetric muscle weakness, elevated levels of muscle enzymes, characteristic muscle biopsy findings, muscle pain, and eventually muscle atrophy. Dermatomyositis may be associated with malignancy, especially in adults.

Clinical Features. The main dermatologic findings in dermatomyositis are the heliotrope rash and Gottron's papules. The heliotrope rash is a distinctive violaceous, slightly edematous periorbital swelling. It is found most often on the upper eyelids. Gottron's papules are discrete purple-red papules over bony prominences such as the knees, knuckles, and elbows. Evolution of these papules into plaques with telangiectasis and pigmentary changes is known as *Gottron's sign.*

Histopathology. The histologic changes may be almost indistinguishable from those seen in systemic lupus erythematosus (SLE). The epidermis is thinned, the basement membrane is fragmented, a sparse lymphocytic infiltrate is found perivascularly, and interstitial mucin is deposited. Severe inflammatory changes may include subepidermal fibrin deposition. Unlike SLE, dermatomyositis is not characterized by immune complexes at the dermal-epidermal junction.

Treatment. Treatment of dermatomyositis is usually with prednisone and bed rest, with tapering initiated once muscle weakness has started to improve. Other modalities used for unresponsive cases include plasmapheresis, cytotoxic drugs, and total-body irradiation. Improvement usually occurs with the use of steroids; however, this is often a very chronic and debilitating disease. Treatment of the underlying malignancy, if present, resolves the symptoms.

Lupus Erythematosus

See Chapter 3.

Scleroderma

Scleroderma is a chronic disease of unknown cause, although it is generally regarded as an immune dysfunction condition. Two basic forms are recognized:

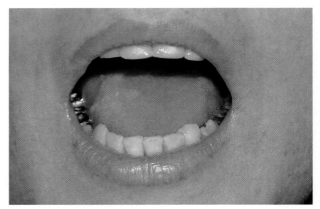

Figure 17-32   Scleroderma; perioral fibrosis limiting the oral opening.

a relatively inconsequential but disfiguring localized cutaneous form known as *morphea* and a potentially life-threatening form known as *systemic scleroderma.* The remainder of this discussion focuses on the systemic type. It often occurs in conjunction with other autoimmune conditions such as rheumatoid arthritis, lupus erythematosus, dermatomyositis, and Sjögren's syndrome. Rheumatoid factor and antinuclear antibodies are typically demonstrable in patients with scleroderma. Hypergammaglobulinemia and an elevated erythrocyte sedimentation rate are also noted. Along with an increased rate of collagen synthesis is the appearance of vascular changes. Inflammatory and obstructive changes are seen microscopically in arterioles and capillaries, supporting the notion that vessel changes are important in the pathogenesis of scleroderma. Also, Raynaud's phenomenon, a peripheral vascular condition, often precedes the other manifestations of the disease. Systemic scleroderma appears usually during middle age (30 to 50 years) and predominantly in women (4 to 1). There is no racial predilection.

Clinical Features. The disease can affect any organ and may progress to affect many organ systems (Figures 17-32 to 17-34). The skin is typically affected first, although joint involvement may provide the initial sign. In time, as fibrosis of organs progresses, signs of organ failure begin to appear.

Cutaneous manifestations are typified by pitting edema early in the disease process, followed by tightness and rigidity of the skin. The skin eventually becomes indurated, smooth, and atrophic, with telangiectasias. The face becomes expressionless and seems masklike. Fibrosis of the fingers leads to stiffness and atrophy of the skin over the digits. Vascular compro-

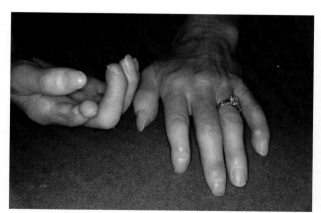

Figure 17-33 **Scleroderma** resulting in thickened and shortened fingertips.

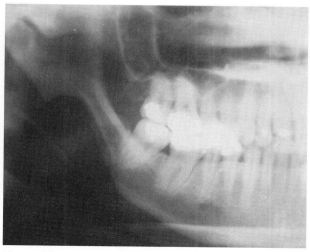

Figure 17-34 **Scleroderma** resulting in resorption of the posterior ramus.

mise may result in ischemia and ulceration of the fingertips—a phenomenon seen in both scleroderma and Raynaud's phenomenon.

The rigidity of the perioral skin causes restriction of the oral orifice. Oral hygiene and routine dental care become difficult. Fibrosis of the salivary glands gives rise to xerostomia and potentially to cervical caries. Mandibular bone resorption and uniformly widened periodontal membranes (as seen in periapical films) are also characteristic oral manifestations of this disease.

Histopathology. The primary histologic feature of scleroderma is the deposition of vast amounts of relatively acellular collagen. Perivascular lymphocytic infiltrates

are also typical. Minor salivary gland changes include pronounced interstitial fibrosis and acinar atrophy.

Treatment. Systemic disease stabilizes in most patients after a time. Patients with progressive disease are likely to succumb to renal, cardiac, or pulmonary failure. Other than supportive therapy, there is no satisfactory treatment for scleroderma. Corticosteroids may provide some benefit early but are not likely to give lasting control in progressive cases. Other drugs such as penicillamine and azathioprine have shown some promise.

BIBLIOGRAPHY

SOLAR LENTIGO

Griffiths CE, Goldfarb MT, Finkel LJ, et al: Topical tretinoin (retinoic acid) treatment of hyperpigmented lesions associated with photoaging in Chinese and Japanese patients: a vehicle-controlled trial, *J Am Acad Dermatol* 30:76-84, 1994.

ERYSIPELAS

Bisno AL, Stevens DL: Streptococcal infections of skin and soft tissues, *N Engl J Med* 334:1478, 1996.

SEBACEOUS HYPERPLASIA

Rosian R, Goslen JB, Brodell RT: The treatment of benign sebaceous hyperplasia with the topical application of bichloracetic acid, *J Dermatol Surg Oncol* 17:876-879, 1991.

ATOPIC DERMATITIS

Cooper KD: Atopic dermatitis: recent trends in pathogenesis and therapy (review), *J Invest Dermatol* 102:128-137, 1994.

Reitamo S, Remitz A, Kyllonen H, et al: Topical noncorticosteroid immunomodulation in the treatment of atopic dermatitis, *Am J Clin Dermatol* 3:381-388, 2002.

ERYTHEMA MULTIFORME

Detjen PF, Patterson R, Noskin GA, et al: Herpes simplex virus associated with recurrent Stevens-Johnson syndrome: a management strategy, *Arch Intern Med* 152:1513-1516, 1992.

Levy M, Shear NH: *Mycoplasma pneumoniae* infections and Stevens-Johnson syndrome: report of eight cases and review of the literature, *Clin Pediatr* 30:42-49, 1991.

DERMATOMYOSITIS

Cronin ME, Plotz PH: Idiopathic inflammatory myopathies, *Rheum Dis Clin North Am* 16:655–665, 1990.

DISCOID LUPUS ERYTHEMATOSUS

Weiss JS: Antimalarial medications in dermatology: a review, *Dermatol Clin* 9:377-385, 1991.

ADVANCED DIAGNOSTIC METHODS IN ORAL AND MAXILLOFACIAL PATHOLOGY

The analysis of DNA, RNA, and proteins, obtained from diagnostic specimens, is currently revolutionizing the practice of surgical pathology and heralds a new era of diagnostic and prognostic tests that will greatly influence our day-to-day clinical decision making. The diagnosis of cancer and many other diseases is fundamentally based on the microscopic study of cells and tissues. This diagnostic method remains the standard by which all other diagnostic tests are measured. Nevertheless, the era in which the pathologist relies entirely on the examination of tissue sections stained by histochemical methods is gradually being replaced by a time when advanced immunologic and molecular techniques (i.e., analysis of DNA, RNA, or protein structure or function) augment the process by which complicated infectious, inflammatory, metabolic, and neoplastic diseases are diagnosed and classified. Many of these molecular advances had their start in basic science research laboratories; following validation, technologic improvements, and automation, they have made their way into applied molecular pathology research and increasingly into the day-to-day practice of pathology. Today the extent to which immunopathologic and molecular pathologic techniques are employed varies greatly, but it is conceivable that in the next decade many of today's most technically advanced methods of molecular analysis will become standard practice.

MOLECULAR METHODS IN DIAGNOSTIC PATHOLOGY

Principles of Molecular Pathology

The basic building blocks for all eukaryotic life reside in the genes of cells. Genes, composed of deoxyribonucleic acid (DNA), encode for proteins that are the principal effector molecules for all biologic processes. The structure of DNA was unknown until 1953, when James Watson and Francis Crick published evidence for the double helix. DNA is a highly coiled, double-stranded molecule located within the nucleus of eukaryotic cells. It is composed of an ordered sequence of nucleotides, each consisting of the sugar deoxyribose, a phosphate group, and one of four bases: adenine (A), thymine (T), guanine (G), or cytosine (C). Each single strand of DNA binds, in a complementary fashion, with its opposing strand by adenine-thymine (A-T) and guanine-cytosine (G-C) pairing. Nucleotide pairing is highly precise; thus information represented by the genetic code is contained in each strand.

Protein synthesis proceeds through a series of defined steps, the first being the transcription of DNA into ribonucleic acid (RNA). *Transcription* is the term describing the base-pairing process that copies DNA into complementary RNA. Unlike DNA, RNA is single stranded, consisting of the sugar ribose, a phosphate group, and the nucleotide bases adenine, guanine, cytosine, and in place of thymine, uracil (U). RNA is formed in the nucleus by complementary binding of RNA nucleotides to a single strand of DNA, which acts as a nucleotide sequence template. With transport of the RNA molecule to the cytoplasm and some modification, the molecule is termed *messenger RNA (mRNA)*. A protein is produced on the mRNA template by the assembly of a string of amino acids—a process termed *translation*. The sequence of nucleotide base triplets (codon) in the mRNA dictates the order of specific amino acids, linked together to form a protein.

Polymerase Chain Reaction–Based Diagnostics. Polymerase chain reaction (PCR) has emerged as one of the most powerful tools for the amplification of genes and their RNA transcripts. Although the technique is relatively new, having first been described in 1985, it was alluded to conceptually at least 30 years ago. The identification of a heat-stable DNA polymerase and the development of machines to automate the repetitive heating and cooling cycles needed for the technique have greatly improved the methodology. Today PCR is one of the most important techniques used to study DNA and RNA obtained from a variety of tissue sources.

PCR typically begins with the isolation of DNA (genomic DNA) from a fresh tissue specimen or from tissue in a paraffin block. If RNA is the object of analysis, it must be isolated and converted to complementary DNA (cDNA) through reverse transcription. Heating separates the cDNA strands into single-stranded forms intended to act as a template for the addition of nucleotide sequences in vitro. Two short oligonucleotide primers are designed to anneal (bind) to the template and flank a region of interest (Figure 18-1). A thermostable DNA polymerase, isolated from the *Thermophilus aquaticus* organism, known as *Taq* polymerase, catalyzes the sequential addition of the four nucleotides (deoxynucleotide triphosphates [dNTPs]) to the primers. Cooling the solution permits the primers to bind to the template DNA, and then the Taq polymerase catalyzes the addition of dNTPs to the template between the primers. This process is then repeated, and with each cycle there is an exponential increase in the quantity of DNA such that after n cycles the amount increases by 2^n. A typical PCR application involves 30 to 40 cycles; therefore after 35 cycles, 3.44×10^{10} copies of the template DNA have been made.

Although PCR is a powerful method to increase the amount of a gene of interest in vitro, it has a number of important limitations. Difficulties can be encountered when studying small quantities of DNA, since the ingredients necessary for PCR (oligonucleotide primers, dNTPs, Taq polymerase) may be exhausted before sufficient target is produced. The specificity of the reaction may be limited and depends on many complex, interrelated factors, including the oligonucleotide primer size, annealing temperature, and buffer salt concentration. Long DNA fragments (>300 base pairs) are difficult to amplify when the starting material is degraded, such as that obtained following formalin fixation. A major limitation of PCR is the susceptibility of the process to contamination, particularly in experiments intended to detect rare DNA

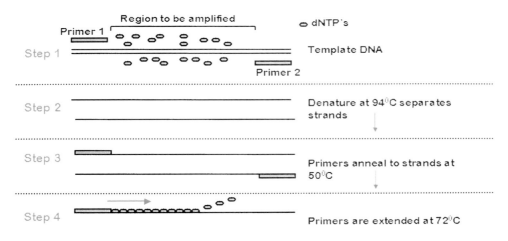

Figure 18-1 The basic steps for a single cycle of PCR. The steps are then repeated n times to generate 2^n copies of the DNA region of interest.

sequences. With "clean" laboratory techniques such as those employing disposable laboratory-wear and with appropriate sample controls, this problem can be overcome. Finally, on occasion the Taq polymerase may produce nucleotide addition errors, since the enzyme has no "proofreading" properties. Moreover, nucleotide sequence errors are more likely when the template DNA is fragmented or degraded, such as that obtained from formalin-fixed, paraffin-embedded tissue sections. This is of particular concern when the target fragment is destined for determination of the nucleotide sequence.

Many different types of clinical samples have been used for PCR analysis, including blood, saliva, sputum, semen, and single hairs. Whereas the traditional methods for genetic analysis, such as Southern blotting (a technique to analyze DNA whereby the DNA is size fractionated by gel electrophoresis, transferred to a nylon membrane, and then hybridized with a labeled probe; see Southern Blotting) and Northern blotting (similar to Southern blotting but for analysis of RNA; see Northern and Western Blotting) require relatively large amounts of high-quality DNA or RNA, PCR can be used to amplify relatively degraded DNA from a variety of sources, including DNA extracted from paraffin-embedded tissue sections.

The tissue fixative 4% neutral buffered formalin causes cross-linking and nicks the DNA. Although proteolytic digestion of tissues produces large quantities of DNA, most is fragmented, thus limiting the size of the target area of the gene that can be subjected to PCR. Precipitating fixatives such as ethanol and acetone do not cross-link or shear the DNA and therefore produce more consistent PCR results. Longer fixation times (>24 hours) may also adversely affect the quality of the DNA extracted from routinely processed tissues and thereby reduce PCR efficiency.

The counterstain used for tissue visualization, before DNA extraction, can also affect the quality of the reaction. For example, methyl green and neutral fast red counterstains produce PCR efficiency comparable to that obtained with unstained sections. By contrast, hematoxylin often produces significantly poorer PCR results than other stains and may be due to the binding of hematoxylin to DNA phosphate groups and to increased resistance to protease digestion.

Applications of Polymerase Chain Reaction

MICROBIOLOGY. The use of PCR has revolutionized the diagnosis and study of infectious diseases and malignancies associated with microorganisms. PCR overcomes many of the problems associated with culture methods and in some cases has replaced traditional pathogen identification methods. The DNA or RNA of an infectious organism can be detected in test material even when the organism number is low or is slowly growing, or when the infectious agent is in material not suitable for culture. Examination of archival material has permitted retrospective studies establishing the role of infectious organisms in the etiology and pathogenesis of many neoplasms, including human papillomavirus (HPV) in cervical carcinoma and in some verrucous carcinomas, Epstein-Barr virus (EBV) in posttransplant malignancies, and human herpesvirus 8 (HHV8) in Kaposi's sarcoma (also known as Kaposi's sarcoma herpesvirus [KSHV]). The list of infectious agents that can be detected by PCR is extensive, and the technique has been used to detect organisms in blood, saliva, sputum, semen, and feces, as well as in fixed tissues.

HUMAN GENETICS. PCR plays an important role in the identification of chromosome disorders and hereditary diseases. These include cystic fibrosis, Gaucher's disease, alpha-1-antitrypsin deficiency, hemophilia, and sickle cell anemia. PCR can also be used to analyze fetal DNA for aneuploidy *(the presence of extra chromosomes or the absence of chromosomes)*, trisomy 21, Turner's syndrome, and Klinefelter's syndrome, as well as for sex determination.

FORENSIC PATHOLOGY. Forensic pathology has employed PCR for a variety of situations, including the identification of mutilated or decomposed human tissues, for sex determination, and for disputed paternity cases. "DNA fingerprinting" is based on the identification of variable tandem repeats (VNTRs)—short, repeating DNA nucleotide sequences—that are located throughout the human genome. This process has proved to be an important tool in the identification of criminals.

TUMOR BIOLOGY. PCR has revolutionized the study of cancer and provided greater insights into the pathobiology of neoplasia. PCR has been used to detect mutations in cancer-associated oncogenes (e.g., K-*ras*, N-*ras*), tumor suppressor genes (e.g., *p53*, *p16*), monoclonality in B- and T-cell lymphomas, chromosome translocations such as the Philadelphia chromosome t(14;18) in chronic myelogenous leukemia, and minimal residual neoplastic disease, as well as the study of genetic alterations in formalin-fixed tissues. Since PCR is ideally suited to the study of low numbers of unique DNA fragments, it has been applied to the detection of malignant cells in urine, sputum, and saliva.

Quantitative Polymerase Chain Reaction. Quantification of DNA by PCR has tremendous potential, since it can permit the determination of gene amplification *(a mutational event whereby a gene is found in greater numbers than the normal numbers of copies)* of a myriad of genes. For example, the technique has been used to quantify *cyclin D1* gene amplification in oral epithelial dysplasia and carcinomas and to determine the gene levels of *CDK4*, *MDM2*, and *SAS* in oral osteosarcomas.

Potentially, quantitative PCR offers a number of advantages over traditional gene quantification methods such as Southern blot analysis. For example, the exponential increase in DNA during PCR cycling permits the use of relatively small amounts of genetic material that may be fragmented or degraded. Moreover, PCR methods can be automated to permit analysis of large sample numbers relatively easily, providing a measure of flexibility not permitted by conventional laborious and time-consuming methods.

In practice, however, a number of technical challenges have had to be overcome to develop reliable, quantitative PCR. One principal challenge is the nature of PCR product accumulation. During the reaction there are two defined phases whereby PCR product increases. At low-cycle numbers, PCR product accumulates exponentially (exponential phase), but at higher-cycle numbers, as template DNA, dNTPs, and primer are consumed, the rate of product formation progressively decreases until none is formed (saturation phase). The detectable exponential phase may be relatively short, lasting only a few cycles. Moreover, the determination of the start and end of this phase may be difficult to determine, since it is affected by many factors, including the amount and quality of template DNA and the kinetics of the reaction. To perform quantitative PCR, measurements of the amount of product must be made during the exponential phase of the reaction, since measurements during the saturated phase will provide inaccurate results.

Currently, the method of choice for quantitative PCR is continuous monitoring of the amount of product at the end of each cycle. There are a number of ways to accomplish this, including the TaqMan PCR 5′ nuclease assay. This technique relies on the 5′ to 3′ endonuclease activity of Taq DNA polymerase to detect target sequences during PCR. Included in the PCR mixture is a short oligonucleotide probe designed to hybridize within the target sequence but not to be extended in the 3′ direction *(by convention, the downstream portion of a DNA strand)*. When the probe is hybridized to the target, no signal is produced, because of the presence of a quencher molecule, which suppresses the fluorescence of a reporter molecule on the probe. During PCR the probe hybridizes to the target DNA, and Taq polymerase cleaves the probe into shorter fragments, thereby releasing the quencher from the reporter molecule. The amount of fluorescence generated is therefore directly proportional to the amount of PCR product generated. By measuring the amount of PCR product produced at the end of each single cycle, PCR growth curves can be plotted and measurements taken from the exponentially expanding region of the reaction.

Reverse Transcriptase Polymerase Chain Reaction. Another important application of PCR has been the detection and quantification of mRNA in cells. Since mRNA is short-lived and unstable, the determination of its relative abundance is often difficult in tissue sections using conventional methods of RNA analysis, such as Northern blotting (see Northern and Western Blotting). Moreover, the proportion of mRNA in the total amount of RNA in a cell (composed of ribosomal RNA, transfer RNA, and mRNA) may be as little as 2%, making the identification of specific mRNA species challenging. The analysis of mRNA is important, since it provides direct evidence of cell transcription and therefore is a measure of cellular function.

The basis of reverse transcriptase (RT)–PCR is the conversion of RNA to DNA. cDNA is that which is transcribed from an RNA template by the enzyme RT. This enzyme functions in an analogous but reverse manner to the way that RNA is made from a DNA template by RNA polymerases. Thus an RNA nucleotide sequence of GGUUA is directly converted by RT to CCAAG in cDNA. This cDNA can then be used as a template for PCR or quantitative PCR. If the starting material was mRNA, then the resultant cDNA will contain only exons *(the parts of the gene that are found in the mRNA molecule that will be used to code for the protein)* and not introns *(the part of the gene that is not found in the transcribed mRNA)*, since these are spliced out when mRNA is made.

An important application of RT-PCR has been the detection and quantification of the transcripts of tumor-associated translocations. Many neoplasms, particularly hematopoietic malignancies, contain specific chromosome translocations. For example, the Philadelphia chromosome is a genetic alteration that is most commonly identified in chronic myeloid leukemias and a subset of acute lymphoblastic

leukemias. This is the result of a reciprocal translocation between chromosome 9 and chromosome 22,
causing the relocation of the protooncogene c-*abl*
(from chromosome 9) adjacent to the c-*bcr* gene on
chromosome 22 [t(9 : 22)]. This produces a hybrid
c-*abl-bcr* transcript (mRNA) that encodes for a chimeric protein with tyrosine kinase activity. RT-PCR can be
used to detect the fusion transcript when PCR primers
are designed to flank the translocation. Quantitative
PCR methods can also be applied to the cDNA of the
fusion transcript to provide a measure of the amount
of mRNA present in a neoplastic cell. This strategy can
also be used for the detection of minimal residual
disease in leukemic patients following treatment. Other
tumor-defining translocations can be detected by RT-
PCR, including t(15;17) in acute promyelocytic
leukemia, t(8;14) in Burkitt's lymphoma, t(2;5) in
anaplastic large cell lymphoma, t(11;22) in Ewing's
sarcoma, t(2;13) in alveolar rhabdomyosarcoma (primitive neuroectodermal tumor), and t(X;18) in synovial
sarcoma.

DNA-Sequencing Methods

The most precise description of a gene is delineation
of its nucleotide sequence. Since a mutational event
is required for inactivation of most tumor suppressor
genes, including *p53* and *CDKN2A*, the goal of many
tumor studies is the determination of the tumor's DNA
sequence. Sequencing methods have been employed
for several decades, but improvements in technology
have reduced testing time to several hours and permitted characterization of genes composed of up to
hundreds of thousands of nucleotides.

Two methods have been developed to sequence
DNA. In 1977 Allan Maxam and Walter Gilbert
described a method involving chemical degradation
of radioisotopically labeled DNA at susceptible sites,
which are then analyzed by gel electrophoresis *(the
movement of charged molecules toward an electrode of the
opposite charge; used to separate DNA, RNA, and protein by
size)*. Today most manual and automated sequencing
methods are based on the method described by Fred
Sanger and co-workers (1997) relying on the genera-
tion of complementary single-stranded DNA using
DNA polymerase. Here, four mixtures are prepared,
each containing DNA polymerase and all the deoxynucleotide triphosphates (adenosine triphosphate,
cytidine triphosphate, thymidine triphosphate, dATP,
dCTP, dTTP, and dGTP, respectively). One of the
nucleotide precursors is labeled with a radioactive or

fluorescent marker in each mixture. In addition, each
of the four reaction mixtures also contains a limiting
amount of one dideoxynucleotide (ddATP, ddCTP,
ddTTP, or ddGTP), which, when incorporated into
the DNA, causes premature chain termination. Therefore in the reaction tube containing the ddGTP,
nucleotides will be added to the complementary strand
until a ddGTP is added. When this occurs, chain elongation ceases, since ddGTP (or ddCTP, ddATP, or
ddTTP, depending on the reaction tube) lacks the
3′-hydroxyl group required for subsequent nucleotide
addition. Thus the reaction tube mixture containing
the ddGTP will generate multiple strands of DNA of
various lengths, all terminating at positions where
ddGTP has been incorporated. Similarly, the other
three tubes will all contain DNA fragments of various
lengths terminating at positions where the respective
dideoxynucleotide has been added. The contents of
each of the four tubes are individually separated via gel
electrophoresis, with each band produced corresponding to the size of the terminated DNA fragments. Since
smaller fragments travel faster in the gel, those fragments that were terminated early by the addition of
the dideoxynucleotide will migrate farthest in the gel.

In the past, DNA sequencing was performed using
laborious and time-consuming manual techniques.
Today this process is often automated by using fluorescence-labeled nucleotides read by a laser during
passage through an electrophoresis sequencing gel.
The fastest methods available involve sequencing analysis by capillary electrophoresis whereby parallel tiny
fiberoptic glass tubes contain a special polyacrylamide
sieving medium for separation of fluorescence-labeled
DNA fragments generated by the sequencing reaction.

Hybridization Methods

Hybridization refers to the pairing of complementary
RNA or DNA strands to produce a double-stranded
nucleic acid. The nucleotide base-pair relationship is
so specific that strands cannot anneal unless the respective nucleotide strand sequences are complementary.
All hybridization methods use a radio- or fluorescence-
labeled DNA or RNA probe that binds to the target
DNA or RNA of interest, permitting visualization. The
target nucleic acids can either be immobilized in a
membrane ("blotting") or examined in tissue sections
(in situ).

Southern Blotting. A widely used method for analyzing
the structure of DNA is that described by Ed Southern in 1975. This involves the transfer or blotting of

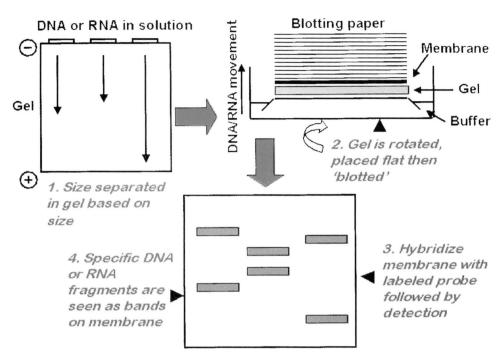

Figure 18-2   The basic steps involved in Northern (RNA) and Southern (DNA) blotting.

DNA fragments onto a membrane (Figure 18-2). DNA is first enzymatically cleaved into smaller pieces by restriction endonucleases (enzymes that are able to cut DNA at specific recognition sites) and then size separated by agarose gel electrophoresis. Smaller fragments travel farther in the gel, moving away from the negatively charged cathode, whereas larger pieces migrate a shorter distance. Thus electrophoresis serves to separate fragments according to size—a process termed *fractionation*. After fragment separation, the DNA is transferred from the gel to a nylon or nitrocellulose membrane through the capillary action of a buffer as it is absorbed by blotting paper. Then the DNA is bound to the membrane by baking the membrane in a vacuum oven or by ultraviolet (UV) light cross-linking. Finally, specific DNA fragments can be identified by hybridizing the membrane with labeled cDNA or RNA probes, followed by detection of the label on an x-ray film by autoradiography (the use of radioactivity to excite photographic emulsion; applied to the detection of gene expression and cell kinetics in tissues) or by chemiluminescence (the emission of light as a product of a chemical reaction).

Northern and Western Blotting. A modification of Southern blot analysis permits the study of RNA from tissues. By analogy to Southern blotting, this method was referred to, initially in a jocular context, as "Northern blotting." The term is now widely accepted. The separation and identification of proteins in a similar fashion is referred to as "Western blotting."

Northern blotting consists of RNA that is size separated via agarose gel electrophoresis, transfer to nylon or nitrocellulose membrane, and hybridization with specific, labeled DNA or RNA probes. RNA is sensitive to degradation by heat-stable ribonucleases that resist common sterilization methods. Single-stranded RNA tends to stabilize by folding into double-stranded configurations known as "hairpin loops," distorting the RNA and interfering with its analysis. To prevent these changes in RNA during analysis, separation gels must be run in the presence of strong, denaturing agents such as formaldehyde or methyl mercury. Laser densitometric scanning of the signal on blots obtained with DNA or RNA extracted from tumors provides a means of quantitative analysis of oncogenes. However, a limitation of these types of investigations is that the genetic material is removed from its topographic surroundings. The genetic material under investigation comes from a heterogeneous collection of stromal and neoplastic cells. This "contamination" with stromal cells dilutes the signal from the neoplastic cells.

In Situ Hybridization. In situ hybridization (ISH) is a technique used to examine DNA and RNA in their normal topographic surroundings. The technical approaches to the identification of DNA and RNA differ slightly but are conceptually similar to blotting techniques previously described whereby a labeled probe is used to hybridize with target nucleic acids.

ISH, using radioactive labeled probes, was first described in 1969. Recombinant DNA technology and isotopic labeling procedures permit demonstration of single-copy genes in metaphase *(the mitotic phase in which the condensed chromosomes are attached to the spindle fibers and line up in the middle of the cell)* chromosome spreads known as fluorescence ISH (FISH) (see Fluorescence in Situ Hybridization). Subsequent developments of ISH have included the use of nonradioactive probe labels, which have improved procedure safety and simplicity and closely approach the sensitivity levels of techniques employing radioactive labels.

ISH has a wide range of applications in pathology. It has been used to detect EBV particles in oral hairy leukoplakia, a lesion often seen in immunosuppressed individuals, such as those infected with the human immunodeficiency virus (HIV). ISH has found other applications in microbiology, embryology, cytogenetics, and neurobiology. Applications of ISH include the study of homeotic gene expression (i.e., "master switch" genes, some of them oncogenes) during embryogenesis, the role of genetic "memory" (sexual imprinting by methylation of DNA) in gene expression, and the effects of neuroendocrine stimuli on gene expression in neurons.

Traditionally viruses have been identified by culture techniques. Although this process is sensitive, it is technically difficult, requires significant time, and is not applicable to all types of viruses. ISH and immunohistochemistry have provided new methods for the identification and study of many viruses. Although ISH analysis for the detection of viral DNA and immunohistochemical analysis for the identification of viral proteins provide equal sensitivity in disclosing evidence of virus, the former technique is often preferable when no antigen is present in the tissue section or when commercially prepared antisera are unavailable.

Other Advanced Technologies

Flow Cytometry. Flow cytometry is an important method used to analyze cell kinetics *(the distribution of cells in different phases of the cell cycle)* and protein expression in normal and tumor cells. For the determination of

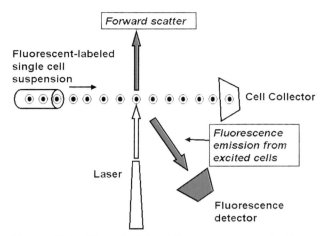

Figure 18-3 The principle of flow cytometry and cell sorting using fluorescence-labeled single-cell suspensions passed through a laser.

cell kinetics, flow cytometry offers many advantages over autoradiography, including speed and automation. In addition, large numbers of cells can be analyzed rapidly, providing a distribution profile of several thousand cells at one time.

Flow cytometry permits analysis of tissue when it is prepared as a single-cell suspension stained with a DNA-binding fluorescent dye (Figure 18-3). The amount of fluorescence thereby corresponds to the amount of DNA present in the cell. The labeled cells are then directed, in single file, along a charged column through a laser beam, which excites the fluorescent dye bound to the cell. The fluorescent emissions from the excited cells are then collected by a fluorescence detector and analyzed. Cell size can also be detected using data from the forward scatter of the excitation laser passing through the stream of single cells.

A number of different dyes have been used in flow cytometry, including ethidium bromide *(a dye that stains DNA orange when viewed under a UV light)*, propidium iodide, acridine orange, mithramycin, and Hoechst 33342. Acridine orange is particularly useful because it permits the separation of cells on the basis of the amount of double-stranded DNA (green fluorescence) and single-stranded RNA (red fluorescence). Fluorescence-labeled antibodies can also be used that bind to specific cellular proteins, which can be detected when the cells pass through the laser.

Flow cytometry can be used to provide information on the distribution of cells in the cell cycle that is based on the proportion with 2N DNA (G_0 and G_1), 4N DNA

(G$_2$ and M phases), and intermediate DNA content (S phase). Computer modeling can then generate a profile of all the cells and the proportion in each phase of the cell cycle. The technique can also be applied to the kinetic study of cells obtained from paraffin blocks. In 1983 David Hedley and colleagues described a technique wherein thick (i.e., 30 μm) sections are cut from tissue blocks and single-cell suspensions are prepared by the incubation of sections in a proteolytic solution, and then the cells are stained. This method is particularly useful for the retrospective study of cell kinetics in archival material such as can be obtained from tumor banks.

Since single-cell suspensions are a prerequisite for flow cytometry, lymphomas and leukemias have lent themselves particularly well to this technology. These cell populations lack intercellular adhesion molecules and can be easily separated into single-cell suspensions. Flow cytometry has been used to define lymphoma and leukemia subtypes and to separate lymphomas from forms of reactive lymphoid hyperplasia. B-cell lymphoma is monoclonal and expresses only one type of immunoglobulin light chain—either kappa (κ) or lambda (λ). Therefore lymphocyte population expression of a mixture of κ- and λ-light chains is strongly suggestive of reactive rather than neoplastic cell proliferation. By contrast, a population of lymphoid cells that expresses only κ or λ (light-chain restricted) is deemed monoclonal and is more likely to represent neoplastic disease. Flow cytometry is very sensitive and can detect a monoclonal population of lymphocytes constituting only 5% to 10% of an otherwise polyclonal population of cells. Flow cytometry can also be used to define the expression profiles of proteins in tumor cells, including growth factors, protein products of oncogenes, and markers of drug resistance, such as P-glycoprotein.

Fluorescence in Situ Hybridization. FISH has been used to map genes on chromosomes and to characterize chromosome abnormalities. Although conceptually identical to ISH (discussed earlier), it differs in several aspects. A DNA probe, labeled with biotin or digoxigenin, specific for a chromosome segment or a whole chromosome, is used. Chromosomes are typically studied in metaphase spread, and the DNA probe is hybridized to chromosomes. After nonspecifically bound probe is washed off, the section is incubated with a fluorescence-labeled *antibody* directed against biotin or digoxigenin.

FISH can be used to order genes and DNA segments on chromosomes to a resolution of two to three megabases. Based on the amount of fluorescence, FISH can be used to determine gene amplification or loss, although the resolution is not high. FISH can also be performed on cells in interphase *(the phase of mitosis in which the chromosomes are condensed)*, where this technique is useful for determining gene amplification by multiple gene copies and numerical changes in chromosomes. Here, FISH is usually combined with confocal microscopy, a computer-assisted imaging method to examine thin serial sections of whole cells in interphase. Chromosome *deletions*, translocations, and breakpoints can also be detected using FISH. The *bcr-abl* rearrangement and *CCND1* (cyclin D1) gene amplification can be rapidly determined using FISH.

Comparative Genomic Hybridization. When the cytogenetic abnormality is unknown, a suitable probe for FISH cannot be selected. Comparative genomic hybridization (CGH) permits the development of a detailed map of chromosome differences between normal and tumor cells by detecting increases (amplifications) or decreases (deletions) of segments of DNA. The technique involves labeling tumor DNA with biotin, which is detected with fluorescein (green), and labeling normal DNA with digoxigenin, which is detected with rhodamine (red). DNA samples from both normal and tumor tissue are then hybridized together onto a metaphase spread of unlabeled normal chromosomes. Regions of gain or loss of DNA, such as deletions, duplications, or amplifications, are seen as changes in the relative ratios of red and green. Thus areas of amplification are represented by green, and areas of loss by red. Subtle changes in color may not be discernible by the naked eye, requiring sophisticated image analysis software for quantification of these gene regions.

A major disadvantage of CGH is its relative insensitivity, since only chromosome changes larger than 5 megabases can be detected. However, the technique is useful for identifying relatively small chromosome translocations that cannot be detected by traditional Giemsa staining of metaphase spreads (karyotyping) and for identifying novel gene amplification or loss in tumors. Balanced rearrangements such as inversions and translocations cannot be detected by CGH.

Microarrays. A major advance in the quantitative study of mRNA expression has been the development of microarray technology, commonly referred to as "DNA chips." Using microarrays, the expression levels of hundreds to thousands of genes can be determined simultaneously, providing a unique profile of increased

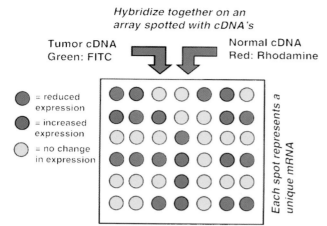

Hybridize together on an array spotted with cDNA's

Tumor cDNA
Green: FITC

Normal cDNA
Red: Rhodamine

● = reduced expression
● = increased expression
○ = no change in expression

Each spot represents a unique mRNA

Figure 18-4 The analysis of gene expression by complementary DNA (cDNA) microarrays involves the hybridization of labeled tumor and normal cDNA onto a "chip" that has been spotted with known cDNA or oligonucleotides. Reduced gene expression is seen as red, whereas increased gene expression is seen as green.

or decreased gene expression in tissues. Although an emerging technology, molecular expression profiles have been examined in forms of lymphoma and melanoma, with findings suggesting alternative taxonomy based on molecular differences in the expression of novel genes.

Conceptually, DNA microarray technology (Figure 18-4) is similar to the underlying principles of blotting. The process relies on the hybridization of a "probe" to multiple defined genomic DNAs, cDNAs, expressed sequence tags (ESTs), or oligonucleotides that have been "printed" onto specific locations of a solid phase, or "chip." The probe is usually composed of cDNA fragments produced by reverse transcription of tumor mRNA and then labeled with a fluorescent marker. The probe and the spotted cDNAs are hybridized, resulting in varying red/green and yellow fluorescent emissions. These emissions are then scanned by a reader consisting of lasers and a scanning fluorescence confocal microscope. The use of computer image analysis permits quantification of the intensity of thousands of different genes on the array, which can then be compared with the expression in normal tissues. Since this is evolving technology, the scope of applications has yet to be defined. Some of the types of studies that have used microarray technology include gene expression studies in tumor versus normal tissue, genotyping of mutations in tumors, functional analyses of genes expressed in yeast, and gene mapping to identify loci of disease susceptibility genes.

Laser Capture Microdissection. One major limitation of the application of molecular biology to pathology has been the heterogeneous nature of available tissue samples. Tissue samples of tumors, inflammatory lesions, infections, and even normal tissues consist of complex, heterogeneous mixtures of cells. To develop useful, reproducible data, it is desirable to study pure populations of cells obtained from actual biopsy or autopsy samples of tissues, both normal and diseased.

Laser capture microdissection (LCM) is a new and exciting technology for rapid preparation of relatively pure cell samples from tissue sections. In large part, the original impetus for this technology appears to have been the need to develop expression libraries *(collections of mRNA from defined cell populations)* from malignant and premalignant lesions. At least two different devices are now available commercially.

The principle on which LCM is based is the preferential adherence of identified cells to a plastic membrane activated by a low-energy infrared laser pulse. The full apparatus consists of (1) an inverted microscope, (2) an infrared laser diode, (3) laser controls, (4) a microscope stage controlled by joysticks, (5) a slide immobilizer by vacuum, (6) a charged couple device (CCD) camera, (7) a color monitor, and (8) a thermoplastic membrane for cell transfer—approximately 6 mm in diameter, mounted on an optically clear cap that fits on standard 0.5-ml microcentrifuge tubes for further analysis.

A mechanical transport arm, on which is suspended the cap, and is placed on the area of interest within a dehydrated section. The cells to be studied are visualized through a microscope, and the area is selected with the use of a positioning beam. Then laser activation is initiated, and focal melting of the plastic membrane follows. The cells adhere to the membrane rather than the glass slide and can now be lifted by raising the cap. The adherent cells are then transferred to a microcentrifuge tube containing appropriate reagents and buffers. The low energy levels of the laser result in a modest temperature rise that does not degrade the DNA, RNA, or proteins of interest. Other commercial systems are available but function along a similar theme.

The method is fast, precise, and adaptable to a wide range of tissues and molecules to be studied. The tissue left behind and the tissue retrieved can be identified, and the morphology of both is excellent. Large numbers of well-characterized cells can be obtained within a few minutes. Both fresh and archived material may be used, although results from stained tissue sections can be challenging, and at times impossible, to interpret. The minimum laser spot size is about 7.5 µm, rendering isolation of single cells difficult, although not impossible. There is also the risk of contamination from adjacent cells, even with careful laser microdissecting or during transfer of tissues to the microcentrifuge tube.

The applications of microdissection in pathology are legion. A few examples include obtaining pure cell populations from fresh, frozen, or fixed tissues, and cytology samples for DNA molecular genetic analysis; gene expression studies involving mRNA, such as RT-PCR; and combined immunohistochemistry or immunofluorescence to better identify cells for mRNA analysis. Other studies have combined immunofluorescence studies with flow cytometry, for example to analyze cell cycle characteristics of nuclei from paraffin sections. In oral disease investigations LCM has been used to identify immunoglobulin genes in plasma cells in salivary glands, to study the expression of differentiation and growth-related genes in oral cancer, and to determine amplification or loss of specific oncogenes and their transcripts.

IMMUNOHISTOCHEMICAL METHODS IN DIAGNOSTIC PATHOLOGY

Fundamentals of Immunohistochemistry

The application of immunologic methods to histopathology has resulted in marked improvement in the microscopic diagnosis of neoplasms. Although histologic analysis of hematoxylin and eosin (H&E)–stained tissue sections remains at the core of the practice of head and neck surgical pathology, immunohistochemistry has become a powerful tool in the armamentarium of the pathologist. It affords a significant advantage in the diagnosis of difficult and equivocal tumors, where it augments traditional tissue histomorphologic, histochemical, and electron microscopic study. Immunohistochemistry has also provided insight into tumor histopathogenesis and has contributed to more accurate determination of patient prognosis.

Predictable tumor expression of many of the same antigens (*a macromolecular protein or polysaccharide that can bind to an antibody molecule*) as their cells of origin or normal tissue counterparts validates the principle of tumor classification by immunohistochemistry. Distinguishing between undifferentiated neoplasms of different origins is achieved through the detection of tumor antigens using known antibodies. Some caution is necessary, since antigens may be shared by several tumor types and on occasion may react with several distinct antigens and antibodies. It is also important to note that this technique does not in itself differentiate between benign and malignant neoplasms, and as yet, no single antibody can consistently identify a specific type of malignant lesion.

Many significant advantages are associated with the use of immunohistochemistry in surgical pathology. First, the technique can be performed on routinely prepared tissue sections, permitting the pathologist to work in a familiar microscopic environment while linking morphology with the immunologic phenotype. Second, it is a very sensitive system that can detect antigens expressed at relatively low levels, and if carefully selected, antibody-antigen binding can be very specific. Third, the technical aspects are most favorable; equipment costs are low, and only a small amount of laboratory space is needed. Furthermore, the technique is relatively straightforward and easily learned.

Of utmost importance is careful interpretation of immunohistochemically stained slides. This is typically subjective in nature, although semiquantitative (e.g., 1+ to 4+) and quantitative scales are sometimes used. Staining intensity, proportion, and morphologic features of positive cells must be considered when evaluating staining reactions. Moreover, the distribution of positive staining relative to cell structure (nucleus, nuclear envelope, cytoplasm, or plasmalemma) must be considered, since nonspecific staining frequently may show incorrect antigen localization. Positive controls are necessary for stain interpretation. Internal positive controls are particularly helpful; when they are not present, external positive controls are needed to confirm staining specificity. In any event, immunohistochemical studies must be interpreted only in the context of the impression made after review of H&E sections.

Principles and Technical Advances

The selection of antibodies for immunohistochemical testing is based on their tumor specificity and the likelihood that they will react with the tumor under evaluation. After tissue sections are incubated with the prospective antibodies, positive reactions (tumor antigen-antibody binding) are identified through the application of one of several detection systems. Those that have the greatest sensitivity use a secondary antibody, reactive against the primary antibody, which is conjugated or linked to an enzyme marker. This system tends to be very sensitive because it allows for the attachment of a relatively large number of enzyme molecules, such as peroxidase, at the antigen site. The color of the reaction is determined by the selection of a precipitating chromogen, usually diaminobenzidine (DAB) (brown) or aminoethylcarbazole (AEC) (red), with which the enzyme reacts.

For a laboratory to produce uniform immunohistochemical results, standardization of immunohistochemical technique is critical. Inconsistencies can often be related directly to improper tissue fixation and processing, inadequate unmasking of antigenic epitopes *(that part of an antigen that combines with the antigen-binding site of an antibody molecule)*, and/or low sensitivity of the detection system.

Tissue Fixation. Although antigens are best preserved in frozen tissue, good, if not excellent, results can be achieved with formalin-fixed tissue through the application of newer antigen retrieval methods and recently developed antibody preparations. Many of these newer antibodies are also effective in the recognition of leukocyte *c*luster of *d*ifferentiation (CD) antigens, giving this technique considerable utility in the classification of lymphoid tumors. Formalin-fixed tissues provide the pathologist with a readily available test material, applicability of familiar and cost-effective laboratory methods, and results characterized by well-preserved microscopic detail.

Immunohistochemical studies are most often performed on specimens fixed in 4% neutral-buffered formalin. However, the effects of fixation, including protein-protein and protein–nucleic acid cross-linking and calcium ion bonding, mask or damage epitopes through alteration of the protein three-dimensional structure. These changes can often be overcome by one of several antigen retrieval methods. Other problems include delayed or extensive fixation times, inadequate tissue dehydration, and/or excessive paraffin-embedding temperatures (>56°C). These preventable factors can contribute significantly to poor staining, resulting in weak or false-negative results.

Assurance of fixative-neutral pH is important, since acidic solutions reduce antigenicity. Delay in the placement of excised tissue into fixative may reduce antigen expression. Ideally, tissue specimens should be small (0.5 cm) and placed in fixative immediately. To ensure complete but not excessive fixation, tissue should be immersed in formalin for approximately 24 hours, but not more than 48 hours. Tissue received from outside sources, as is the case for many outpatient biopsy services, may suffer significant antigenic compromise, necessitating careful selection of antibodies, an effective unmasking procedure matched to the antibody, and selection of a sensitive detection system.

Antigen Retrieval. Antigen retrieval is the process by which antigenic epitopes, made unavailable because of fixation-associated protein cross-linking, are rendered accessible to antibodies for binding. Antigen retrieval (epitope unmasking) in formalin-fixed tissue can be achieved through either enzyme digestion or heating of sections. The method of choice depends on the antigen and antibody under study and is usually determined by trial-and-error testing to observe which method gives the best staining result. Automated immunostainers have reduced some of the vagaries of immunohistochemistry. Unfortunately, technique protocols for available antibodies necessarily vary from one laboratory to another, making interlaboratory standardization and reproducibility difficult to attain.

Enzymatic digestion of tissue sections for epitope unmasking is typically accomplished via incubation in a solution of protease, trypsin, or pepsin. All are effective but may result in increased background staining. Generally, enzyme digestion provides less intense staining results than heating. There are several methods to heat sections, and all require a calcium chelating buffer, such as sodium citrate or ethylenediaminetetraacetic acid (EDTA), to keep tissue moist and stabilize antigens. Sections may be heated in a microwave oven, pressure cooker, or waterbath.

Antigen Amplification. Several systems are available for detecting antigen-antibody reactions. Those that have the greatest sensitivity require the attachment or conjugation of an enzyme marker to a secondary antibody, and a tertiary complex. Traditionally, alkaline phosphatase-antialkaline phosphatase and avidin-biotin-peroxidase systems, in which there are three linkage layers (primary antibody–secondary antibody–marker enzyme complex), have been widely used with excellent results. A large number of enzyme molecules (peroxidase or alkaline phosphatase), as well as numerous secondary antibody molecules, are conjugated to a dextran backbone and used as the second link to the primary antibody.

The object of layering or linkage of primary and secondary antibodies is to achieve attachment of as many enzyme molecules at the antigenic site as possible, thus increasing the intensity of the color reaction in the tissue section. Peroxidase is the most widely used enzyme marker because of convenience and clarity of reaction. Alkaline phosphatase is sometimes used, especially when it is desirable to stain for two antigens in the same section. The color of the antigen-antibody reaction is determined by the selection of chromogen or substrate with which the enzyme reacts. DAB, which is water insoluble, produces a brown color, and water-soluble AEC produces a red color. These are the two most common chromogens used in this technique.

Antibodies. Cytoplasmic, nuclear, and cell membrane proteins represent the targets for antibodies used in immunohistochemical tumor classification. Whether or not polyclonal or monoclonal antibodies are used depends on the availability and effectiveness of individual antibody preparations. The high specificity, intense staining, and low background obtained with monoclonal preparations are usually desirable but may occasionally be a detriment because of reactivity with only a single antigenic epitope. If the epitope to which the monoclonal antibody reacts is damaged or altered in the neoplastic cells, a false-negative result may occur. Polyclonal antibodies, by contrast, react with more than one epitope, potentially increasing the odds of a positive reaction. However, occasional cross-reaction with unrelated antigens and increased background staining may render interpretations of test results problematic.

Immunohistochemical Applications: Diagnostically Challenging Oral Malignant Neoplasms

Immunohistochemistry has been shown to be an effective adjunct to H&E diagnosis in a majority of equivocal tumor cases, through the establishment of a definitive diagnosis or through confirmation of H&E section impression. Immunohistochemistry is applied typically to cases when the definitive diagnosis cannot be established solely on the basis of findings in H&E sections. Diagnostically difficult tumors generally fall into one of the morphologic subsets listed in Table 18-1.

Most head and neck neoplasms listed in Table 18-1 can be identified by their pattern of reactivity with several antibodies, some of which are more specific than others. It is logical and cost-effective to begin an immunohistochemical study with a small panel of antibodies that serves to distinguish between major groups of neoplasms (e.g., epithelial, connective tissue, melanocytic). On the basis of these results, a more focused sequence of immunostaining with specific antibody preparations can be performed for precise tumor classification. For example, an initial panel for round cell tumors might include anti–S-100 protein, an anti-keratin cocktail, an anti–leukocyte common antigen (anti-LCA; CD45) cocktail, desmin, and possibly chromogranin to separate melanocytic, epithelial, lymphoid, skeletal muscle, and neuroendocrine neoplasms. An initial panel for spindle cell tumors might include anti–S-100 protein, anti–muscle actin, and anti-CD34 to assist in the separation of neural/melanocytic, smooth muscle, and endothelial neoplasms. Oral neoplasms and the antibodies most commonly used to confirm their diagnosis by immunohistochemistry are listed in Table 18-2.

Molecular Marker Descriptions

Epithelial Marker. Immunohistochemical staining for cytokeratins, known generically as keratins, is frequently done to help confirm the epithelial lineage

---

TABLE 18-1   **Subsets of Diagnostically Difficult Head and Neck Tumors**

Subsets	Tumors
Small round cell tumors	Squamous cell carcinoma, adenocarcinoma, rhabdomyosarcoma, melanoma, Langerhans cell disease, neuroendocrine carcinomas, olfactory neuroblastoma, Ewing's tumor/PNETs, Merkel cell tumor, lymphoid tumors
Large round cell tumors	Squamous cell carcinoma, adenocarcinoma, rhabdomyosarcoma, melanoma, lymphoid tumors, paraganglioma
Spindle cell tumors	Spindle cell carcinoma, rhabdomyosarcoma, leiomyosarcoma, neurosarcoma, fibroblastic and myofibroblastic tumors, Kaposi's sarcoma
Metastatic jaw tumors	Lung, gastrointestinal tract, breast, kidney, prostate
Minor salivary gland tumors	Polymorphous low-grade adenocarcinoma, adenoid cystic carcinoma, mixed tumor, monomorphic adenoma

PNETs, Primitive neuroectodermal tumors.

of a poorly differentiated carcinoma, adenocarcinoma, or spindle cell carcinoma (Figures 18-5 and 18-6). Thus keratin antibodies, used as an antikeratin cocktail (mixture of antibodies to low- and high-molecular-weight keratins), are typically used as part of a general screening panel for undifferentiated tumors.

The cytokeratins represent a group of structurally related intermediate filament proteins. They are subdivided into 19 subsets, depending on their molecular weight (M_r), which varies from 40,000 to 68,000. Cytokeratins are identified either by molecular weight or by numerical designation 1 through 19. Generally, keratin subtypes expressed by epithelial neoplasms are similar but not identical to those expressed by their presumed cells of origin. However, as dedifferentiation occurs, there may be a general shift to the pro-

TABLE 18-2 Tumor-Associated Antigens That Are Useful in Immunohistochemical Diagnosis

Neoplasm	Antigens
Carcinomas	Keratins
Adenocarcinomas	Keratins
Salivary gland tumors	S-100 protein, actins, calponin
Rhabdomyosarcoma	Desmin, myoglobin, actins, myogenin
Leiomyosarcoma	Smooth muscle actin, muscle specific actin
Leiomyoma	Smooth muscle actin, muscle specific actin, desmin
Myofibroblastic tumors	Smooth muscle actin, muscle specific actin (desmin negative)
Neurosarcoma	Neurofilaments, S-100
Angiosarcoma and Kaposi's sarcoma	CD31, CD34, factor VIII–related antigen
Melanoma	HMB45, S-100 protein, MART-1 (Melan-A)
Langerhans cell disease	CD1a, S-100
Lymphomas	CD45, CD45RB isoform
B-cell lymphomas	CD20, CD79a, CD45RA isoform
T-cell lymphomas	CD3, CD43, CD45RO isoform
Anaplastic large cell	CD30 (Ber-H2 clone), ALK-1
Hodgkin's disease (RS cells)	CD15, CD30
Plasma cell myeloma	κ/λ Light chains
Leukemic infiltrates	TdT, myeloperoxidase
Paraganglioma and neuroendocrine carcinoma	Synaptophysin, chromogranin, neurofilaments
Olfactory neuroblastoma	Synaptophysin, chromogranin, neurofilament
Merkel cell tumor	Synaptophysin, chromogranin
Ewing's sarcoma and PNET	CD99
Solitary fibrous tumor	CD34, CD99, Bcl-2

RS, Reed-Sternberg cells; *TdT*, terminal deoxynucleotidyl transferase; *PNET*, peripheral neuroendocrine tumor.

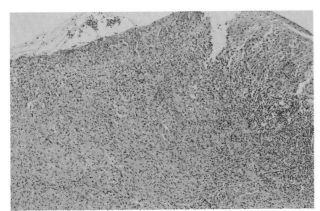

Figure 18-5 Spindle cell carcinoma from the palate of a 79-year-old woman (hematoxylin and eosin stain).

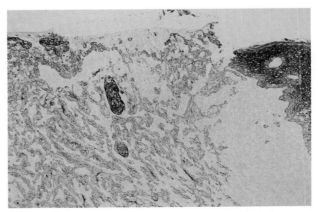

Figure 18-6 Positive immunohistochemical staining with an antikeratin "cocktail." Note normal epithelium to the right and invasive neoplasm at the center and to the left.

duction of lower-molecular-weight subtypes, or more of one subtype may be produced at the expense of another. Abnormal expression of subtypes has been described in epithelial cells of dysplastic and in situ carcinoma lesions of the oral mucosa, suggesting the possibility of markers of premalignancy. Metastatic epithelial cells generally express keratin profiles that are similar to those of the primary tumor. This antigen fidelity may be exploited to gain insight to the primary site of lesions metastatic to the jaws (see Metastatic Tumor Markers).

As squamous cell carcinomas produce a wide range of keratin subtypes, it is necessary to use a broadly reactive antikeratin cocktail in the identification of carcinomas. Antibodies to low-molecular-weight keratins are invaluable in identifying undifferentiated carcinomas and adenocarcinomas. It is important to note that antibodies to keratins, as well as to other tissue antigens, appear to have limited potential in separating benign from malignant lesions, because expression of these antigens may be independent of tumor differentiation and clinical behavior.

In general, keratin typing of salivary gland tumors by immunohistochemistry has been of little value in tumor diagnosis because all tumors, benign and malignant, contain keratin filaments. Once antibodies to the 19 specific keratin subtypes become available, studies may reveal diagnostically useful information. Currently, antibodies to glial fibrillary acidic protein (GFAP), actin proteins, and S-100 protein are of some help in salivary gland tumor diagnosis, although the H&E microscopic pattern is still the most important diagnostic criterion.

Cross-reactive keratin expression may also be evident in moderately to well-differentiated neuroectodermal carcinomas, but not in paragangliomas. Also, synovial sarcomas may stain positive for keratins.

General Mesenchymal Marker. Staining for cytoplasmic filaments, including vimentin, desmin, GFAP, and neurofilaments, can aid in the precise identification of connective tissue tumors, including sarcomas. Vimentin, an M_r 57,000 intermediate filament, is found in most mesenchymal cells, lymphoid cells, and neural crest cells, including melanocytes, Langerhans cells, and nevus cells, as well as in their neoplastic counterparts. However, coexpression of vimentin with other intermediate filaments is not uncommon in head and neck tumors, such as spindle cell carcinoma. Because of this coexpression and the wide variety of neoplasms that demonstrate antibody reactivity to vimentin, these intermediate filaments tend to be of only limited value in the diagnosis of tumors by immunohistochemistry.

Muscle Markers. Muscle differentiation in a neoplasm can be established by demonstrating the expression of desmin, actin, or myoglobin proteins. Desmin is an intermediate filament of approximately M_r 53,000 that is found in muscle cells. Desmin and myoglobin immunoreactivity are helpful in the diagnosis of tumors of muscle origin, especially rhabdomyosarcoma. Antibody to myogenin, one of several myogenic differentiation proteins, may be of value in the identification of rhabdomyosarcoma. Actin is a small cytoplasmic filament, approximately 5 nm in diameter, that has contractile properties. Six actin isotypes differentiate smooth muscle, striated muscle, and nonmuscle cells. Anti–muscle-specific actin and anti-smooth muscle actin generally provide good sensitivity and intensity for the detection of leiomyosarcoma. Staining for desmin is less reliable as it is positive in about two thirds of cases. Myofibroblastic tumors are positive for smooth muscle actin and muscle specific actin, but negative for desmin. Anti–muscle-specific actin is effective in staining myoepithelium of salivary glands. Because most salivary gland neoplasms contain myoepithelial cells, this antibody is of limited value in the classification of these lesions. However, newly developed antibodies against smooth muscle proteins α-smooth muscle actin, smooth muscle myosin heavy chains, and calponin) have been shown to be effective in separating positively staining adenoid cystic carcinoma from negatively staining polymorphous low-grade adenocarcinoma.

Neural Markers. S-100 protein, once thought to be unique to the central nervous system, has been identified in numerous other cells outside the central nervous system, including Schwann cells, chondrocytes, Langerhans cells, and some nevus cells.

The antibody to S-100 protein stains a wide array of unrelated neoplasms, including neural tumors, paraganglioma, some salivary gland tumors, granular cell tumor, Langerhans cell disease (LCD), chondrosarcoma, some muscle tumors, and approximately 95% of melanomas. It should be noted that CD1a is a specific marker for normal Langerhans cells and the pathologic cells in LCD. A monoclonal antibody reactive to CD1a is now available and is effective for immunohistochemical analysis of formalin-fixed tissue, replacing the less specific anti–S-100 protein for the confirmation of LCD.

Neural differentiation of a tumor can be confirmed with antibodies to either GFAP or neurofilaments. GFAP is an intermediate filament of M_r 51,000 that is typically found in glial cells and their neoplastic counterparts. Occasionally, GFAP immunoreactivity may be demonstrated in cells of the peripheral nervous system, particularly in Schwann cells. Correspondingly, tumors such as neurofibroma and neurosarcoma may also contain these filaments. Myoepithelial cells of salivary glands and salivary gland neoplasms, in particular mixed tumor, also express GFAP. By contrast, neurofilaments are found in neurons. These intermediate filaments may be encountered in neoplasms of the central nervous system, as well as of the peripheral nervous system. Neuroblastoma (also identified by antibody NB84), olfactory neuroblastoma, ganglioneuroma, paraganglioma, and Merkel cell tumor also express neurofilament antigens.

CD57 is expressed by natural killer cells but also somewhat inconsistently in some neural tumors, such as neurofibroma and granular cell tumor. Anti-CD57 cross-reacts with myelin-associated glycoprotein. This antibody may have some utility in confirming the neural origin of some benign and malignant tumors.

Endothelial Markers. Vascular differentiation of a tumor can be established with the antibodies to CD31, CD34, and factor VIII–related antigen. In diagnostic problems in which Kaposi's sarcoma or other neoplasms of vascular origin are being considered, any of these three antibodies may be used, although anti-CD34 seems to be the most consistent marker of endothelial cells in Kaposi's sarcoma. Anti-CD34 is also useful in confirming solitary fibrous tumors.

Melanocytic Markers. Melanoma, especially when amelanotic, can histologically mimic other malignancies and is often included in the histopathologic differential diagnosis of poorly differentiated neoplasms. Three reliable antibodies that react with proteins expressed by melanoma are HMB45, MART-1, and anti–S-100 protein. These reactions do not involve antigens directly linked to melanin formation, making such immunohistochemical analysis effective in distinguishing pigment-poor melanomas from other tumors with similar microscopic appearance. Staining with these antibodies may also be useful in locating occult tumor cells in tissue sections, aiding in the evaluation of the depth of invasion and detection of metastasis.

HMB45 reacts with an intracellular antigen in a variable number of cells in approximately 90% of melanomas. Although highly specific for melanoma, some nevi may be reactive. Normal melanocytes are typically nonreactive. Recently some nonmelanoma tumors (lymphoma, adenocarcinoma, angiomyolipoma) have also been shown to react to HMB45.

A recently developed antibody to a transmembrane protein on melanoma cells recognized by T cells (anti–MART-1, or melanin-A) has been shown to be useful in the diagnosis of melanoma. Because this antigen (protein) is preserved in formalin-fixed tissue, it can be used when S-100 and HMB 45 stains are equivocal or in lieu of HMB 45.

Lymphoid Markers. The diagnosis of B-cell differentiated lymphomas, especially plasmacytoid forms, can be confirmed through the identification of a monoclonal κ or λ population (Figure 18-7). Although this is most easily done on frozen sections, it is often possible immunohistochemically to stain cytoplasmic light chains in paraffin-embedded tissues. Significant alteration in the normal **light chain** ratio would be strong evidence of a monoclonal population of cells. Predominance of one form of light chain is termed light-chain restriction.

Leukocyte CD markers are typically used to subtype lymphomas. Until recently, lymphocyte subtypes could be identified only in frozen tissue, but several new antibodies directed against various lymphocyte antigens have recently been developed for use in routinely processed tissue. Although these antibodies cannot distinguish benign from malignant proliferations, they can be used to differentiate B- and T-cell lymphomas. Because these new markers are not completely lineage specific, some cross-reactions may occur, making the use of antibody panels necessary to avoid misinterpretation of false-positive reactions.

The antibodies most widely used to determine T- and B-cell differentiation are CD3 and CD20 (clone L26), respectively (see Table 18-2). The most commonly used CD3 antibody is a polyclonal preparation reactive with an epitope located on the cytoplasmic domain of the CD3 protein. CD43, also a T-cell marker with some cross-reactivity with B cells, is sometimes used to confirm lymphomas of T-cell lineage. CD20 is a highly reliable B-cell marker, and L26 is generally regarded as an effective antibody for identification of normal B cells, staining approximately 95% of these cells. L26 is highly useful in identification of B-cell lymphoma and some lymphomas that are nonreactive to anti-LCA (CD45). L26 is believed to be reactive to an intracellular membrane–associated epitope of the CD20 antigen. In unusual B-cell lymphoma cases,

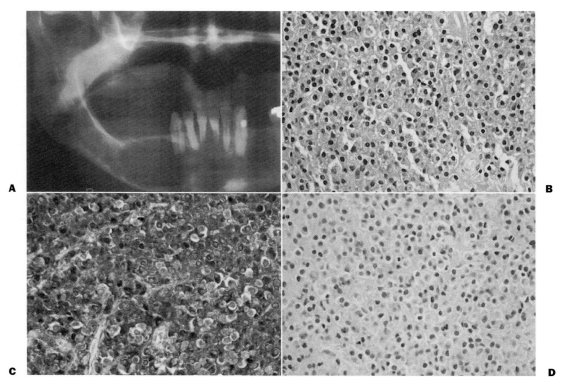

Figure 18-7 **A,** Multiple jaw radiolucencies in a 61-year-old woman representing previously undiagnosed multiple myeloma. **B,** Histologic section showing atypical plasmacytoid cells. **C,** Positive immunohistochemical staining for light chains. **D,** Negative staining for light chains. (**A** courtesy Dr. Steven Rowan.)

where there is no detectable expression of CD20, CD79a may be detected and can be used for confirmation of B-cell lineage. CD79a is a dimeric protein that is part of the B-cell receptor complex. It is expressed early in B-cell development and persists to the plasma cell stage.

Leukocytes typically can be stained with antibodies to CD45. CD45 and its three isotypes—RA (clone 4KB5), RB, and RO (clone UCHL1)—show reactivity to antibodies in formalin-fixed tissue. The CD45RA isoform is found on B cells, CD45RB is found on both B and T cells, and CD45RO is found on T cells. Most T-cell lymphomas can be identified with antibody to CD45RO; fewer than 1% of B-cell lymphomas are reactive. The anti-CD45 cocktail is particularly useful in the evaluation of undifferentiated "round cell" tumors, since it stains lymphoma but not carcinoma, sarcoma, or melanoma. In contrast to anti-κ and anti-λ antibodies, anti-CD45 findings do not distinguish between benign and malignant proliferations.

Antigens CD15 and CD30 can be expressed by Reed-Sternberg cells in Hodgkin's disease. More important is the membrane expression of CD30 by tumor cells of anaplastic large cell lymphomas (ALCLs). These tumors also express cytoplasmic aberrant tyrosine kinase related to chromosome translocations, usually t(2;5). Antibody (ALK-1) to this enzyme is also useful in identifying a majority of ALCLs.

Terminal deoxynucleotidyl transferase (TdT) is an enzyme that may be expressed by acute leukemia cells, especially those of acute myeloid and acute lymphoblastic leukemias. Immunohistochemical staining for this enzyme can be helpful in identifying leukemic infiltrates in oral tissues, and it may aid in separating leukemias from lymphomas. However, some caution must be exercised in the interpretation of TdT-stained slides, since not all acute leukemias will express TdT. A correlation between TdT expression and prognosis has not been shown. Granulocyte differentiation can be confirmed with antibody to myeloperoxidase or with a histochemical stain for chloroacetate esterase (Leder stain).

Traditional methods for identification of macrophages in paraffin-embedded tissue have included the use of polyclonal antibodies reactive to intracellular enzymes such as lysozyme, antitrypsin, and antichymotrypsin. Newer monoclonal antibodies are reactive to macrophage membrane antigens and are proving to be desirable alternatives to the traditional polyclonal antibodies. These antibodies are helpful in separating macrophages from neoplastic cells. CD68, a glycoprotein found in lysosomes and to a lesser extent on surface membranes, is highly expressed by macrophages and neutrophils. KP1 seems to be the most reliable antibody for detection of the antigen. Other macrophage-associated antibodies (MAC 387, HAM-57, PG-M1) are less commonly used but are available for confirmation, if necessary.

Neuroendocrine Markers. Catecholamine production is a common characteristic of neuroendocrine cells. These neurotransmitter substances are found in cytoplasmic neurosecretory granules (dense core granules) and provide morphologic and chemical evidence of cell origin. Synaptophysin and chromogranin are neurosecretory-associated proteins that have been used for the development of monoclonal antibodies specific for paraganglioma, neuroendocrine carcinomas, Merkel cell tumor, medullary carcinoma of the thyroid, and olfactory neuroblastoma.

Ewing's Tumor and Primitive Neuroectodermal Tumor Marker. Ewing's tumor and primitive neuroectodermal tumors (PNETs) are closely related, if not identical, neoplasms. They share similar chromosome translocations, predominantly t(11;22)—translocations that result in a novel fusion gene encoding for a chimeric oncoprotein that appears to act as a transcription factor. These tumors also express cell surface glycoprotein p30/32 (CD99) encoded by the *MIC2* gene. The monoclonal antibody O13, which binds this glycoprotein, is helpful in identifying this rare group of tumors when analyzing formalin-fixed tissues. Interpretation of round cell tumors must be made with the knowledge that some lymphomas and rhabdomyosarcomas may also stain positive with this antibody, although LCA and muscle markers can be used for separating these cases. (It should be noted that solitary fibrous tumors also stain positive for CD99.) Definitive diagnosis of Ewing's tumor/PNETs can be made with either cytogenetic, FISH, or RT-PCR analyses to identify the characteristic chromosome/molecular defects in these tumors.

Metastatic Tumor Markers. The application of immunohistochemistry can on occasion be helpful in deter-

TABLE 18-3 Immunohistochemical Staining Profile of Metastatic Epithelial Malignancies

Tumor	Antigenic Profile
Lung (adenocarcinoma)	CK7+/CK20–/villin+
Lung (squamous cell carcinoma)	CK7–/CK20–
Colon	CK7–/CK20+/villin+
Breast	CK7+/CK20–/villin–
Kidney	CK7–/CK20–/villin–
Prostate	CK7–/CK20–/PSA+

mining the organ from which epithelial neoplasms metastatic to the jaws originated. By using stains for cytokeratins 7, 20, and villin (actin-binding protein in microvilli), primary sites of origin can be reasonably well predicted. The scheme in Table 18-3 has been substantiated in several studies. Also, monoclonal antibody to prostate-specific antigen (PSA) may be effective in the identification of metastatic adenocarcinoma of the prostate in formalin-fixed sections.

Minor Salivary Gland Tumor Markers, S-100 Protein, Actins. Immunohistochemistry is presently of minimal value in the microscopic diagnosis of minor salivary gland tumors, due in part to the varying participation of cells with both epithelial and myoepithelial differentiation in all of the tumors. Antigenic markers lack specificity in these tumors; however, there are some quantitative differences that occasionally may be diagnostically helpful. S-100 protein is typically expressed to a greater degree in polymorphous low-grade adenocarcinoma than in adenoid cystic carcinomas. On the other hand, muscle-specific actins are expressed to a greater degree in adenoid cystic carcinoma than in polymorphous low-grade adenocarcinoma, reflecting greater myoepithelial differentiation in adenoid cystic carcinomas. Newly developed antibodies reactive to smooth muscle proteins, such as calponin, may prove to be of considerable value in helping to distinguish these tumors. Actins are also expressed in mixed tumor (pleomorphic adenoma), but minimally so in monomorphic adenoma.

Knowing the principles and practice of applied immunohistochemistry makes the pathologist more competent and effective through greater understanding of tumor differentiation and classification. Immunohistochemistry adds an important tool in the microscopic diagnosis of difficult tumors and in tumor research.

DIRECT IMMUNOFLUORESCENCE IN DIAGNOSTIC PATHOLOGY

Fundamentals

Like immunohistochemistry, direct immunofluorescence (DIF) uses known prepared antibodies to identify antigens in tissue sections. The antigens typically stained with DIF are autoantibodies (immunoglobulins G, A, and M [IgG, IgA, and IgM]) and inflammatory proteins. For practical purposes, this method is used predominantly in the confirmation of microscopic diagnosis of a small number of vesiculobullous-ulcerative diseases that often have overlapping clinical and histologic features.

The method requires unfixed frozen tissue because the antigenic determinates become almost undetectable because of the protein cross-linking associated with tissue fixation. Tissue sections are incubated with the known antibody, to which is conjugated a fluorescent molecule. The sections are then washed, covered, and viewed through a fluorescent microscope. Positive reactions, in which the conjugated antibody remains, appear as bright green fluorescence in a dark background.

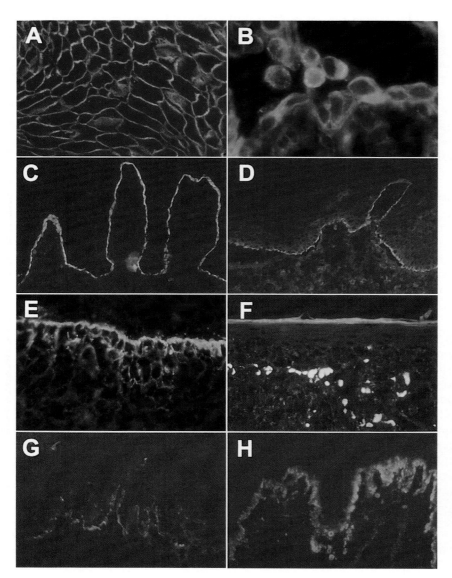

Figure 18-8 Direct immunofluorescence images. **A** and **B, Pemphigus vulgaris** showing intercellular staining for IgG and C3. **C** and **D, Mucous membrane pemphigoid** showing basement membrane zone fluorescence for C3. **E** and **F, Lichen planus** showing basement membrane zone and superficial lamina propria fluorescence for fibrinogen and apoptotic body fluorescence for IgM. **G, Erythema multiforme** showing nonspecific fine granular basement membrane zone fluorescence for C3. **H, Lupus erythematosus** showing coarse-granular basement membrane zone fluorescence for IgM. (Courtesy Dr. Troy E. Daniels, University of California San Francisco.)

Immunofluorescence Applications

With DIF (see also Chapters 1 and 2), distinctive staining patterns can be seen in pemphigus vulgaris, mucous membrane pemphigoid, linear IgA disease, lupus erythematosus, and lichen planus (Figure 18-8). DIF examination of pemphigus shows an intercellular staining pattern that is due to deposition of IgG (autoantibody) and complement (C3). In pemphigoid the DIF staining pattern is linear along the basement membrane as a result of deposits of IgG, IgA, and C3. In linear IgA disease, only IgA is deposited along the basement membrane in a linear pattern. DIF examination of lupus biopsy specimens results in coarse granular basement membrane staining due to deposition of IgG, IgM, and C3. In lichen planus, fibrinogen deposition can be detected in the basement membrane zone and superficial lamina propria with DIF examination, and immunoglobulins may be evident in apoptotic keratinocytes. Erythema multiforme exhibits nonspecific staining, but a negative or nonspecific DIF examination can sometimes be helpful to separate erythema multiforme from pemphigus vulgaris, mucous membrane pemphigoid, linear IgA disease, lupus erythematosus, and lichen planus, which can occasionally exhibit similar clinical pathologic features.

BIBLIOGRAPHY

ADVANCED MOLECULAR METHODS

DeRisi J, Penland L, Brown PO, et al: Use of a cDNA microarray to analyse gene expression patterns in human cancer, *Nat Genet* 14:457-460, 1996.

Emmert-Buck MR, Bonner RF, Smith PD, et al: Laser capture microdissection, *Science* 274:998-1001, 1996.

Jordan RC, Diss TC, Lench NJ, et al: Immunoglobulin gene rearrangements in lymphoplasmacytic infiltrates of labial salivary glands in Sjögren's syndrome: a possible predictor of lymphoma development, *Oral Surg Oral Med Oral Pathol Oral Radiol Endod* 79:723-729, 1995.

Jordan RC, Pringle JH, Speight PM: High frequency of light chain restriction in labial gland biopsies of Sjögren's syndrome detected by *in situ* hybridization, *J Pathol* 177:35-40, 1995.

Kallioniemi A, Kallioniemi OP, Waldman FM, et al: Detection of retinoblastoma gene copy number in metaphase chromosomes and interphase nuclei by fluorescence in situ hybridization, *Cytogenet Cell Genet* 60:190-193, 1992.

Leethanakul C, Patel V, Gillespie J, et al: Distinct pattern of expression of differentiation and growth-related genes in squamous cell carcinomas of the head and neck revealed by the use of laser capture microdissection and cDNA arrays, *Oncogene* 19:3220-3224, 2000.

Schneeberger C, Eder S, Swoboda H, et al: A differential PCR system for the determination of CCND1 (cyclin D1) gene amplification in head and neck squamous cell carcinomas, *Oral Oncol* 34:257-260, 1998.

Shahnavaz SA, Bradley G, Regezi JA, et al: Patterns of CDKN2A gene loss in sequential oral epithelial dysplasias and carcinomas, *Cancer Res* 61:2371-2375, 2001.

Sidransky D, Tokino T, Hamilton SR, et al: Identification of ras oncogene mutations in the stool of patients with curable colorectal tumors, *Science* 256:102-105, 1992.

ADVANCED IMMUNOHISTOCHEMICAL AND IMMUNOFLUORESCENCE METHODS

Chrysomali E, Papanicolaou SI, Dekker NP, et al: Benign neural tumors of the oral cavity: a comparative immunohistochemical study, *Oral Surg Oral Med Oral Pathol Oral Radiol Endod* 84:381-390, 1997.

Dabelsteen E: Molecular biological aspects of acquired bullous diseases, *Crit Rev Oral Biol Med* 9:162-178, 1998.

Guo B, Cao S, Toth K, et al: Overexpression of Bax enhances antitumor activity of chemotherapeutic agents in head and neck squamous cell carcinoma, *Clin Cancer Res* 6:718-724, 2000.

Helander SD, Rogers RS III: The sensitivity and specificity of direct immunofluorescence testing in disorders of mucous membranes, *J Am Acad Dermatol* 30:65-75, 1994.

Perez-Ordonez B, Koutlas IG, Strich E, et al: Solitary fibrous tumor of the oral cavity: an uncommon location for a ubiquitous neoplasm, *Oral Surg Oral Med Oral Pathol Oral Radiol Endod* 87:589-593, 1999.

Prasad AR, Savera AT, Gown AM, et al: The myoepithelial immunophenotype in 135 benign and malignant salivary gland tumors other than pleomorphic adenoma, *Arch Pathol Lab Med* 123:801-806, 1999.

Regezi JA, Zarbo RJ, Stewart JC: Extra-nodal oral lymphomas: histologic subtypes and immunophenotypes (in routinely processed tissue), *Oral Surg Oral Med Oral Pathol* 72:702-708, 1991.

Scully C, Carrozzo M, Gandolfo S, et al: Update on mucous membrane pemphigoid: a heterogeneous immune-mediated subepithelial blistering entity, *Oral Surg Oral Med Oral Pathol Oral Radiol Endod* 88:56-68, 1999.

Shi SR, Chaiwun B, Young L, et al: Antigen retrieval technique utilizing citrate buffer or urea solution for immunohistochemical demonstration of androgen receptor in formalin-fixed paraffin sections, *J Histochem Cytochem* 41:1599-1604, 1993.

Index

Note: Page numbers followed by "f" refer to illustrations; page numbers followed by "t" refer to tables; page numbers followed by "b" refer to boxes. Page numbers preceded by "O-" refer to overview section.